Handbook of Renal Replacement

Handbook of Renal Replacement

Editor: Penny Summers

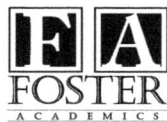

FA FOSTER
ACADEMICS

www.fosteracademics.com

www.fosteracademics.com

FA
FOSTER
A C A D E M I C S

Cataloging-in-Publication Data

Handbook of renal replacement / edited by Penny Summers.
    p. cm.
Includes bibliographical references and index.
ISBN 978-1-63242-816-5
1. Kidneys--Transplantation. 2. Hemodialysis. 3. Chronic renal failure--Treatment.
4. Transplantation of organs, tissues, etc. I. Summers, Penny.
RD575 .H35 2019
617461 059 2--dc23

Foster Academics,
118-35 Queens Blvd., Suite 400,
Forest Hills, NY 11375, USA

ISBN 978-1-63242-816-5 (Hardback)

Contents

Permissions

List of Contributors

Index

Preface

Over the recent decade, advancements and applications have progressed exponentially. This has led to the increased interest in this field and projects are being conducted to enhance knowledge. The main objective of this book is to present some of the critical challenges and provide insights into possible solutions. This book will answer the varied questions that arise in the field and also provide an increased scope for furthering studies.

A form of therapy which is used to replace the normal blood-filtering function of the kidneys is known as renal replacement therapy. It is used in cases like acute kidney injury, chronic kidney disease and renal failure. Renal replacement therapy involves several ways of filtration of blood such as dialysis, hemofiltration, hemodiafiltration and kidney transplantation. The process of artificially removing excess water and toxins from the blood is known as dialysis. It is performed in cases where the patient's kidneys are no longer able to perform these functions naturally. This book brings forth some of the most innovative concepts and elucidates the unexplored aspects of renal replacement. Different approaches, evaluations, methodologies and advanced studies on renal replacement have been included herein. As this field is emerging at a rapid pace, the contents of this book will help the readers understand the modern concepts and applications of the subject.

I hope that this book, with its visionary approach, will be a valuable addition and will promote interest among readers. Each of the authors has provided their extraordinary competence in their specific fields by providing different perspectives as they come from diverse nations and regions. I thank them for their contributions.

Editor

Heterogeneity of clinical indices among the older dialysis population—a study on Japanese dialysis population

Norio Hanafusa[1]* (iD), Satoko Sakurai[2] and Masaomi Nangaku[2]

Abstract

Background: The older dialysis population is increasing, and several studies have investigated the effect of actual age on the relationship between clinical parameters or clinical practice and prognosis. There is concern that biological age does not necessarily reflect the actual effects of aging, and it is important to take heterogeneity into account when considering the older population. In this study, we investigated whether such heterogeneities exist in a large number of clinical parameters and how any disparities might be affected by the domains of clinical indices.

Methods: We investigated the published, summarized results of the Japanese Society for Dialysis Therapy Renal Data Registry, a nationwide survey of the Japanese dialysis population, for the year 2013.

Results: The potential population comprised 306,925 dialysis patients. We investigated coefficient of variations (CVs) of 25 clinical indices across age groups and compared them with the CVs of the 45–59 years age group as a reference group, using tests for homogeneity of variances. Almost all variables showed some heterogeneity by age. The domain for muscle mass or visceral protein exhibited greater heterogeneity in older patients, but surprisingly, the domain for body mass or physique exhibited less heterogeneity. The mean values of most parameters declined in the older population.

Conclusions: This study demonstrated that variations exist in clinical indices in the older dialysis population. Apart from biological age, we should take these heterogeneities into account when interpreting the findings of clinical studies involving older dialysis patients and in their individualized management.

Keywords: Aging phenotype, Biological age, Coefficient of variances, Heterogeneity, Older patients, Wasting

Background

The dialysis population has become much older in recent years, and the proportion of elderly patients is increasing in many registries [1, 2]. There are several clinical problems to overcome in the older hemodialysis population. One of the most important involves malnutrition-related syndromes, such as sarcopenia [3], protein energy wasting [4], and frailty [5]. These syndromes are in fact associated with a worse prognosis in the dialysis population as a whole [6, 7]; these phenotypes are considered to be most important in the management of the older population.

Strategies against complications for older dialysis patients sometimes differ from those for their younger counterparts [8]. However, the definition of "older" patients varies in different reports [9–11]. The reason for this may be due to the heterogeneity among the elderly population in terms of phenotype. Some patients look younger than their actual age, while some look older. Moss et al. reported that the "surprise" question, "Would I be surprised if this patient died in the next year?" correlated well with 1 year survival [12], indicating that the phenotype, presumably wasting or malnutrition, seems important for survival.

We speculated that such phenotype of the "older" population does matter and that it is important to take the heterogeneities of such patients into account, which

* Correspondence: hanafusa@kc.twmu.ac.jp
[1]Department of Blood Purification, Kidney Center, Tokyo Women's Medical University, 8-1 Kawada-cho, Shinjuku-ku, Tokyo 162-8666, Japan
Full list of author information is available at the end of the article

might affect the older phenotype. However, there have been no reports on the heterogeneity of the elderly population. Therefore, here, we focused on the heterogeneity of the older dialysis population and investigated which clinical indices exhibited large heterogeneity and were potentially related to a poor prognosis, using national registry data compiled by the Japanese Society for Dialysis Therapy (JSDT). It is anticipated that our results will help the clinician to undertake individualized management of older dialysis patients.

Methods

Population

Data from the annual Japanese Society for Dialysis Therapy Renal Data Registry (JRDR) survey run by JSDT were used for this analysis. The details of this registry have been described previously [13]. We analyzed the data collected in 2013. The summarized tables are recorded in CD-ROM or are reported on the internet. In this analysis, we used data that appears on JSDT's website [14].

The potential population for this study was the entire dialysis population as of December 31, 2013, namely 306,925 patients. The population was divided by 15-year age groups. We excluded patients with missing data on age ($n = 12$) and patients who were younger than 15 years ($n = 116$).

Clinical indices

The following clinical indices were investigated: (1) mineral and bone disorder markers (corrected calcium and phosphate); (2) malnutrition-related factors (total cholesterol, high-density lipoprotein (HDL) cholesterol, non-HDL cholesterol, percent creatinine generation rate (%CGR) [15], normalized protein catabolic rate (nPCR) [16], and albumin); (3) body mass and volume status (body height, postdialytic body weight (BW), body mass index (BMI), BW change, and fractional BW change); (4) dialysis prescription and its consequences (dialysis duration, spKt/V [16], eqKt/V [17], blood flow rate, predialytic blood urea, and creatinine); (5) circulatory factors (systolic blood pressure, diastolic blood pressure, and pulse rate); and (6) other factors (hemoglobin (Hb) level, glycoalbumin, and HbA1c). Postdialytic BW, dialysis duration, and blood flow rate were investigated among the patients who were treated by hemodialysis, hemodiafiltration, or hemoperfusion. The values of%CGR, nPCR, BW change, fractional BW change, spKt/V, eqKt/V, and creatinine were investigated only in patients who were treated by hemodialysis, hemodiafiltration, or hemoperfusion three times weekly with a dialysis history of ≥2 years. Glycoalbumin and HbA1c were investigated among those who had history of diabetes or were on glucose-lowering therapies. Parameters other than those described above were studied in the entire dialysis population.

Statistical analysis

This analysis consists of two parts: one is to determine the heterogeneities of age populations, and the other is to compare them with the standard of 45–59 year-old group.

The heterogeneity was measured by coefficient of variations (CV) in this analysis, because standard deviation (SD) does not necessarily express the degree of heterogeneity when the averages vary. The tables of the JRDR summarized data give the number of patients and mean values and SD for each parameter in all age groups. CVs were calculated by dividing the SD by the mean for each age category. The larger CV is more heterogenic or heteroscedastic the population can be considered.

Relative CVs were calculated by dividing the CVs of each age group by that of the 45–59 years age group. If the value is larger than one, the index is more heterogenic in older population than the younger counterpart. Relative means were also calculated as the ratio of the mean of each age group to that of the 45–59 years age group, similarly to relative CVs.

Finally, we statistically compared the heterogeneities across age groups by investigating the homogeneity of variances. In details, we calculated variances by squaring standard deviations. The tests for homogeneity of variances were performed on the squared relative CVs using Bartlett's test among overall groups and F tests for each pair of age groups. The former investigated the homogeneity of the variances by age groups as a whole. When the test indicated statistical significance, it shows that the clinical index is heterogenic across age groups. On the other hand, the latter tested statistical significance by comparing the CV of each age group with that of the reference group of ages 45–59. When a test was significant, it indicates that the clinical index is more heterogenic in that age group compared to that in the 45–59-year-old age group. Post hoc adjustment for multiple comparisons was done by Bonferroni correction. The p values less than 0.05 were considered significant. For multiple comparisons, p values less than 0.01 were considered significant because five pairs of comparisons were performed with the 45–59 years age group as the reference group. All statistical calculations and analyses were performed using Microsoft Excel 2013 (Microsoft Corporation, Redmond, WA).

Ethical issues

This study is the secondary analyses of the summarized and published data and does not deal with any personal information. Therefore, we consider that this study is deemed exempt from the Institutional Review Board or Ethics Committee approval. This study adhered to the Declaration of Helsinki.

Results

The demographics and characteristics of the total population who underwent dialysis therapy in 2013 are shown in Table 1 [1]. Mean age was 67.21 ± 12.51 years (mean ± SD). The age groups 15–29, 30–44, 45–59, 60–74, 75–89, and ≥90 years accounted for 0.37, 4.91, 18.56, 45.87, 28.72, and 1.54% of the total population, respectively.

Table 2 shows the number of patients and their proportion of sex, vintage, and primary diagnoses for each age category. In the older age groups, there was a higher proportion of female patients and a higher proportion of patients with the primary diagnosis of nephrosclerosis; less predominant were the proportion of patients with a long history of dialysis and the proportion with diabetes as the primary diagnosis.

Table 3 shows the SDs and means of the variables investigated as well as the number of the patients. Table 4 shows the CVs relative to those of the 45–59 years age group, which is used as the reference group. The overall differences of variances, including chi-square values and p values calculated with the Bartlett test, are shown, as well as p values for the differences of variances of the age groups, taking the variance of the 45–59 years age group as the references. For almost all variables, the variances differed by age group. However, the trends themselves differed by index. We can categorize these indices according to the relative CV for the 75–89 years age group into four categories: (1) relative CVs of more than 1.1 (indicating the most heteroscedastic indices), namely for %CGR, albumin, creatinine, fractional BW reduction, blood urea nitrogen, and diastolic blood pressure; (2)

relative CVs of 1.0–1.1 (mildly heterogeneous), namely for phosphate, total cholesterol, nPCR, body height, BW reduction, blood flow rate, systolic blood pressure, pulse rate, and Hb; (3) relative CVs of 0.9–1.0 (less heterogeneous), namely for corrected calcium, non-HDL, HDL, session duration, spKt/V, and eqKt/V; and (4) relative CVs of less than 0.9 (least heterogeneous), namely for BW, BMI, glycoalbumin, and HbA1c.

Figure 1 indicates that the disparities in representative indices between several domains differ significantly across the age groups. The relative CVs of indicators relating to the muscle mass or visceral proteins increased steadily with age, becoming more heteroscedastic. The parameters related to dietary intake showed a modest relationship across the age groups. On the other hand, indices of body mass demonstrated that the dispersion progressively decreased with the age of the population.

Figure 1 was designated to demonstrate the CVs by themselves so that the heteroscedasticity can be recognized easily. On the other hand, the CVs were calculated from the SDs and means. The means are also subjected to change by age groups, and the relative means indicate the trend of the distributions of the absolute values as a whole by age groups. Therefore, in Fig. 2, we added the information about the relative means to the results shown in Fig. 1 so that information about whether the absolute values tended to become smaller among the older population as well as the information about the heteroscedasticity. This figure indicates that the mean values of all indices included in Fig. 1 were lower in the older age groups, irrespective of relative CVs. This fact might indicate that the normal aging process accompanies universal declines in clinical indices.

Discussion

Heterogeneity as determined by CV increased with age in some domains, especially that of muscle mass or visceral proteins. However, in some other domains such as body mass, the disparities seem to be diminished in the older population. This is the first study investigating the heteroscedasticity of clinical indices, using nationwide registry data.

There were differences among the domains of indices; factors related to sarcopenia or wasting were most prominently dispersed. Moreover, the mean values of these parameters declined with age. Therefore, muscle mass and albumin level generally decreases with age, but their speed of decline varies among individuals. The decrease in these parameters, as discussed above, reportedly relates to poor survival relating to wasting [6, 7]. Therefore, the heterogeneity of these clinical indices might reflect the diversity of the older population in terms of "old" phenotypes and relate to a worse prognosis. Moreover, the mean values of CGR and albumin decreased less in older population,

Table 1 Background characteristics of the patients

Number of patients	306,925	
Sex (male/female)	194,965/111,960	
Age (mean ± SD)	67.21 ± 12.51	
Vintage (years, number of patients, %)		
<2	68,475	(22.3)
2–4	76,589	(25.0)
5–9	77,197	(25.2)
10–14	39,490	(12.9)
15–19	20,874	(6.8)
20–24	11,421	(3.7)
25–29	6611	(2.2)
30+	6155	(2.0)
Primary diagnoses (numbers, %)		
Diabetes	115,484	(37.6)
Glomerulonephritis	99,492	(32.4)
Nephrosclerosis	26,569	(8.7)
Polycystic kidney	10,683	(3.5)
Others or unknown	54,697	(17.8)

Table 2 Patient characteristics by age group

Age groups	15–29	30–44	45–59	60–74	75–89	90+
Sex						
Male	749 (66.8)	10,315 (68.4)	38,610 (67.8)	91,189 (64.8)	51,997 (59.0)	2032 (42.9)
Female	372 (33.2)	4756 (31.6)	18,340 (32.2)	49,583 (35.2)	36,150 (41.0)	2704 (57.1)
Vintage (years, number of patients, %)						
<2	383 (34.2)	3556 (23.6)	11,484 (20.2)	28,358 (20.2)	23,464 (26.6)	1163 (24.6)
2–4	323 (28.8)	3756 (24.9)	12,996 (22.8)	32,734 (23.3)	25,177 (28.6)	1565 (33.1)
5–9	263 (23.5)	3564 (23.7)	13,807 (24.3)	35,296 (25.1)	22,800 (25.9)	1447 (30.6)
10–14	103 (9.2)	2134 (14.2)	7782 (13.7)	19,446 (13.8)	9598 (10.9)	425 (9.0)
15–19	34 (3.0)	1176 (7.8)	4673 (8.2)	10,882 (7.7)	4007 (4.5)	102 (2.2)
20–24	11 (1.0)	605 (4.0)	2890 (5.1)	6174 (4.4)	1715 (1.9)	26 (0.5)
25–29	4 (0.4)	206 (1.4)	1734 (3.0)	3890 (2.8)	774 (0.9)	3 (0.1)
30+	0 (0.0)	69 (0.5)	1564 (2.7)	3948 (2.8)	572 (0.6)	2 (0.0)
Primary diagnoses (numbers, %)						
Diabetes	61 (5.4)	4268 (28.3)	21,653 (38.0)	57,903 (41.1)	30,672 (34.8)	920 (19.4)
Glomerulonephritis	389 (34.7)	5635 (37.4)	20,180 (35.4)	46,654 (33.1)	25,273 (28.7)	1344 (28.4)
Nephrosclerosis	34 (3.0)	614 (4.1)	2411 (4.2)	8917 (6.3)	13,311 (15.1)	1279 (27.0)
Polycystic kidney	21 (1.9)	433 (2.9)	2738 (4.8)	5373 (3.8)	2050 (2.3)	63 (1.3)
Others or unknown	615 (54.9)	4119 (27.3)	9967 (17.5)	21,917 (15.6)	16,832 (19.1)	1130 (23.9)

The number of patients (percentage) in each age group is shown. Patients with missing or unknown values for age or background characteristics were excluded. Therefore, the sum of the numbers is not equal to the total population shown in Table 1

compared to other indices as shown in Fig. 2. This fact might reflect that CGR and albumin are less affected by aging and they could be good markers of aging phenotype. In this analysis, we investigated the disparity in muscle mass in terms of CGR. However, muscle strength is reported to relate to survival to a greater degree [6]. The concept of dynapenia has been proposed [18, 19]. Future studies investigating the heterogeneity of muscular strength and its relation to survival are required.

Albumin has been used as a marker of malnutrition, but many other factors also affect albumin levels [20]. Dietary restriction only does not decrease the albumin level and it is now regarded as a factor of wasting [20]. The 2013 annual JRDR survey, the source of the data analyzed in this study, also investigated C-reactive protein (CRP). However, the distribution of CRP does not follow a normal distribution, and its heterogeneity cannot be assessed by SD or CV as we performed on other variables because the variables that do not follow normal distribution cannot be summarized by SDs or means. Therefore, we could not investigate the heterogeneity of CPR, and we cannot draw the conclusion that the disparity of albumin relates to inflammation status.

Dietary intake is reduced in the elderly population because of reduced appetite [21]. Moreover, the degree of appetite itself relates to prognosis [21]. In this study, we used nPCR as a surrogate of dietary intake. On the other hand, phosphate is contained in foods that contain much protein [22]. Phosphate binders and dialysis

dosage, especially session length, also affect the level of phosphate [22]. It is interesting to note then that nPCR and phosphate exhibited similar trends. Intradialytic BW reduction can be related to sodium intake during interdialytic periods [23], which also followed a similar trend to that of nPCR and phosphate levels. Therefore, these clinical indices can be considered as surrogate markers of dietary intake in patients.

Surprisingly, the distribution of body mass tended to be smaller in the older population even though the disparities of muscle mass become wide among the elderly population. An inverse relationship can be observed in the dialysis population [24]; patients with larger BMI experience better survival [25]. However, in the Asian population, such relationship might be weaker than in the white or black populations [25]. Female patients tend to have better survival among the Japanese population, and the average age of female patients is higher than their male counterparts [1]. Actually, Table 2 shows that the proportion of female patients was larger among the older age groups. Obviously, female patients have a smaller physique than male patients. Therefore, the present results might be attributed to the predominance of female patients in the older age groups. On the other hand, it is possible that the findings of the smaller and relatively homogeneous physique in older patients merely reflect the trend in the general population because this study did not examine variances in the general population.

Table 3 Details of investigated clinical indices by age group

Age groups	15–29			30–44			45–59			60–74			75–89			90+		
	n	Mean	SD	n	Mean	SD	n	Mean	SD	n	Mean	SD	n	Mean	SD	n	Mean	SD
Corrected calcium (mg/dl)	982	9.23	1.01	13,372	9.21	0.95	50,910	9.28	0.95	125,857	9.29	0.92	78,390	9.28	0.89	4159	9.32	0.88
Phosphate (mg/dl)	982	6.20	1.75	13,395	5.94	1.70	51,003	5.66	1.51	126,082	5.24	1.38	78,480	4.86	1.35	4163	4.58	1.35
Total cholesterol (mg/dl)	733	151.42	34.05	10,072	161.17	36.00	38,259	161.91	36.68	94,475	156.90	35.81	58,543	152.40	34.76	3074	152.01	34.89
Non-HDL (mg/dl)	572	98.53	30.52	8163	110.54	34.88	30,913	111.28	35.04	75,683	107.96	33.74	46,507	105.29	32.34	2386	105.10	31.91
HDL cholesterol (mg/dl)	649	51.96	15.40	9291	50.68	17.81	35,085	50.48	18.04	85,526	48.81	16.71	52,604	47.17	15.33	2707	47.06	14.59
%Creatinine generation rate (%)	576	97.84	22.30	9279	102.51	22.47	37,051	101.84	23.50	92,017	100.60	25.51	52,501	96.04	27.78	2763	89.88	30.00
Normalized protein catabolic rate (g/kg/day)	576	0.96	0.19	9283	0.93	0.18	37,071	0.90	0.18	92,080	0.88	0.18	52,547	0.83	0.17	2768	0.81	0.18
Albumin (g/dl)	957	3.94	0.46	13,123	3.86	0.40	49,868	3.76	0.39	123,713	3.62	0.41	77,239	3.44	0.44	4082	3.26	0.45
Body height (cm)	951	160.35	12.28	12,879	165.28	9.76	49,316	164.41	9.00	121,116	160.36	8.77	74,553	155.74	8.97	3895	150.46	9.31
Postdialytic body weight (kg)	904	55.07	15.10	12,921	64.44	17.75	49,320	62.10	14.59	123,611	55.35	11.02	77,661	49.86	9.67	4130	43.68	8.29
Body mass index (kg/m²)	907	20.96	4.33	12,468	23.40	5.26	47,739	22.89	4.49	117,550	21.51	3.55	72,249	20.56	3.24	3751	19.36	3.22
Body weight reduction (kg)	598	2.84	1.20	9692	3.19	1.22	38,748	2.95	1.10	96,978	2.52	0.91	55,482	2.17	0.83	2954	1.84	0.78
Fractional body weight reduction (%)	588	5.23	1.75	9627	5.09	1.67	38,616	4.83	1.57	96,725	4.61	1.56	55,325	4.41	1.61	2945	4.26	1.70
Session duration (h)	928	4.11	0.60	13,153	4.15	0.61	50,237	4.11	0.56	125,686	4.00	0.50	79,179	3.84	0.51	4228	3.68	0.54
spKt/V	576	1.55	0.33	9260	1.47	0.32	36,997	1.47	0.31	91,943	1.50	0.29	52,461	1.48	0.30	2759	1.45	0.31
eqKt/V	576	1.35	0.30	9270	1.29	0.30	37,018	1.29	0.28	91,982	1.31	0.27	52,478	1.29	0.27	2762	1.25	0.29
Blood flow rate (ml/min)	910	215.90	40.58	12,992	223.89	39.60	49,599	218.83	37.45	124,081	206.67	34.32	78,016	192.68	33.07	4149	179.45	32.49
Predialytic blood urea (mg/dl)	601	69.22	16.40	9729	67.31	15.90	38,895	64.89	15.54	97,289	62.47	15.51	55,647	58.45	15.43	2956	56.73	15.77
Creatinine (mg/dl)	601	13.83	3.12	9727	13.38	2.79	38,905	11.99	2.62	97,292	10.48	2.46	55,646	8.88	2.30	2955	7.42	2.15
Systolic blood pressure (torr)	844	147.58	22.58	11,584	152.31	24.84	43,661	153.49	24.07	108,150	152.08	23.81	67,379	148.93	24.16	3586	145.85	25.04
Diastolic blood pressure (torr)	843	87.65	16.31	11,557	88.44	15.51	43,545	84.86	14.03	107,857	77.84	13.33	67,193	72.10	13.14	3576	68.01	13.34
Pulse rate (/min)	785	80.69	13.35	11,009	81.29	12.92	41,376	78.50	12.58	102,757	74.40	12.46	64,244	72.38	12.63	3396	71.16	12.49
Hemoglobin (g/dl)	971	10.83	1.31	13,204	10.90	1.27	50,256	10.85	1.26	124,487	10.70	1.24	77,553	10.52	1.27	4096	10.37	1.25
Glycoalbumin (%)	25	21.38	7.09	1692	21.41	7.01	8742	20.82	5.82	23,723	21.24	5.21	13,001	21.35	4.93	420	21.41	5.31
A1c (%)	39	6.34	1.51	2363	6.64	1.51	12,166	6.40	1.29	32,540	6.18	1.12	17,481	6.00	1.05	544	5.83	0.99

HDL high-density lipoproteins, spKt/V single pool Kt/V, eqKt/V equilibrated Kt/V, HbA1c hemoglobin A1c, n number of patients, SD standard deviations

Table 4 Trends in relative and standardized standard deviations of all clinical indices by age group

Age groups	15–29		30–44		45–59		60–74		75–89		90+		Trend analysis	
	Relative CV	p value	Relative CV	p value	Relative CV	p value	Relative CV	p value	Relative CV	p value	Relative CV	p value	Chi-square values	p value
Corrected calcium (mg/dl)	1.069	0.001	1.008	0.134	1	Ref	0.967	<0.001	0.937	<0.001	0.922	<0.001	356.9	<0.001
Phosphate (mg/dl)	1.058	0.006	1.073	<0.001	1	Ref	0.987	0.000	1.041	<0.001	1.105	<0.001	463.8	<0.001
Total cholesterol (mg/dl)	0.993	0.396	0.986	0.038	1	Ref	1.007	0.042	1.007	0.073	1.013	0.160	11.3	0.080
Non-HDL (mg/dl)	0.984	0.299	1.002	0.405	1	Ref	0.993	0.057	0.975	<0.001	0.964	0.008	32.9	<0.001
HDL cholesterol (mg/dl)	0.829	<0.001	0.983	0.021	1	Ref	0.958	<0.001	0.909	<0.001	0.868	<0.001	482.4	<0.001
%creatinine generation rate (%)	0.988	0.347	0.950	<0.001	1	Ref	1.099	<0.001	1.254	<0.001	1.446	<0.001	3282.4	<0.001
Normalized protein catabolic rate (g/kg/day)	0.990	0.370	0.968	<0.001	1	Ref	1.023	<0.001	1.024	<0.001	1.111	<0.001	122.8	<0.001
Albumin (g/dl)	1.126	<0.001	0.999	0.448	1	Ref	1.092	<0.001	1.233	<0.001	1.331	<0.001	3463.1	<0.001
Body height (cm)	1.399	<0.001	1.079	<0.001	1	Ref	0.999	0.401	1.052	<0.001	1.130	<0.001	693.7	<0.001
Postdialytic body weight (kg)	1.167	<0.001	1.172	<0.001	1	Ref	0.847	<0.001	0.825	<0.001	0.808	<0.001	5473.5	<0.001
Body mass index (kg/m^2)	1.053	0.013	1.146	<0.001	1	Ref	0.841	<0.001	0.803	<0.001	0.848	<0.001	5456.5	<0.001
Body weight reduction (kg)	1.133	<0.001	1.026	0.001	1	Ref	0.968	<0.001	1.026	<0.001	1.137	<0.001	401.1	<0.001
Fractional body weight reduction (%)	1.029	0.155	1.009	0.123	1	Ref	1.041	<0.001	1.123	<0.001	1.228	<0.001	884.0	<0.001
Session duration (h)	1.071	0.001	1.079	<0.001	1	Ref	0.917	<0.001	0.975	<0.001	1.077	<0.001	1243.2	<0.001
spKt/V	1.010	0.367	1.032	<0.001	1	Ref	0.917	<0.001	0.961	<0.001	1.014	0.160	604.6	<0.001
eqkt/V	1.024	0.207	1.071	<0.001	1	Ref	0.950	<0.001	0.964	<0.001	1.069	<0.001	410.3	<0.001
Blood flow rate (ml/min)	1.098	<0.001	1.034	0.044	1	Ref	0.970	<0.001	1.003	0.239	1.058	<0.001	243.6	<0.001
Predialytic blood urea (mg/dl)	0.989	0.364	0.986	<0.001	1	Ref	1.037	<0.001	1.102	<0.001	1.161	<0.001	620.9	<0.001
Creatinine (mg/dl)	1.032	0.130	0.954	<0.001	1	Ref	1.074	<0.001	1.185	<0.001	1.326	<0.001	1992.9	<0.001
Systolic blood pressure (torr)	0.976	0.164	1.040	<0.001	1	Ref	0.998	0.342	1.034	<0.001	1.095	<0.001	184.0	<0.001
Diastolic blood pressure (torr)	1.126	<0.001	1.061	<0.001	1	Ref	1.036	<0.001	1.102	<0.001	1.186	<0.001	692.0	<0.001
Pulse rate (/min)	1.032	0.100	0.992	0.139	1	Ref	1.045	<0.001	1.089	<0.001	1.095	<0.001	449.3	<0.001
Hemoglobin (g/dl)	1.042	0.035	1.003	0.315	1	Ref	0.998	0.289	1.040	<0.001	1.038	0.001	185.3	<0.001
Glycoalbumin (%)	1.186	0.089	1.171	<0.001	1	Ref	0.877	<0.001	0.826	<0.001	0.887	<0.001	703.6	<0.001
A1c (%)	1.182	0.054	1.128	<0.001	1	Ref	0.899	<0.001	0.868	<0.001	0.842	<0.001	564.6	<0.001

Indicated CVs were relative (i.e., SD of the 45–59 years age group was set as 1) CV. The p values for each age group were calculated from F tests compared with those of the 45 and 59 years age group. Trend analysis was performed using Bartlett's test; chi-square and p values are shown. HDL high-density lipoproteins, spKt/V single pool Kt/V, eqkt/V equilibrated Kt/V, HbA1c hemoglobin A1c, n number of patients, SD standard deviation, ref reference

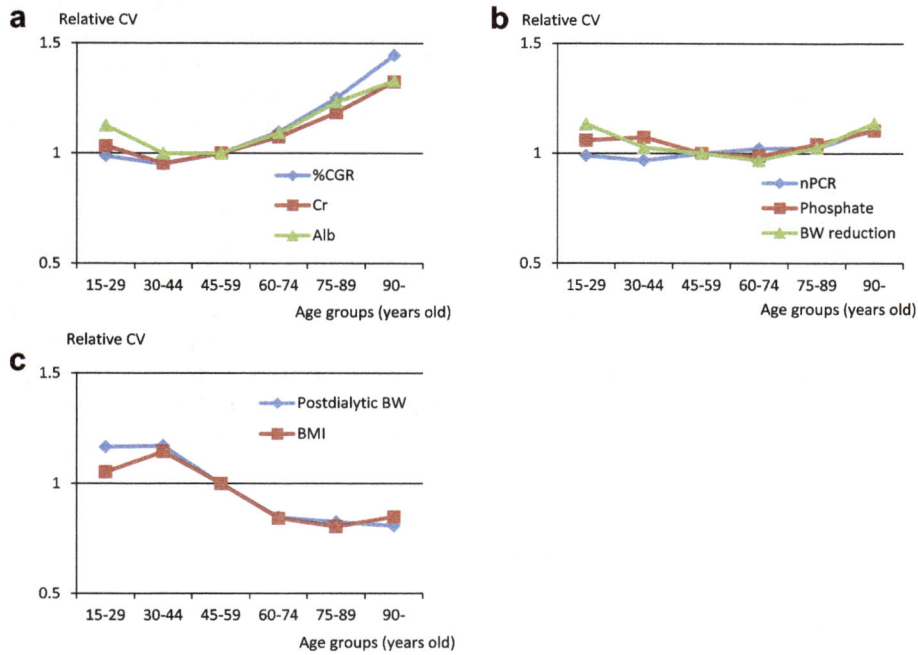

Fig. 1 Heterogeneity of representative clinical parameters by age group. The figure shows the trends in relative coefficient of variations (CV) (i.e., the CV of the 45–59 years age group was set as 1) for the clinical parameters related to **a** muscle mass or visceral proteins, **b** dietary intake, and **c** body mass or physique. The CVs for indices of muscle mass or visceral proteins became larger among the older population, whereas the CVs for those of body mass became smaller. Indices for dietary intake tended to be dispersed in the very old population. *CV* coefficient of variance, *%CGR* percent creatinine generation ratio, a surrogate marker of muscle mass, *Cr* creatinine, *Alb* albumin, *nPCR* normalized protein catabolic rate, *BW* body weight, *BMI* body mass index, *ref* reference

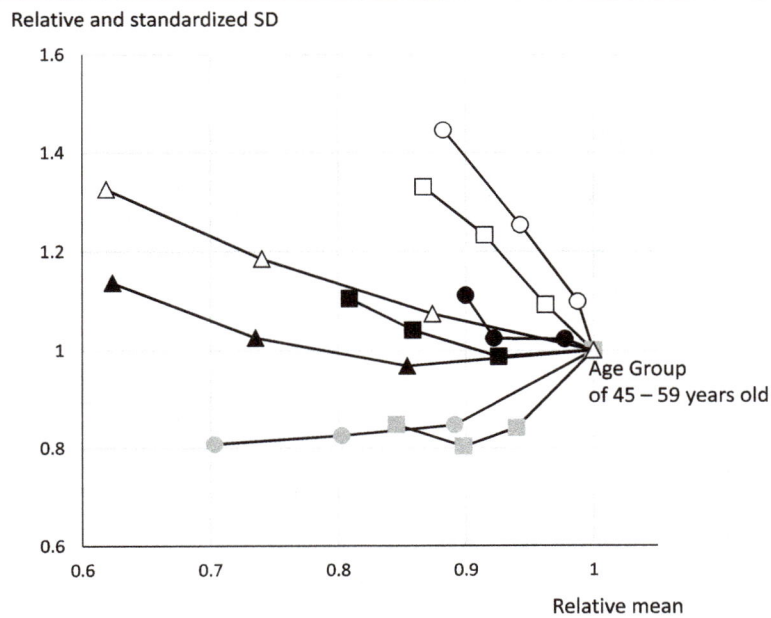

Fig. 2 Evolution of the relationship between mean and SD for representative indices among age groups ≥45 years. The relationship between the set of relative coefficients of variations (CV) and relative mean values are shown. The 45–59 years age group was set as a standard for both CV and means. The mean of all the indices decreased to a large degree in the older population. Each point indicates the age groups of 45–59, 60–74, 75–89, and ≥90 years. *Open circles*, %CGR; *open squares*, Alb; *open triangles*, Cr; *closed circles*, nPCR; *closed squares*, phosphate; *closed triangles*, body weight reduction; *gray circles*, body weight; and *gray squares*, body mass index

Moreover, there was a discrepancy in terms of heteroscedasticity between the indices regarding body mass such as BMI or BW and the indices regarding muscle mass such as %CGR or creatinine. The former showed to be less heterogenic, while the latter showed to be more heterogenic in older population. BMI is one of the simplest indices to describe the physiques. However, it cannot distinguish fat mass from muscle mass. The dialysis patients are shown to reduce muscle mass, while they often lose less amount of fat or even gain it during the course of dialysis therapy [26]. Therefore, BMI can underestimate the changes in muscle mass [27]. This point might cause the discrepancy of heteroscedasticity between body mass and muscle mass. On the other hand, body height can contribute to BMI. However, as Table 4 shows, the heterogeneity of height remained small even in the older population. Moreover, the mean values of body height were less in older population. Several recent studies demonstrated that taller dialysis patients might experience worse survival [28, 29]. Thus, the smaller and less heterogenic older population in terms of their body height might be due to the survival effects partly.

Nonetheless, we should pay attention to the clinical indices which exhibited large heterogeneity, such as creatinine generation rate, creatinine, and albumin, when we perform clinical practice on the older population. The deterioration of these indices might reflect the degree of the morbid conditions among older population. Future study will be required to investigate the relationship to the clinical outcomes, such as mortality, quality of life (QOL), and activity of daily living (ADL). After that, the interventions to the indices are warranted to improve the outcomes of the patients.

This study has several limitations. The first is its cross-sectional and observational nature. Therefore, we cannot draw any conclusions about the time course or cause-effect relationship. The second is that this study was based on results that appeared in summarized tables, and therefore, detailed investigations, such as further stratification by sex or primary diagnoses, could not be performed. The third is that the data that we used did not contain the data for clinical outcomes. Therefore, we could not investigate the effect of heterogeneity observed on mortality, QOL, or ADL. The fourth is that the JRDR data were almost exclusively derived from Japanese people. Therefore, the applicability of our findings to other ethnicities is unclear. Lastly, data was missing on some parameters in some patients. Although the number of the patients was sufficiently large, which is the most important advantage of this study, it is possible that errors exist.

Although there are several limitations in this study, the strengths of this study are the large number of patients and parameters that were examined. These results may contribute to the individualized management of the older dialysis population. Further studies on the cause of disparities and the relationship to the prognosis of the patients are required. We anticipate that the findings of such studies will provide a better understanding of phenotypes in the older dialysis population.

Conclusions
This is the first study to investigate heterogeneity in the older dialysis population. There were some disparities in heterogeneity across the parameters. Clinical parameters related to muscle mass or wasting exhibited larger heterogeneity, while those related to body mass or BW exhibited less heterogeneity. Individualized management for older dialysis patients with these heterogeneities might contribute to better outcomes in this population.

Abbreviations
%CGR: Percent creatinine generation rate; ADL: Activity of daily living; BMI: Body mass index; BW: Body weight; CD-ROM: Compact disk read-only memory; CRP: C-reactive protein; CV: Coefficient of variation; eqKt/V: Equilibrated Kt/V; Hb: Hemoglobin; HbA1c: Hemoglobin A1c; HDL: High-density lipoprotein; JRDR: The Japanese Society for Dialysis Therapy Renal Data Registry; JSDT: The Japanese Society for Dialysis Therapy; nPCR: Normalized protein catabolic rate; QOL: Quality of life; SD: Standard deviation; spKt/V: Single pool Kt/V

Acknowledgements
The data reported here were provided by the JSDT. The interpretation and reporting of these data are the responsibility of the authors and do not reflect the official interpretation or views of the JSDT.

Funding
The authors did not have specific funding source to be disclosed.

Authors' contributions
NH conceived of the study design, analyzed the data, and wrote the manuscript. SS and MN made the critical revisions to the manuscript and helped to finalize the article. All authors read and approved the final manuscript.

Competing interests
NH has received research consulting fees from Kyowa Hakko Kirin Co., Ltd.; lecture fees from Bayer Yakuhin, Ltd., Chugai Pharmaceutical Co., Ltd., Kyowa Hakko Kirin Co., Ltd., and Nikkiso Co., Ltd.; and grant support from Chugai Pharmaceutical Co., Ltd. and Kyowa Hakko Kirin Co., Ltd. NH was also a member of a division that is funded by Terumo Corporation. The other authors declare that they have no competing interests.

Author details
[1]Department of Blood Purification, Kidney Center, Tokyo Women's Medical University, 8-1 Kawada-cho, Shinjuku-ku, Tokyo 162-8666, Japan. [2]Division of Nephrology and Endocrinology, The University of Tokyo School of Medicine, Tokyo, Japan.

References

1. Masakane I, Nakai S, Ogata S, Kimata N, Hanafusa N, Hamano T, Wakai K, Wada A, Nitta K. An overview of regular dialysis treatment in Japan (as of 31 December 2013). Ther Apher Dial. 2015;19:540–74.
2. Saran R, Li Y, Robinson B, Ayanian J, Balkrishnan R, Bragg-Gresham J, Chen JT, Cope E, Gipson D, He K, et al. US renal data system 2014 annual data report: epidemiology of kidney disease in the United States. Am J Kidney Dis. 2015;66:Svii. S1-305.
3. Fielding RA, Vellas B, Evans WJ, Bhasin S, Morley JE, Newman AB, Abellan van Kan G, Andrieu S, Bauer J, Breuille D, et al. Sarcopenia: an undiagnosed condition in older adults. Current consensus definition: prevalence, etiology, and consequences. International working group on sarcopenia. J Am Med Dir Assoc. 2011;12:249–56.
4. Fouque D, Kalantar-Zadeh K, Kopple J, Cano N, Chauveau P, Cuppari L, Franch H, Guarnieri G, Ikizler TA, Kaysen G, et al. A proposed nomenclature and diagnostic criteria for protein-energy wasting in acute and chronic kidney disease. Kidney Int. 2008;73:391–8.
5. Fried LP, Tangen CM, Walston J, Newman AB, Hirsch C, Gottdiener J, Seeman T, Tracy R, Kop WJ, Burke G, et al. Frailty in older adults: evidence for a phenotype. J Gerontol A Biol Sci Med Sci. 2001;56:M146–56.
6. Isoyama N, Qureshi AR, Avesani CM, Lindholm B, Barany P, Heimburger O, Cederholm T, Stenvinkel P, Carrero JJ. Comparative associations of muscle mass and muscle strength with mortality in dialysis patients. Clin J Am Soc Nephrol. 2014;9:1720–8.
7. Johansen KL, Chertow GM, Jin C, Kutner NG. Significance of frailty among dialysis patients. J Am Soc Nephrol. 2007;18:2960–7.
8. Hanafusa N, Nomura T, Hasegawa T, Nangaku M. Age and anemia management: relationship of hemoglobin levels with mortality might differ between elderly and nonelderly hemodialysis patients. Nephrol Dial Transplant. 2014;29:2316–26.
9. Locatelli F, Pisoni RL, Combe C, Bommer J, Andreucci VE, Piera L, Greenwood R, Feldman HI, Port FK, Held PJ. Anaemia in haemodialysis patients of five European countries: association with morbidity and mortality in the Dialysis Outcomes and Practice Patterns Study (DOPPS). Nephrol Dial Transplant. 2004;19:121–32.
10. Canaud B, Tong L, Tentori F, Akiba T, Karaboyas A, Gillespie B, Akizawa T, Pisoni RL, Bommer J, Port FK. Clinical practices and outcomes in elderly hemodialysis patients: results from the Dialysis Outcomes and Practice Patterns Study (DOPPS). Clin J Am Soc Nephrol. 2011;6:1651–62.
11. Foote C, Ninomiya T, Gallagher M, Perkovic V, Cass A, McDonald SP, Jardine M. Survival of elderly dialysis patients is predicted by both patient and practice characteristics. Nephrol Dial Transplant. 2012;27:3581–7.
12. Moss AH, Ganjoo J, Sharma S, Gansor J, Senft S, Weaner B, Dalton C, MacKay K, Pellegrino B, Anantharaman P, Schmidt R. Utility of the "surprise" question to identify dialysis patients with high mortality. Clin J Am Soc Nephrol. 2008;3:1379–84.
13. Hanafusa N, Nakai S, Iseki K, Tsubakihara Y. Japanese society for dialysis therapy renal data registry—a window through which we can view the details of Japanese dialysis population. Kidney Int Suppl. 2015;5:15–22.
14. An Overview of Regular Dialysis Treatment in Japan [http://member.jsdt.or.jp/member/contents/cdrom/2013/main.html]. Accessed 17 Apr 2016.
15. Shinzato T, Nakai S, Miwa M, Iwayama N, Takai I, Matsumoto Y, Morita H, Maeda K. New method to calculate creatinine generation rate using pre- and postdialysis creatinine concentrations. Artif Organs. 1997;21:864–72.
16. Shinzato T, Nakai S, Fujita Y, Takai I, Morita H, Nakane K, Maeda K. Determination of Kt/V and protein catabolic rate using pre- and postdialysis blood urea nitrogen concentrations. Nephron. 1994;67:280–90.
17. Daugirdas JT. Simplified equations for monitoring Kt/V, PCRn, eKt/V, and ePCRn. Adv Ren Replace Ther. 1995;2:295–304.
18. Clark BC, Manini TM. Sarcopenia =/= dynapenia. J Gerontol A Biol Sci Med Sci. 2008;63:829–34.
19. Kim JC, Kalantar-Zadeh K, Kopple JD. Frailty and protein-energy wasting in elderly patients with end stage kidney disease. J Am Soc Nephrol. 2013;24:337–51.
20. Friedman AN, Fadem SZ. Reassessment of albumin as a nutritional marker in kidney disease. J Am Soc Nephrol. 2010;21:223–30.
21. Lopes AA, Elder SJ, Ginsberg N, Andreucci VE, Cruz JM, Fukuhara S, Mapes DL, Saito A, Pisoni RL, Saran R, Port FK. Lack of appetite in haemodialysis patients—associations with patient characteristics, indicators of nutritional status and outcomes in the international DOPPS. Nephrol Dial Transplant. 2007;22:3538–46.
22. Kalantar-Zadeh K, Gutekunst L, Mehrotra R, Kovesdy CP, Bross R, Shinaberger CS, Noori N, Hirschberg R, Benner D, Nissenson AR, Kopple JD. Understanding sources of dietary phosphorus in the treatment of patients with chronic kidney disease. Clin J Am Soc Nephrol. 2010;5:519–30.
23. Levin NW, Kotanko P, Eckardt KU, Kasiske BL, Chazot C, Cheung AK, Redon J, Wheeler DC, Zoccali C, London GM. Blood pressure in chronic kidney disease stage 5D-report from a kidney disease: improving global outcomes controversies conference. Kidney Int. 2010;77:273–84.
24. Kalantar-Zadeh K, Block G, Humphreys MH, Kopple JD. Reverse epidemiology of cardiovascular risk factors in maintenance dialysis patients. Kidney Int. 2003;63:793–808.
25. Kalantar-Zadeh K, Kopple JD, Kilpatrick RD, McAllister CJ, Shinaberger CS, Gjertson DW, Greenland S. Association of morbid obesity and weight change over time with cardiovascular survival in hemodialysis population. Am J Kidney Dis. 2005;46:489–500.
26. Marcelli D, Brand K, Ponce P, Milkowski A, Marelli C, Ok E, Merello Godino JI, Gurevich K, Jirka T, Rosenberger J, et al. Longitudinal changes in body composition in patients after initiation of hemodialysis therapy: results from an international cohort. J Ren Nutr. 2016;26:72–80.
27. Abramowitz MK, Sharma D, Folkert VW. Hidden obesity in dialysis patients: clinical implications. Semin Dial. 2016;29:391–5.
28. Shapiro BB, Streja E, Ravel VA, Kalantar-Zadeh K, Kopple JD. Association of height with mortality in patients undergoing maintenance hemodialysis. Clin J Am Soc Nephrol. 2015;10:965–74.
29. Elsayed ME, Ferguson JP, Stack AG. Association of height with elevated mortality risk in ESRD: variation by race and gender. J Am Soc Nephrol. 2016;27:580–93.

2

Causative organisms and outcomes of peritoneal dialysis-related peritonitis in Sarawak General Hospital, Kuching, Malaysia: a 3-year analysis

Vui Eng Phui[1*], Clare Hui Hong Tan[1], Chee Kean Chen[2], Kee Hoe Lai[3], Kwek Foong Chew[1], Hock Hin Chua[1], Laura Lui Sian Ngu[1] and Lawrence Wei Soon Hii[1]

Abstract

Background: Peritoneal dialysis peritonitis remains a significant cause of morbidity for peritoneal dialysis patients and the main reason for conversion from peritoneal dialysis to hemodialysis. As the characteristics of patients and microbial susceptibility vary from center to center, the aim of this study is to evaluate the microbiology and the clinical outcomes among continuous ambulatory peritoneal dialysis patients in Kuching, Malaysia.

Methods: This is a retrospective record review of 82 continuous ambulatory peritoneal dialysis patients who developed peritonitis during 2013 to 2015. Data examined included patients' demographic data, causative organisms, and outcomes.

Results: A total of 124 episodes of peritonitis were recorded, and the overall peritonitis rate was 0.40 episodes per patient-year. There was an increasing incidence in continuous ambulatory peritoneal dialysis peritonitis over the 3-year study period (0.35 to 0.47 episodes per patient-year). The gram-negative peritonitis rate increased over the period until towards the end of the study period, when gram-positive and gram-negative organisms accounted for almost equal proportions of peritonitis. *Streptococcus* sp. was the most common organism among the gram-positive peritonitis while *Pseudomonas* sp. was the most common organism in gram-negative peritonitis. The culture-negative peritonitis rate was 25.8%. The peritoneal dialysis catheter was removed in 32 episodes (26.6%). The catheter loss rate was significantly higher in gram-negative peritonitis, as compared to gram-positive peritonitis (38.9 vs 16.7%, $p = 0.027$).

Conclusions: The increasing trend of peritonitis and high rates of culture negativity and peritoneal dialysis catheter removal are areas that need further evaluation and improvement in the future. Study on risk factors of continuous ambulatory peritoneal dialysis peritonitis, detailed microbiology, and antimicrobial treatment and response are warranted to further improve the outcomes of continuous ambulatory peritoneal dialysis patients.

Keywords: Continuous ambulating peritoneal dialysis, Peritonitis, Microorganisms, Catheter removal

* Correspondence: leshally@hotmail.com
[1]Department of Medicine, Sarawak General Hospital, Jalan Hospital, 93586 Kuching, Sarawak, Malaysia
Full list of author information is available at the end of the article

Background

Peritoneal dialysis (PD) is an important treatment modality for patients with end-stage renal disease (ESRD) [1–4]. Despite the introduction of improved connection systems and PD solutions, peritonitis remains a significant cause of morbidity for PD patients and the main reason for conversion from PD to hemodialysis [4–7].

The clinical outcome of PD peritonitis is determined greatly by the causative organism [8, 9]. Empirical treatment usually covers both gram-positive and gram-negative organisms. However, the causative organism may vary depending on the area and the environment and social background of patients. Treatment guidelines should be modified from time to time based on knowledge of recent, local epidemiological trends and susceptibility to antimicrobial agents, to try to improve patient outcomes [10].

Sarawak is a state in Malaysia with a big geographical area and widely varied population characteristics. There is currently no published data on the causative organisms in continuous ambulatory peritoneal dialysis (CAPD) peritonitis and their outcomes in Sarawak. Hence, we studied the incidence, the microbiological characteristics, and the eventual clinical outcomes of CAPD peritonitis for all CAPD patients followed up at Sarawak General Hospital, between January 2013 and December 2015.

Methods

This is a retrospective record review of all CAPD patients on follow-up at the Nephrology Unit, Sarawak General Hospital, Kuching, Malaysia, who developed peritonitis between January 2013 and December 2015. A total of 82 CAPD patients developed peritonitis during this study period, and 124 episodes of peritonitis were recorded.

For all CAPD patients in our center, a double-cuffed straight Tenckhoff catheter was inserted by surgical technique by one of the three urologists. CAPD was started after a break-in period of 12 ± 4 days. All patients had routine screening for *Staphylococcus aureus* nasal carriage, and eradication of carriers was done by intranasal mupirocin before catheter insertion. Eight of the patients were carriers and needed the eradication. Intravenous cefoperazon and cefazolin were given as prophylactic antibiotics immediately prior to catheter insertion. All patients or their assistants underwent a structured 10 to 14 days of training at the start of CAPD. This included basic principles of CAPD, types of PD solutions and consumables, handwashing techniques and hygiene, CAPD exchange procedures and exit-site care, recording of BP, weight and ultrafiltration, peritonitis recognition and management, and diet and medication counseling. Subsequently, they were started on a disconnect system using PD solution

with three 2-L exchanges daily. Forty-six patients (56.1%) were on the Baxter system and 36 patients (43.9%) on the Fresenius system. Either mupirocin or gentamicin cream was used on the exit site as a daily routine, and the choice was left to the discretion of the treating nephrologist.

Demographic data collected included age at time of peritonitis, sex, body mass index, education level and causes of ESRD. Clinical data pertaining to peritonitis collected included causative organisms, antimicrobial therapy, serum albumin and potassium level, intraperitoneal leucocyte count at the beginning of peritonitis, susceptibility of each organism, and date of catheter removal.

The diagnosis of PD peritonitis was made when at least two of the following three criteria were fulfilled: (i) signs and symptoms of peritonitis, (ii) cloudy dialysate with white blood cell count of >100/µL. and (iii) demonstration of organism either by smear examination or by culture of peritoneal dialysate. All 82 patients fulfilled the first and second criteria as they presented with abdominal symptoms and had cloudy dialysate with white cell count of >100/µL. An episode of peritonitis within 4 weeks after the treatment of a previous episode was considered a relapse and was not classified as a new infection. A peritonitis episode which occurred within 7 days after catheter placement was also excluded in this study. Refractory peritonitis was defined as peritonitis that did not respond to second-line antimicrobial treatment and resulted in catheter removal. The culture of PD fluid and antimicrobial sensitivity were obtained from the microbiology department of this hospital, based on hospital standard operating procedure. The causative organisms were divided into gram-positive, gram-negative, polybacterial, fungal, mycobacterium, and culture-negative.

Our first-line therapy for CAPD peritonitis was a combination of intraperitoneal cefazolin and ceftazidime. The antibiotics were adjusted later once culture and sensitivity results became available. If the peritonitis did not improve within 72 h and culture was negative, treatment would be escalated to IP meropenam and vancomycin. If the peritonitis still failed to respond, then the PD catheter would be removed. All patients with peritonitis also received oral nystatin or fluconazole empirically during antibiotic therapy.

Outcomes of peritonitis were classified as initial cure, catheter loss, conversion to hemodialysis, and patient death. Initial cure was defined as total resolution of peritonitis with only antimicrobial treatment. Catheter loss was defined as removal of catheter due to non-resolution of peritonitis. Patient death included any mortality within 4 weeks of presentation of peritonitis when all other possible causes of mortality had been excluded.

Peritonitis rate was calculated by totaling all the peritonitis episodes that occurred during the entire time at risk on CAPD for all the patients in the program during the period of the study. This total was then divided by the time at risk in years. The time at risk for peritonitis was counted from the first day of training till the occurrence of peritonitis.

Data were expressed as episodes per patient-year, percent, and mean ± standard deviation (SD). Differences in the proportion of causative organisms were analyzed according to each calendar year. Antimicrobial susceptibilities and catheter removal rates according to the pathogens were analyzed using chi-square analysis or Fischer's exact test. Statistical significance was determined as p value less than 0.05.

Results

Population characteristics

During the study period, 124 episodes of peritonitis were detected among 82 CAPD patients. Fifty-four patients had a single episode, 18 patients had two episodes, 7 patients had three episodes, and 3 patients had four episodes of peritonitis. Gender distribution was equal with 41 male and female patients. Their mean age at the time of peritonitis was 45.4 ± 15.8 years. 18.3% of patients had diabetes mellitus. Twenty-eight patients (34.1%) were on exit-site mupirocin while the remaining 54 patients (65.9%) were on exit-site gentamicin. The baseline characteristics of patients and the underlying causes of renal impairment are shown in Table 1.

Peritonitis and microbiology

The overall peritonitis rate during the 3-year period was 0.40 episodes per patient-year. The peritonitis rate showed an increasing trend over time (Table 2). About one third (33.9%) of the peritonitis was caused by gram-positive organisms, 29.0% by gram-negative bacteria, 3.2% were fungal infection, and 1.6% were *Mycobacterium tuberculosis*. Culture was sterile in 28.2% of the cases and polymicrobial in five cases (4%).

During the 3-year period, there was an increase in peritonitis due to gram-negative organisms, from 18.8% in 2013 to 32.5% in 2014 and 32.7% in 2015. By 2015, gram-positive and gram-negative organisms accounted for almost equal proportions of peritonitis at our center. Culture-negative peritonitis has reduced from 37.5% in 2013 to 26.9% in 2015. Peritonitis episodes secondary to fungal, *M. tuberculosis*, and polybacterial infection did not change significantly over the 3-year period.

The most common gram-positive organism responsible for CAPD peritonitis at our center was *Streptococcus* sp., accounting for more than one third of the gram-positive episodes, followed in descending order of frequency by coagulase-negative *Staphylococcus* (CoNS), *S. aureus*, and *Enterococci*. *Pseudomonas aeruginosa* (PAE) was the most commonly identified gram-negative organism, followed by

Escherichia coli (*E. coli*), *Acinetobacter* spp., *Klebsiella* spp. (KPN), and *Enterobacter*.

There were four episodes (3.2%) of fungal and two episodes (1.6%) of *M. tuberculosis* (TB) infections during the 3-year period. Five episodes of polymicrobial peritonitis were isolated, and the combinations of infection were *M. tuberculosis* and CoNs, PAE and fungal infection, *Acinetobacter app* and *Streptococcus viridans*, PAE and *Achromobacter spp.*, and KPN, *E. coli*, and *Enterobacter*. The causative organisms of peritonitis over the 3-year study period are listed in Table 3.

Table 1 Characteristics of patients

	Total
Patients (*n*)	82
Sex (male/female) (%)	41 (50.0):41 (50.0)
Age (years)	45.4 (±15.8)
Body mass index (kg/cm²)	22.1 (±3.8)
Ethnicity (%)	
Malay	32 (39.0)
Chinese	15 (18.3)
Iban	20 (24.4)
Bidayuh	13 (15.9)
Others	2 (2.4)
Living area (%)	
Urban	40 (48.4)
Suburban	42 (51.6)
Education level (%)	
Illiterate	12 (14.6)
Primary	31 (37.8)
Secondary	32 (39.0)
Tertiary	7 (8.6)
Underlying disease (%)	
Hypertension	34 (41.5)
Diabetes mellitus	15 (18.3)
Obstructive nephropathy	8 (9.8)
Systemic lupus erythematosus	2 (2.4)
Glomerulonephritis	8 (9.8)
Unknown	15 (18.3)
Exit-site cream (mupirocin/gentamicin) (%)	28 (34.1):54 (65.9)

Table 2 Peritonitis rate per patient-year, 2013–2015

	2013	2014	2015
Cumulative patient-days	32,177	39,233	41,289
Cumulative episodes	31	40	53
Cumulative patient-months	1057.9	1289.9	1357.4
Cumulative patient case	34.1	32.3	25.6
Peritonitis episode per patient-year	0.350	0.370	0.468

Table 3 The microbiology of peritonitis episodes

	Number isolated in 2013	Number isolated in 2014	Number isolated in 2015	Total number isolated (n = 124)	Percentage of total episode
Gram-positive organism	10 (31.3%)	14 (35%)	18 (34.6%)	42	33.9
Streptococcus sp.	4	4	10	18	14.5
Coagulase-negative Staphylococcus (CoNS)	4	5	5	14	13.7
Staphylococcus aureus	1	3	3	7	4.0
Other gram-positive organisms	1	2	0	3	1.6
Gram-negative organism	6 (18.8%)	13 (32.5%)	17 (32.7%)	36	29.0
Pseudomonas sp.	3	4	7	14	11.3
Escherichia coli (E. coli)	1	1	4	6	4.0
Acinetobacter sp.	1	2	2	5	4.0
Klebsiella sp.	1	2	1	4	4.0
Enterobacter sp.	0	1	1	2	1.6
Other gram-negative organisms	0	3	2	5	6.5
Fungi	2	1	1	4	3.2
Mycobacterium tuberculosis	1	0	1	2	1.6
Polymicrobial	1	3	1	5	4.0
Culture-negative	12 (37.5%)	9 (22.5%)	14 (26.9%)	35	28.2
Total	32	40	52	124	100.0

Outcome

The PD catheter was removed in 33 (26.6%) peritonitis episodes after failing to respond to antimicrobial treatment. Twenty-three patients were converted to hemodialysis due to the peritonitis during the study period. No death was reported in current study. Tables 4 and 5 show various causative organisms which resulted in catheter loss. The catheter loss was significantly higher in gram-negative peritonitis episodes ($p < 0.05$). Polybacterial infection also had a high rate of catheter loss (60%). 27.8% of gram-negative peritonitis resulted in conversion to HD vs 14.3% of gram-positive peritonitis, but this did not reach statistical significance.

Among 14 episodes of *Pseudomonas* peritonitis, eight were on mupirocin cream, and six were on gentamicin cream. Among the six gentamicin users, four (66.4%) gentamicin users compared with only three (37.5%) mupirocin users needed catheter removal, as shown in Table 6.

Discussion

Peritonitis is an important cause of morbidity and mortality for CAPD patients. The epidemiology, treatment, prevention, and outcome of CAPD peritonitis have been the subject of interest among clinicians and researchers since a few decades ago [3–5]. Despite the widespread availability and awareness of both local and international guidelines for its prevention and treatment, there is still substantial variation in CAPD peritonitis microbiology and outcome among different centers and regions.

The overall CAPD peritonitis rate of 0.40 episodes per patient-year in this study is comparable to that of other centers in this region, e.g., Japan 0.195 [11], Australia 0.60 [9], Northern India 0.41 [12], Korea 0.40 [13], Thailand 0.47 [14], Singapore 0.59 [15], and Indonesia 0.25 [16]. This is however higher than the national average of 0.28 in 2014 [17]. The possible reasons could include lower educational level among our study population as 52.4% of them were either illiterate or only obtained primary education, and 51.6% were from suburban area. This may result in poorer adherence to aseptic techniques during PD exchange, suboptimal home

Table 4 Removal of PD catheter in various causative agents in peritonitis

	Removal of catheter		Total
	Yes	No	
Gram-positive	7 (16.7%)	35 (83.3%)	42
Gram-negative	14 (38.9%)	22 (61.1%)	36
Fungal	3 (75.0%)	1 (25.0%)	4
Tuberculosis	2 (100%)	0 (0.0%)	2
Polybacterial	3 (60.0%)	2 (40.0%)	5
Culture-negative	3 (8.6%)	32 (91.4%)	35
Total	32 (26.6%)	92 (73.4%)	124

Table 5 Comparison of outcomes in gram-positive and gram-negative peritonitis

Outcome	Gram-positive (n = 42)	Gram-negative (n = 36)	p
Catheter loss	7 (16.7%)	14 (38.9%)	0.027*
Shift to hemodialysis	7 (16.7%)	10 (27.8%)	0.236

* p < 0.05

environment for PD including irregular clean water supply, and delay in seeking treatment or medical advice. This is consistent with our national registry report where the higher income group has lower risk of peritonitis [17]. Other factors such as bowel flora migration and chronic malnutrition seem less likely as most patients had normal serum albumin and potassium during initial presentation of PD peritonitis (mean of 32.19 ± 6.45 mmol/L and 3.45 ± 0.75 mmol/L, respectively).

The current study has allowed us to evaluate the evolution of microbiology in CAPD peritonitis in our population. Over the 3-year study period, there was an increasing incidence in CAPD peritonitis in contrary to other centers which showed significant decreasing trend in incidence over years [12, 13]. This is worrying and may be contributed by the reasons stated below but needs further analysis so that the rate of peritonitis can be reduced. We have increased intake of CAPD patients over the 3-year study period. There were 17 new patients in 2013, 28 new patients in 2014, and 42 new patients in 2015. Many of our patients are from suburban areas where the home environment may not be ideal for CAPD and a clean water supply may not be available all the time. They may also present late or do not seek advice promptly from our CAPD staff when needed. Some patients have to resort to rain water or mountain water supply at times, and some patients reported dirty water from the pipe prior to onset of peritonitis. To overcome this problem, we have started installing water filters for some of the patients. In 2013–2015, we installed water filters for three patients per year and this has increased to seven patients in 2016. Our CAPD nurses also tried to do more home visits to see how to improve patients' home environment for CAPD. This may be quite difficult and time-consuming as some of our patients live very far away in the rural areas. In 2013, 10 home visits were done and this has increased

to 18 in 2014 and 29 in 2015. All patients or their assistants were trained for 10 days to 2 weeks prior to the start of CAPD. Some of them, however, did not follow instructions strictly after discharge, and some assistants subsequently passed the "job" to other family members when they were busy. We noted quite a number of cases of peritonitis due to CAPD being performed by non-trained personnel. We have re-emphasized this during training and have done reassessment or re-training of the patients or their assistants during hospital admissions, clinic visits, or home visits. Similar problems with different magnitude have been reported in previous studies from developing countries involving CAPD in rural area [18, 19].

The increase in overall peritonitis rate in the current study was mainly due to the increase in gram-negative peritonitis while the episodes of gram-positive peritonitis remained the same. At the end of the 3-year period, gram-positive and gram-negative organisms accounted for almost equal proportions of peritonitis at our center. This trend is also noted in our national registry [17] and similar to those reported by Prasad et al. [12] and other studies [20, 21]. Most of the previous series, however, reported that gram-positive bacteria accounted for approximately two thirds of the peritonitis episodes with gram-negative bacteria accounting for one third or less of peritonitis episodes [4, 9, 11, 13].

In gram-positive single-organism peritonitis, CoNS was the most common organism isolated in many previous reports [3, 9, 12, 13]. However, in our study, *Streptococcus* sp. was the most common among the gram-positive organisms, a finding which is quite similar to those from Spanish [8], Japanese [11], and Taiwanese [22] cohorts.

Pseudomonas sp. was the most commonly isolated organism in gram-negative peritonitis episodes in our study. This is in contrast with our national registry data and other series where *E. coli* was the most common pathogen in gram-negative peritonitis [4, 9, 11, 12, 17]. Such findings could be related to the water source among our CAPD patients. More than half of our patients lived in suburban areas where a clean water supply may not be universal and consistent, and some may be using untreated water from natural resources when the need arises.

Daily application of mupirocin or gentamicin cream to the exit site was routine practice in our patients. Overall, about one third of our CAPD patients used mupirocin and two thirds used gentamicin cream. As we did not collect data for those patients without peritonitis, we are unable to analyze whether there was any difference in the incidence of peritonitis between mupirocin or gentamicin cream users. It is interesting to note that among those patients with peritonitis, mupirocin use or gentamicin use was

Table 6 Association of PD catheter removal and exit-site cream among 14 episodes of Pseudomonas peritonitis

Exit-site cream	PD catheter removal		Total
	Yes	No	
Mupirocin	3	5	8
Gentamycin	4	2	6
	7	7	14

associated with almost equal proportion of gram-positive and gram-negative peritonitis.

When we explore further into these 14 episodes of *Pseudomonas* peritonitis, current data suggests that gentamicin cream may be associated with lower incidence of *Pseudomonas* infection as the majority (two thirds) of our CAPD patients used gentamicin cream. However, the higher rate of catheter removal (66.4%) among the gentamicin users vs 37.5% of mupirocin users in this subpopulation may suggest resistance of *Pseudomonas* to gentamicin. As the number of patients with *Pseudomonas* peritonitis in current study was small, this remains an interesting observation and may be an area of future research. The superiority of either exit-site mupirocin or gentamicin in preventing PD peritonitis remains the subject of further investigation even though there are more evidence showing exit-site gentamicin to be associated with lower overall peritonitis rate [23, 24].

Our culture-negative peritonitis rate was 25.8% which was comparable with the national average of 25.6% [17]. This is however high by the International Society for Peritoneal Dialysis (ISPD) standard [10]. Isolation of microorganism depends upon various factors, namely culture technique, previous antibiotic exposure, concentration of dialysate effluent, and lag times between sample collection and culturing [25, 26]. In our center. CAPD staff took PD fluid for culture for all cases with suspected peritonitis immediately before antibiotic administration. Delay in culturing might have contributed to culture-negative peritonitis as there was a small portion of patients with peritonitis who presented to the hospital after office hour. PD fluid for culture was taken, but the PD fluid was kept in the refrigerator and was sent to the laboratory the following morning. The high incidence of culture-negative peritonitis in this center could also be explained by previous antibiotic exposure. As over half of our patients came from suburban areas, they presented to the nearest district hospitals first when they were unwell and often intravenous antibiotics were started before they were transferred to our center. Hence, PD fluid culture was done after the start of antibiotics in these cases. Similar observations were reported by Kim et al. [13] and Szeto et al. [27], where the incidence of culture-negative peritonitis was high in the respective centers. PD fluid culture method is another aspect that we need to stress here as during the period of study conducted, the culture method in our hospital has not been standardized. PD fluid culture was carried out by either one of the three methods, namely direct inoculation of PD fluid into a blood culture bottle (BACTEC), direct culturing of PD fluid on an agar plate, or culturing the sediment after centrifuging PD fluid on an agar plate. The last method is the ISPD-recommended method [10], and we will encourage this method in order to decrease culture-negative peritonitis rate in the future.

The catheter loss rate in this study was 26.6%, a rate which was high compared to previous series in which the catheter loss rate ranged between 9.8 and 20.4% [9, 11–13, 28]. We believe that the higher rate of catheter loss in our study was mainly due to the high proportion of gram-negative peritonitis (29% of total peritonitis episodes) especially *Pseudomonas* peritonitis. From our renal registry, *Pseudomonas* peritonitis was associated with the highest catheter loss rate excluding fungal and TB peritonitis [17]. Other contributing factors may include late presentation and treatment. Our study also confirmed that catheter loss was significantly higher in gram-negative peritonitis, as compared to gram-positive peritonitis (38.9 vs 16.7%, $p = 0.027$). This has been reported in many previous series, where gram-negative peritonitis was associated with a higher rate of antimicrobial resistance, catheter loss, shift of PD to hemodialysis, and mortality [12, 29, 30].

Some limitations of the study must be stressed. The most obvious limitation of the current study is that it is retrospective in design, and therefore, it has all the flaws and problems associated with such studies. This study was carried out on CAPD patients with peritonitis only. Therefore, the risk factors associated with developing peritonitis cannot be determined as data of CAPD patients without peritonitis were not collected. Due to various degrees of incomplete data collection, analysis on antimicrobial treatment and response was not possible, an aspect which is important in developing future guidelines in management of peritonitis. Lastly, this is a single-center study and the outcomes described here are unique to this study population.

Conclusions

In summary, this study provides timely data on emerging trends of epidemiology and microbiology of CAPD peritonitis in our population. Despite some similarities, there are also significant differences in the microbiological profiles and outcomes of our CAPD peritonitis from those of other centers. Increasing trend of peritonitis, high rates of culture negativity and PD catheter removal, and the role of exit-site cream in developing antimicrobial resistance are areas that need further evaluation and improvement in the future. Studies on risk factors of CAPD peritonitis, detailed microbiology, and antimicrobial treatment and response are warranted to further improve the outcome of CAPD patients.

Abbreviations

CAPD: Continuous ambulatory peritoneal dialysis; CoNS: Coagulase-negative *Staphylococcus*; ESRD: End-stage renal disease; KPN: *Klebsiella pneumoniae*; PAE: *Pseudomonas aeruginosa*; PD: Peritoneal dialysis; SD: Standard deviation

Acknowledgements

The authors would like to thank Dr. Goh Kiang Hua, MBBS, FRCS, for the critical review and editing support of this manuscript.

Funding

The authors declare no financial disclosure.

Authors' contributions

VEP was responsible for the data collection and drafted the entire manuscript. KHL and KFC participated in the design of the study and were involved in data the collection. LLSN and LWSH interpreted the results and contributed to the manuscript writing. HHC was involved in developing the study protocol and study implementation. CKC performed the data analysis and contributed to the manuscript writing. CHHT overviewed the research. All authors read and approved the final manuscript.

Competing interests

The authors declare that they have no competing interests.

Author details

[1]Department of Medicine, Sarawak General Hospital, Jalan Hospital, 93586 Kuching, Sarawak, Malaysia. [2]Department of Anaesthesiology, Kuching Specialist Hospital, Kuching, Sarawak, Malaysia. [3]Department of Medicine, University Malaysia Sarawak, Kota Samarahan, Sarawak, Malaysia.

References

1. Bargman JM. Advances in peritoneal dialysis: a review. Semin Dial. 2012;25:545–9.
2. USRDS: the United States Real Data System. Am J Kidney Dis. 2003; 42: Suppl 5:1-230
3. Szeto CC, Wong TY, Chow KM, Leung CB, Law MC, Wang AY. Impact of dialysis adequacy on the mortality and morbidity of anuric Chinese patients receiving continuous ambulatory peritoneal dialysis. J Am Soc Nephrol. 2001;12:355–60.
4. Han SH, Lee SC, Ahn SV, Lee JE, Choi HY, Kim BS, et al. Improving outcome of CAPD: twenty-five years' experience in a single Korean center. Perit Dial Int. 2007;27:432–40.
5. Perez Font M, Rodriguez-Carmona A, Garcia-Naveiro R, Rosales M, Villaverde P, Valdes F. Peritonitis-related mortality in patients undergoing chronic peritoneal dialysis. Perit Dial Int. 2005;25:274–84.
6. Boudville N, Kemp A, Clayton P, Lim W, Badve SV, Hawley CM, et al. Recent peritonitis associates with mortality among patients treated with peritoneal dialysis. J Am Soc Nephrol. 2012;23:1398–405.
7. van Esch S, Krediet RT, Struijk DG. 32 years' experience of peritoneal dialysis-related peritonitis in a university hospital. Perit Dial Int. 2014;34:162–70.
8. Lartundo JAQ, Palomar R, Dominguez-Diez A, Salas C, Ruiz-Criado J, Rodrigo E, et al. Microbiological profile of peritoneal dialysis peritonitis and predictors of hospitalization. Adv Perit Dial. 2011;27:38–42.
9. Ghali JR, Bannister KM, Brown FG, Rosman JB, Wiggins KJ, Johnson DW, et al. Microbiology and outcomes of peritonitis in Australian peritoneal dialysis patients. Perit Dial Int. 2011;31:651–62.
10. Li PK, Szeto CC, Piraino B, Arteaga J, Fan S, Figueiredo AE, et al. ISPD peritonitis recommendations: 2016 update on prevention and treatment. Perit Dial Int. 2016;36:481–508.
11. Higuchi C, Ito M, Masakane I, Sakura H. Peritonitis in peritoneal dialysis patients in Japan: a 2013 retrospective questionnaire survey of Japanese Society for Peritoneal Dialysis member institutions. Renal Replacement Therapy. 2016;2(2):1–8.
12. Prasad KN, Singh K, Rizwan A, Mishra P, Tiwari D, Prasad N, et al. Microbiology and outcomes of peritonitis in northern India. Perit Dial Int. 2014;34:188–94.
13. Kim DK, Yoo TH, Ryu DR, Xu ZG, Kim HJ, Choi KH, et al. Changes in causative organisms and their antimicrobial susceptibilities in CAPD peritonitis: a single center's experience over one decade. Perit Dial Int. 2004;24:424–32.
14. Kanjanabuch T, Chancharoenthana W, Katavetin P, Sritippayawan S, Praditpornsilpa K, Ariyapitipan S, et al. The incidence of peritoneal dialysis-related infection in Thailand: a nationwide survey. J Med Assoc Thai. 2011;94:7–12.
15. Lee GS, Woo KT. Infection in continuous ambulatory peritoneal dialysis (CAPD): aetiology, complications and risk factors. Ann Acad Med Singapore. 1992;21:354–60.
16. Suhardjono. The development of a continuous ambulatory peritoneal dialysis program in Indonesia. Perit Dial Int. 2008;28 Suppl 3:59–62.
17. Goh BL, Ong LM, editors. Twenty second report of the Malaysian dialysis and transplant 2014, Kuala Lumpur. 2015.
18. Hyodo T, Hirawa N, Hayashi M, Than KMM, Tuyen DG, Pattanasittangkur K, et al. Present status of renal replacement therapy at 2015 in Asian countries (Myanmar, Vietnam, Thailand, China and Japan). Ren Replace Ther. 2017;3(11):1–14.
19. Nayak KS, Sinoj KA, Subhramanyam SV, Mary B, Rao NV. Our experience of home visits in city and rural areas. Perit Dial Int. 2007;27 Suppl 2:27–31.
20. Zelenitsky S, Barns L, Findlay I, Alfa M, Ariano R, Fine A, Harding G. Analysis of microbiological trends in peritoneal dialysis-related peritonitis from 1991 to 1998. Am J Kidney Dis. 2000;36:1009–13.
21. Verger C, Ryckelynck JP, Duman M, Veniez G, Lobbedez T, Boulanger E, et al. French peritoneal dialysis registry (RDPLF): outline and main results. Kidney Int Suppl. 2006;103:S12–20.
22. Hsieh YP, Chang CC, Wang SC, Wen YK, Chiu PF, Yang Y. Predictor for and impact of high peritonitis rate in Taiwanese continuous ambulatory peritoneal dialysis patients. Int Urol Nephrol. 2015;47:183–9.
23. Bernardini J, Bender F, Florio T, Sloand J, Palmmontalbano L, Fried L, et al. Randomized, double-blind trial of antibiotic exit site cream for prevention of exit site infection in peritoneal dialysis patients. J Am Soc Nephrol. 2005;16:539–45.
24. Burkhalter F, Clemenger M, Haddoub SS, McGrory J, Hisole N, Brown E. Pseudomonas exit-site infection: treatment outcomes with topical gentamicin in addition to systemic antibiotics. Clin Kidney J. 2015;8(6):781–4.
25. Kocyigit I, Unal A, Karademir D, Bahcebasi S, Sipahioglu MH, Tokgoz B, et al. Improvement in culture-negative peritoneal dialysis-related peritonitis: a single center's experience. Perit Dial Int. 2012;32:476–8.
26. Sewell DL, Golper TA, Hulman PB, Thomas CM, West LM, Kubey WY, et al. Comparison of large volume culture to other methods for isolation of microorganisms from dialysate. Perit Dial Int. 1990;10:49–52.
27. Szeto CC, Wong TYH, Chow KM, Leung CB, Li PKT. The clinical course of culture-negative peritonitis complicating peritoneal dialysis. Am J Kidney Dis. 2003;42:567–74.
28. Lee S, Kim H, Kim KH, Hann HJ, Ahn HS, Kim SJ, Kang DH, Choi KB, Ryu DR. Technique failure in Korean incident peritoneal dialysis patients: a national population-based study. Kidney Res Clin Pract. 2016;35:245–51.
29. Siva B, Hawley CM, McDonald SP, Brown FG, Rosman JB, Wiggins KJ, et al. Pseudomonas peritonitis in Australia: predictors, treatment, and outcomes in 191 cases. Clin J Am Soc Nephrol. 2009;4(5):957–64.
30. Jarvis EM, Hawley CM, McDonald SP, Brown FG, Rosman JB, Wiggins KJ, et al. Predictors, treatment, and outcomes of non-Pseudomonas Gram-negative peritonitis. Kidney Int. 2010;78(4):408–14.

3

Efficacy of Saxagliptin versus Mitiglinid in patients with type 2 diabetes and end-stage renal disease

Yukinao Sakai[1,3*], Saori Sakai[2], Koji Mugishima[1], Anna Katayama[1], Yuichiro Sumi[1], Yusuke Otsuka[1], Tomoyuki Otsuka[1] and Shuichi Tsuruoka[3]

Abstract

Background: There are very few oral antidiabetic drugs recommended for patients on dialysis. Saxagliptin is known for its potent effect and long duration of action. In this study, we compared the efficacy of Saxagliptin with Mitiglinid for diabetes control and renal anemia in hemodialysis patients with type 2 diabetes mellitus.

Methods: We performed a 6-month prospective, open-label, parallel group study of 41 patients with type 2 diabetes mellitus undergoing hemodialysis who took alpha-glucosidase inhibitors or meglitinides and did not use insulin. Saxagliptin and Mitiglinid were administered at 2.5 and 5 mg/day, respectively. The primary outcomes were changes in hemoglobin A1c (HbA1c) and glycated albumin (GA). Other efficacy assessments included changes in Hb, darbepoetin alpha (DA) dose, and erythropoietin responsiveness index (ERI).

Results: No patient required an increase in Saxagliptin or Mitiglinid dose, and there were no cases of hypoglycemia with symptoms. HbA1c and GA values were not significantly different between both groups. For HbA1c, the gradient of the regression line of the Saxagliptin and Mitiglinid groups were $Y = -7.144\text{e-}005*X + 6.023$ and $Y = -0.02604*X + 6.292$, respectively, and no significant difference was found ($p = 0.3281$). However, for GA, the regression line of the Saxagliptin group significantly decreased ($Y = -0.5036*X + 19.34$ and $Y = -0.2346*X + 18.79$, $p = 0.0371$). Both groups did not have a significant change in the DA dose through the observation period. However, the DA dose of the Saxagliptin group significantly decreased when we compared the regression lines ($Y = -0.8304*X + 21.06$ and $Y = 0.6286*X + 16.12$, $p = 0.0019$) of both groups. Furthermore, ERI did not change significantly but showed a significant difference when regression lines were compared ($Y = -0.2030*X + 6.654$ and $Y = 0.1116*X + 5.288$, $p = 0.0082$).

Conclusions: The present study showed that Saxagliptin was not inferior to Mitiglinid in the glycemic control of ESRD patients with type 2 diabetes mellitus, and it is well tolerated and safe. Saxagliptin may also improve bioavailability of iron compared to Mitiglinid, but long-term follow-up in a large scale study with more precise ferrokinetic marker measurements are necessary to confirm these results.

Keywords: End-stage renal disease, Diabetes mellitus, Hemodialysis, DPP-4 inhibitor, Saxagliptin, Glycated albumin

* Correspondence: y-sakai@nms.ac.jp
[1]Department of Nephrology, Nippon Medical School Musashikosugi Hospital, 1-396 kosugi-cho, Nakahara-ku, Kawasaki, Japan
[3]Department of Nephrology, Graduate School of Medicine, Nippon Medical School, 1-1-5 Sendagi, Bunkyo-ku, Tokyo 113-8603, Japan
Full list of author information is available at the end of the article

Background

Type 2 diabetes mellitus is on a rapid increase globally, especially in Asia [1, 2]. In Japan, the number of hemodialysis patients where diabetic nephropathy is a primary disease is increasing. Currently, diabetic nephropathy is the primary disease for approximately 40% of all patients on dialysis [3].

The National Kidney Foundation–Kidney Disease Outcomes Quality Initiative (NKF-KDOQI) guidelines recommend standard hemoglobin A1c (HbA1c) targets for patients with type 2 diabetes mellitus and end-stage renal disease (ESRD) to potentially reduce the risk of other microvascular complications (neuropathy and retinopathy) [4, 5]. However, treatment options available for these patients are limited due to safety and tolerability issues [6]. Oral medications recommended in the Japanese guidelines include only alpha-glucosidase inhibitors, meglitinides, and dipeptidyl peptidase-4 (DPP-4) inhibitors [7]. These three drug types in combination and insulin preparation are used in treatment. However, there is no evidence indicating which drug is ideal.

The DPP-4 inhibitor has few hypoglycemic side effects [8]. Also, it is hard to cause the weight gain too [9]. It has been reported to exert a kidney protection effect and is expected as the new drug of choice in diabetes treatment where there is decreased renal function [10–16]. Recently, DPP-4 inhibits hemopoietic factors such as granulocyte-colony stimulating factor (G-CSF) or erythropoietin, and it is reported that the antagonism is inhibited by DPP-4 inhibitors [17–19]. However, the clinical effect on renal anemia treatment is unknown. Meglitinides are a class of oral hypoglycaemic agents that increase insulin secretion in the pancreas. Their effect is to produce a rapid, short-lived insulin output [20].

Saxagliptin is a selective DPP-4 inhibitor specifically designed for extended inhibition of the DPP-4 enzyme that is primarily metabolized by cytochrome P450 (CYP) 3A4/5 to form an active metabolite, 5-hydroxy Saxagliptin, which is cleared by the kidney [21, 22]. Saxagliptin is eliminated by both renal and hepatic routes [23, 24]. Recent studies have shown that Saxagliptin is a well-tolerated treatment option for patients with type 2 diabetes mellitus and renal impairment [13, 25–27].

To further characterize the use of Saxagliptin in patients with kidney disease, the present study compared the efficacy of Saxagliptin with that of Mitiglinid monotherapy for diabetes control and renal anemia administered over 6 months in patients with type 2 diabetes mellitus and ESRD requiring hemodialysis.

Methods

Patients

The inclusion criteria was intended for patients who took alpha-glucosidase inhibitors or meglitinides, among patients who were on hemodialysis in an outpatient setting for chronic renal failure due to type 2 diabetes mellitus and who were not on insulin.

Patients were on hemodialysis therapy for at least 6 months and were 20 years or older at the screening visit. Exclusion criteria were as follows: (1) age <20 years; (2) a history of severe heart failure, angina, myocardial infarction, or stroke within the past 6 months; (3) the presence of infectious disease, liver dysfunction, thyroid disease, malignant tumors, or treatment with steroids or immunosuppressants; and (4) treatment with any DPP-4 inhibitor within the past 6 months.

Hemodialysis

All patients underwent dialysis for 4 or 5 h. Blood flow rate was 200 mL/min and a dialysate flow rate was 500 mL/min. All centers used the high-flux membrane, and the size of the dialyzer was decided according to the physique of the patient. The ultrafiltration-rate was decided according to the dry weight. The glucose concentration of the dialysate was 125 mg/dL. Heparin was administered at a dose of 2500–6000 U per dialysis session for anticoagulation.

Study design

This was a 6-month, prospective, open-label, parallel-group, bi-center study and was conducted between May 2014 and April 2015. Before randomization, patients stopped alpha-glucosidase inhibitors or meglitinides intake and entered a 1-month drug washout.

The patients were subsequently randomly assigned to the Saxagliptin or Mitiglinid group (open-label random assignment). For the randomization method, we performed simple randomization with alternate assignment. In the Saxagliptin group, patients received 2.5 mg of Saxagliptin once a day. In the mitiglinide group, patients received 5 mg of mitiglinide three times a day.

Downtitration, including interruption of treatment, could occur if a patient had unexplained hypoglycemia or at the clinical judgment of the investigator, to reduce the risk of hypoglycemia. Treatment adherence was assessed by patient query at prespecified visits throughout the study.

Blood samples were obtained before the first hemodialysis session of the week. Postprandial plasma glucose, complete blood cell counts, and other biochemical measurements were performed every month. All patients received Darbepoetin alpha (DA) and DA dose was adjusted according to the severity of anemia. The erythropoietin responsiveness index (ERI) was defined as the mean weekly erythropoiesis stimulating agents (ESA) dose divided by the clinical dry weight and mean blood hemoglobin [i.e., ERI = weekly ESA dose (units)/dry weight (kg)/hemoglobin (g/dL), DA (µg): ESA (units) = 1: 200] [28].

Efficacy endpoints

The primary efficacy endpoint was changes in HbA1c and GA values and comparison between the two groups. Other efficacy assessments included changes in Hb, DA dose, and ERI. Patients could be withdrawn from the study in the event of drug intolerance, if either the serum transaminase concentration or creatine kinase concentration increased to more than two times the upper limit of the normal range or other adverse events, based on the investigator's judgment.

Statistical analyses

Measurement values are shown as mean +/− standard deviation (mean +/− SD). Continuous variables were compared using the Student's t test, and one-way ANOVA was performed on the longitudinal data to address its multiplicity. Tukey's multiple comparison test was used as the post-hoc test. P values less than 0.05 were regarded as statistically significant. Regression lines were separately determined for the data collected during the 6-month period and compared. All analyses were performed using Prism software version 6 (GraphPad Software, Inc., La Jolla, CA, USA).

Results

Patient characteristics

A total of 94 patients were initially screened, and 41 patients were randomly assigned to the Saxagliptin ($n = 21$) or Mitiglinid ($n = 20$) group. Colorectal cancer was detected during an observation period, and one case in the Saxagliptin group was excluded. There was a final of 20 subjects in each group. For the premedication in both groups, there were 6 acarbose, 6 voglibose, and 8 mitiglinide in the Saxagliptin group and 8 acarbose, 5 voglibose, and 6 mitiglinide in the mitiglinide group. There was also one Glimepiride recipient in the mitiglinide group. The patient profiles are shown in Table 1. There were no significant differences in the baseline age, anthropometric variables, and laboratory data between the two groups except for serum Ca concentration.

Glycemic control

No parameter showed any significant changes during the period of examination. There were no changes in the doses of Saxagliptin and Mitiglinid.

No significant change was found in postprandial plasma glucose values over the study duration. Mean postprandial plasma glucose value 6 months after Saxagliptin administration was 152.4 +/− 74.71 mg/dL (ANOVA; $p = 0.0938$), and the regression line gradient was $Y = -0.5571*X + 150.6$ (Fig. 1), while mean postprandial plasma glucose value

Table 1 Patients' baseline profiles ($N = 40$)

Number	Saxagliptin	Mitiglinide	P value
	20	20	
Female (n)	2	5	0.4075
Age	68.6 ± 10.1	63.0 ± 13.1	0.1288
BMI	22.5 ± 2.7	24.2 ± 3.5	0.0973
HD dulation (months)	42.8 ± 36.3	70.4 ± 58.2	0.0745
DM dulation (years)	14.5 ± 6.2	15.7 ± 7.4	0.5853
Acarbose (mg/day)	225.0 ± 82.2	187.5 ± 69.4	0.3728
Voglibose (mg/day)	0.75 ± 0.16	0.66 ± 0.13	0.3527
Mitiglinide (mg/day)	16.9 ± 5.3	15.0 ± 0.0	0.4082
Glimepiride (mg/day)	–	0.50 ± 0.0	–
HbA1c (%)	6.0 ± 0.9	6.3 ± 1.4	0.5219
GA (%)	19.2 ± 3.2	18.9 ± 4.4	0.8372
BUN (mg/dL)	59.7 ± 11.9	64.4 ± 14.6	0.2724
Cr (mg/dL)	9.36 ± 2.63	10.81 ± 3.47	0.1396
UA (mg/dL)	5.8 ± 1.4	6.5 ± 1.5	0.1427
Na (mEq/L)	133.9 ± 2.2	138.4 ± 2.7	0.384
K (mEq/L)	5.0 ± 0.7	4.7 ± 0.7	0.1736
Cl (mEq/L)	107.3 ± 3.3	95.0 ± 3.2	0.0898
Ca (mg/dL)	8.2 ± 0.4	8.6 ± 0.7	0.0285
P (mg/dL)	5.1 ± 1.0	5.4 ± 1.1	0.246
TP (g/dL)	6.8 ± 0.5	6.7 ± 0.4	0.5831
Glu (mg/dL)	163.0 ± 59.8	158.2 ± 55.9	0.7934
AST (U/L)	13.9 ± 6.1	11.5 ± 5.2	0.2023
ALT (U/L)	10.3 ± 5.4	9.8 ± 4.6	0.7818
LDH (U/L)	208.4 ± 45.8	179.7 ± 44.3	0.0515
ALP (U/L)	238.5 ± 68.2	256.3 ± 146.5	0.6199
GTP (U/L)	34.5 ± 78.2	23.3 ± 14.1	0.5437
iPTH (pg/mL)	191.0 ± 101.3	204.2 ± 151.0	0.7457

BMI body mass index, *HD* hemodialysis, *DM* diabetes mellitus, *HbA1c* hemoglobin A1c, *GA* glycated albumin, *BUN* blood urea nitrogen, *Cr* creatinine, *UA* uric acid, *TP* total protein, *Glu* glucose, *AST* aspartate aminotransferase, *ALT* alanine aminotransferase, *GTP* γ-glutamyl transpeptidase, *iPTH* intact parathyroid hormone

6 months after Mitiglinid administration was 138.1 +/− 71.77 mg/dL (ANOVA; $p = 0.9357$), and the regression line gradient was $Y = -2.404*X + 149.3$. No significant difference was found when the regression line gradient of Saxagliptin and Mitiglinid was compared ($p = 0.5252$).

No significant change was found in HbA1c values over the study duration. Mean HbA1c value 6 months after Saxagliptin administration was 5.905 +/− 0.9770% (ANOVA; $p = 0.9099$), and the gradient of the regression line was $Y = -7.144e\text{-}005*X + 6.023$ (Fig. 2), while mean HbA1c value of the Mitiglinid group was 6.145 +/− 1.1540 (ANOVA; $p = 0.9994$), and the gradient of the regression line was $Y = -0.02604*X + 6.292$. No significant

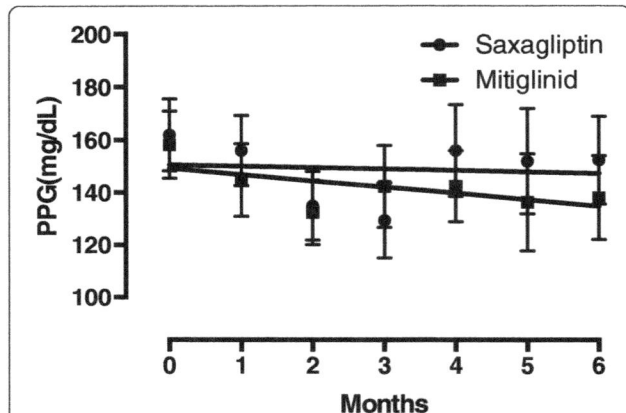

Fig. 1 Comparison of regression line gradients of postprandial plasma glucose between Saxagliptin and Mitiglinid groups. Saxagliptin group $Y = -0.5571 \ast X + 150.6$, Mitiglinid group $Y = -2.404 \ast X + 149.3$. *PPG* postprandial plasma glucose

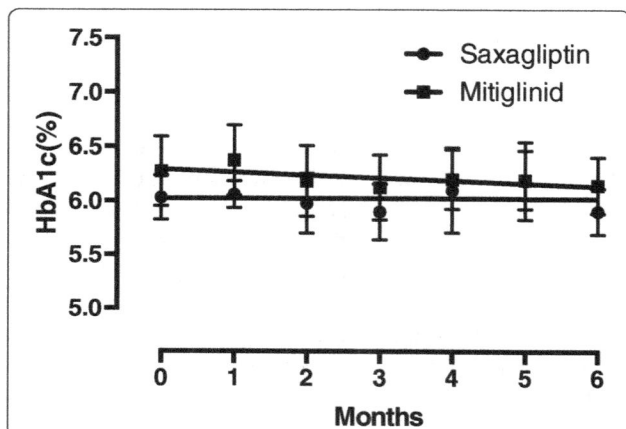

Fig. 3 Comparison of regression line gradients of GA between Saxagliptin and Mitiglinid groups. Saxagliptin group: $Y = -0.5036 \ast X + 19.34$, Mitiglinid group $Y = -0.2346 \ast X + 18.79$, $p = 0.0371$

difference was found when the slope of regression lines of Saxagliptin and Mitiglinid was compared ($p = 0.3281$).

Mean GA value 6 months after Saxagliptin administration was 16.45 +/− 2.981% (ANOVA; $p = 0.0883$), and the gradient of the regression line was $Y = -0.5036 \ast X + 19.34$, while mean GA value of the Mitiglinid group was 17.12 +/− 4.383% (ANOVA; $p = 0.9552$), and the gradient of the regression line was $Y = -0.2346 \ast X + 18.79$. There was a significant difference in the slope of regression lines between the two groups ($p = 0.0371$) (Fig. 3).

ESA dose and laboratory variables

Renal anemia was well controlled in both groups. After 6 months, in Saxagliptin group mean DA dose was 16.75 +/− 22.08 µg/w, and in Mitiglinid group was 19.50 +/− 11.46 µg/w. Both groups did not have a significant change through the observation period

(Saxagliptin group, ANOVA $p = 0.4333$; Mitiglinid group, ANOVA, $p = 0.3768$). However, the slope of the regression lines of both groups had a significant difference (Saxagliptin group, $Y = -0.8304 \ast X + 21.06$; Mitiglinid group, $Y = 0.6286 \ast X + 16.12$, $p = 0.0019$) (Fig. 4).

Both groups also did not have a significant change in ERI over the study duration (Saxagliptin group, from 6.891 +/− 6.958 to 5.561 +/− 8.330, ANOVA $p = 0.5856$; Mitiglinid group, from 4.982 +/− 4.107 to 5.842 +/− 3.766, ANOVA $p = 0.9910$), but a significant difference was observed when the slope of regression lines were compared between the two groups (Saxagliptin group, $Y = -0.2030 \ast X + 6.654$; Mitiglinid group, $Y = 0.1116 \ast X + 5.288$, $p = 0.0082$) (Fig. 5).

Baseline parameters were not different between the two groups (Table 1), but subjects administered Saxagliptin showed a significant increase in transferrin saturation (TSAT) ($p = 0.0148$) and serum Fe level ($p =$

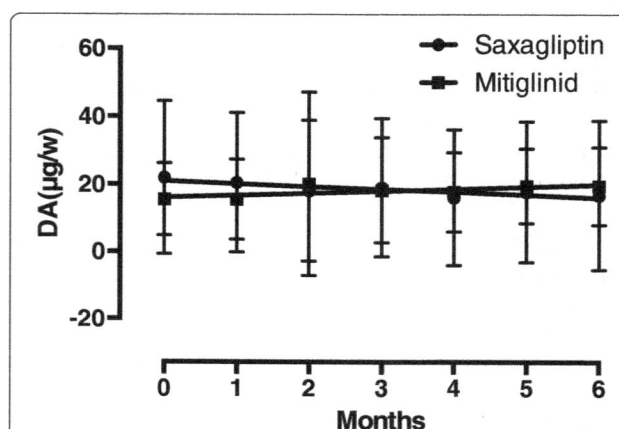

Fig. 2 Comparison of regression line gradients of HbA1c between Saxagliptin and Mitiglinid groups. Saxagliptin group $Y = -7.144\mathrm{e}\text{-}005 \ast X + 6.023$, Mitiglinid group $Y = -0.02604 \ast X + 6.292$, $p = 0.3281$

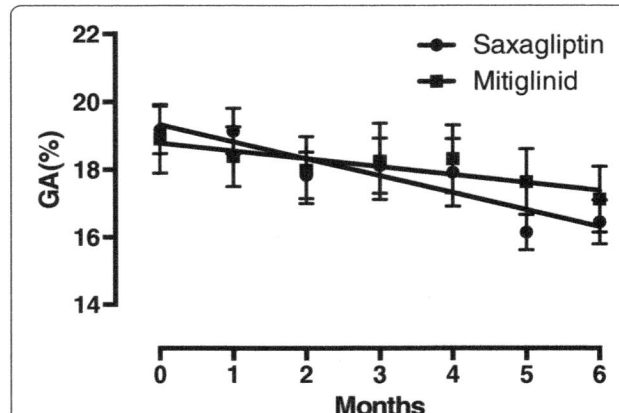

Fig. 4 Comparison of regression line gradients of DA dose between Saxagliptin and Mitiglinid groups. Saxagliptin group $Y = -0.8304 \ast X + 21.06$, Mitiglinid group $Y = 0.6286 \ast X + 16.12$, $p = 0.0019$

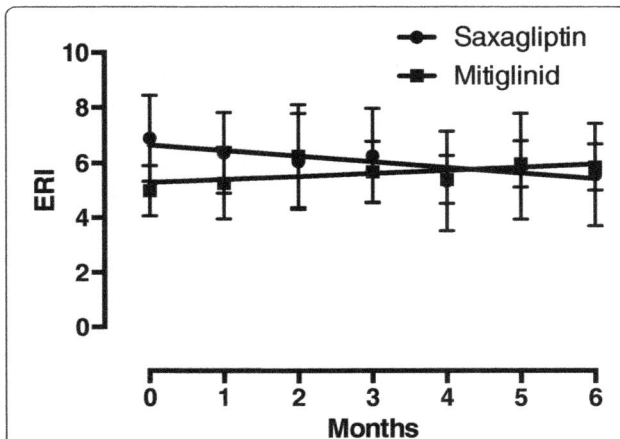

Fig. 5 Comparison of regression line gradients of ERI between Saxagliptin and Mitiglinid groups. Saxagliptin group:$Y = -0.2030 * X + 6.654$, Mitiglinid group $Y = 0.1116 * X + 5.288$, $p = 0.0082$

0.0085) when these were compared during the observation period. Ferritin showed a tendency to decrease. These trends observed in subjects in the Saxagliptin group were reversed in the Mitiglinid group, but significant changes in parameters such as the serum Fe level were not found (Table 2).

Also, during the observation period, the Mitiglinid group received saccharated ferric oxide more than the Saxagliptin group (188.6 +/− 117.1 mg versus 131.4 +/− 79.04 mg), but there was no significant difference ($p = 0.3056$) (Fig. 5).

No significant changes were found between both groups for the nutrition index-related marker and inflammatory reaction marker (e.g., CRP) (Table 2).

Adverse event

In this study, no patients experienced liver dysfunction. No cases required an increase in Saxagliptin or Mitiglinid dose over the study duration. There were also no recognized cases of hypoglycemia with symptoms or abnormal liver function. There were no patients who stopped medicine. During the study period, neoplasm was reported for one patient in the Saxagliptin group and none in the Mitiglinid group. However, as it was a colorectal cancer detected during the early phase of this study, the relationship with the drug is thought to be low.

Discussion

Patients with type 2 diabetes mellitus and ESRD have limited therapeutic options to manage hyperglycemia [7, 29]. Furthermore, few randomized controlled trials have compared antihyperglycemic agents in these patients [30].

In this study, we demonstrate that Saxagliptin can be used safely in diabetic patients undergoing hemodialysis, but cannot significantly reduce HbA1c and GA levels during a 6-month treatment period. Analysis of this study's results demonstrated that Saxagliptin was not inferior to Mitiglinid in the glycemic control of ESRD patients with type 2 diabetes mellitus.

The usefulness of Mitiglinid in dialysis patients is usually reported as a meglitinide preparation with

Table 2 Effect on renal anemia during study period and changes in nutritional status and CRP

	Saxagliptin			Mitiglinide		
	Pre	Post	P value	Pre	Post	P value
Hb (g/dL)	10.5 ± 0.8	10.9 ± 0.8	0.1523	10.7 ± 0.9	10.7 ± 0.7	0.9855
DA (μg/w)	22.0 ± 22.6	16.8 ± 22.1	0.2238	15.5 ± 10.7	19.5 ± 11.5	0.1343
Fe (mg/dL)	58.1 ± 21.0	73.9 ± 25.0	0.0085	70.8 ± 34.2	68.5 ± 25.9	0.733
TIBC (mg/dL)	295.8 ± 58.5	296.6 ± 62.1	0.921	285.4 ± 34.7	286.7 ± 50.5	0.8657
TSAT (%)	20.2 ± 7.7	25.9 ± 10.5	0.0148	25.3 ± 12.8	24.5 ± 9.5	0.7349
Ferritin (ng/mL)	58.8 ± 145.0	40.3 ± 37.7	0.5738	33.5 ± 29.7	54.1 ± 99.2	0.3343
DW (kg)	62.4 ± 9.6	62.1 ± 9.9	0.3695	67.7 ± 18.4	68.0 ± 18.6	0.7227
ERI	6.9 ± 7.0	5.6 ± 8.3	0.3769	5.0 ± 4.1	5.8 ± 3.8	0.3522
Alb (g/dL)	3.7 ± 0.3	3.8 ± 0.3	0.2698	3.7 ± 0.3	3.7 ± 0.2	0.5929
TC (mg/dL)	148.9 ± 38.2	148.2 ± 39.7	0.852	148.4 ± 41.2	147.4 ± 41.9	0.8656
HDL-C (mg/dL)	43.4 ± 10.9	46.0 ± 11.2	0.1802	38.8 ± 12.0	39.3 ± 12.7	0.6884
LDL-C (mg/dL)	83.6 ± 26.7	83.1 ± 27.8	0.8805	76.9 ± 24.4	81.8 ± 33.3	0.276
TG (mg/dL)	126.0 ± 85.0	126.6 ± 89.6	0.9351	187.6 ± 178.4	163.2 ± 123.1	0.2044
CRP (mg/dL)	0.16 ± 0.17	0.17 ± 0.18	0.6847	0.20 ± 0.26	0.33 ± 0.31	0.1201

Hb hemoglobin, *DA* darbepoetin alfa, *TIBC* total iron binding capacity, *TSAT* transferrin saturation, *DW* dry weight, *ERI* erythropoietin responsiveness index, *Alb* albumin, *TC* total cholesterol, *HDL-C* high-density lipoprotein cholesterol, *LDL-C* low-density lipoprotein cholesterol, *TG* triglyceride, *CRP* C-reactive protein

accommodation to a patient on dialysis, and it has become the drug of choice in glycemic control for patients on dialysis who have few treatment options [31–33]. Saxagliptin, in contrast, has been reported for use in patients with moderate CKD with type 2 diabetes mellitus and ESRD [13, 27, 30]. In particular, the SAVOR-TIMI53 study, which included large-scale clinical trials that followed approximately 16,000 patients for an average of 2.1 years, reported that the safety of Saxagliptin is not significantly different from placebo in chronic kidney disease (CKD) patients not on dialysis [34].

No changes in HbA1c in comparison with GA were found in this study. This may be due to our target population where patients having difficulty in glycemic control and using insulin were excluded from this study, and only patients who could control blood glucose with oral medication only were included. Therefore, the baseline GA and HbA1c values were low, and it seems that there was no difference in value at the end of the study. Based on a report using a different DPP-4 inhibitor, the rate of HbA1c decline may depend on the baseline value [9, 35]. GA is recognized as a more reliable marker than HbA1c for monitoring glycemic control in ESRD patients with diabetes [36, 37]. In this study, there was a significant difference in the regression line gradient in GA but not HbA1c in the Saxagliptin group. Our data also suggest that GA is a better marker for glycemic control in diabetic patients with ESRD compared to HbA1c.

Meglitinides and DPP-4 inhibitors are both medicines classified as insulin secretagogue, but their duration of action is different [29, 38]. Meglitinide is a drug aimed at primarily correcting postprandial hyperglycemia to avoid a delay in insulin secretion and the concomitant protraction of the hyperglycemic state and therefore has a relatively short duration of action [33, 39]. However, DPP-4 inhibitors exert a hypoglycemic effect through incretin effects that lasts for 24 h [23]. This difference in duration of action may explain the difference in glycemic control profile, and the likelihood that GA is decreased more in the Saxagliptin group has been considered.

In this study, increase in serum iron concentrations and transferrin saturation (TSAT) were significant in the Saxagliptin but not the Mitiglinid group. The ferritin was not significantly altered in both group, but a decrease trend was found in the Saxagliptin group, adversely an upward trend was found in the Mitiglinid group. For Hb, no significant alteration was found in both groups, but a decrease in the DA dose and improvement of the ERI was found in the Saxagliptin group. Though there was less consumption of saccharated ferric oxide in the Saxagliptin group, thus, bioavailability of the iron might be improved in the Saxagliptin group. However, it is necessary to measure a more precise ferrokinetic marker such as hepciden 25 or ferroportin [40–44].

DPP-4 inhibits hemopoietic factors such as G-CSF or erythropoietin, and it has been reported that the antagonism is inhibited by a DPP-4 inhibitor [16–18]. Several reports suggest that DPP-4 inhibitors have antiinflammatory effects and can improve bone marrow function [45, 46]. The possibility of scission protection by DPP-4 with anti-inflammatory agents such as BNP/ANP (brain natriuretic peptide/atrial natriuretic peptide) or NPY (neuropeptide), which are substrates of DPP-4, is suggested, and an intracorporeal inflammation condition is therefore thought to be ameliorated by DPP-4 inhibitor [47–50]. This may explain the improved iron bioavailability.

No significant alteration was found in the marker used to indicate inflammatory status in this study during the study period. We used C-reactive protein (CRP), a common laboratory examination item, as the inflammatory associated marker. A difference between both groups might be detected if a high-precision inflammatory marker, such as high-sensitivity CRP or interleukin-6 (IL-6), was used instead. These possibilities need to be addressed in future studies.

Limitations

There are some limitations to this study. First, it was conducted at just two centers; therefore, subject numbers were limited. This trial also did not have a double-blind design, and results might have been biased. While this study was too small to allow robust statistical analysis, it demonstrated obvious contrasts between the two groups in renal anemia and Fe movement parameters at each evaluation.

Conclusions

The present study showed that Saxagliptin was not inferior to Mitiglinid in the glycemic control of ESRD patients with type 2 diabetes mellitus, and it is well tolerated and safe. Furthermore, Saxagliptin may improve iron bioavailability compared to Mitiglinid. However, long-term follow-up in a larger scale study with more precise ferrokinetic markers is necessary to confirm its efficacy and safety.

Acknowledgements
The authors thank all the participants and the dialysis staffs.

Funding
The authors have received no research funds.

Authors' contributions
Y Sakai designed and performed the study, analyzed the data, and wrote the paper. SS, KM, AK, Y Sumi, YO, and TO performed the study and acquired the laboratory data with Y Sakai. ST supervised the study. All authors read and approved the final manuscript.

Competing interests

The authors declare that they have no competing interests.

Author details

[1]Department of Nephrology, Nippon Medical School Musashikosugi Hospital, 1-396 kosugi-cho, Nakahara-ku, Kawasaki, Japan. [2]Department of Internal Medicine, Zenjinkai Maruko-Clinic, 1-840 Shinmaruko-higashi, Nakahara-ku, Kawasaki, Japan. [3]Department of Nephrology, Graduate School of Medicine, Nippon Medical School, 1-1-5 Sendagi, Bunkyo-ku, Tokyo 113-8603, Japan.

References

1. Thomas MC, Cooper ME, Zimmet P. Changing epidemiology of type 2 diabetes mellitus and associated chronic kidney disease. Nat Rev Nephrol. 2015;12(2):73–81.
2. NCD-RisC NRFC. Articles: worldwide trends in diabetes since 1980: a pooled analysis of 751 population-based studies with 4·4 million participants. Lancet. 2016;387(10027):1513–30.
3. Masakane I, Nakai S, Ogata S, Kimata N, Hanafusa N, Hamano T, Wakai K, Wada A, Nitta K. An overview of regular dialysis treatment in Japan (as of 31 December 2013). Ther Apher Dial. 2015;19(6):540–74.
4. Slinin Y, Ishani A, Rector T, Fitzgerald P, MacDonald R, Tacklind J, Rutks I, Wilt TJ. Management of hyperglycemia, dyslipidemia, and albuminuria in patients with diabetes and CKD: a systematic review for a KDOQI clinical practice guideline. Am J Kidney Dis. 2012;60(5):747–69.
5. Foundation NK. KDOQI clinical practice guideline for diabetes and CKD: 2012 update. Am J Kidney Dis. 2012;60(5):850–86.
6. Rossing P, de Zeeuw D. Need for better diabetes treatment for improved renal outcome. Kidney Int. 2011;79(S120):S28–32.
7. Nakao T, Inaba M, Abe M, Kaizu K, Shima K, Babazono T, Tomo T, Hirakata H, Akizawa T, Therapy JSfD. Best practice for diabetic patients on hemodialysis 2012. Ther Apher Dial. 2015;19:40–66.
8. Monami M, Ahrén B, Dicembrini I, Mannucci E. Dipeptidyl peptidase-4 inhibitors and cardiovascular risk: a meta-analysis of randomized clinical trials. Diabetes Obes Metab. 2012;15(2):112–20.
9. Rosenstock J, Rendell MS, Gross JL, Fleck PR, Wilson CA, Mekki Q. Alogliptin added to insulin therapy in patients with type 2 diabetes reduces HbA1c without causing weight gain or increased hypoglycaemia. Diabetes Obes Metab. 2009;11(12):1145–52.
10. Sakai Y, Suzuki A, Mugishima K, Sumi Y, Otsuka Y, Otsuka T, Ohno D, Murasawa T, Tsuruoka S. Effects of alogliptin in chronic kidney disease patients with type 2 diabetes. Intern Med. 2014;53(3):195–203.
11. McGill JB, Sloan L, Newman J, Patel S, Sauce C, von Eynatten M, Woerle H-J. Long-term efficacy and safety of linagliptin in patients with type 2 diabetes and severe renal impairment: a 1-year, randomized, double-blind, placebo-controlled study. Diabetes Care. 2013;36(2):237–44.
12. Ramirez G, Morrison A, Bittle P. Clinical practice considerations and review of the literature for the use of DPP-4 inhibitors in patients with type 2 diabetes and chronic kidney disease. Endocr Pract. 2013;19(6):1025–34.
13. Nowicki M, Rychlik I, Haller H, Warren ML, Suchower L, Gause-Nilsson I. Saxagliptin improves glycaemic control and is well tolerated in patients with type 2 diabetes mellitus and renal impairment. Diabetes Obes Metab. 2011;13(6):523–32.
14. Graefe-Mody U, Friedrich C, Port A, Ring A, Retlich S, Heise T, Halabi A, Woerle HJ. Effect of renal impairment on the pharmacokinetics of the dipeptidyl peptidase-4 inhibitor linagliptin. Diabetes Obes Metab. 2011; 13(10):939–46.
15. Lukashevich V, Schweizer A, Shao Q, Groop PH, Kothny W. Safety and efficacy of vildagliptin versus placebo in patients with type 2 diabetes and moderate or severe renal impairment: a prospective 24-week randomized placebo-controlled trial. Diabetes Obes Metab. 2011;13(10):947–54.
16. Tanaka T, Higashijima Y, Wada T, Nangaku M. The potential for renoprotection with incretin-based drugs. Kidney Int. 2014;86(4):701–11.
17. Broxmeyer HE, Hoggatt J, O'Leary HA, Mantel C, Chitteti BR, Cooper S, Messina-Graham S, Hangoc G, Farag S, Rohrabaugh SL, et al. Dipeptidylpeptidase 4 negatively regulates colony-stimulating factor activity and stress hematopoiesis. Nat Med. 2012;18(12):1786–96.
18. O'Leary H, Ou X, Broxmeyer HE. The role of dipeptidyl peptidase 4 in hematopoiesis and transplantation. Curr Opin Hematol. 2013;20(4):314–9.
19. Ou X, O'Leary HA, Broxmeyer HE. Implications of DPP4 modification of proteins that regulate stem/progenitor and more mature cell types. Blood. 2013;122(2):161–9.
20. Abe M, Okada K, Soma M. Antidiabetic agents in patients with chronic kidney disease and end-stage renal disease on dialysis: metabolism and clinical practice. Curr Drug Metab. 2011;12(1):57–69.
21. Scheen AJ. Pharmacokinetics of dipeptidylpeptidase-4 inhibitors. Diabetes Obes Metab. 2010;12(8):648–58.
22. Neumiller JJ, Campbell RK. Saxagliptin: a dipeptidyl peptidase-4 inhibitor for the treatment of type 2 diabetes mellitus. Am J Health Syst Pharm. 2010; 67(18):1515–25.
23. Baetta R, Corsini A. Pharmacology of dipeptidyl peptidase-4 inhibitors: similarities and differences. Drugs. 2011;71(11):1441–67.
24. Yang LPH. Saxagliptin: a review of its use as combination therapy in the management of type 2 diabetes mellitus in the EU. Drugs. 2012; 72(2):229–48.
25. Scheen AJ. Saxagliptin plus metformin combination in patients with type 2 diabetes and renal impairment. Expert Opin Drug Metab Toxicol. 2012;8(3):383–94.
26. Aschner PJ. The role for saxagliptin within the management of type 2 diabetes mellitus: an update from the 2010 European Association for the Study of Diabetes (EASD) 46th annual meeting and the American Diabetes Association (ADA) 70th scientific session. Diabetol Metab Syndr. 2010;2:69.
27. Nowicki M, Rychlik I, Haller H, Warren M, Suchower L, Gause-Nilsson I, Schützer K-M. Long-term treatment with the dipeptidyl peptidase-4 inhibitor saxagliptin in patients with type 2 diabetes mellitus and renal impairment: a randomised controlled 52-week efficacy and safety study. Int J Clin Pract. 2011;65(12):1230–9.
28. Marcelli D, Bayh I, Merello JI, Ponce P, Heaton A, Kircelli F, Chazot C, Di Benedetto A, Marelli C, Ladanyi E, et al. Dynamics of the erythropoiesis stimulating agent resistance index in incident hemodiafiltration and high-flux hemodialysis patients. Kidney Int. 2016;90(1):192–202.
29. Nakamura Y. Diabetes therapies in hemodialysis patients: dipeptidase-4 inhibitors. World J Diabetes. 2015;6(6):840–9.
30. Abe M, Higuchi T, Moriuchi M, Okamura M, Tei R, Nagura C, Takashima H, Kikuchi F, Tomita H, Okada K. Efficacy and safety of saxagliptin, a dipeptidyl peptidase-4 inhibitor, in hemodialysis patients with diabetic nephropathy: a randomized open-label prospective trial. Diabetes Res Clin Pract. 2016;116(C):244–52.
31. Abe M, Okada K, Maruyama T, Maruyama N, Matsumoto K. Efficacy and safety of mitiglinide in diabetic patients on maintenance hemodialysis. Endocr J. 2010;57(7):579–86.
32. Abe M, Okada K, Maruyama T, Maruyama N, Matsumoto K. Combination therapy with mitiglinide and voglibose improves glycemic control in type 2 diabetic patients on hemodialysis. Expert Opin Pharmacother. 2010;11(2):169–76.
33. Black C, Donnelly P, McIntyre L, Royle PL, Shepherd JP, Thomas S. Meglitinide analogues for type 2 diabetes mellitus. Cochrane Database Syst Rev. 2007;2:CD004654.
34. Scirica BM, Bhatt DL, Braunwald E, Steg PG, Davidson J, Hirshberg B, Ohman P, Frederich R, Wiviott SD, Hoffman EB, et al. Saxagliptin and cardiovascular outcomes in patients with type 2 diabetes mellitus. N Engl J Med. 2013; 369(14):1317–26.
35. Pratley RE, Kipnes MS, Fleck PR, Wilson C, Mekki Q, Group AS. Efficacy and safety of the dipeptidyl peptidase-4 inhibitor alogliptin in patients with type 2 diabetes inadequately controlled by glyburide monotherapy. Diabetes Obes Metab. 2009;11(2):167–76.
36. Inaba M, Okuno S, Kumeda Y, Yamada S, Imanishi Y, Tabata T, Okamura M, Okada S, Yamakawa T, Ishimura E, et al. Glycated albumin is a better glycemic indicator than glycated hemoglobin values in hemodialysis patients with diabetes: effect of anemia and erythropoietin injection. J Am Soc Nephrol. 2007;18(3):896–903.
37. Peacock TP, Shihabi ZK, Bleyer AJ, Dolbare EL, Byers JR, Knovich MA, Calles-Escandon J, Russell GB, Freedman BI. Comparison of glycated albumin and hemoglobin A1c levels in diabetic subjects on hemodialysis. Kidney Int. 2008;73(9):1062–8.
38. Guardado-Mendoza R, Prioletta A, Jimenez-Ceja LM, Sosale A, Folli F. The role of nateglinide and repaglinide, derivatives of meglitinide, in the treatment of type 2 diabetes mellitus. Arch Med Sci. 2013;9(5):936–43.
39. Phillippe HM, Wargo KA. Mitiglinide: a novel agent for the treatment of type 2 diabetes mellitus. Ann Pharmacother. 2010;44(10):1615–23.

40. Vermeulen E, Vermeersch P. Hepcidin as a biomarker for the diagnosis of iron metabolism disorders: a review. Acta Clin Belg. 2012;67(3):190–7.
41. Poggiali E, Migone De Amicis M, Motta I. Anemia of chronic disease: a unique defect of iron recycling for many different chronic diseases. Eur J Intern Med. 2014;25(1):12–7.
42. Konz T, Montes-Bayon M, Vaulont S. Hepcidin quantification: methods and utility in diagnosis. Metallomics. 2014;6(9):1583–90.
43. Ganz T, Nemeth E. Iron balance and the role of hepcidin in chronic kidney disease. Semin Nephrol. 2016;36(2):87–93.
44. Sebastiani G, Wilkinson N, Pantopoulos K. Pharmacological targeting of the hepcidin/ferroportin axis. Front Pharmacol. 2016;7:160.
45. Avogaro A, Fadini GP. The effects of dipeptidyl peptidase-4 inhibition on microvascular diabetes complications. Diabetes Care. 2014;37(10):2884–94.
46. Satoh-Asahara N, Sasaki Y, Wada H, Tochiya M, Iguchi A, Nakagawachi R, Odori S, Kono S, Hasegawa K, Shimatsu A. A dipeptidyl peptidase-4 inhibitor, sitagliptin, exerts anti-inflammatory effects in type 2 diabetic patients. Metab Clin Exp. 2013;62(3):347–51.
47. Mima A, Hiraoka-Yamomoto J, Li Q, Kitada M, Li C, Geraldes P, Matsumoto M, Mizutani K, Park K, Cahill C. Protective effects of GLP-1 on glomerular endothelium and its inhibition by PKCβ activation in diabetes. Diabetes. 2012;61(11):2967–79.
48. Hocher B, Reichetzeder C, Alter ML. Renal and cardiac effects of DPP4 inhibitors—from preclinical development to clinical research. Kidney Blood Press Res. 2012;36(1):65–84.
49. Muskiet MHA, Smits MM, Morsink LM, Diamant M. The gut-renal axis: do incretin-based agents confer renoprotection in diabetes? Nat Rev Nephrol. 2014;10(2):88–103.
50. Panchapakesan U, Mather A, Pollock C. Role of GLP-1 and DPP-4 in diabetic nephropathy and cardiovascular disease. Clin Sci. 2013;124(1):17–26.

4

Timing-adjusted iron dosing enhances erythropoiesis-stimulating agent-induced erythropoiesis response and iron utilization

Tomoyuki Kawano[1,2], Tadashi Kuji[1,3], Tetsuya Fujikawa[1,4*], Eiko Ueda[1], Midori Shino[1], Satoshi Yamaguchi[5], Toshimasa Ohnishi[6], Kouichi Tamura[1], Nobuhito Hirawa[1] and Yoshiyuki Toya[1]

Abstract

Background: We recently demonstrated, using an index of recently synthesized hemoglobin, reticulocyte hemoglobin (Ret-Hb), that iron administration remarkably improves hemoglobin (Hb) synthesis during the period of high activation of erythropoiesis induced by the administration of a continuous erythropoietin receptor activator (CERA). We aimed to investigate whether repetition of iron dosing sustains effective erythropoiesis and suppresses iron storage.

Methods: In a 3-month comparison of monthly CERA administration, 104 hemodialysis patients were randomized into two groups that received 40 mg iron intravenously 3 times; the first-week iron group [$n = 51$], given iron in the first week after CERA administration, during the period of high activation of erythropoiesis, and the third-week iron group [$n = 53$], given iron in the third week at the time of mild erythropoiesis activation.

Results: Initial mean CERA dosages were 123.5 ± 67.5 μg/month and did not differ between the groups. Hb levels were not different between the groups throughout the study. One-week increases in Ret-Hb levels after CERA administration were higher, during the first and the third month, in the group given iron in the first week compared with the third-week iron group (241.9 ± 63.3 vs. 196.2 ± 82.8 mg/dL, $P = 0.004$; 227.2 ± 83.5 vs. 187.9 ± 88.7 mg/dL, $P = 0.037$, respectively). The increase in ferritin levels was suppressed 3 months later in the first-week iron group compared with that of the third-week iron group (22.3 ± 64.0 vs. 69.0 ± 76.6 ng/mL, $P = 0.002$). Hepcidin levels decreased 1 week after CERA administration in both groups and were not different between the groups.

Conclusions: Timing-adjusted iron administration increased the levels of recently produced Hb and iron utilization and suppressed the ferritin levels. The iron administration timing deserves consideration when optimizing the efficiency of erythropoiesis-stimulating agents in patients undergoing hemodialysis.

Keywords: Hemodialysis, Renal anemia, Iron supplementation method, Continuous erythropoietin receptor activator

Background

Anemia is a common comorbidity among patients with end-stage renal disease requiring dialysis therapy and is a major cause of morbidity and mortality among hemodialysis (HD) patients [1]. Recombinant human erythropoietin is an effective treatment agent for renal anemia. Although anemia can be effectively corrected by erythropoiesis-stimulating agents (ESA) [2], responses to ESA vary widely among individuals [3, 4]. ESA response is a clinically important issue because a hampered response per se and anemia are risk factors for morbidity and mortality [3, 4]. Many factors, including iron deficiency, inflammation, and malnutrition, are related to responsiveness to ESA [5]. In particular, iron deficiency is a major cause of resistance to ESA therapy [6].

* Correspondence: tftf@yokohama-cu.ac.jp
[1]Department of Medical Science and Cardiorenal Medicine, Yokohama City University Graduate School of Medicine and School of Medicine, Yokohama, Kanagawa, Japan
[4]Center for Health Service Sciences, Yokohama National University, Yokohama, Kanagawa, Japan
Full list of author information is available at the end of the article

Ferritin and transferrin saturation (TSAT) are commonly used in routine clinical practice as indicators of iron storage and iron availability. The appropriate range is described in the Kidney Disease: Improving Global Outcomes guidelines [7], European Best Practice Guidelines [8], and Japanese guidelines [9]. Excessive iron supplementation has toxic effects [10], and observational studies have linked higher iron doses with mortality [11]. Nevertheless, the recommended range of ferritin, a marker of iron storage in the body, differs among guidelines around the world.

Ferritin levels are decreased by iron utilization during erythropoiesis [12–14]. The rate of decline in ferritin depends on the degree of stimulation of erythropoiesis. In a previous study, using epoetin beta pegol or continuous erythropoietin receptor activator (CERA), we showed that ferritin and TSAT levels decrease remarkably, associated with the increase in ESA-stimulated erythropoiesis, with a maximal response at 1 week [13]. Iron deficiency disturbs the ESA response [6]. The results imply that iron may be deficient during the transient ferritin drop.

Reticulocyte hemoglobin (Ret-Hb) is a specific, short-term indicator for recently synthesized hemoglobin (Hb), which is a valid index for the erythropoiesis response as compared with the Hb level. The Hb level comprises pre-existing Hb that is affected by multiple factors over approximately 3 months prior to the measurement, equivalent to the life span of red blood cells, implying that the erythropoiesis response is difficult to evaluate accurately using this index. In a subsequent study that utilized Ret-Hb levels, we showed that iron administration during a period of high stimulation of erythropoiesis was associated with a decline in the ferritin level in the first week after CERA administration, as well as remarkably improved Hb synthesis, compared with iron administration during the third week after CERA administration, during a period of mild activation of erythropoiesis [14]. The timing of iron dosing can be an important factor to achieve the optimal erythropoiesis by ESA.

However, the potential advantage by repetition of the time-adjusted iron dosing during highly stimulated erythropoiesis is unknown. We aimed to investigate whether repeated iron administration further enhances erythropoiesis and iron utilization, leading to suppression of iron storage in the body.

Methods

Participants

Study patients were recruited from outpatients undergoing HD at the Kohsaikai Bunkojin Clinic and Kohsaikai Kamioooka Jinsei Clinic in Yokohama, Japan. Patients were included if they underwent HD for >12 weeks, received ESA treatment for ≥12 weeks before recruitment,

and had ferritin levels below 200 ng/mL. Patient exclusion criteria included patients with congestive heart failure, uncontrolled hypertension (diastolic blood pressure above 110 mmHg), malignancy, that has undergone major surgery within the previous 6 months, with gastrointestinal bleeding, the need for erythrocyte transfusion in the 12 weeks prior to the study, with systemic inflammatory disease and/or C-reactive protein levels >3 mg/dL, or receiving oral iron therapy and/or iron containing phosphate binder. After assessment, 104 patients were eligible for enrollment in the study (Fig. 1). The procedures followed were in accordance with the Helsinki Declaration. The institutional review board of Yokohama City University and the local ethics committee approved the protocol. This study was registered in the UMIN Clinical Trials Registry (registration ID number UMIN000016375). All patients provided written informed consent before enrollment.

Study protocol

This was a randomized, controlled, parallel-group study of 3 months duration. The previous study was a 1-month study using a short-term indicator of Hb synthesis; therefore, longer study duration was desirable to confirm the significance of the acceleration of Hb by time-adjusted iron dosing. A centralized allocation method was used to randomize eligible patients to receive intravenous iron during the first week or the third week after monthly CERA administration. The activation of erythropoiesis is high during the first week and mild during the third week after CERA dosing [13, 14]. After inclusion in the study, CERA was not administered for a period of at least 4 weeks and iron implementation was continued as needed at each clinic. At the start of the study, demographic, clinical, and laboratory data were recorded for each patient. CERA (Mircera®; Chugai Pharmaceutical Co., Tokyo, Japan) was administered monthly (days 0, 28,

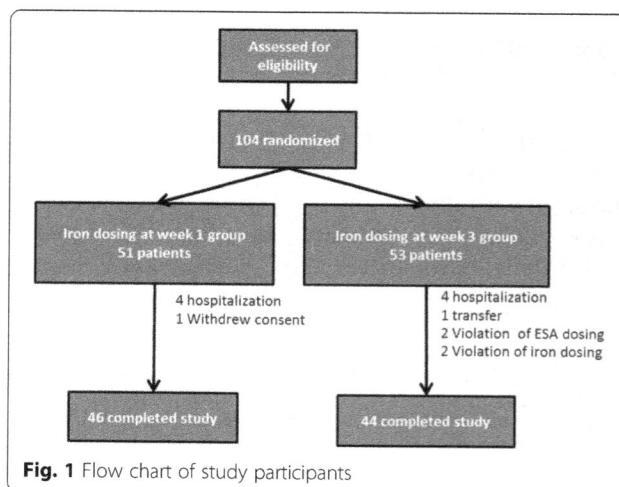

Fig. 1 Flow chart of study participants

and 56) to maintain the target Hb level of 10–11 g/dL, according to the 2008 Guidelines for Renal Anemia in Chronic Kidney Disease of the Japanese Society for Dialysis Therapy [9]. CERA doses were adjusted as needed at the discretion of attending physicians. Each patient received 40 mg intravenous elemental iron (Fesin®; Nichi-Iko Pharmaceutical Co., Ltd., Toyoma City, Japan) at all 3 HD sessions during the first week after monthly CERA administration (days 0, 2, 4, 28, 30, 32, 56, 58, and 60; the first-week iron group; $n = 51$) or at all 3 sessions during the third week after monthly CERA administration (days 14, 16, 18, 42, 44, 46, 70, 72, and 74; the third-week iron group; $n = 53$). Hb and reticulocyte Hb equivalent (Ret-He) levels were examined immediately before and 1 week after the HD session at which CERA was administered (days 0, 7, 28, 35, 56, 63, and 84). TSAT and ferritin levels were examined before the HD session at which CERA was administered every 4 weeks (days 0, 28, 56, and 84). During the first month, hepcidin, ferritin, and TSAT were evaluated weekly (days 0, 7, 14, 21, and 28). TSAT was calculated using the following formula: TSAT (%) = serum iron (µg/dL)/total iron-binding capacity (µg/dL) × 100. HD was performed 3 times per week regularly for 3–6 h with a dialysate flow rate of 400 mL/min in most patients, and the blood flow rate ranged from 150 to 280 mL/min. Dry weight was determined for each patient using the pre-dialysis cardiothoracic ratio. Before the study, intravenous doses of 40 mg of elemental iron per week were administered if the serum ferritin level was below 100 ng/mL and transferrin saturation was less than 20%.

Analytical methods

Ret-He shows the Hb amount per reticulocyte and has been proved to be a direct indicator of iron utilization as well as reticulocyte Hb content or CHr [15, 16]. Conventional erythrocyte parameters and Ret-He were measured using an XE-5000 hematology analyzer (XE RET MASTER; Sysmex, Kobe, Japan). Ret-He was analyzed using a fluorescent flow cytometry technique. In the reticulocyte channel, using a polymethine dye, this technique also determines the mean value of forward light scatter intensity derived from mature erythrocytes and reticulocytes [15]. The Hb concentration is a measure of the total amount of Hb, including pre-synthesized Hb, whereas the Ret-Hb concentration is a specific index of recently synthesized Hb. The Ret-Hb level enables estimates to be made of the efficiency in erythropoiesis during the previous 3–4 days. Ret-Hb (mg/dL) was calculated by multiplying Ret-He (pg) per cell by the reticulocyte count (10^9 cells/L), as described previously [14, 17]. CERA-induced erythropoiesis is the most highly activated in the first week after CERA administration [13, 14], and iron dosing enhances erythropoiesis

efficiency, especially in the first week [14]. To assess the peak activation of erythropoiesis induced by CERA, the 1-week increase in Ret-Hb was applied, defined as the increase in Ret-Hb levels from day 0 to day 7 after CERA administration.

Statistical analysis

Sample size was estimated based on a previous report [14] with the following assumptions: α was set at 0.05, the expected power was 80%, a difference between groups in changes of ferritin of 17%, and a standard deviation of 30%. Unless otherwise specified, data are presented as mean ± standard deviation. Differences between the groups were analyzed using the unpaired Student's t test for parametric variables or the Wilcoxon sum rank test for non-parametric valuables, with the χ^2 test used to determine proportions. P values of <0.05 were considered to be statistically significant. Statistical analyses were performed using SPSS for Windows version 19.0 (SPSS, Inc., Chicago, IL, USA).

Results

Figure 1 displays a flow chart of the study patients. During the 3-month comparison period, 5 patients from the first-week iron group withdrew from the study, owing to hospital admission ($n = 4$) and withdrawal of consent ($n = 1$). Nine patients in the third-week iron group withdrew because of hospital admission ($n = 4$), clinic transfer ($n = 1$), extra ESA administration ($n = 2$), and iron dosing violations ($n = 2$) (Fig. 1). The baseline characteristics of the 104 patients (the first-week iron group, $n = 51$; the third-week iron group, n = 53) are shown in Table 1. No significant differences in baseline characteristics were evident between the groups.

Ninety participants (the first-week iron group, $n = 46$; the third-week iron group, $n = 44$) were included in the final analysis. No significant differences in baseline characteristics were detected between the groups included in the final analysis. Initial CERA dosages were 130.4 ± 67.3 µg/month in the first-week iron group and 116.5 ± 69.0 µg/month in the third-week iron group ($P = 0.334$). There were no significant differences in the CERA dosages over the 3-month comparison period between the first-week and third-week iron groups (1st month, 1.09 ± 1.22 µg vs. 2.84 ± 24.8 µg, $P = 0.637$; 2nd month, −9.78 ± 31.4 µg vs. −5.11 ± 42.7 µg, $P = 0.413$; 3rd month, −21.2 ± 38.0 µg vs. −14.8 ± 45.9 µg, $P = 0.312$). The mean Hb levels during the 3 month comparison period were 10.1 ± 0.8 g/dL in the first-week iron group and 10.2 ± 0.7 g/dL in the third-week iron group ($P = 0.901$). No patients required blood transfusion during the study period.

Changes in Hb levels, compared with baseline, Ret-Hb levels, TSAT, and ferritin levels are shown in Fig. 2. The increases seen in Hb levels at 1, 2, and 3 months were

Table 1 Baseline characteristics of patients between first-week iron and third-week iron groups

Variables	First-week iron group	Third-week iron group	P value
	n = 51	n = 53	
Age, years	67.8 ± 10.2	67.6 ± 11.6	0.919
Male, %	60.8	52.8	0.413
Body mass index, kg/m2	21.9 ± 3.6	21.8 ± 3.2	0.815
Hemodialysis vintage, months	94.7 ± 89.0	108.0 ± 75.5	0.158
Single-pool Kt/V	1.05 ± 0.20	1.12 ± 0.24	0.113
Mean CERA dose, µg/4 weeks	129.6 ± 66.9	117.9 ± 68.2	0.344
Arteriovenous fistula, %	96.1	98.1	0.465
Renin-angiotensin system inhibitors, %	49.0	58.5	0.333
Diabetes mellitus, %	35.3	41.5	0.515
Hypertension, %	96.1	98.1	0.485
Cardio vascular disease, %	25.5	24.5	0.910
Hematologic disease, %	5.9	1.9	0.294
Hemoglobin, g/dl	10.7 ± 0.7	10.8 ± 0.9	0.767
Creatinin, mg/dl	11.0 ± 2.2	1.0 ± 2.5	0.906
Blood urea nitrogen, mg/dl	71.6 ± 17.1	72.3 ± 14.6	0.844
Albumin, g/dl	3.85 ± 0.22	3.85 ± 0.31	0.969
C-reactive protein, mg/dl	0.32 ± 0.54	0.22 ± 0.34	0.865
Intact-parathyroid hormon, pg/ml	164.7 ± 78.8	180.1 ± 108.2	0.797
Serum iron, µg/dl	96.4 ± 30.1	89.6 ± 25.9	0.248
Total Iron binding capacity, µg/dl	236.7 ± 34.1	237.1 ± 42.7	0.955
Transferrin saturation, %	40.9 ± 14.2	40.2 ± 14.8	0.826
Ferritin, ng/ml	163.3 ± 63.7	169.6 ± 63.1	0.623

Data are mean ± SD. P values for the difference between the two groups
CERA continuous erythropoietin receptor activator

not significantly different between the groups (Fig. 2a). The 1-week increases in Ret-Hb levels after CERA administration were higher, during the first and the third month, in the group given iron in the first week compared with the third-week iron group (241.9 ± 63.3 mg/dL vs. 196.2 ± 82.8 mg/dL, $P = 0.004$; 227.2 ± 83.5 mg/dL vs. 187.9 ± 88.7 mg/dL, $P = 0.037$; Fig. 2b). Changes in TSAT did not differ at 1, 2, and 3 months between the groups (Fig. 2c). The ferritin levels increased to a lesser degree in the first-week iron group at 1, 2, and 3 months, compared with the third-week iron group (−5.37 ± 32.9 vs. 37.1 ± 46.4 ng/mL, $P < 0.001$; 16.5 ± 60.0 vs. 56.4 ± 56.9 ng/mL, $P = 0.002$; 22.3 ± 64.0 vs. 69.0 ± 76.6 ng/mL, $P = 0.002$, respectively; Fig. 2d).

Hepcidin and iron-related parameters were measured weekly during the first month. Hepcidin levels decreased at 1-week post-treatment in both groups, and changes in hepcidin levels were not significantly different between the groups (Fig. 3a). Changes in iron-related parameters from week 0 were evaluated in the same way as in the previous study [14]. Changes in TSAT levels were not different between the groups (Fig. 3b). At 1 and 2 weeks

after CERA administration, the decreases seen in ferritin levels were not as pronounced in the first-week iron group compared with the third-week iron group (5.1 ± 23.7 vs. −59.2 ± 23.9 ng/mL, $P < 0.001$; −39.6 ± 35.6 vs. −78.8 ± 37.6 ng/mL, $P < 0.001$, respectively. Fig. 3c). The ferritin levels increased to a lesser degree at 3 and 4 weeks after CERA administration in the first-week iron group compared with the third-week iron group (−26.1 ± 35.7 vs. 84.2 ± 315.2 ng/mL, $P = 0.023$; −5.4 ± 32.9 vs. 37.1 ± 46.6 ng/mL, $P < 0.001$, respectively. Fig. 3c).

Discussion

This study compared erythropoiesis efficiency and iron-related parameters between two schedules of iron administration, during highly stimulated erythropoiesis and mildly stimulated erythropoiesis, and found an increase in Hb synthesis and inhibition of ferritin levels when iron was administered during highly stimulated erythropoiesis.

Ret-Hb is a reticulocyte-related marker that is a measure of recently generated Hb. Iron administration during the activation of erythropoiesis leads to increased Ret-Hb levels, and a benefit was observed from repeated iron

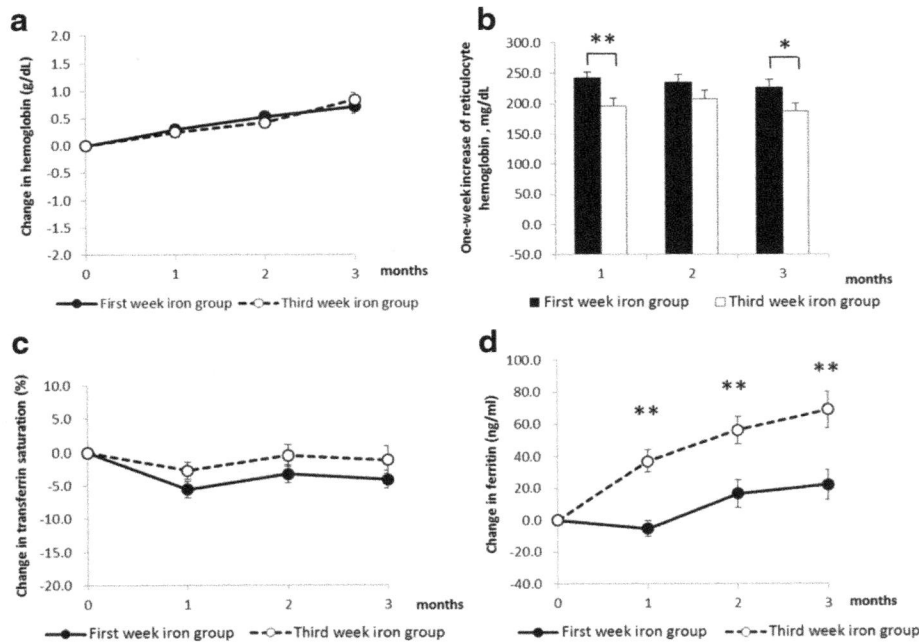

Fig. 2 Changes in **a** hemoglobin levels, **c** transferrin saturation, and **d** ferritin levels, and **b** 1-week increase in reticulocyte hemoglobin levels between groups that received iron administration in the first week or the third week following CERA administration. CERA was administered every month. Data are presented as means ± standard error of mean. *$P < 0.01$, **$P < 0.05$, for comparisons between the groups

administration on a monthly basis. The result has confirmed that the iron administration improves erythropoiesis efficiency by enhancing erythropoiesis. This suggests that iron should be administered according to the increase in iron requirement during erythropoiesis.

In this 3-month comparison, the increase in ferritin levels was not as large when iron was administered during the period of high stimulation of erythropoiesis, compared with administration during mild erythropoiesis stimulation. This is the first report to show a difference in the degree of ferritin induction, dependent on the timing of iron administration, in a study with a randomized controlled trial design. Our result suggests that iron administration during highly activated erythropoiesis enhances iron utilization and erythropoiesis, leading to inhibition of iron storage. It is worth examining whether an improvement in iron utilization maintains a low ferritin level and contributes to a favorable prognosis.

Intravenous iron dosing causes a transient excessive increase in serum non-transferrin-bound iron and evokes inflammation [18, 19]. Inflammation increases ferritin levels [20]. The increase in non-transferrin-bound iron may enhance the rise in ferritin levels after intravenous iron dosing. Iron administration during activated erythropoiesis increased newly produced Hb. Enhanced iron utilization might have suppressed the increase in the peak level of the transient non-transferrin-bound iron. Further research is needed to investigate whether the

transient increase in non-transferrin-bound iron is suppressed and whether the suppression is a key mechanism accounting for the difference in ferritin levels between the groups.

Intravenous iron causes a transient rapid increase in ferritin within 1 week, exceeding real storage [21]. Therefore, in this study, ferritin level was measured at least 10 days after iron dosing. Although ferritin levels were measured in the standard manner, long-term follow-up is needed to further confirm the suppression of ferritin levels after iron dosing during highly stimulated erythropoiesis and to assess body iron stores in patients with a suppressed ferritin level.

Iron dosing reportedly increases hepcidin levels [22]. In our study, iron was not administered at the same time but at different times in the two groups. This allowed us to compare the reactions of hepcidin during the presence and absence of iron dosing. However, our data did not show a difference in hepcidin levels, measured weekly, associated with iron dosing during the first week and the third week. Hepcidin levels decrease according to the iron requirement during activated erythropoiesis [13]. The effect of activated erythropoiesis on decreasing hepcidin levels might suppress the effect of iron administration in increasing hepcidin levels. Hepcidin is an important factor that hinders iron intake into reticulocytes [23]. It remains to be determined whether iron dosing during the activation of erythropoiesis can prevent a rise in hepcidin levels.

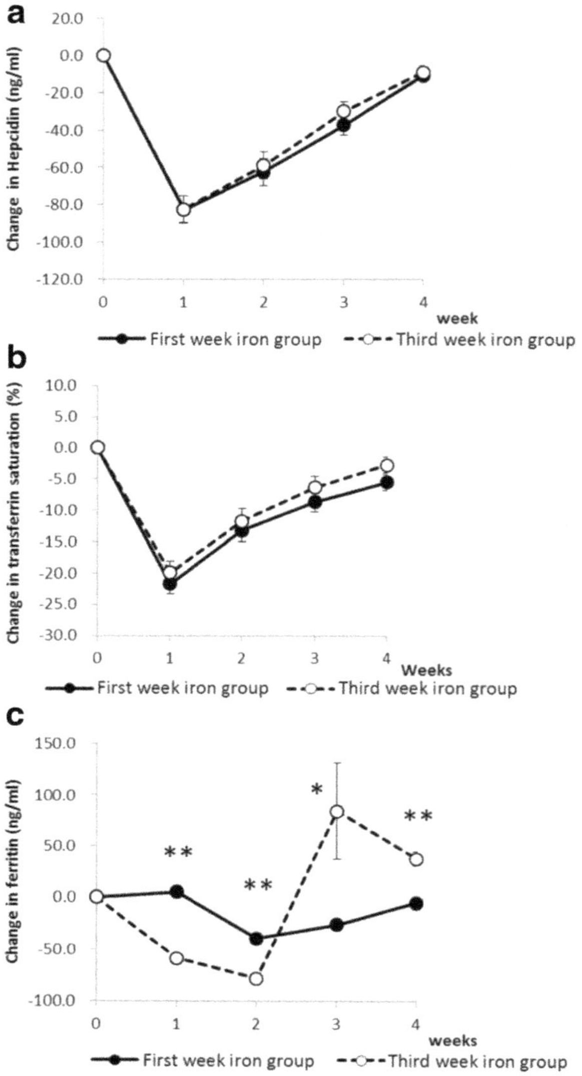

Fig. 3 Changes in **a** hepcidin levels, **b** transferrin saturation, and **c** ferritin levels between groups that received iron administration in the first week or the third week following CERA administration. CERA was administered on day 0. Data are presented as means ± standard error of mean. *$P < 0.01$, **$P < 0.05$, for comparison between the groups

Limitations

There were limitations in this study. Firstly, the number of study participants was not adequate and a number of patients withdrew from the study; there is further scope to investigate the effect of timing-adjusted iron administration on the balance between ESA and Hb levels achieved. Secondly, the patient exclusion criteria had the potential to introduce a selection bias. This study did not include patients with baseline ferritin levels over 200 ng/mL. The patients with high ESA resistance often have high ferritin levels and need more effective therapy for anemia. It is worth examining whether our results apply to these populations. Furthermore, the excluded patients with severe conditions may have a notable benefit from timing-adjusted iron administration methods. Further study is needed to examine the characteristics of patients that benefit the most from receiving timing-adjusted iron administration. Thirdly, this study was not designed to investigate the optimal dose of iron supplementation during the activation of erythropoiesis. It is still necessary to elucidate what amount of iron supplementation, given with adjusted timing, is required during ESA therapy.

Conclusions

These results suggest that timing-adjusted iron administration leads to an increase in recently produced Hb and iron utilization and suppresses ferritin levels. Iron administration timing deserves consideration when optimizing ESA efficiency in HD patients.

Abbreviations
CERA: Continuous erythropoietin receptor activator; ESA: Erythropoiesis-stimulating agents; Hb: Hemoglobin; HD: Hemodialysis; Ret-Hb: Reticulocyte hemoglobin; Ret-He: Reticulocyte hemoglobin equivalent; TSAT: Transferrin saturation

Acknowledgements
The authors thank the medical staff who supported this study in the Kohsaikai Bunkojin Clinic and Kohsaikai Kamioooka Jinsei Clinic.

Funding
There was no funding.

Authors' contributions
TK was involved in the study design, study procedure implementation, data collection, and article writing of the manuscript. TK, TF, and YT contributed to the study design, data analysis, and article writing of the manuscript. EU and MK contributed to the study design, data collection, and data analysis. SY, TO, KT, and NH reviewed the study design and interpretation of results. All authors read and approved the final manuscript.

Competing interests
The authors declare that they have no competing interests.

There was no significant difference in Hb levels between the groups, probably because ESA dose adjustments were conducted appropriately to maintain target levels. The scale and duration of this study did not allow the detection of ESA dose differences between the groups. However, iron dosing during activated erythropoiesis increased the efficiency of erythropoiesis and suppressed iron storage. It is possible that the ESA dose required to maintain targeted Hb levels might be reduced by timing the administration of iron during activated erythropoiesis.

Author details
[1]Department of Medical Science and Cardiorenal Medicine, Yokohama City University Graduate School of Medicine and School of Medicine, Yokohama, Kanagawa, Japan. [2]Kohsaikai Bunkojin Clinic, Yokohama, Kanagawa, Japan. [3]Yokodai Central Clinic, Yokohama, Kanagawa, Japan. [4]Center for Health Service Sciences, Yokohama National University, Yokohama, Kanagawa, Japan. [5]Kohsaikai Yokohama Jinsei Hospital, Yokohama, Kanagawa, Japan. [6]Kohsaikai Kamioooka Jinsei Clinic, Yokohama, Kanagawa, Japan.

References
1. Foley RN, Parfrey PS, Harnett JD, Kent GM, Murray DC, Barre PE. The impact of anemia on cardiomyopathy, morbidity and mortality in end-stage renal disease. Am J Kidney Dis. 1996;28:53–61.
2. Eschbach JW, Egrie JC, Downing MR, Browne JK, Adamson JW. Correction of the anemia of end stage renal disease with recombinant human erythropoietin. Results of a combined phase I and II clinical trial. N Engl J Med. 1987;316:73–8.
3. López-Gómez JM, Portolés JM, Aljama P. Factors that condition the response to erythropoietin in patients on hemodialysis and their relation to mortality. Kidney Int Suppl. 2008;111:S75–81.
4. Fujikawa T, Ikeda Y, Fukuhara S, Akiba T, Akizawa T, Kurokawa K, Saito A. Time-dependent resistance to erythropoiesis-stimulating agent and mortality in hemodialysis patients in the Japan Dialysis Outcomes and Practice Patterns Study. Nephron Clin Pract. 2012;122(1-2):24–32.
5. Richardson D. Clinical factors influencing sensitivity and response to epoetin. Nephrol Dial Transplant. 2002;l7(Suppl):53–9.
6. Drüeke T. Hyporesponsiveness to recombinant human erythropoietin. Nephrol Dial Transplant. 2001;16:25–8.
7. Kidney Disease: Improving Global Outcomes (KDIGO) Anemia Work Group. KDIGO clinical practice guideline for anemia in chronic kidney disease. Kidney Int. 2012;2:279–335.
8. Locatelli F, Bárány P, Covic A, De Francisco A, Del Vecchio L, Goldsmith D, Hörl W, London G, Vanholder R, Van Biesen W, ERA-EDTA ERBP Advisory Board. Kidney Disease: Improving Global Outcomes guidelines on anaemia management in chronic kidney disease: a European Renal Best Practice position statement. Nephrol Dial Transplant. 2013;28(6):1346–59.
9. Tsubakihara Y, Nishi S, Akiba T, Hirakata H, Iseki K, Kubota M, Kuriyama S, Komatsu Y, Suzuki M, Nakai S, Hattori M, Babazono T, Hiramatsu M, Yamamoto H, Bessho M, Akizawa T. 2008 Japanese Society for Dialysis Therapy: guidelines for renal anemia in chronic kidney disease. Ther Apher Dial. 2010;14(3):240–75.
10. Brewster UC. Intravenous iron therapy in end-stage renal disease. Semin Dial. 2006;19(4):285–90.
11. Kalantar-Zadeh K, Regidor DL, McAllister CJ, Michael B, Warnock DG. Time-dependent associations between iron and mortality in hemodialysis patients. J Am Soc Nephrol. 2005;16(10):3070–80.
12. Major A, Mathez–Loic F, Rohling R, Gautschi K, Brugnara C. The effect of intravenous iron on the reticulocyte response to recombinant human erythropoietin. Br J Haematol. 1997;98:292–4.
13. Kakimoto-Shino M, Toya Y, Kuji T, Fujikawa T, Umemura S. Changes in hepcidin and reticulocyte hemoglobin equivalent levels in response to continuous erythropoietin receptor activator administration in hemodialysis patients: a randomized study. Ther Apher Dial. 2014;18(5):421–6.
14. Kuji T, Toya Y, Fujikawa T, Kakimoto-Shino M, Nishihara M, Shibata K, Tamura K, Hirawa N, Satta H, Kawata S, Kouguchi N, Umemura S. Acceleration of iron utilization after intravenous iron administration during activated erythropoiesis in hemodialysis patients: a randomized study. Ther Apher Dial. 2015;19(2):131–7.
15. Thomas L, Franck S, Messinger M, Linssen J, Thome M, Thomas C. Reticulocyte hemoglobin measurement—comparison of two methods in the diagnosis of iron-restricted erythropoiesis. Clin Chem Lab Med. 2005;43:1193–202.
16. Fishbane S, Galgano C, Langley Jr RC, Canfield W, Maesaka JK. Reticulocyte hemoglobin content in the evaluation of iron status of hemodialysis patients. Kidney Int. 1997;52:217–22.
17. Goodnough LT, Skikne B, Brugnara C. Erythropoietin, iron, and erythropoiesis. Blood. 2000;96(3):823–33.
18. Besarab A, Kaiser JW. Frinak S A study of parenteral iron regimens in hemodialysis patients. Am J Kidney Dis. 1999;34(1):21–8.
19. Pai AB, Conner T, McQuade CR, Olp J, Hicks P. Non-transferrin bound iron, cytokine activation and intracellular reactive oxygen species generation in hemodialysis patients receiving intravenous iron dextran or iron sucrose. Biometals. 2011;24(4):603–13.
20. Nakanishi T, Kuragano T, Nanami M, Otaki Y, Nonoguchi H, Hasuike Y. Importance of ferritin for optimizing anemia therapy in chronic kidney disease. Am J Nephrol. 2010;32:439–46.
21. Locatelli F, Aljama P, Bárány P, Canaud B, Carrera F, Eckardt KU, Hörl WH, Macdougal IC, Macleod A, Wiecek A, Cameron S. European Best Practice Guidelines Working Group. Revised European best practice guidelines for the management of anaemia in patients with chronic renal failure. Nephrol Dial Transplant. 2004;19(Suppl 2):ii1–47.
22. Ghoti H, Rachmilewitz EA, Simon-Lopez R, Gaber R, Katzir Z, Konen E, Kushnir T, Girelli D, Campostrini N, Fibach E, Goitein O. Evidence for tissue iron overload in long-term hemodialysis patients and the impact of withdrawing parenteral iron. Eur J Haematol. 2012;89(1):87–93.
23. Swinkels DW, Wetzels JF. Hepcidin: a new tool in the management of anaemia in patients with chronic kidney disease? Nephrol Dial Transplant. 2008;23(8):2450–3.

5

The optimal timing of continuous renal replacement therapy according to the modified RIFLE classification in critically ill patients with acute kidney injury: a retrospective observational study

Jun Suzuki[1], Tetsu Ohnuma[2], Hidenori Sanayama[3], Kiyonori Ito[4], Takayuki Fujiwara[5], Hodaka Yamada[6], Alan Kawarai Lefor[7] and Masamitsu Sanui[2]*

Abstract

Background: Acute kidney injury (AKI) requiring continuous renal replacement therapy (CRRT) is associated with high mortality in critically ill patients. However, the optimal timing to initiate CRRT in patients with AKI is unknown. The purpose of this study is to investigate whether the timing of initiation of CRRT according to severity of AKI is associated with in-hospital mortality.

Methods: We retrospectively reviewed 189 patients treated with CRRT for AKI in the intensive care unit between January 2009 and February 2013. Patients aged <18 years or receiving renal replacement therapy for end-stage renal disease were excluded. The modified RIFLE classification was used to stratify patients into two groups at initiation of CRRT, including early (no AKI or risk) and late (injury or failure).

Results: There were 52 (28%) patients in the early group and 137 (72%) patients in the late group. The median age was 72 (range 61–78) years, including 70% males. The median intensive care unit and hospital stays were 10 (4–18) and 26 (13–58) days, respectively. Crude early vs. late group intensive care unit mortality was 50 vs. 44% ($P = 0.51$), and in-hospital mortality was 64 vs. 50% ($P = 0.10$), respectively. Logistic regression analysis showed that late initiation (OR, 0.30; 95% CI, 0.13–0.71; $P = 0.006$) and lower SAPS score (OR, 1.04; 95% CI, 1.02–1.06; $P < 0.001$) were independently associated with decreased mortality.

Conclusions: This study suggests that late initiation of CRRT is associated with a lower risk of in-hospital mortality in patients with AKI. Further studies are needed to confirm the optimal timing for initiation of CRRT.

Keywords: Acute kidney injury, Continuous renal replacement therapy, Timing, RIFLE classification

Background

Acute kidney injury (AKI) is a life-threatening complication with an incidence of 36–67% in critically ill patients [1, 2]. Approximately 4–5% of patients with AKI in the intensive care unit (ICU) require continuous renal replacement therapy (CRRT), resulting in a mortality rate greater than 50% [3, 4].

* Correspondence: msanui@mac.com
[2]Department of Anesthesiology and Critical Care Medicine, Jichi Medical University Saitama Medical Center, 1-847 Amanuma, Omiya-ku, Saitama City, Saitama 330-8503, Japan
Full list of author information is available at the end of the article

Although a consensus does not exist for the timing of initiation of renal replacement therapy (RRT) in patients with AKI, early initiation of RRT tended to improve mortality. A recent systematic review and meta-analysis concluded that early RRT initiation in critically ill patients with AKI may result in a survival benefit [5]. However, the study included only two small randomized clinical trials evaluating the timing of RRT initiation, and the definitions of classification of AKI and RRT initiation as "early" or "late" RRT varied significantly between the studies. Although two recent prospective randomized trials were reported [6, 7], the results were conflicting.

The RIFLE classification, developed by the Acute Dialysis Quality Initiative in 2004, classifies AKI patients into five groups according to creatinine and urine output criteria. The groups include Risk, Injury, Failure, Loss, and End-stage renal disease [8]. This classification was reported to be a useful system for predicting AKI severity and in-hospital mortality in patients with AKI [1, 9, 10]. Recent retrospective and prospective observational studies used the modified RIFLE classification as a marker for the optimal timing of RRT initiation for postoperative or septic patients with AKI [11–14].

The aim of this study was to evaluate whether early or late initiation of CRRT defined by the modified RIFLE classification is associated with in-hospital mortality in medical and surgical critically ill patients with AKI. We hypothesized that early initiation of CRRT is associated with lower in-hospital mortality than the late initiation.

Methods
Study population
We retrospectively reviewed the records of patients admitted to the combined medical–surgical intensive care unit (ICU) at Jichi Medical University Saitama Medical Center between January 2009 and February 2013. This study was approved by the Institutional Review Board of Jichi Medical University Saitama Medical Center. Patients aged less than 18 years with end-stage renal disease treated with chronic hemodialysis were excluded. If multiple CRRT treatments were performed on one patient in the ICU, only the first CRRT treatment was considered in this analysis. The diagnosis of AKI was made according to the modified RIFLE classification (Table 1) defined using only estimated glomerular filtration rate (eGFR) criteria comparing pre-admission baseline serum creatinine levels with those at the time of initiating CRRT. If the pre-admission baseline creatinine was unknown, a baseline eGFR of 75 ml/min/1.73 cm^2 was used based on a calculation from the abbreviated Modification of Diet in Renal Disease, as suggested by the Acute Dialysis Quality Initiative [15].

Table 1 Categorization of patients based on the Modified RIFLE classification ($n = 189$)

Modified RIFLE classification	eGFR criteria (%)	n (%)
Non-acute kidney injury	eGFR decrease ≤25	16 (9)
Risk	eGFR decrease >25	36 (19)
Injury	eGFR decrease >50	70 (37)
Failure	eGFR decrease >75	67 (35)

Abbreviations: eGFR estimated glomerular filtration rate

Data collection
Chart reviews including baseline characteristics and laboratory data were performed in eligible patients. The characteristics reviewed included age, gender, primary diagnosis, creatinine at baseline and at ICU admission, and pre-existing comorbidities, including hypertension, diabetes mellitus, chronic kidney disease (CKD), and congestive heart failure. CKD is defined as an eGFR less than 60 ml/min/1.73 cm^2 over 3 months or previously diagnosed. CKD is classified into five groups defined by the CKD guidelines [16]. The Simplified Acute Physiology Score (SAPS) II was calculated on the day of ICU admission [17]. We recorded the use of mechanical ventilation, vasopressors, diuretics, PaO$_2$/FiO$_2$ ratio, Glasgow Coma Scale, bilirubin, platelets, albumin, urine output, creatinine, eGFR, and blood urea nitrogen (BUN) at the time of CRRT initiation. Continuous venovenous hemodiafiltration was used in all patients. We used dialysis membranes composed of polysulfone, polymethylmethacrylate, and polyacrylonitrile. Continuous veno-venous hemodiafiltration was performed with blood flow rates ranging from 80 to 120 ml/min, a dialysis flow rate ranging from 500 to 3950 ml/h, and a replacement flow rate ranging from 0 to 3800 ml/h.

The following general indications for RRT were used: (1) metabolic acidosis (pH <7.2 and serum bicarbonate <16 mEq/l in arterial blood gas), (2) hyperkalemia (serum K$^+$ >5.5 mmol/l), (3) azotemia (BUN >150 mg/dl) with uremic symptoms, (4) oliguria/anuria (urine output <100 ml/12 h), or otherwise (5) the indications were at the discretion of the treating physician.

Patients were categorized into four groups (non-AKI, risk, injury, and failure) according to the modified RIFLE classification (Table 1). Early initiation was defined as initiation of CRRT in patients in the non-AKI or risk groups, whereas patients classified in the injury or failure group constituted the late initiation group (8). Factors contributing to AKI were selected from a list of the following choices: septic shock, cardiogenic shock, drug-induced AKI, hypovolemia, major surgery, and others (4). In each case, one or more contributing factors could be selected. Sepsis was defined based on systemic inflammation syndrome and consensus guidelines [18].

As a primary outcome, we compared in-hospital mortality between the groups. We also reviewed the duration of CRRT, ICU length of stay, post-RRT hospital length of stay, hospital length of stay, time interval from ICU admission to RRT initiation, and ICU mortality as secondary outcomes.

Statistical analysis
Data are presented as medians and interquartile ranges (25th to 75th percentiles) or percentages, as appropriate.

The chi-square test or Fisher's exact test were used for nominal variables and the Mann–Whitney test was used for continuous variables. A P value <0.05 was considered statistically significant. Single variables with a P value of less than 0.12 were then applied into multivariable logistic regression analysis, which was performed to evaluate risk factors for hospital mortality. The following variables were included as covariates in a logistic regression analysis: age, gender, hypertension, CKD, SAPS II, vasopressor use, mechanical ventilation use, hypovolemia, PaO_2/FiO_2 ratio at CRRT initiation, urine output at CRRT initiation, BUN at CRRT initiation, albumin at CRRT initiation, and early vs. late CRRT initiation. All statistical analyses were performed with EZR which is a graphical user interface for R (The R Foundation for Statistical Computing, Vienna, Austria, version 2.13.0) [19]. EZR is a modified version of the R commander designed to add statistical functions frequently used in biostatistics.

Results

A total of 189 patients were included in this analysis. There were 16 patients (9%) in the non-AKI group, 36

(19%) in the risk group, 70 (37%) in the injury group, and 67 (35%) in the failure group, according to the modified RIFLE classification (Table 1). In the early and late CRRT initiation groups, there were 52 (28%) and 137 patients (72%), respectively.

Baseline characteristics and comorbidities are shown in Table 2. The median age was 72 (61–78) years, and 70% were male. Pre-admission baseline creatinine was available for 124 (66%) patients, and the median creatinine was 1.0 (0.7–1.5) mg/dl. CKD was present in 47%, and hypertension represented 61% of comorbidities. The proportion of patients with CKD in stages 2, 3, 4, and 5 were 7, 40, 18, and 13%, respectively. The median SAPS II score on admission to the ICU was 57 (range 44–72).

A summary of demographic data at the time of CRRT initiation is shown in Table 3. Mechanical ventilation, vasopressor, and diuretic use among patients was 79, 53, and 37%, respectively. Renal data were as follows: serum creatinine at CRRT initiation was 2.7 (1.9–4.0) mg/dl, eGFR was 18 (12–28) ml/min/1.73 m^2, urine output before CRRT initiation was 19 (8–35) ml/h, and BUN was 50 (31–72) mg/dl. Factors contributing to the development of AKI included sepsis (39%), cardiogenic shock

Table 2 Baseline characteristics of the early and late CRRT groups

	All patients (n = 189)	Early patients (n = 52)	Late patients (n = 137)	P value
Baseline data				
Age (years), median (IQR)	72 (61–78)	74 (62–78)	71 (61–77)	0.37
Gender (male), n (%)	133 (70)	36 (69)	97 (71)	0.86
Baseline serum creatinine (mg/dl), median (IQR)	1.0 (0.7–1.5)[a]	1.5 (0.9–2.9)[a]	0.9 (0.7–1.2)[a]	<0.001
Comorbidities				
Hypertension, n (%)	116 (61)	36 (69)	80 (58)	0.19
Diabetes mellitus, n (%)	56 (30)	17 (33)	39 (29)	0.6
Chronic kidney disease, n (%)	89 (47)	33 (63)	56 (41)	0.009
Stage 2, n (%)	6 (7)	2 (4)	4 (3)	0.69
Stage 3, n (%)	36 (40)	10 (19)	26 (19)	1
Stage 4, n (%)	16 (18)	10 (19)	6 (4)	0.002
Stage 5, n (%)	12 (13)	10 (19)	2 (2)	<0.001
Unknown, n (%)	19 (21)	1 (2)	18 (16)	0.04
Congestive heart failure, n (%)	34 (18)	10 (19)	24 (18)	0.83
Data on admission to ICU				
Serum creatinine (mg/dl), median (IQR)	2.0 (1.2–3.4)	1.5 (1.1–2.9)	2.1 (1.3–3.5)	0.047
Bilirubin (mg/dl), median (IQR)	0.8 (0.5–1.6)	0.8 (0.5–1.3)	0.8 (0.5–1.7)	0.42
Platelets (cells/10^3), median (IQR)	146 (66–211)	124 (66–207)	146 (68–214)	0.98
PaO$_2$/FiO$_2$ ratio (Torr), median (IQR)	200 (117–329)	195 (117–297)	200 (119–329)	0.91
SAPS II, median (IQR)	57 (44–72)	57 (40–68)	57 (45–72)	0.5
Glasgow Coma Scale, median (IQR)	14 (6–15)	14 (3–15)	14 (6–15)	0.24

Abbreviations: CRRT continuous renal replacement therapy, *ICU* intensive care unit, *IQR* interquartile range, *BUN* blood urea nitrogen, *eGFR* estimated glomerular filtration rate, *SAPS II* Simplified Acute Physiology Score II
[a]Sixty-five, six, and fifty-nine patients with unknown baseline creatinine were not included

Table 3 Comparisons of demographic date at CRRT initiation and outcomes in early and late groups

	All patients (n = 189)	Early group (n = 52)	Late group (n = 137)	P value
Demographic data at CRRT initiation				
Mechanical ventilation, n (%)	150 (79)	45 (87)	105(77)	0.16
Vasopressor, n (%)	101 (53)	26 (50)	75 (55)	0.63
Diuretic use, n (%)	70 (37)	21 (40)	49 (36)	0.61
Creatinine (mg/dl), median (IQR)	2.7 (1.9–4.0)	1.8 (1.2–3.0)	2.8 (2.2–4.2)	<0.001
eGFR (ml/min/1.73 m^2)	18 (12–28)	30 (15–44)	18 (11–25)	<0.001
BUN (mg/dl), median (IQR)	50 (31–72)	37 (29–59)	54 (34–87)	<0.001
Urine Output (ml/h), median (IQR)	19 (8–35)	21 (10–46)	17 (7.6–33)	0.09
Bilirubin (mg/dl), median (IQR)	1.0 (0.6–2.3)	1.8 (0.7–3.7)	1.0 (0.6–2.5)	0.83
Platelets (cells/10^3), median (IQR)	112 (63–188)	107 (65–159)	118 (62–194)	0.84
Albumin (g/dl), median (IQR)	2.5 (2.0–3.1)	2.5 (2.1–3.1)	2.5 (2.0–3.1)	0.87
PiO$_2$/FiO$_2$, (Torr), median (IQR)	181 (117–293)	198 (139–338)	200 (119–329)	0.16
Glasgow Coma Scale, median (IQR)	13 (6–15)	13 (6–15)	13 (6–15)	0.69
Factors contributing to AKI				
Sepsis, n (%)	74 (39)	21 (40)	53 (39)	0.87
Cardiogenic shock, n (%)	59 (31)	20 (39)	39 (29)	0.22
Drug-induced AKI, n (%)	4 (2)	1 (2)	3 (2)	1
Hypovolemia, n (%)	15 (8)	1 (2)	14 (10)	0.07
Post-operative, n (%)	35 (19)	10 (19)	25 (18)	0.87
Post-renal failure, n (%)	1 (2)	0 (0)	1 (1)	1
Others, n (%)	7 (4)	2 (4)	5 (4)	1
Outcomes				
Duration of CRRT (day), median (IQR)	3 (1–8)	3 (1–6)	3 (1–9)	0.3
ICU length of stay (day), median (IQR)	10 (4–18)	8(3–16)	10 (5–18)	0.34
Post-CRRT hospital length of stay (day), median (IQR)	11 (1–32)	13 (1–32)	11 (1–32)	0.81
Hospital length of stay (days), median, median (IQR)	26 (13–57)	29 (14–43)	26 (11–62)	0.81
Time interval from ICU admission to CRRT initiation (day), median (IQR)	0.8 (0.1–1.9)	0.8 (0.2–2.0)	0.8 (0.1–1.9)	0.89
ICU mortality, n (%)	86 (47)	26 (50)	60 (44)	0.51
Hospital mortality, n (%)	101 (53)	33 (64)	68 (50)	0.1

Others: hyperkalemia (two patients), acute pancreatitis, Goodpasture syndrome, mixed acidosis, acute renal stroke, and catastrophic anti-phospholipid syndrome

Abbreviations: CRRT continuous renal replacement therapy, IQR interquartile range, BUN blood urea nitrogen, eGFR estimated glomerular filtration rate, AKI acute kidney injury, ICU intensive care unit

(31%), drug-induced AKI (2%), hypovolemia (8%), post-operative (19%), post-renal failure (2%), and others (4%). The "others" group included hyperkalemia (two patients), acute pancreatitis, Goodpasture syndrome, mixed acidosis, acute renal stroke, and catastrophic anti-phospholipid syndrome.

For the primary outcome, crude early vs. late group in-hospital mortality was 64 vs. 50% (P = 0.10). For the secondary outcomes, the median CRRT length (3 vs. 3 days, P = 0.3), the median post-CRRT hospital length of stay (13 vs. 11 days, P = 0.81), the median hospital length of stay (29 vs. 26 days, P = 0.81), the median ICU length of stay (8 vs. 8 days, P = 0.34), the median time

interval from ICU admission to CRRT initiation, and intensive care unit mortality (50 vs. 44%, P = 0.51) were not significant statistically.

As shown in Table 4, logistic regression analysis showed that late initiation of CRRT [odds ratio (OR), 0.30; 95% confidence interval (CI), 0.13–0.71; P = 0.006] and lower SAPS II score (OR, 1.04; 95% CI, 1.02–1.06; P < 0.001) were associated with lower in-hospital mortality.

Discussion

This is a single-center retrospective study evaluating the optimal timing for initiation of CRRT, as defined by the

Table 4 Independent predictors of in-hospital mortality using logistic regression analysis

Variables	Odds ratio	95% confidence interval	P value
Timing of RRT initiation			
Early initiation	1.0[a]		
Late initiation	0.30	0.13–0.71	0.006
SAPS II score	1.04	1.02–1.06	<0.001

Abbreviations: *RRT* renal replacement therapy, *SAPS II* Simplified Acute Physiology Score II
[a]Reference indicator variable

modified RIFLE classification in a mixed medical–surgical ICU. The major finding of this study is that late CRRT initiation, as defined by the modified RIFLE classification and lower SAPS scores, was associated with lower in-hospital mortality.

The optimal timing of RRT initiation for patients with AKI remains controversial because initiation of RRT can be influenced by the following factors: (1) patient-specific factors including renal function, co-morbid diseases, and primary diagnosis; (2) clinician-specific factors, including goals of therapy and local practice patterns; and (3) organizational factors including health costs, ICU type, and nursing availability [20]. Well-accepted indications for initiating RRT in patients with AKI include volume overload, hyperkalemia, uremia, severe metabolic acidosis, and drug intoxication. However, since there is currently no consensus regarding the optimal timing of initiating RRT, some clinicians initiate RRT in patients with non-AKI or early-stage AKI to prevent the development of complications induced by AKI.

A previous report showed that earlier RRT initiation reduced mortality and contributed to better renal recovery [5]. A recent single-center randomized trial showed that early RRT initiation reduced the 90-day mortality compared with delayed RRT initiation (39.3 vs. 54.7%, $P = 0.003$) [6]. In this study, the early group consisted of patients within 8 h of diagnosis with stage 2 AKI in Kidney Disease Improving Global Outcome (KDIGO) criteria, while the late group consisted of patients after 12 h of diagnosis with stage 3 AKI. However, Bagshaw et al performed a prospective multicenter observational study at 54 centers in 23 countries enrolling 1238 patients, which showed that late initiation of RRT classified by creatinine was associated with lower mortality (OR, 0.46; 95% CI, 0.36–0.58; $P < 0.0001$) [21]. Another recent prospective multicenter randomized trial showed no apparent benefit from the early initiation strategy [7]. A recent systematic review and meta-analysis reported by Wierstra et al. concluded that early RRT initiation in critically ill patients with AKI did not result in a survival benefit [22]. A systematic review and meta-analysis of randomized controlled trials reported by Xu et al. showed similar results [23]. The data in the current

study may support the results of previous studies, suggesting that early initiation strategy has no clinical benefit.

Differences in etiological background between the two groups including contributing factors to AKI and distribution of CKD deserve mention. First, in the early group, substantial numbers of patients might have had fluid overload, reflected by lower serum creatinine levels. In fact, studies suggest lower creatinine may reflect a state of fluid overload that can cause higher mortality [24, 25]. Bouchard et al. conducted a prospective multicenter observational study including critically ill patients with AKI who needed RRT to assess whether fluid accumulation was associated with mortality with positive results (OR 2.07 [95% CI 1.27–3.37]) and non-recovery of kidney function [26]. In our study, the number of patients with cardiogenic shock in the early group appeared larger than the late group (39 vs. 29%). Those patients with cardiogenic shock may have well been complicated with fluid overload (Table 3). Physicians might not have recognized the true degree of AKI due to the apparent lower serum creatinine.

Second, more patients with CKD were included in the early group compared with the late group ($p = 0.009$). AKI in patients with CKD may be associated with a higher risk of mortality [27]. Wu et al. reported a multicenter observational study of 9425 patients for diagnosis of AKI after major surgery and evaluated mortality risk from post-operative AKI with or without CKD. The results showed that patients with a past history of CKD had higher mortality (HR, 3.94; 95% CI, 2.79–5.28, $P < 0.001$) compared with the patients without CKD [28]. In this study, the mortality of patients with end-stage renal disease was higher than in patients with or without prior CKD. In the present study, there are fewer patients with CKD in the late RRT group than in the early RRT group. Also, the number of patients with CKD stages 4 and 5 were greater in the early RRT group than in the late RRT group (Table 2). For these hypothetical reasons, late RRT initiation was associated with a better prognosis in our study.

Finally, late RRT initiation policy has a potential to avoid unnecessary RRT. In a recent multicenter randomized controlled trial comparing the early vs. late policy, Gaudry et al. reported that renal function was more rapidly recovered and less frequency of catheter related blood stream infections occurred in late RRT initiation [7]. Patients with higher creatinine may undergo earlier treatment, and their prognosis would be better than that of patients with lower creatinine [29]. In our study, although there were no statistically significant differences regarding the time interval from ICU admission to RRT initiation in both early and late groups, more rapidly increasing creatinine appeared in the late group (Tables 2 and 3). It is possible that early treatment, including antibiotics, fluid challenges, nephrology consultation, and vasopressor use may have contributed to a better prognosis for patients with higher serum creatinine levels.

This study has several limitations. First, this study may have excluded a large number of AKI patients who met the criteria for RRT initiation but did not undergo CRRT. Second, this study was a single-center retrospective analysis with a relatively small sample size. Therefore, we cannot exclude the potential effects of unknown confounding factors. Third, we defined AKI according to the modified RIFLE classification and did not use urine criteria instead of the standard RIFLE classification. However, Haase et al. suggested that urine output criteria are not a more important predictive factor for in-hospital mortality than creatinine criteria [30]. Fourth, there was a lack of baseline creatinine data in approximately 34% of patients for whom we estimated the eGFR based on calculations. Therefore, the exact prevalence of CKD in the study population is unknown. Finally, some of the late group who started CRRT within 24 h of admission to ICU may have been early starters if laboratory testing had not been delayed, and there is potential for crossover of patients between the assigned groups.

Conclusions

The late initiation of CRRT, as defined by the modified RIFLE classification, is associated with a lower risk of in-hospital mortality in critically ill patients with AKI. Further studies are needed to confirm the optimal timing for the initiation of CRRT.

Abbreviations

AKI: Acute kidney injury; BUN: Blood urea nitrogen; CKD: Chronic kidney disease; CRRT: Continuous renal replacement therapy; eGFR: Estimated glomerular filtration rate; HR: Hazard ratio; ICU: Intensive care unit; IQR: Interquartile range; KDIGO: Kidney Disease Improving Global Outcome; OR: Odds ratio; RRT: Renal replacement therapy; SAPS II: Simplified Acute Physiology Score II

Acknowledgements

All work was performed at the Jichi Medical University Saitama Medical Center. We thank Katsunobu Ando, Tsukasa Higuchi, and Makoto Hashimoto for clinical assistance. Part of this research was presented at the 26th Annual Meeting of the European Society of Intensive Care Medicine in Paris, 2013.

Funding

The authors declare that they have no funding for this study.

Authors' contributions

All authors contributed the design of the study. JS participated in the data collection and drafted the manuscript. TO helped and revised the manuscript. HS, KI, TF, HY, AL, and MS participated in the data collection and manuscript writing. All authors read and approved the final manuscript.

Competing interests

The authors declare that they have no competing interests.

Author details

[1]Division of Infectious Diseases, Jichi Medical University Hospital, 3311-1 Yakushiji, Shimotsuke, Tochigi 329-0498, Japan. [2]Department of Anesthesiology and Critical Care Medicine, Jichi Medical University Saitama Medical Center, 1-847 Amanuma, Omiya-ku, Saitama City, Saitama 330-8503, Japan. [3]Division of General Medicine, The First Department of Comprehensive Medicine, Jichi Medical University Saitama Medical Center, 1-847 Amanuma, Omiya-ku, Saitama City, Saitama 330-8503, Japan. [4]Division of Nephrology, The First Department of Comprehensive Medicine, Jichi Medical University Saitama Medical Center, 1-847 Amanuma, Omiya-ku, Saitama City, Saitama 330-8503, Japan. [5]Division of Cardiology, The First Department of Comprehensive Medicine, Jichi Medical University Saitama Medical Center, 1-847 Amanuma, Omiya-ku, Saitama City, Saitama 330-8503, Japan. [6]Division of Endocrinology and Metabolism, The First Department of Comprehensive Medicine, Jichi Medical University Saitama Medical Center, 1-847 Amanuma, Omiya-ku, Saitama City, Saitama 330-8503, Japan. [7]Department of Surgery, Jichi Medical University, 3311-1 Yakushiji, Shimotsuke, Tochigi 329-0498, Japan.

Reference

1. Ostermann M, Chang RW. Acute kidney injury in the intensive care unit according to RIFLE. Crit Care Med. 2007;35:1837–43.
2. Hoste EA, Clermont G, Kersten A, Venkataraman R, Angus DC, De Bacquer D, et al. RIFLE criteria for acute kidney injury are associated with hospital mortality in critically ill patients: a cohort analysis. Crit Care. 2006;10:R73.
3. Metnitz PG, Krenn CG, Steltzer H, Lang T, Ploder J, Lenz K, et al. Effect of acute renal failure requiring renal replacement therapy on outcome in critically ill patients. Crit Care Med. 2002;30:2051–8.
4. Uchino S, Kellum JA, Bellomo R, Doig GS, Morimatsu H, Morgera S, et al. Acute renal failure in critically ill patients: a multinational, multicenter study. JAMA. 2005;294:813–8.
5. Karvellas CJ, Farhat MR, Sajjad I, Mogensen SS, Leung AA, Wald R, et al. A comparison of early versus late initiation of renal replacement therapy in critically ill patients with acute kidney injury: a systematic review and meta-analysis. Crit Care. 2011;15:R72.
6. Zarbock A, Kellum JA, Schmidt C, Van Aken H, Wempe C, Pavenstädt H, et al. Effect of early vs delayed initiation of renal replacement therapy on mortality in critically ill patients with acute kidney injury: the ELAIN Randomized Clinical Trial. JAMA. 2016;315:2190–9.
7. Gaudry S, Hajage D, Schortgen F, Martin-Lefevre L, Pons B, Boulet E, et al. Initiation strategies for renal-replacement therapy in the intensive care unit. N Engl J Med. 2016;375:122–33.
8. Bellomo R, Ronco C, Kellum JA, Mehta RL, Palevsky P. Acute renal failure—definition, outcome measures, animal models, fluid therapy and information technology needs: the Second International Consensus Conference of the Acute Dialysis Quality Initiative (ADQI) Group. Crit Care. 2004;8:R204–12.
9. Bagshaw SM, George C, Bellomo R. A comparison of the RIFLE and AKIN criteria for acute kidney injury in critically ill patients. Nephrol Dial Transplant. 2008;23:1569–74.
10. Uchino S, Bellomo R, Goldsmith D, Bates S, Ronco C. An assessment of the RIFLE criteria for acute renal failure in hospitalized patients. Crit Care Med. 2006;34:1913–7.
11. Shiao CC, Wu VC, Li WY, Lin YF, Hu FC, Young GH, et al. Late initiation of renal replacement therapy is associated with worse outcomes in acute kidney injury after major abdominal surgery. Crit Care. 2009;13:R171.
12. Shum HP, Chan KC, Kwan MC, Yeung AW, Cheung EW, Yan WW. Timing for initiation of continuous renal replacement therapy in patients with septic shock and acute kidney injury. Ther Apher Dial. 2013;17:305–10.
13. Wu SC, Fu CY, Lin HH, Chen RJ, Hsieh CH, Wang YC, et al. Late initiation of continuous veno-venous hemofiltration therapy is associated with a lower survival rate in surgical critically ill patients with postoperative acute kidney injury. Am Surg. 2012;78:235–42.
14. Chou YH, Huang TM, Wu VC, Wang CY, Shiao CC, Lai CF, et al. Impact of

timing of renal replacement therapy initiation on outcome of septic acute kidney injury. Crit Care. 2011;15:R134.

15. National Kidney Foundation. K/DOQI clinical practice guidelines for chronic kidney disease: evaluation, classification, and stratification. Am J Kidney Dis. 2002;39:S1–26.

16. Inker LA, Astor BC, Fox CH, Isakova T, Lash JP, Peralta CA, et al. KDOQI US commentary on the 2012 KDIGO clinical practice guideline for the evaluation and management of CKD. Am J Kidney Dis. 2014;63:713–35.

17. Le Gall JR, Lemeshow S, Saulnier F. A new Simplified Acute Physiology Score (SAPS II) based on a European/North American multicenter study. JAMA. 1993;270:2957–63.

18. Levy MM, Fink MP, Marshall JC, Abraham E, Angus D, Cook D, et al. 2001 SCCM/ESICM/ACCP/ATS/SIS International Sepsis Definitions Conference. Crit Care Med. 2003;31:1250–6.

19. Kanda Y. Investigation of the freely available easy-to-use software "EZR" for medical statistics. Bone Marrow Transplant. 2013;48:452–8.

20. Vesconi S, Cruz DN, Fumagalli R, Kindgen-Milles D, Monti G, Marinho A, et al. Delivered dose of renal replacement therapy and mortality in critically ill patients with acute kidney injury. Crit Care. 2009;13:R57.

21. Bagshaw SM, Uchino S, Bellomo R, Morimatsu H, Morgera S, Schetz M, et al. Timing of renal replacement therapy and clinical outcomes in critically ill patients with severe acute kidney injury. J Crit Care. 2009;24:129–40.

22. Wierstra BT, Kadri S, Alomar S, Burbano X, Barrisford GW, Kao RLC. The impact of "early" versus "late" initiation of renal replacement therapy in critical care patients with acute kidney injury: a systematic review and evidence synthesis. Crit Care. 2016;20:122.

23. Xu Y, Gao J, Zheng X, Zhong B, Na Y, Wei J. Timing of initiation of renal replacement therapy for acute kidney injury: a systematic review and meta-analysis of randomized-controlled trials. Clin Exp Nephrol. 2016; Epub ahead of print.

24. Biesen Van W, Yegenaga I, Vanholder R, Verbeke F, Hoste E, Colardyn F, et al. Relationship between fluid status and its management on acute renal failure (ARF) in intensive care unit (ICU) patients with sepsis: a prospective analysis. J Nephrol. 2005;18(1):54–60.

25. Sakr Y, Vincent JL, Reinhart K, Groeneveld J, Michalopoulos A, Sprung CL, et al. High tidal volume and positive fluid balance are associated with worse outcome in acute lung injury. Chest. 2005;128:3098–108.

26. Bouchard J, Soroko SB, Chertow GM, Himmelfarb J, Ikizler TA, Paganini EP, et al. Fluid accumulation, survival and recovery of kidney function in critically ill patients with acute kidney injury. Kidney Int. 2009;76:422–7.

27. Rocha E, Soares M, Valente C, Nogueira L, Bonomo H, Godinho M, et al. Outcomes of critically ill patients with acute kidney injury and end-stage renal disease requiring renal replacement therapy: a case-control study. Nephrol Dial Transplant. 2009;24:1925–30.

28. Wu V-C, Huang T-M, Lai C-F, Shiao C-C, Lin Y-F, Chu T-S, et al. Acute-on-chronic kidney injury at hospital discharge is associated with long-term dialysis and mortality. Kidney Int. 2011;80:1222–30.

29. Cerda J, Cerda M, Kilcullen P, Prendergast J. In severe acute kidney injury, a higher serum creatinine is paradoxically associated with better patient survival. Nephrol Dial Transpl. 2007;22:2781–4.

30. Haase M, Bellomo R, Matalanis G, Calzavacca P, Dragun D, Haase-Fielitz A. A comparison of the RIFLE and Acute Kidney Injury Network classifications for cardiac surgery-associated acute kidney injury: a prospective cohort study. J Thorac Cardiovasc Surg. 2009;138:1370–6.

6

Virological response to daclatasvir and asunaprevir combination therapy for chronic hepatitis C virus genotype 1b infection in dialysis patients: a prospective, multicenter study

Haruki Uojima[1,2*], Shuzo Kobayashi[3], Hisashi Hidaka[2], Shuichi Matsumoto[4], Takayasu Ohtake[3], Takeshi Kinbara[1], Machiko Oka[3], Yasuhiro Yamanouchi[5], Takehiko Kunieda[6], Hiroki Yamanoue[7], Takayuki Kanemaru[8], Kazuhiko Tsutsumi[9], Tomoaki Fujikawa[10], Ji Hyun Sung[1] and Makoto Kako[1]

Abstract

Background: The introduction of direct-acting antiviral agents (DAAs) for the treatment of chronic hepatitis C virus (HCV) infection in patients undergoing hemodialysis (HD) has improved sustained virological response (SVR) rates. Our aim was to assess the characteristics of the virological response to daclatasvir (DCV) and asunaprevir (ASV) combination therapy for HCV in HD patients.

Methods: A multicenter prospective study was conducted at eight centers in Japan. Patients on HD with chronic genotype 1b HCV infections were orally administered DCV and ASV for 24 weeks at doses of a 60-mg capsule once daily and a 100-mg tablet twice daily, respectively. The primary endpoint of this trial was the proportion of patients with a sustained virological response at 24 weeks after the treatment ended (SVR24). We also investigated the characteristics associated with the virological response to combination therapy.

Results: Thirty patients were enrolled in this study, and the proportion that achieved an SVR24 after treatment was 83.3% (25/30). Virological failure was observed in 4 patients (13.3%). Two exhibited virological breakthrough at weeks 16 and 20 of drug administration, and viral relapse occurred in 2 patients at weeks 4 and 8 after the end of treatment. Virological failure was defined as HCV-RNA levels exceeding 5.5 $\log_{10}$ IU/mL, and resistance-associated variants (RAVs) NS5A-L31M/V and Y93H were not exhibited at baseline.

Conclusions: DCV and ASV therapy for chronic HCV on HD was significantly effective. Most importantly, patients with the low viral loads undergoing HD demonstrated a higher response to combination therapy regardless of RAV.

Keywords: Daclatasvir, Asunaprevir, Chronic kidney disease, Hepatitis C virus

* Correspondence: kiruha555@yahoo.co.jp
[1]Department of Gastroenterology, Shonan Kamakura General Hospital, 1370-1 Okamoto, Kamakura, Kanagawa 247-8533, Japan
[2]Department of Gastroenterology, Internal Medicine, Kitasato University School of Medicine, Sagamihara, Kanagawa, Japan
Full list of author information is available at the end of the article

Background

Hepatitis C virus (HCV) has been recognized as the most important causative agent of liver disease in patients receiving long-term hemodialysis (HD) in both developed and less-developed countries [1]. There are six distinguishable HCV genotypes, and the use of conventional interferon (IFN), pegylated IFN-α, or a combination of IFN with ribavirin for treatment depends on the genotype of the HCV virus [2]. Although treatment options for patients on HD are the same as for the general population, it is important to consider that treatment-related toxicity with IFN and ribavirin occurs frequently in patients on HD [3, 4]. According to the KDIGO (Kidney Disease Improving Global Outcome) guidelines, monotherapy with standard IFN is the therapy of choice for HCV-infected patients on maintenance HD [5]. Although IFN-related therapy achieves a sustained virological response (SVR) in 33–45% of HD patients with genotype 1, alternative therapies are required [4].

Presently, direct-acting antiviral agents (DAAs) have assumed a more prominent role in the treatment of patients with HCV [6–10]. The introduction of DAAs has improved SVR rates and shortened treatment durations. DAAs also enabled successful treatment without IFN therapy [7]. In Japan, a phase III study demonstrated that a 24-week combined regimen of daclatasvir (DCV) and asunaprevir (ASV) was highly effective in patients with HCV genotype 1b infections [10]. DCV was the first nonstructural protein 5A (NS5A) replication complex inhibitor to show potential efficacy against all HCV genotypes [11–14]. ASV is a second-generation NS3 (nonstructural protein 3) protease inhibitor that exhibited strong antiviral activity against HCV genotypes 1 and 4. It has been shown to act by inhibiting the viral nonstructural 3/4A serine protease required for viral replication [15, 16]. The pharmacokinetics of DCV and ASV, which are eliminated primarily by hepatic metabolism, have been assessed in patients with end-stage renal disease, which indicated that dose adjustments of either drug were unnecessary in cases of severe renal dysfunction. Recently, two prospective studies reported the efficacy of DCV and ASV combination therapy for the treatment of chronic HCV in patients undergoing HD, showing dramatically improved rates of sustained virological response at 12 weeks after treatment (SVR12) compared with monotherapy with standard IFN [17, 18]. However, it remains unclear whether end-stage renal disease, including those in patients on HD, affects the viral response to DAA-based antiviral therapy for HCV. Therefore, we studied the characteristics associated with the virological response to DCV and ASV combination therapy for HCV on HD patients.

Methods

Study design and patients

A multicenter prospective study was conducted at eight centers in Japan. The enrollment commenced in February 2015, and the study was completed in August 2016. Patients with chronic genotype 1b HCV infection undergoing HD received DCV and ASV for 24 weeks. DCV and ASV were administered orally at doses of a 60-mg capsule once daily and a 100-mg tablet twice daily, respectively, according to the manufacturer's prescribing information for both medications. The discontinuance criteria for the enrolled patients included (1) viral breakthrough occurrence (increase in plasma HCV-RNA levels exceeding 1 $\log_{10}$ IU/mL compared with the lowest recorded on-treatment value), (2) a lower than 2 $\log_{10}$ IU/mL decrease in HCV-RNA levels compared with those at the baseline and at week 8, (3) occurrence of severe adverse events ($\geq$grade 3) according the National Cancer Institute Common Terminology Criteria for Adverse Events (CTCAE), version 4.0, and (4) the patient's desire to terminate.

Eligibility criteria

This study enrolled patients with chronic HCV genotype 1b infection for at least 6 months and plasma HCV-RNA levels exceeding 2 $\log_{10}$ IU/mL. Eligible patients consisted of men and women who were treatment-naïve or treatment-experienced (previously treated with an IFN-based therapy), over 20 years of age, and currently undergoing HD.

The main exclusion criteria included the presence of (1) decompensated liver cirrhosis (Child-pugh B and C), (2) hepatocellular carcinoma, (3) infection/co-infection with hepatitis B virus (HBV) or human immunodeficiency virus (HIV), (4) previous exposure to IFN-based therapy within 1 month before drug administration, (5) previous exposure to DAA inhibitors, and (6) defined laboratory abnormalities during screening. Furthermore, patients with alanine aminotransferase (ALT) levels greater than five times the upper limit of the normal range, platelet, and white blood cell (WBC) counts lower than 50,000 and 4000/mm^3, respectively, and hemoglobin levels less than 8.5 g/dL, were also excluded.

Clinical parameters

The clinical characteristics evaluated were the demographic information, plasma HCV-RNA levels, and baseline laboratory data before and after the study drug administration. Blood samples were collected at each study visit before a dialysis, and the plasma HCV-RNA levels were quantified using the Cobas TaqMan version 2.0 assay (Roche Diagnostics, Tokyo, Japan); the lower limits of quantification were 1.2 $\log_{10}$ IU/mL. The HCV-RNA levels were measured at baseline and at weeks 0, 2,

4, 8, 12, 16, 20, and 24, as well as at posttreatment weeks 4, 8, 12, and 24. The resistance-associated variants (RAVs) of NS5A-Y93H and L31M/V were identified using direct sequencing [19], which was conducted on all enrolled patients. The laboratory tests performed were the analysis of hemoglobin, WBC count, neutrophils, platelets, serum albumin, blood urea nitrogen (BUN), creatinine, total bilirubin, aspartate aminotransferase (AST), ALT, and α-fetoprotein levels.

Efficacy

The primary endpoint of this trial was the proportion of patients with a sustained virological response 24 weeks after the treatment ended (SVR24) as determined by using intention-to-treat analysis. The secondary endpoints were the proportion of patients with undetectable HCV-RNA levels at weeks 4, 8, 12, 16, 20, and 24, at the end of the treatment, and at weeks 4, 8, and 12 after the treatment ended. We also investigated the characteristics associated with the virological response to the combination therapy. To study the pharmacological effects of combination therapy, laboratory data on blood biomarkers were assessed.

Safety assessment

To evaluate drug safety during the trial period, we assessed the adverse events that occurred after the commencement of trial drug administration at each study visit. The data on all adverse events were collected from the start of study drug administration to up to 30 days after the last study drug dosing. The severity of any serious or nonserious adverse events was graded using CTCAE, version 4.0.

Statistical evaluation

Our estimation of the SVR24 rates in patients undergoing HD was 85% based on previous studies [10]. With an alpha of 0.05 and power of 80%, 30 patients were required for this trial. Under the principles of intent to treat, the population analyzed consisted of all patients who signed informed consent forms. The data were analyzed using the statistical software JMP 11.0.1 (Statistical Analysis Software, SAS Institute). All the data were expressed as mean ± standard deviation, and the Wilcoxon signed-rank test was used for the analysis of the paired data. All differences with a P value <0.05 were considered significant.

Results
Characteristics of patients

A total of 33 patients were assessed in February 2015, and the study was completed in August 2016 (Fig. 1). Of these 33 patients, 3 patients dropped out during the run-in period due to failure to meet the criteria to commence treatment. The remaining 30 patients received the combination therapy, and of these, only 1 patient did not complete the study due to nontreatment-related death (sudden death at week 13 of drug administration). The enrolled patients' demographics and other baseline clinical characteristics are summarized in Table 1. All patients who were enrolled in the trial were included in the analyses. The patients' mean age was 65.5 ± 7.7 years

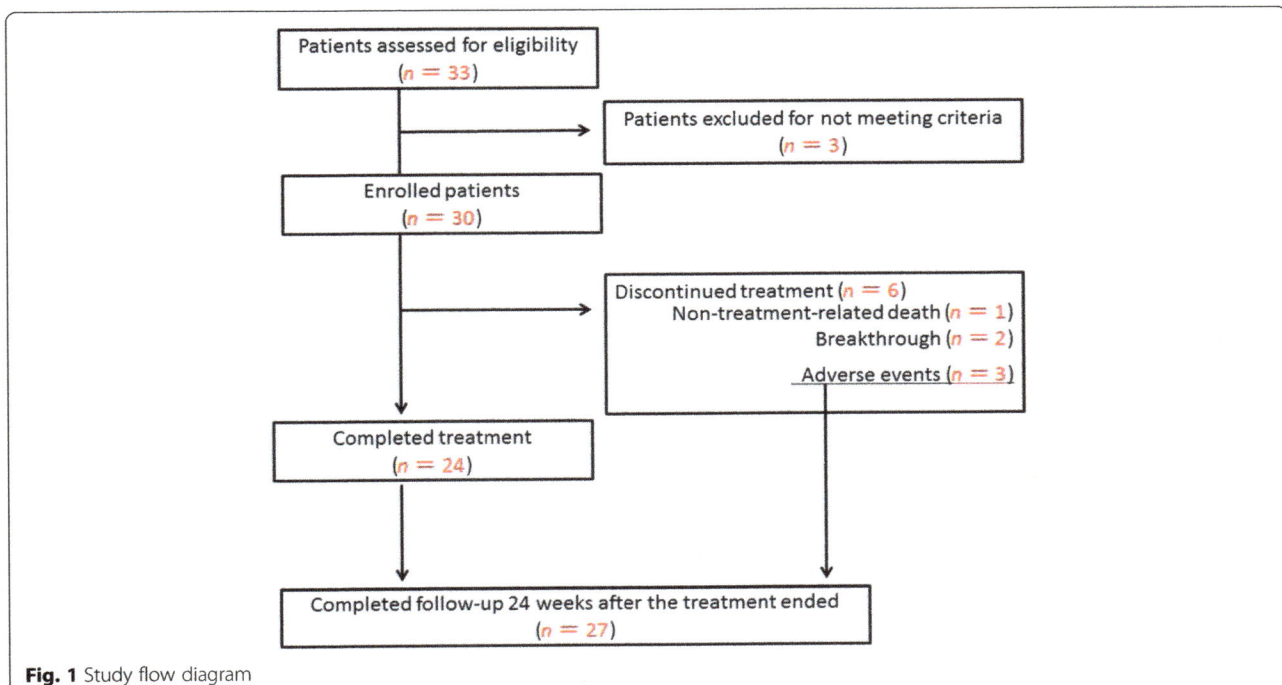

Fig. 1 Study flow diagram

Table 1 Patient baseline clinical characteristics

Characteristics		All patients
N		30
Age, years		65.5 ± 7.7
Sex, male	n (%)	23 (76.7)
Duration of hemodialysis	years	15.4 ± 10.5
Etiology of end-stage renal disease	n (%)	
Diabetic nephropathy		13 (43.3)
Polycystic kidney disease		2 (6.7)
Interstitial nephritis		3 (10.0)
Glomerulonephritis		7 (23.3)
Others		5 (16.7)
Weight	kg	51.2 ± 10.1
Previous treatment	n (%)	
Naïve		21 (70.0)
Relapse		5 (16.6)
Non-viral response		4 (13.3)
Liver cirrhosis	n (%)	9 (30.0)
Serum HCV-RNA levels	$\log_{10}$IU/mL	5.15 ± 0.95
NS5A inhibitor RAVs	n (%)	2 (6.7)
Laboratory data		
Hemoglobin	g/dL	10.6 ± 1.50
WBC	/μL	5484 ± 1760
Neutrophils	/μL	3718 ± 1381
Platelets	$\times 10^4$/μL	16.5 ± 6.38
Serum AST	IU/L	20.1 ± 13.1
Serum ALT	IU/L	16.1 ± 8.21
Serum albumin	g/dL	3.40 ± 0.35
BUN	mg/dL	51.9 ± 16.5
Serum creatinine	mg/dL	9.31 ± 2.39
Serum total bilirubin	mg/dL	0.36 ± 0.16
Alpha-fetoprotein	ng/mL	2.39 ± 0.98

Data are expressed as median, number (%), or mean ± standard deviation
RAVs resistance-associated variants, BUN blood urea nitrogen, PT-INR international normalized ratio of prothrombin time

(range 53–82 years), and 23 patients (76.7%) were male. Furthermore, 9 patients (30%) had liver cirrhosis and received previous treatment. The duration of HD was 15.4 ± 10.5 years (range 0.5–35 years), and the cause of end-stage renal dysfunction was diabetic nephropathy in 13 patients, polycystic kidney disease in 2 patients, and glomerulonephritis in 7 patients. The mean HCV level was 5.15 ± 0.95 $\log_{10}$ IU/mL (range, 3.2–6.9 $\log_{10}$ IU/mL). The mean serum albumin, creatinine, and ALT levels were 3.40 ± 0.35 g/dL, 9.31 ± 2.39 mg/dL, and 16.1 ± 8.21 IU/L, respectively (ranges 2.5–4.0 g/dL, 7.9–15.1 mg/dL, and 4–44 IU/L, respectively). Furthermore, the RAV NS5A-Y93H was detected in 2 patients (6.9%) while L31M/V was not detected at baseline.

Virological response
The patient plasma HCV-RNA levels declined following administration of the combination therapy (Fig. 2), and the mean decrease from baseline was 4.4 $\log_{10}$ IU/mL at week 4. The results of the primary endpoint determination revealed an SVR24 rate of 83.3% (25/30). The proportions of patients with undetectable HCV-RNA levels at treatment weeks 4, 8, and 12, and at the treatment end were 26/30, 30/30, 30/30, and 27/30 (86.7, 100, 100, and 90.0%), respectively, while at weeks 4, 8, and 12 after the treatment ended, the proportions were all 25/30 (83.3%). Furthermore, the 3 patients who were followed up to the discontinuation of the combination therapy, due to adverse events and laboratory abnormalities, achieved SVR24.

Virological failure
The demographics of the patients with virological failure and other baseline clinical characteristics are summarized in Table 2. Virological failure was observed in 4 patients (13.3%), 2 patients exhibiting virological breakthrough, one of those at week 16 and the other at week 20 of drug administration, respectively, and viral relapse occurred in 2 patients, one at week 4 and the other at week 8 after the treatment ended.

Virological failure had HCV-RNA levels exceeding 5.5 $\log_{10}$ IU/mL, although there were no significant differences with the virological response and failure group in the mean viral load. There were no significant differences with the virological response or failure group in age, sex, duration of hemodialysis, liver cirrhosis, or previous treatment.

We also investigated the influence of pretreatment RAVs of NS5A-L31M/V and Y93H. We discovered that the patients who showed virological failure did not exhibit RAVs at baseline, while NS5A-L31M/V and Y93H were observed at the time of failure.

Pharmacological effects
Following drug administration, a decrease in the mean ALT level from 16.1 ± 8.21 to 10.2 ± 10.6 IU/IU was observed at the end of the treatment (P = 0.0475). The baseline and posttreatment serum creatinine levels were indistinguishable (9.31 ± 2.39 vs. 9.31 ± 3.82 mg/dL, P = 0.481). The baseline and posttreatment hemoglobin levels were indistinguishable (10.6 ± 1.50 vs. 10.5 ± 1.82, P = 0.736). There were no significant differences in the levels of WBC counts, neutrophils, platelets, serum albumin, BUN, total bilirubin, or α-fetoprotein.

Safety assessment
The observed adverse events are summarized in Table 3. Adverse events were observed in 10 patients (33.3%) receiving treatment, and there were no treatment-related

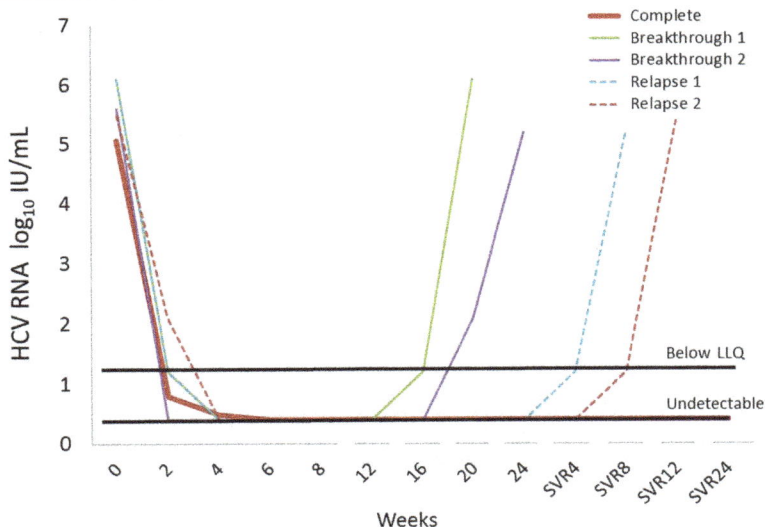

Fig. 2 Change in HCV-RNA levels during treatment with daclatasvir and asunaprevir in complete, relapse, and breakthrough patients. HCV-RNA levels at baseline, at weeks 0, 2, 4, 8, 12, 16, 20, and 24, and posttreatment at weeks 4, 8, 12, and 24. *LLQ* lower limit of quantification (IU/mL). Complete indicates patients with a mean sustained virological response at 24 weeks after the treatment ended

deaths. Incidences of headache, diarrhea, and fatigue were reported in 9 patients (30.0%) during the treatment. Although serious adverse events (≥grade 3) were not reported, there were three adverse events that led to the discontinuation of the combination therapy. Two patients, who discontinued therapy, exhibited fatigue at week 14 and had diarrhea at week 20. Another patient showed increased ALT levels (grade 2), leading to the discontinuation of the combination therapy at week 13 due to the physician's decision (Fig. 3).

Discussion

We evaluated the DCV and ASV combination therapy for the treatment of chronic HCV genotype 1b infection

in patients undergoing HD. In this multiple prospective study, we demonstrated that the achievement of an SVR24 in HCV genotype 1b infection in patients on HD was significantly higher following combination therapy, and there were a number of virological failures in patients who had HCV-RNA levels exceeding 5.5 $\log_{10}$ IU/mL without the RAVs NS5A-L31M/V and Y93H. It is commonly known that the most important factor related to the viral response to DAAs is the presence of RAVs [20]. In a phase III study of a 24-week regimen of DCV plus ASV, multivariate analysis confirmed that the RAVs, NS5A-Y93H, and L31M/V were independent of the factors affecting the response to this combination therapy (overall response (OR) 17.81; 95% confidence interval (CI) 7.17–44.25; and OR 26.81; 95% CI 4.61–155.7, respectively). Therefore, the high SVR rate of 83.3% achieved in this study was assumed to be attributable to the lower proportion of RAVs, where NS5A-Y93H was detected in only two cases and L31M/V was not detected at the baseline. The patients with the RAV NS5A-Y93H fortunately also achieved SVR12.

Table 2 Virological failure baseline clinical characteristics

Characteristics	Complete (n = 25)	Failure (n = 4)	P value
Age, years	64.9 ± 8.19	69.5 ± 2.69	0.182
Sex, male (n) [%]	21/25 (80.7)	2/4 (50.0)	0.180[†]
Duration of hemodialysis (years)	16.1 ± 9.5	15.3 ± 10.4	0.393*
Previous treatment (n) [%]			
Naïve	19/25 (76.0)	1/4 (25.0)	0.076[†]
Relapse and non-viral response	6/25 (24.0)	3/4 (75.0)	
Liver cirrhosis (n) [%]	6/25 (24.0)	3/4 (75.0)	0.076[†]
Serum HCV-RNA levels ($\log_{10}$ IU/mL)	5.06 ± 0.99	5.88 ± 0.28	0.158*
≥5.0 $\log_{10}$ IU/mL (n) [%]	16/25 (64.0)	4/4 (100)	0.280[†]
≥5.5 $\log_{10}$ IU/mL (n) [%]	9/25 (36)	4/4 (100)	0.030[†]
NS5A inhibitor RAVs (n) [%]	2/25 (8)	0/4 (0)	1.000[†]

Data are expressed as median, number (%), or mean ± standard deviation
*Mann-Whitney *U* test, [†]Fisher's exact test

Table 3 Adverse events and laboratory abnormality during the treatment period

Adverse events	Clinical events (n = 10)	[n (%)]
	Any grade	≥Grade 3
Diarrhea	4 (13.3)	0
Headache	2 (6.7)	0
Bloating	2 (6.7)	0
Fatigue	1 (3.3)	0
ALT increased	1 (3.3)	0

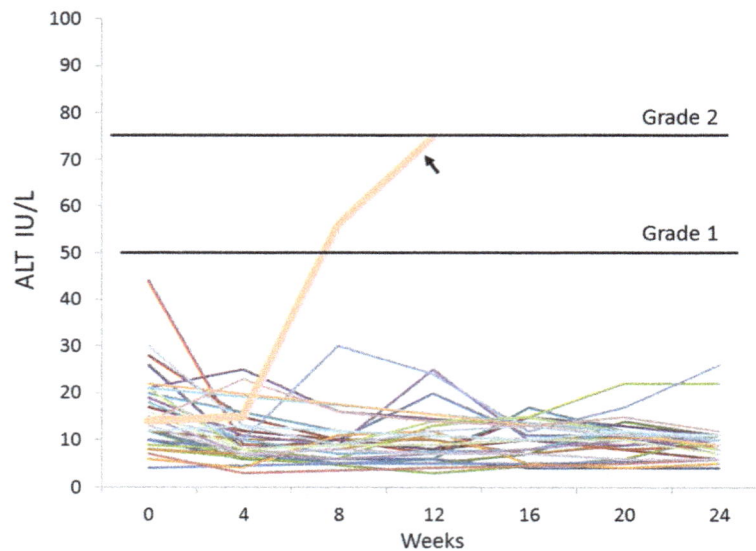

Fig. 3 Individual patient serum ALT levels at weeks 0, 4, 8, 12, 16, 20, and 24 after the administration of daclatasvir and asunaprevir. Only 1 patient discontinued treatment 12 weeks after commencing therapy due to elevation of serum ALT to 75 IU/l (*black arrow*). All the other patients continued through week 24

On the other hand, the present study demonstrated a number of characteristics of treatment failure in patients undergoing HD. All of the virological failures occurred in patients without the RAVs NS5A-Y93H and L31 M/V, and all patients had HCV-RNA levels exceeding 5.5 log_{10} IU/mL even though the HCV-RNA quantity was not correlated with the response to the combination therapy in patients without renal dysfunction [10]. We suggested that high viral loads on HD affected the viral response to direct-acting antiviral agents regardless of RAVs. According to a recent study, maintenance HD decreased the HCV-RNA levels in HD patients with chronic HCV infections [21, 22]. The influence of high viral loads in patients on HD might be significantly higher than that on non-uremic patients. Consequently, hemodialysis, which decreased the HCV-RNA levels, may affect the viral response of direct antiviral agents.

Furthermore, the SVR rate in the present study was considerably lower than those in other articles [17, 18]. Another factor that differs from other studies was that the present study was conducted under the principles of intent to treat and did not elucidate RAVs NS3 D168. We also consider that serum concentrations and drug activity of DCV and ASV combination therapy on hemodialysis may affect the viral response. Although DCV and ASV undergo hepatic biotransformation to more polar but less pharmacologically active compounds that require intact renal function for their efficient elimination [23], it has been reported that renal impairment affects the non-renal clearance of many drugs through mechanisms that appear to include downregulation/

inhibition of cytochrome P450 activity by blood uremic components [23–26]. However, this mechanism is not clear because there is little data presented to support this conclusion.

The administration of the combination therapy was well tolerated in patients with chronic kidney disease (CKD) undergoing HD, relative to IFN- or ribavirin-related therapies. It is noteworthy that hemoglobin declines were not frequent because this regimen was managed without interruption of ribavirin. The study of DAAs with ribavirin in stages 4 or 5 CKD including those in patients on HD demonstrated that declines in hemoglobin levels were frequent [27]. The absence of ribavirin could be an advantage in avoiding severe side effects. However, in the present study, four clinical events that led to the discontinuation of the combination therapy must not be ignored. In particular, 1 patient died of unknown causes during the study period. This patient had an ischemic heart disease, and he was found dead at his home. We determined that the sudden death had been probably due to shock and sudden failure of the heart's action, and this clinical event was a nontreatment-related death. It is well known that the predominant cause of death in patients on regular dialysis is cardiovascular, and sudden cardiac death frequently occurs in CKD patients [28]. HCV infection in patients undergoing HD was also reported as a cardiovascular risk factor [29, 30]. We need to consider that HCV patients on dialysis have a high risk of sudden death due to cardiac disease during combination therapy.

This study has four limitations. First, it was conducted with a relatively small number of patients and a selection bias. Second, we postulated that the achievement of a high SVR rate following treatment with the DCV and ASV combination therapy was likely due to effects of the RAVs in the patients on HD. However, the evidence to support the involvement of the RAVs was insufficient, and further research is warranted to elucidate the other predictors in combination with RAVs, including NS3 D168. Third, although our results suggested that the elimination of HCV in patients undergoing HD may decrease cardiovascular mortality risk, it is not clear whether or not the DAAs improved the long-term prognosis of these patients. Finally, more detailed in vivo pharmacokinetic studies of DCV and ASV combination therapy should be performed and subsequently used to predict serum concentrations and drug activity.

Conclusions

We demonstrated that DCV and ASV combination DAA therapy for chronic HCV genotype 1b infection in patients undergoing HD was significantly effective. Higher responses to the combination therapy in patients with low viral loads can be expected. Therefore, hemodialysis, by decreasing the HCV-RNA levels, could likely affect the viral response of direct antiviral agents.

Abbreviations

ALT: Alanine aminotransferase; AST: Aspartate aminotransferase; ASV: Asunaprevir; BUN: Blood urea nitrogen; CKD: Chronic kidney disease; CTCAE: Common Terminology Criteria for Adverse Events; DAA: Direct-acting antiviral agent; DCV: Daclatasvir; HCV: Hepatitis C virus; HD: Hemodialysis; IFN: Interferon; KDIGO: Kidney Disease Improving Global Outcome; LLQ: Lower limit of quantification; NS3: Nonstructural protein 3; NS5A: Nonstructural protein 5A; RAVs: Resistance-associated variants; SVR: Sustained virological response; SVR24: Sustained virological response 24 weeks after the treatment ended; WBC: White blood cells

Acknowledgements

We thank the Mirai Iryo Research Center, Tokyo, for the assistance with the research and Robert E. Brandt, Founder, CEO, and CME of MedEd Japan, for editing and formatting the manuscript.

Funding

There was no funding for this research.

Authors' contributions

HU and TK contributed equally to this work. HU, SK, TO, and TK designed the research. SM, MO, YY, TK, HY, TK, KT, TF, JHS, and MK performed the research. HU analyzed the data. HU and HH wrote the manuscript. All authors read and approved the final manuscript.

Competing interests

The authors declare that they have no competing interests.

Author details

[1]Department of Gastroenterology, Shonan Kamakura General Hospital, 1370-1 Okamoto, Kamakura, Kanagawa 247-8533, Japan. [2]Department of Gastroenterology, Internal Medicine, Kitasato University School of Medicine, Sagamihara, Kanagawa, Japan. [3]Department of Kidney Disease and Transplant Center, Shonan Kamakura General Hospital, Kamakura, Kanagawa, Japan. [4]Department of General Internal Medicine, Fukuoka Tokushukai Medical Center, Kasuga, Fukuoka, Japan. [5]Department of Kidney Disease, Shinfuji Hospital, Fuji, Shizuoka, Japan. [6]Department of Kidney Disease, Shonan Clinic, Kamakura, Kanagawa, Japan. [7]Department of General Internal Medicine, Shizuoka Tokushukai Hospital, Suruga, Shizuoka, Japan. [8]Department of Surgery, Haibara General Hospital, Makinohara, Shizuoka, Japan. [9]Department of Surgery, Sanpoku Tokushukai Hospital, Murakami, Niigata, Japan. [10]Department of Gastroenterology, Shonan Fujisawa Tokushukai Hospital, Fujisawa, Kanagawa, Japan.

References

1. Latt N, Alachkar N, Gurakar A. Hepatitis C virus and its renal manifestations: a review and update. Gastroenterol Hepatol (N Y). 2012;8:434–45.
2. Uhl P, Fricker G, Haberkorn U, Mier W. Current status in the therapy of liver diseases. Int J Mol Sci. 2014;15:7500–12.
3. Pol S, Jadoul M, Vallet-Pichard A. An update on the management of hepatitis C virus-infected patients with stage 4–5 chronic kidney disease while awaiting the revised KDIGO guidelines. Nephrol Dial Transplant. 2016; (Epub ahead of print).
4. Fabrizi F. Hepatitis C virus infection and dialysis: 2012 update. ISRN Nephrol. 2012. doi:10.5402/2013/159760. eCollection 2013.
5. Alseiari M, Meyer KB, Wong JB. Evidence underlying KDIGO (Kidney Disease: Improving Global Outcomes) guideline recommendations: a systematic review. Am J Kidney Dis. 2016;67:417–22.
6. Holmes JA, Thompson AJ. Interferon-free combination therapies for the treatment of hepatitis C: current insights. Hepat Med. 2015;7:51–70.
7. Elbaz T, El-kassas M, Esmat G. New era for management of chronic hepatitis C virus using direct antiviral agents: A review. J Adv Res. 2015;6:301–10.
8. Chayama K, Hayes CN, Ohishi W, Kawakami Y. Treatment of chronic hepatitis C virus infection in Japan: update on therapy and guidelines. J Gastroenterol. 2013;48:1–12.
9. Ahmed A, Felmlee DJ. Mechanisms of hepatitis C viral resistance to direct acting antivirals. Viruses. 2015;7:6716–29.
10. Kumada H, Suzuki Y, Ikeda K, Toyota J, Karino Y, Chayama K, et al. Daclatasvir plus asunaprevir for chronic HCV genotype 1b infection. Hepatology. 2014;59: 2083–91.
11. Chayama K, Takahashi S, Toyota J, Karino Y, Ikeda K, Ishikawa H, et al. Dual therapy with the nonstructural protein 5A inhibitor, daclatasvir, and the nonstructural protein 3 protease inhibitor, asunaprevir, in hepatitis C virus genotype 1b-infected null responders. Hepatology. 2012;55:742–8.
12. Smith MA, Regal RE, Mohammad RA. Daclatasvir: a NS5A replication complex inhibitor for hepatitis C infection. Ann Pharmacother. 2016;50:39–46.
13. Lee C. Daclatasvir: potential role in hepatitis C. Drug Des Devel Ther. 2013;7: 1223–33.
14. Pelosi LA, Voss S, Liu M, Gao M, Lemm JA. Effect on hepatitis C virus replication of combinations of direct-acting antivirals, including NS5A inhibitor daclatasvir. Antimicrob Agents Chemother. 2012;56:5230–9.
15. Zeuli JD, Adie SK, Rizza SA, Temesgen Z. Asunaprevir plus daclatasvir for the treatment of chronic hepatitis C virus infection. Drugs Today (Barc). 2015;51: 629–43.
16. Akamatsu N, Sugawara Y, Kokudo N. Asunaprevir (BMS-650032) for the treatment of hepatitis C virus. Expert Rev Anti Infect Ther. 2015;13:1307–17.
17. Suda G, Kudo M, Nagasaka A, Furuya K, Yamamoto Y, Kobayashi T, et al. Efficacy and safety of daclatasvir and asunaprevir combination therapy in chronic hemodialysis patients with chronic hepatitis C. J Gastroenterol. 2016;51:733–40.
18. Toyoda H, Kumada T, Tada T, Takaguchi K, Ishikawa T, Tsuji K, et al. Safety and efficacy of dual direct-acting antiviral therapy (daclatasvir and asunaprevir) for chronic hepatitis C virus genotype 1 infection in patients on hemodialysis. J Gastroenterol. 2016;51:741–7.
19. Uchida Y, Kouyama J, Naiki K, Mochida S. A novel simple assay system to quantify the percent HCV RNA levels of NS5A Y93H mutant strains and Y93 wild-type strains relative to the total HCV-RNA levels to determine the indication for antiviral therapy with NS5A inhibitors. PLoS One. 2014;9:e112647.
20. Costilla V, Mathur N, Gutierrez JA. Mechanisms of virologic failure with direct-acting antivirals in hepatitis C and strategies for retreatment. Clin Liver Dis. 2015;19:641–56.

21. Furusyo N, Hayashi J, Ariyama I, Sawayama Y, Etoh Y, Shigematsu M, et al. Maintenance hemodialysis decreases serum hepatitis C virus (HCV) RNA levels in hemodialysis patients with chronic HCV infection. Am J Gastroenterol. 2000;95:490–6.

22. Ozer Etik D, Ocal S, Boyacioglu AS. Hepatitis C infection in hemodialysis patients: a review. World J Hepatol. 2015;7:885–95.

23. Garimella T, Wang R, Luo WL, Hwang C, Sherman D, Kandoussi H, et al. Single-dose pharmacokinetics and safety of daclatasvir in subjects with renal function impairment. Antivir Ther. 2015;20:535–43.

24. Yeung CK, Shen DD, Thummel KE, Himmelfarb J. Effects of chronic kidney disease and uremia on hepatic drug metabolism and transport. Kidney Int. 2014;85:522–8.

25. Dreisbach AW, Lertora JJ. The effect of chronic renal failure on drug metabolism and transport. Expert Opin Drug Metab Toxicol. 2008;4:1065–74.

26. Michaud J, Nolin TD, Naud J, Dani M, Lafrance JP, Leblond FA, et al. Effect of hemodialysis on hepatic cytochrome P450 functional expression. J Pharmacol Sci. 2008;108:157–63.

27. Pockros PJ, Reddy KR, Mantry PS, Cohen E, Bennett M, Sulkowski MS, et al. Efficacy of direct-acting antiviral combination for patients with hepatitis C virus genotype 1 infection and severe renal impairment or end-stage renal disease. Gastroenterology. 2016;150:1590–8.

28. Franczyk-Skóra B, Gluba-Brzózka A, Wranicz JK, Banach M, Olszewski R, Rysz J. Sudden cardiac death in CKD patients. Int Urol Nephrol. 2015;47:971–82.

29. Marinaki S, Boletis JN, Sakellariou S, Delladetsima IK. Hepatitis C in hemodialysis patients. World J Hepatol. 2015;7:548–58.

30. Noiri E, Nakao A, Oya A, Fujita T, Kimura S. Hepatitis C virus in blood and dialysate in hemodialysis. Am J Kidney Dis. 2001;37:38–42.

7

Comparative analysis of the phosphate-binding effects of sucroferric oxyhydroxide, ferric citrate, and lanthanum carbonate

Takeo Ishii[1,2*], Yukiko Nakajima[3] and Kunio Oyama[1]

Abstract

Background: Iron-based phosphate binders are widely used in hemodialysis, to avoid the increased mortality associated with high serum phosphate in dialysis patients. However, comparative studies on the effects of phosphate binders are currently limited. In the present study, a comparative analysis of ferric citrate (FC), sucroferric oxyhydroxide (SF), and lanthanum carbonate (LC) was performed to assess their primary phosphate-binding and secondary iron uptake capacities.

Methods: Patients on maintenance hemodialysis visit our group clinics regularly. The FC, SF, and LC groups comprised 101, 82, and 126 patients, respectively. Subjects were observed from December 2015 to April 2016 (5 months). Serum phosphate levels and other markers were measured in the three medication groups, and changes in phosphate levels and other clinical markers were compared. A drug treatment was considered to be effective if the serum phosphate levels of the patient decreased from baseline in each of the drugs. We evaluated the phosphate-binding capacity compared with each drug using a mixed effect model, for adjusted repeated measured analysis.

Results: SF showed higher phosphate-binding capacity than FC and LC. FC, SF, and LC showed no significant difference in phosphate-binding capacity in the adjusted mixed effect model. However, patients in the FC group exhibited iron accumulation.

Conclusion: Sucroferric oxyhydroxide possesses better phosphate-binding efficacies than ferric citrate and lanthanum carbonate. In addition, ferric citrate showed a strong iron-cumulative effect.

Keywords: Phosphate binder, Hemodialysis, Iron-cumulative effect, Sucroferric oxyhydroxide, Ferric citrate, Lanthanum carbonate, Iron based

Background

High serum phosphate levels in hemodialysis patients are associated with higher mortality, necessitating the use of iron-based phosphate binders with hemodialysis. Ferric citrate (FC) exerts its phosphate-binding effect through ionic interactions and is removed from the body as $FePiPO_4$. Sucroferric oxyhydroxide (SF) binds phosphate as a polymer and causes the excretion of the phosphate. Iron-based phosphate binders are expected to exhibit better phosphate-binding capacity compared to other molecules. In addition, iron is biocompatible and thus possesses high therapeutic potential. However, metals vary in their phosphate-binding capacities and extent of iron release. In this study, we investigated the phosphate-binding capacities and iron absorption effects of SF, FC, and lanthanum carbonate (LC).

Methods

Study subjects

We identified patients who used phosphate binders and visited the Zenjinkai group hospital thrice a week from December 2015 to April 2016. Patients with available electronic medical records were selected for the study. Subjects were categorized into FC, SF, and LC medication groups, which comprised 101, 82, and 126 cases,

* Correspondence: takeo.ishii@grp.zenjinkai.or.jp
[1]Internal Medicine, Zenjinkai group, Yokohama Daiichi Hospital, 2-5-15 Takashima Nishi-ku, Yokohama City, Kanagawa 220-0011, Japan
[2]Department of Medical Science and Cardiorenal Medicine, Graduate School of Medicine, Yokohama City University, Yokohama, Kanagawa, Japan
Full list of author information is available at the end of the article

respectively. SF and FC were administered to circumvent the difficulty in maintaining serum phosphate (Pi) levels below 6.0 mg/dL or unfavorable drug compliance and occurrence of digestion-related symptoms. SF and FC were administered with the starting dose at the baseline week. LC was prescribed continuously and persistently; however, the dosage was increased or decreased to maintain serum Pi under 6.0 mg/dL.

Prescription dose

The Japan Ministry of Health, Labor, and Welfare and the Pharmaceuticals and Medical Devices Agency (PMDA) defined the starting doses of these drugs as SF 750 mg/day (three tablets), FC 1500 mg/day (six tablets), and LC 750 mg/day (three tablets). We prescribed each drug according to these guidelines, and the prescription doses were increased or decreased to regulate serum phosphate levels between 3.5 and 6.0 mg/dL, according to the guidelines of the Japanese Society for Dialysis Therapy and the Japanese Society of Nephrology [1]. The phosphate change rate was defined by the following formula: $(Pi\_week\_n - Pi\_week\_0) \times 100/Pi\_week\_0$. The total prescription dose was defined as the total dose in milligrams during the 5-month observation period, during which each patient visited the hospital 22 times.

Collection of clinical data

For data collection, the STEPII® data system was used to identify patient laboratory data, drug usage, and demographic data. In addition to phosphate, we also analyzed the serum levels of hemoglobin (Hb), STAT (%), and ferritin, as well as the dose of erythropoiesis-stimulating agent (ESA), during each patient visit. The ESA dose for each visit was converted based on the epoetin beta pegol:darbepoetin:epoetin beta ratio of 1:1:200, which is generally used in clinical studies. This study was approved by the facility ethics committee.

Patient characteristics

Three hundred nine patients on maintenance hemodialysis regularly visited our group clinics. The FC, SF, and LC medication groups comprised 101, 82, and 126 cases, respectively (Table 1).

The mean age at the onset of the study was 62.9 years, mean body mass index was 23.2, hemodialysis (HD) vintage was 67.3 months, mean serum Hb was 10.9 g/dL, Pi was 6.1 mg/dL, and percentage of combined phosphate binders (sevelamer and calcium carbonate) was 43.4% (Table 1).

Statistical analysis

We calculated the mean and standard deviation for each parameter and drug dosage and the least square mean for phosphate change rate. We used the least square

Table 1 Baseline characteristics of patients involved in the study

	$n = 309$ (FC = 101, SF = 82, LC = 126)	Mean ± SD	
Age (years)	FC	62.9 ± 12.8	
	SF	63.6 ± 13.3	
	LC	61.7 ± 11.4	
	Total	62.6 ± 12.4	
BMI (kg/m²)	FC	23.1 ± 4.4	
	SF	22.7 ± 4.6	
	LC	23.7 ± 3.8	
	Total	23.2 ± 4.2	
HD duration (months)	FC	59.5 ± 55.0	
	SF	70.6 ± 78.9	
	LC	71.4 ± 54.9	
	Total	67.3 ± 62.1	
Hb g/dL	FC	10.7 ± 1.0	
	SF	11.0 ± 1.2	
	LC	10.9 ± 0.9	
	Total	10.9 ± 1.0	
Pi mg/dL	FC	6.172 ± 1.6339	
	SF	6.216 ± 1.2109	
	LC	5.948 ± 1.4938	
	Total	6.093 ± 1.4726	
Gender		F	M
	FC	27.7%	72.3%
	SF	37.8%	62.2%
	LC	27.0%	73.0%
DM/non-DM		Non-DM	DM
	FC	68.3%	31.7%
	SF	62.2%	37.8%
	LC	57.1%	42.9%
Combined drug	FC	65/101	64.4%
	SF	57/82	69.5%
	LC	54/126	42.9%
	Total	176/311	57.0%

Combined drug: includes sevelamer and a Ca-containing drug
DM diabetes mellitus, BMI body mass index, HD hemodialysis

mean in the phosphate change rate to adjust for the systematic error in the relatively small number of cases analyzed in this study. To evaluate the effect of phosphate binders on phosphate change rate, we fitted the data to the mixed effect model for adjusted repeated measured analysis. The dependent variable was the phosphate change rate, whereas the fixed effect was a combination of drug, age, gender, and phosphate binders. Patients constituted the random effect. The phosphate change rate was calculated and repeatedly measured in this mixed effect model. The estimated differences of the phosphate change rate between FC versus SF, SF versus LC, and FC versus LC were calculated. All statistical analysis were performed using SAS® 9.3 software.

Results

The total usage dose in the LC group was significantly higher than those in the SF and FC groups (Table 2).

The total phosphate change rates for FC, SF, and LC were 2.9, −10.8, and −3.2% (not adjusted), respectively. The time taken to reach serum ferritin levels ≥300 ng/mL was significantly longer in the SF group. The total dose of the ESA was 387.5 IU, and the SF group significantly showed the lowest ESA value among the three medication groups (Table 2).

The least square means of phosphate change rate and the difference from the baseline of the three drugs are described in Table 3. The total least square means of the phosphate change rates are also provided (see Table 3). Figure 1 shows that the mean serum phosphate level decreased, especially with SF and LC.

Table 3 shows that in the SF group, the phosphate change rate significantly decreased after 11 weeks

described by a decrease of the least square mean. However, the change was not significant except on week 12 for the FC group.

The mixed effect model analysis indicated that there were no significant differences in phosphate change rates in FC versus SF, SF versus LC, and FC versus LC.

Changes in serum phosphate levels in 5 months

Figure 1 shows the mean phosphate level of each phosphate binder with standard error. Phosphate levels decreased in the FC group in the first 3 months but returned to initial levels in the latter half period. In the SF group, phosphate levels decreased significantly from the baseline in each week. In the LC group, phosphate levels were relatively low throughout the observation period. Table 3 provides the least square mean and standard error of the phosphate change rate for the three drugs. There was a reduction from the baseline after 12 weeks in the case of the FC treatment. In the SF group, weeks 6 and 7 increased but week 11 to last decreased significantly. In the LC group, the phosphate change rates decreased significantly across several weeks, but the change rates were relatively smaller than those of FC and SF.

Table 2 Effect of prescription doses of phosphate binders and ESA after 5 months of observation

		Mean	SD	SE	ANOVA	95% CI		Minimum	Maximum
						Lower limit	Upper limit		
Total amount of prescription dose (per 5 months)	FC	142.9	80.2	8.0	*	127.0	158.7	10.5	437.8
	SF	132.1	84.0	9.3	*	113.6	150.5	5.3	399.0
	LC	208.7	89.9	8.0	*	192.8	224.5	35.0	462.0
	Total	166.8	91.9	5.2		156.5	177.1	5.3	462.0
Total prescription dose/starting dose	FC	0.6	0.4	0.0	*	0.6	0.7	0.0	2.0
	SF	1.1	0.7	0.1	*	1.0	1.3	0.0	3.4
	LC	1.8	0.8	0.1	*	1.7	1.9	0.3	4.0
	Total	1.2	0.8	0.0		1.2	1.3	0.0	4.0
Phosphate change rate (%) $[(Pi\_end - Pi\_week\_0) \times 100/Pi\_week\_0]$	FC	2.9	31.5	3.1		−3.4	9.1	−45.1	116.3
	SF	−10.8	22.6	2.5	*	−15.8	−5.9	−54.0	48.8
	LC	−3.2	27.8	2.5		−8.1	1.7	−59.5	152.4
	Total	−3.3	28.3	1.6		−6.4	−0.1	−59.5	152.4
Number of times ferritin ≥300 ng/mL	FC	0.1	0.4	0.0		0.0	0.2	0.0	4.0
	SF	2.3	1.5	0.2	*	1.9	2.6	0.0	5.0
	LC	0.0	0.2	0.0		0.0	0.1	0.0	2.0
	Total	0.6	1.3	0.1		0.5	0.8	0.0	5.0
Total amount of ESA dose (μg) #	FC	440.0	567.6	56.5		327.9	552.0	0.0	3960.0
	SF	265.7	339.2	37.5	*	191.2	340.2	0.0	1880.0
	LC	424.7	445.4	39.7		346.2	503.2	0.0	2640.0
	Total	387.5	469.9	26.7		334.9	440.1	0.0	3960.0

Total amount of ESA dose was calculated using an epoetin:darbepoetin:CERA conversion ratio of 200:1:1
SD standard deviation, SE standard error
*used as indicators for p values

Table 3 Phosphate change rates compared to patient baseline

FC	Estimate %	Standard Error	p	SF	Estimate %	Standard Error	p	LC	Estimate %	Standard Error	p
Total vs BaseLine	−1.10	1.86	0.56	Total vs BaseLine	−3.33	1.48	0.03*	Total vs BaseLine	−5.36	1.76	0.00*
1	3.16	2.78	0.26	1	1.78	2.43	0.46	1	−0.30	2.46	0.90*
2	1.60	2.78	0.57	2	3.78	2.43	0.12	2	−5.63	2.46	0.02*
3	−1.17	2.78	0.67	3	2.50	2.43	0.30	3	−7.37	2.46	0.00
4	1.18	2.78	0.67	4	2.58	2.43	0.29	4	−4.27	2.46	0.08*
5	−2.89	2.78	0.30	5	2.25	2.43	0.35	5	−6.85	2.46	0.01*
6	−4.08	2.78	0.14	6	5.50	2.43	0.02*	6	−6.92	2.46	0.01*
7	−5.21	2.78	0.06	7	5.61	2.43	0.02*	7	−5.39	2.46	0.03
8	−0.48	2.78	0.86	8	1.10	2.43	0.65	8	−4.80	2.46	0.05
9	−2.36	2.78	0.40	9	1.98	2.43	0.41	9	−3.24	2.46	0.19*
10	−3.12	2.78	0.26	10	−1.11	2.43	0.65	10	−8.79	2.46	0.00*
11	−4.59	2.78	0.10	11	−6.89	2.43	0.00*	11	−6.30	2.46	0.01*
12	−6.69	2.78	0.02*	12	−7.04	2.43	0.00*	12	−5.12	2.46	0.04*
13	−1.26	2.78	0.65	13	−9.88	2.43	<.0001*	13	−7.31	2.46	0.00*
14	−3.11	2.78	0.26	14	−12.61	2.43	<.0001*	14	−12.02	2.46	<.0001*
15	−0.95	2.78	0.73	15	−10.24	2.43	<.0001*	15	−9.00	2.46	0.00*
16	−1.11	2.78	0.69	16	−11.48	2.43	<.0001*	16	−5.68	2.46	0.02*
17	0.37	2.78	0.90	17	−7.65	2.43	0.00*	17	−5.56	2.46	0.02
18	−1.91	2.78	0.49	18	−7.61	2.43	0.00*	18	−4.04	2.46	0.10*
19	−1.06	2.78	0.70	19	−10.30	2.43	<.0001*	19	−6.23	2.46	0.01
20	0.63	2.78	0.82	20	−10.35	2.43	<.0001*	20	−4.79	2.46	0.05
21	2.81	2.78	0.31	21	−11.33	2.43	<.0001*	21	−4.35	2.46	0.08

* $p < 0.05$; *SE* standard error

Phosphate change rate per cumulative prescription dose (5 months)

Figure 2 shows the relationship between the cumulative prescription dose of each phosphate binder and the phosphate change rates. The cumulative prescription dose was calculated at each visit by adding the prescription dose from the baseline to the observation visit and dividing by the starting dose of each phosphate binder. The phosphate change rate decreased when the values obtained after dividing the prescription dose by the starting dose increased. The phosphate change rate decreased rapidly, especially in the SF group.

Changes in serum Hb levels in 5 months

Figure 3 presents the changes in mean serum Hb in 5 months for each prescription group. Hb levels increased in the FC and SF groups, but not in the LC group.

Changes in serum ferritin levels in 5 months

Figure 4 presents the mean ferritin change in 5 months for each prescription group. FC and SF were administered in the low and moderate serum ferritin groups, respectively, after which the serum ferritin levels increased in both the groups. Ferritin levels did not increase in the LC group.

Changes in transferrin saturation in 5 months

Figure 5 presents the changes in transferrin saturation (TSAT) in 5 months for the three prescription groups. TSAT increased considerably in the FC group and negligibly in the SF group and remained unchanged in the LC group.

Table 4 shows the effectiveness of FC versus SF, FC versus LC, and SF versus LC treatments. In the mixed effect model analysis, the phosphate-lowering effect adjusted to the fixed and random effects of the phosphate change rate were not significantly different within each group.

Discussion

High serum phosphate levels are associated with higher mortality [2]. After adjustment with nutritional markers, hemodialysis patients with phosphate levels ≥5.6 mg/dL had a higher risk of mortality; this risk was reduced with the use of phosphate binders [2].

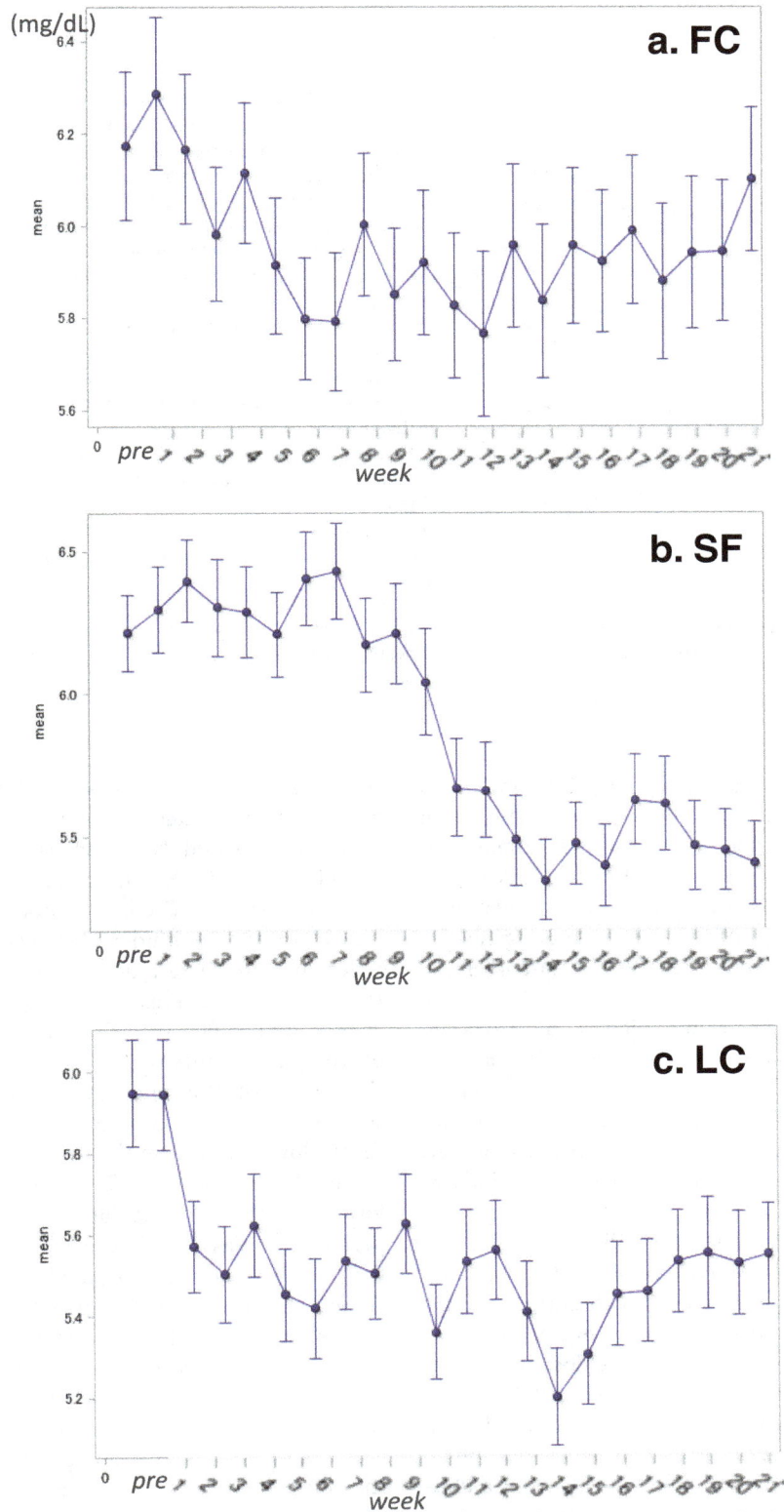

Fig. 1 Changes in serum phosphate levels with phosphate-binder treatment. Mean phosphate levels plus standard error (SE) for the **a** ferric citrate (*FC*) group, **b** sucroferric oxyhydroxide (*SF*) group, and the **c** lanthanum carbonate (*LC*) group

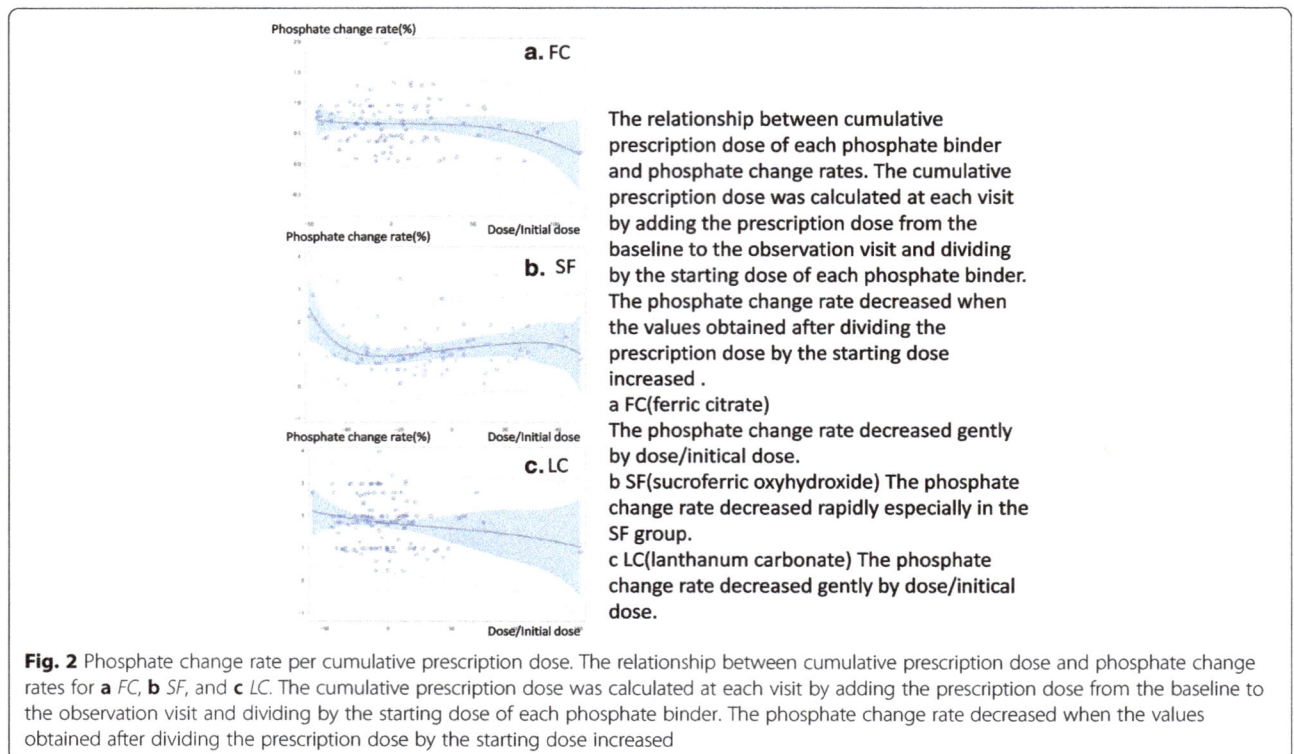

The relationship between cumulative prescription dose of each phosphate binder and phosphate change rates. The cumulative prescription dose was calculated at each visit by adding the prescription dose from the baseline to the observation visit and dividing by the starting dose of each phosphate binder. The phosphate change rate decreased when the values obtained after dividing the prescription dose by the starting dose increased .
a FC(ferric citrate)
The phosphate change rate decreased gently by dose/initical dose.
b SF(sucroferric oxyhydroxide) The phosphate change rate decreased rapidly especially in the SF group.
c LC(lanthanum carbonate) The phosphate change rate decreased gently by dose/initical dose.

Fig. 2 Phosphate change rate per cumulative prescription dose. The relationship between cumulative prescription dose and phosphate change rates for **a** *FC*, **b** *SF*, and **c** *LC*. The cumulative prescription dose was calculated at each visit by adding the prescription dose from the baseline to the observation visit and dividing by the starting dose of each phosphate binder. The phosphate change rate decreased when the values obtained after dividing the prescription dose by the starting dose increased

Based on data from a dialysis cohort, Cannata-Andia et al. [3] reported that the use of phosphate-binding agents was associated with lower mortality. A pronounced HR-lowering effect was observed by sevelamer plus lanthanum treatment compared to those of other drug combinations containing phosphate-binding agents. A meta-analysis indicated that the use of Ca-containing phosphate binders resulted in elevated risk of all-cause mortality and cardiovascular mortality [4, 5]. However, arterial media calcification was observed in patients undergoing hemodialysis who consumed Ca-containing phosphate binders [6]. Randomized controlled trials on sevelamer and lanthanum in Japanese patients indicated identical levels of phosphate-binding efficacy [7]. Isakova et al. also reported that treatment with phosphorus binders independently decreased mortality in patients [8]. Recently, three randomized controlled trials were performed using FC [9–11] on patients with chronic kidney disease [12]. Iida et al. reported that FC prevented vascular calcification in rats and demonstrated the dose-dependent efficacy of FC [13]. Rodby et al. reported that FC treatment reduced hospitalization costs by an estimated 3002 USD per patient per year [14]. Iron-based phosphate binders that are currently used include Velphoro, Ca-containing phosphate binders, Zerenex, FC, Alpharen Fermagate SBR-759, and PT20 [15]. In particular, PA21 was administered to patients undergoing hemodialysis in 2016. A phase III study was performed to compare PA21 with sevelamer [16], and results showed that PA21 had a lower pill burden and better adherence.

We investigated two iron-based phosphate binders, namely FC and SF, and compared their effectiveness with lanthanum (LC), another metal (lanthanum)-based phosphate binder. However, FC and SF have different phosphate-binding mechanisms—FC acts via ionic binding, whereas SF causes polymer adsorption effects. Thus, FC and SF cannot be compared based on their iron content.

Analysis of the phosphate-binding efficiency using the difference of least square mean showed significantly lower values exclusively in week 12 for the FC group. Meanwhile, the SF group showed a significant lowering effect in the latter half of the observation period, whereas LC showed a relatively significant effect throughout the period (Table 4, Fig. 1). We assumed that the reduction in effect of FC in the latter half of the observation period could be caused by unfavorable gastrointestinal symptoms and occurrence of colored feces. Secondly, elevated serum ferritin level (Fig. 4) and increased percentage of TSAT% (Fig. 5) might also reduce the dosage of FC. In contrast, SF showed a relatively weak iron-cumulative effect, especially indicated in TSAT% (Fig. 5), which could result from a carryover of FC to SF in certain cases. In the SF group, serum Hb was maintained in the latter half of the observation period (Fig. 3), ferritin was

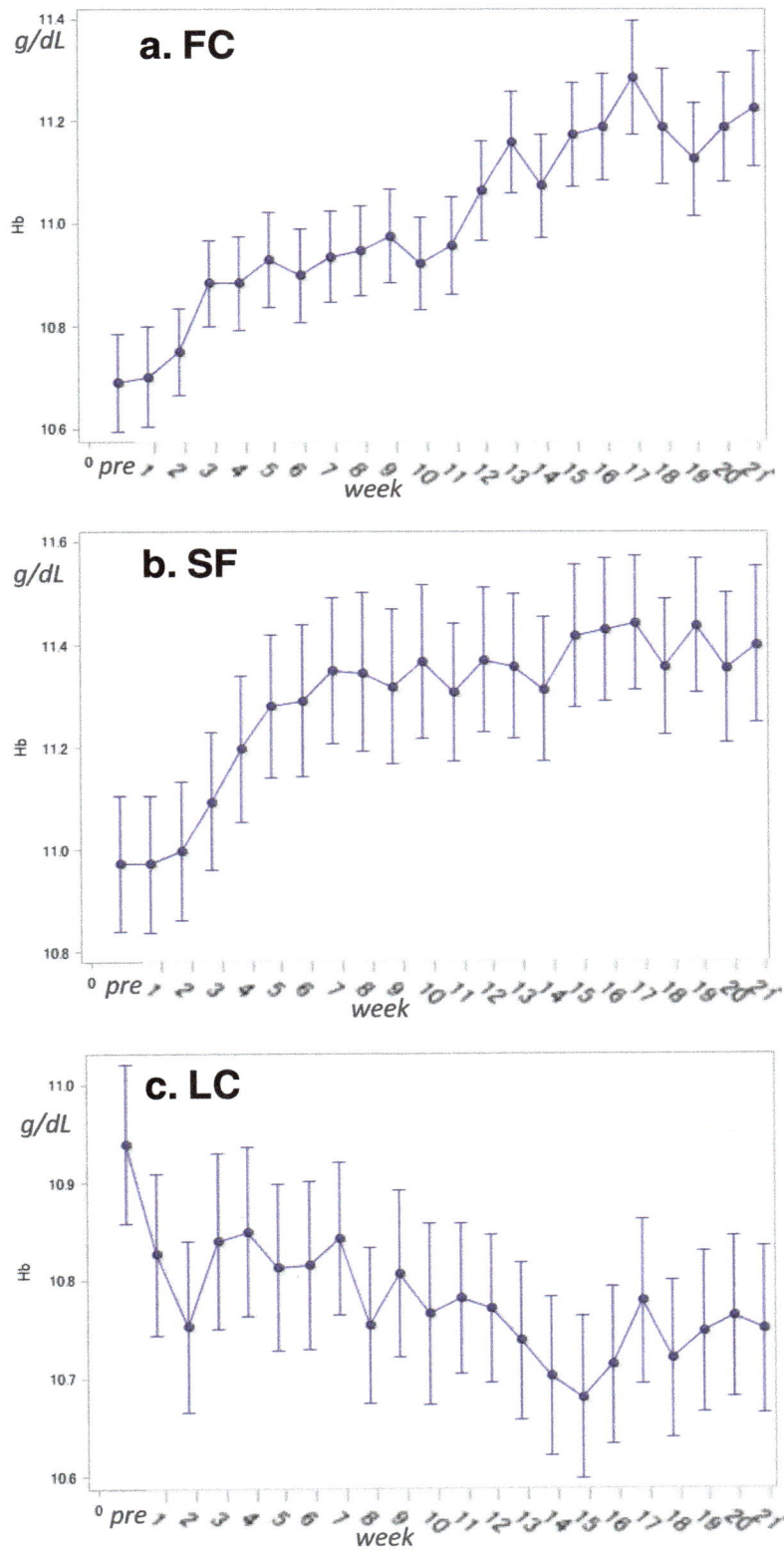

Fig. 3 Changes in serum Hb levels with phosphate-binder treatment. Mean serum hemoglobin (Hb) level plus standard error (SE) for **a** *FC*, **b** *SF*, and **c** *LC*

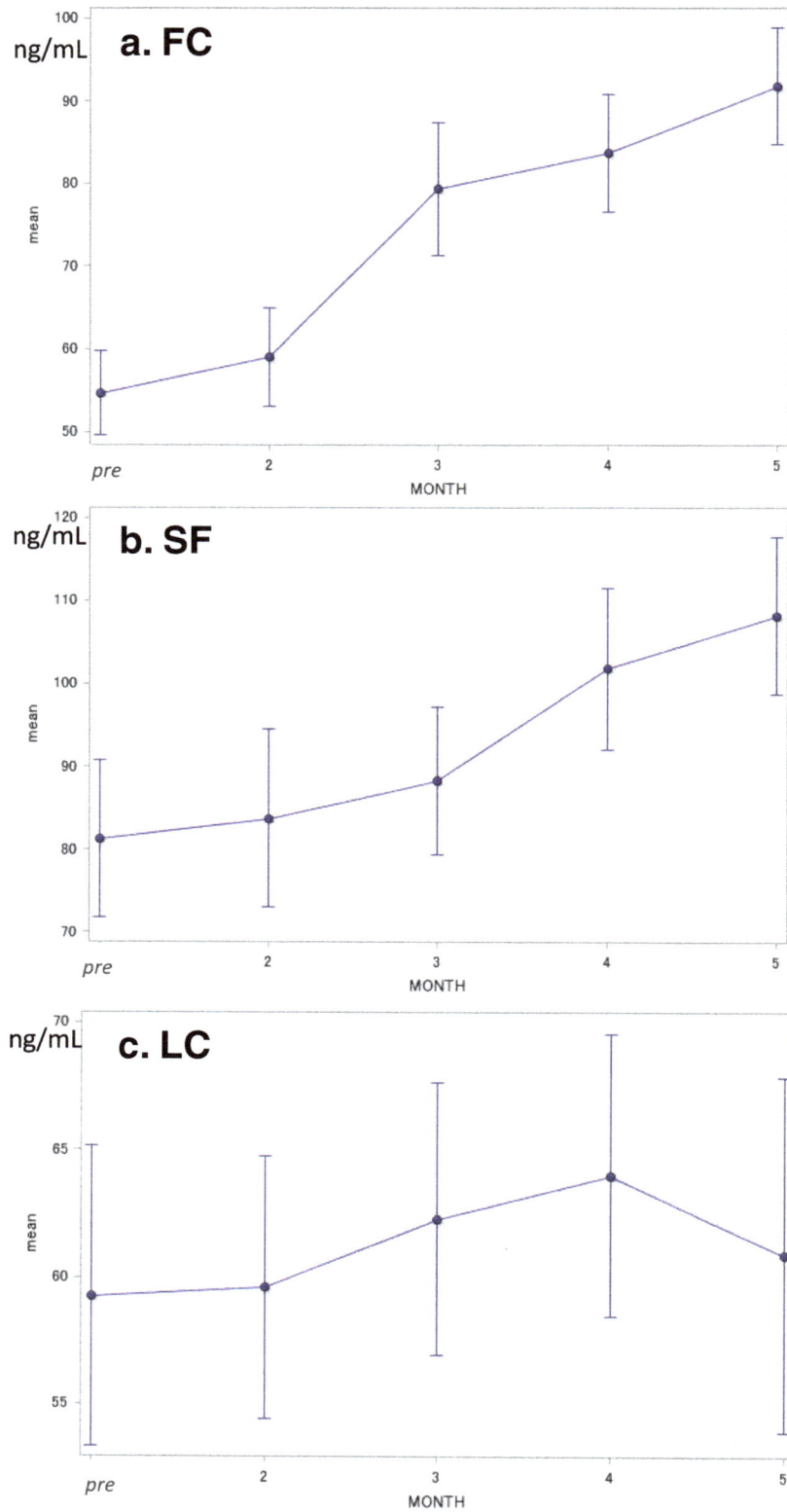

Fig. 4 Changes in ferritin levels with phosphate-binder treatment. Mean serum ferritin (ng/mL) level plus standard error (SE) for **a** *FC*, **b** *SF*, and **c** *LC*

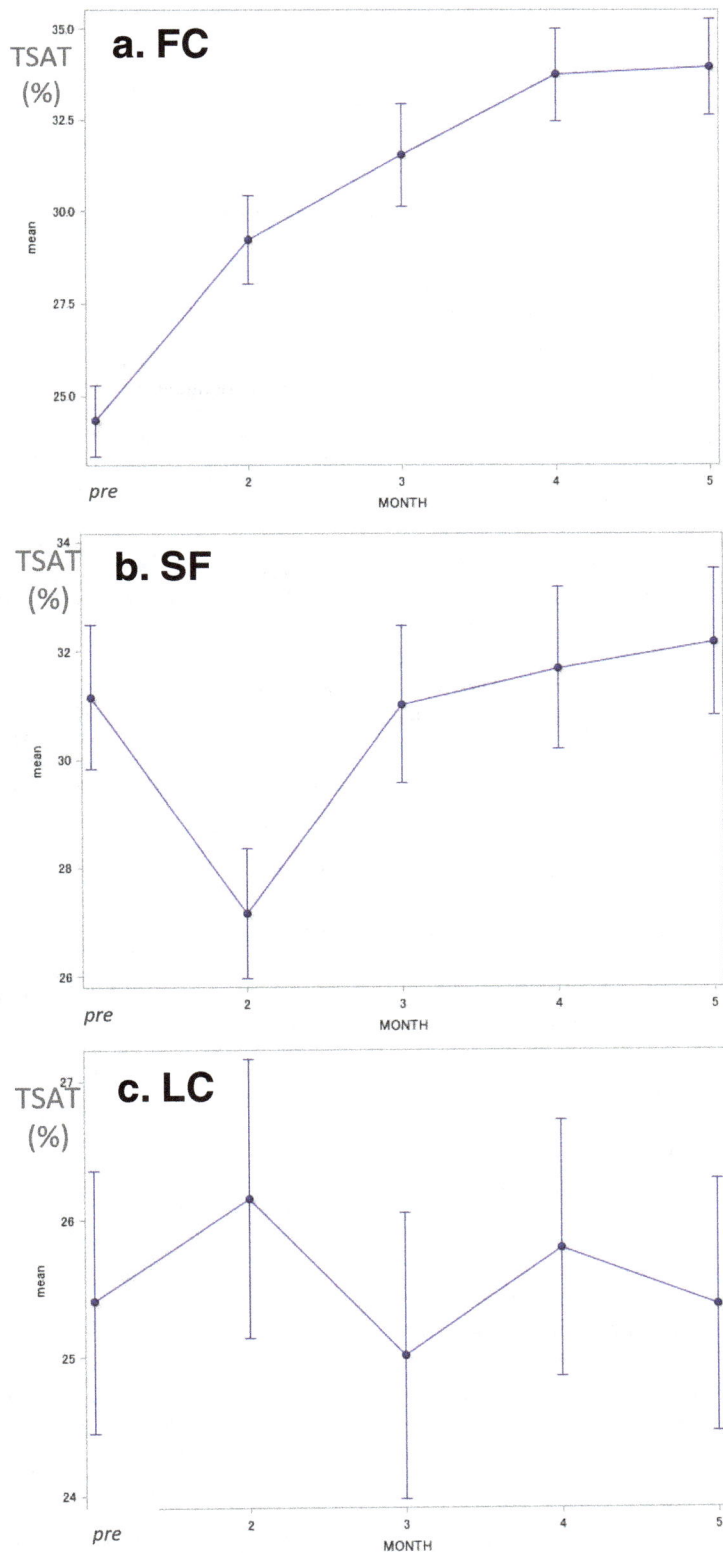

Fig. 5 Change in TSAT percentages with phosphate-binder treatment. Mean transferrin saturation rate (TSAT%) plus standard error (SE) for **a** *FC*, **b** *SF*, and **c** *LC*

Table 4 Mix effect model

| | Result of mixed effect model | | | | | |
	Estimate	Standard error	p	Alfa	Lower Limit	Upper Limit
FC vs SF	−1.0334	1.4716	0.4826	0.05	−3.9187	1.8519
SF vs LC	−1.5953	1.4077	0.2572	0.05	−4.3551	1.1645
FC vs LC	0.6262	1.451	0.6661	0.05	−2.2184	3.4708

Fixed effect was treatment (FC, SF, LC), combined phosphate binder, age or gender. Patients were defined as random effect

elevated from the average level (Fig. 4), and TSAT was slightly increased in the observation period (Fig. 5). The ferritin content of the FC group was ≤60 ng/mL at the baseline (Fig. 4), and therefore, FC might be administrated in cases of iron deficiency anemia. Comparison of the first and last phosphate levels during estimation of the phosphate-binding effect of the three phosphate binders was insufficient because original phosphate levels were regained, which was further confounded with combined drug treatment and other demographic data. To partially avoid these confounders and estimate the repeated measured value, we fitted the date to the mixed effect model [17, 18]. Repeated measured serum phosphate levels were adjusted with combined phosphate binder, age, or gender. Patients were defined as the random effect in the multilevel structure of this mixed effect model. The result of the mixed effect model analysis indicated that SF had relatively strong phosphate-binding effect in these newly developed drugs, but there were no significant differences in the phosphate-binding effect among the three drugs, which might be reflected in the actual medical care response during dialysis therapy.

A limitation of this study is that except for LC, the prescription data of FC and SF were flawed. The LC group was prescribed consistently; however, certain patients in the SF group were prescribed FC before SF. Nevertheless, phosphate change rates and fluctuations and changes of other markers could be evaluated and compared.

Conclusion

Among the newly developed drugs, sucroferric oxyhydroxide exhibited a stronger phosphate-lowering effect than ferric citrate. In addition, ferric citrate showed a stronger iron-cumulative effect than sucroferric oxyhydroxide and thus required adjustment based on iron administration in these iron-based phosphate binders.

Abbreviations
FC: Ferric citrate; LC: Lanthanum carbonate; SF: Sucroferric oxyhydroxide

Acknowledgements
The authors thank all the staff members working at Zenjinkai Clinics and data collecting staff.

Funding
No funding.

Authors' contributions
TI participated in the design of this study, drafted the manuscript, and performed the statistical analysis. YN contributed on data collection. KO kindly reviewed and revised this manuscript. All authors read and approved the final manuscript.

Competing interests
The authors declare that they have no competing interests.

Author details
[1]Internal Medicine, Zenjinkai group, Yokohama Daiichi Hospital, 2-5-15 Takashima Nishi-ku, Yokohama City, Kanagawa 220-0011, Japan. [2]Department of Medical Science and Cardiorenal Medicine, Graduate School of Medicine, Yokohama City University, Yokohama, Kanagawa, Japan. [3]Department of System and Safety, Zenjinkai group, 2-6-32 Takashima Nishi-ku, Yokohama City, Kanagawa, Japan.

References
1. Fukagawa M, Yokoyama K, Koiwa F, Taniguchi M, Shoji T, Kazama JJ, et al. Clinical practice guideline for the management of chronic kidney disease-mineral and bone disorder. Ther Apher Dial. 2013;17:247–88.
2. Lopes AA, Tong L, Thumma J, Li Y, Fuller DS, Morgenstern H, et al. Phosphate binder use and mortality among hemodialysis patients in the Dialysis Outcomes and Practice Patterns Study (DOPPS): evaluation of possible confounding by nutritional status. Am J Kidney Dis. 2012;60:90–101.
3. Cannata-Andia JB, Fernandez-Martin JL, Locatelli F, London G, Gorriz JL, Floege J, et al. Use of phosphate-binding agents is associated with a lower risk of mortality. Kidney Int. 2013;84:998–1008.
4. Jamal SA, Vandermerr B, Raggi P, Mendelssohn DC, Chatterley T, Dorgan M, et al. Effect of calcium-based versus non-calcium-based phosphate binders on mortality in patients with chronic kidney disease: an updated systematic review and meta-analysis. Lancet. 2013;38:1268–77.
5. Jamal SA, Fitchett D, Lok CE, Mendelssohn DC, Tsuyuki RT. The effects of calcium-based versus non-calcium-based phosphate binders on mortality among patients with chronic kidney disease: a meta-analysis. Nephrol Dial Transplant. 2009;24:3168–74.
6. London GM, Guerin AP, Marchais SJ, Metivier F, Pannier B, Adda H. Arterial media calcification in end-stage renal disease: impact on all-cause and cardiovascular mortality. Nephrol Dial Transplant. 2003;18:1731–40.
7. Kasai S, Sato K, Murata Y, Kinoshita Y. Randomized crossover study of the efficacy and safety of sevelamer hydrochloride and lanthanum carbonate in Japanese patients undergoing hemodialysis. Ther Apher Dial. 2012;16:341–9.
8. Isakova T, Gutierrez OM, Chang Y, Shar A, Tamez H, Smith K, et al. Phosphorus binders and survival on hemodialysis. J Am Soc Nephrol. 2009;20:388–96.
9. Yokoyama K, Hirakata H, Akiba T, Sawada K, Kumagai Y. Effect of Rora JTT-751(ferric citrate) on hyperphosphatemia in hemodialysis patients: results of a randomized, double-blind, placebo-controlled trial. Nephrology. 2012;36:478–87.
10. Dwyer JP, Sika M, Schulman G, Chang IJ, Anger M, Smith M, et al. Dose-response and efficacy of ferric citrate to treat hyperphosphatemia in

hemodialysis patients: a short-term randomized trial. Am J Kidney Dis. 2013;61:759–66.

11. Yokoyama K, Akiba T, Fukagawa M, Nakayama M, Sawada K, Kumagai Y, et al. A randomized trial of JTT-751 versus sevelamer hydrochloride in patients on hemodialysis. Am J Nephrol Dial Transplant. 2014;29:1053–60.

12. Block GA, Fishbane S, Rodriguez M, Smits G, Shemesh S, Pergola PE, et al. A 12-week, double-blind, placebo-controlled trial of ferric citrate for the treatment of iron deficiency anemia and reduction of serum phosphate in patients with CKD stages 3-5. Am J Kidney Dis. 2015;65:728–36.

13. Iida A, Kemmochi Y, Kakimoto K, Tanimoto M, Mimura T, Shinozaki Y, et al. Ferric citrate hydrate, a new phosphate binder, prevents the complications of secondary hyperparathyroidism and vascular calcification. Am J Nephrol. 2013;37:346–58.

14. Rodby R, Umanath K, Niecestro R, Jackson JH, Sika M, Lewis JB, et al. Phosphorus binding with ferric citrate is associated with fewer hospitalizations and reduced hospitalization costs. Expert Rev Pharmacoecon Outcomes Res. 2015;15:545–50.

15. Negri AL, Urena-Torres PA. Iron-based phosphate binders: do they offer advantages over currently available phosphate binders? Clin Kidney J. 2015;8:161–7.

16. Floege J, Covic AC, Ketteler M, Mann JFE, Rastogi A, Spinowitz B, et al. Long-term effect of the iron-based phosphate binder, sucroferric oxyhydroxide, in dialysis patients. Nephrol Dial Transplant. 2015;30:1037–46.

17. Laird NM, Ware JH. Random-effects models for longitudinal data. Biometrics. 1982;38:963–74.

18. Breslow NE, Clayton DG. Approximate inference in generalized linear mixed models. JASA. 1993;88:9–25.

8

Microparticles in kidney diseases: focus on kidney transplantation

Fateme Shamekhi Amiri

Abstract

Background: Microparticles are small (0.1–1 μm), extracellular vesicles that are used as diagnostic and prognostics markers of kidney diseases and kidney transplantation. They contain cytoplasm and surface markers of their cells of origin. The aim of this review is to describe the functional capabilities of microparticles in kidney diseases with focus on kidney transplantion.

Main body: Microparticles represent a novel and potentially important method of cell–cell communication, regulating a number of physiological/pathophysiological processes. Increased levels of circulating microparticles, mainly originating from platelets and endothelial cells, have been proposed as causing vascular and endothelial dysfunction in renal diseases. Furthermore, higher levels of endothelial MPs that are observed in hemodialyzed patients reached to normal values after graft. Circulating microparticles have been used in kidney rejection and transplant vasculopathy. The genetic content of circulating microvesicles may have great use for diagnostic and prognostic purposes after organ transplantation.

Conclusion: Microparticles may be a novel marker for creation and diagnosis of different diseases in kidney diseases especially kidney transplantion that imply for further research.

Keywords: Cardiovascular disease, Circulating endothelial cells, Kidney diseases, Kidney transplantion, Microparticles

Background

Intercellular communication is vital for the regulation and coordination of many different processes within multicellular organisms. Extracellular membrane-bound vesicles are emerging as a novel and significant mechanism of cell signaling and communication [1]. Extracellular vesicles are a heteregenous population of particles released from various cell types into the extracellular spaces under both normal and stressed condition. Research on extracellular vesicles (EVs) is not only focused on their potential role as source of biomarkers but also as new therapeutic tools. In the context of acute kidney injury (AKI), only a few studies have tested different sources of EVs for their therapeutic potential. The microRNA (miRNA) content of these vesicles seems to have a positive effect in tubular cells, reducing apoptosis and promoting cell proliferation. Ischemia-reperfusion is characterized by the overexpression of the adhesion molecule of monocyte chemoattractant

protein-1(MCP-1). During this process, transcriptional repressor activating transcription factor 3 (ATF3), which has an anti-apoptotic and anti-inflammatory effect, is induced.

This paper has written based on searching PubMed and Google Scholar to identify potentially relevant articles or abstracts. The mentioned search included the following search terms: Microparticles, microparticles in renal transplantation, and microparticles in kidney transplantation. Search terms were used both discretely and combined with each other using the Boolean operator AND. The author reviewed the bibliographies of all selected articles to identify additional relevant studies. The search retrieved 308 articles; after evaluating the abstracts, 184 articles were excluded. The manuscripts of the remaining 124 articles were completely read and, of these, 109 were excluded due to unrelated subject to kidney transplantation and non-original investigation. Finally, 15 original studies were included in this review (Fig. 1). The aim of this review is to describe the functional capabilities of microparticles in kidney transplantation. In this regard, at first, microparticles and the methods of measuring of these biomarkers and

Correspondence: fa.shamekhi@gmail.com
Division of Nephrology, Imam Khomeini Hospital, Faculty of Medicine, Tehran University of Medical Sciences, Tehran, Iran

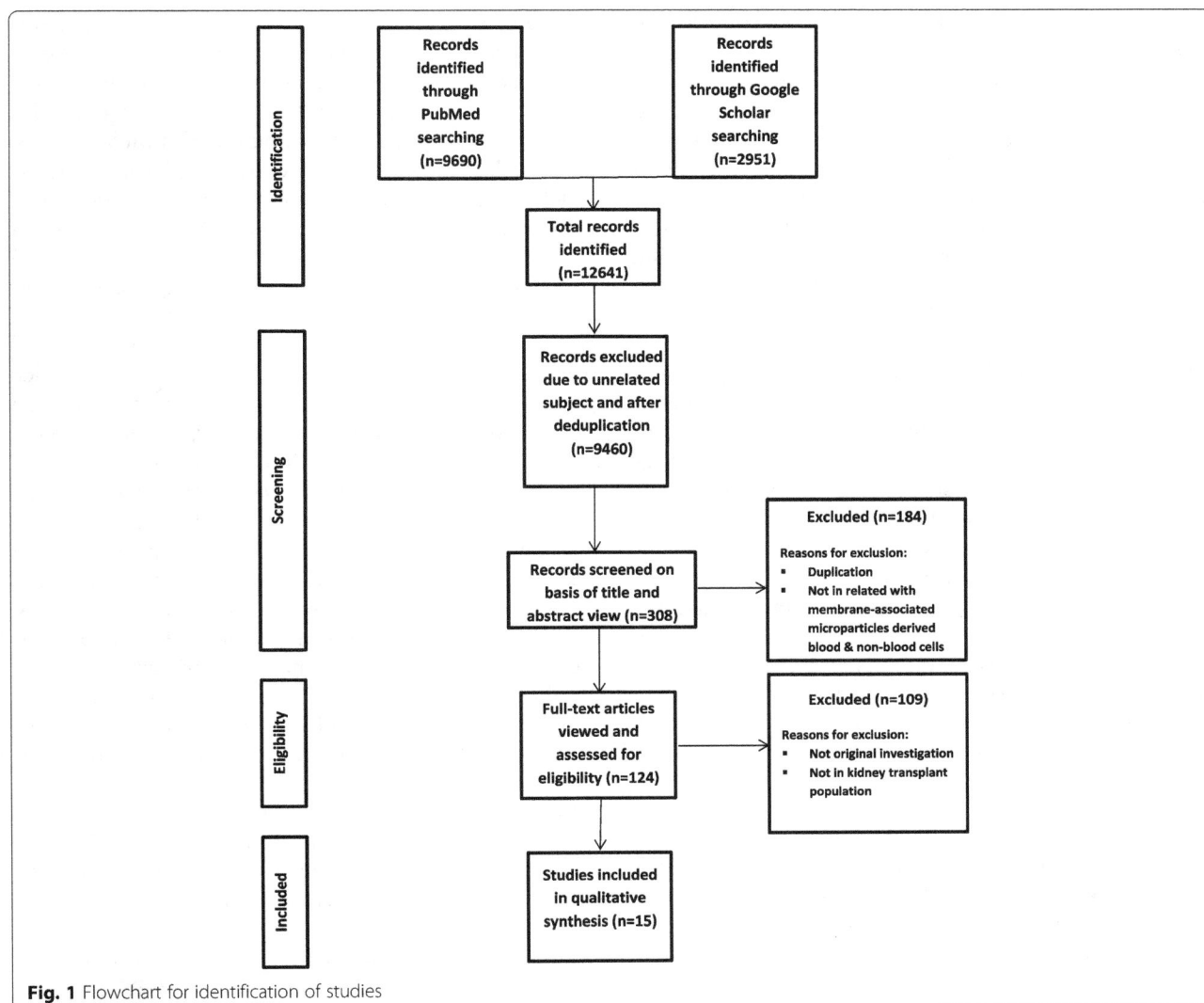

Fig. 1 Flowchart for identification of studies

then pathophysiological processes of kidney diseases relating with microparticles are discussed, briefly. Finally, the discussion is focused on deleterious effects that are caused by microparticles in kidney transplantation.

Microparticles

Extracellular vesicles are divided into three categories—exosomes, apoptotic bodies, and microparticles or microvesicles—on the basis of their size, content, and mechanism of formation [2]. Less common terms for extracellular vesicles, such as exosome-like vesicles (implying 20–50-nm particles similar to exososomes but lacking lipid-rich domains) and membrane particles (which refer to 50–100 nm) membrane fragments enriched in CD133/prominin-1, are more poorly defined and infrequently used [3]. Among the various types of extracellular vesicles formed, membrane microparticles (also referred to as

ectosomes or more broadly, microvesicles) are emerging as both indices of vascular injury and as circulating biologically active entities. Cells in human blood generate a variety of membrane microparticles (MPs), and determination of the cellular origin of MP relies on the expression of specific antigens. First identified by wolf in 1967, MPs (shedding vesicles) are cell plasma membrane-derived small vesicles which are 0.1–1 μm in diameter. MPs are generated from a variety of different vascular cell types, including endothelial cells, monocytes, platelets, red blood cells, and granulocytes. Early studies on MPs focused on platelets because these cells readily generated MPs on activation. Indeed, the original term for MPs was "platelet dust" and platelets are the major source of MPs in the blood of healthy individuals [4]. When stimulated by various environmental factors including serine proteases, inflammatory cytokines, growth factors, and stress inducers, nearly all kinds of mammalian cells can generate MPs [5]. Most studies have shown that microparticles are heterogeneous and vary in phospholipids, surface antigens, and protein contents. MP release is a controlled process triggered by various stimuli including pro-apoptotic stimulation, shear stress, agonists, or damage [6]. By general consensus, MPs are small in size, expose the anionic phospholipid (PL) phosphatidylserine (PS) on the outer leaflet of their membrane, and bear surface membrane antigens reflecting their cell of origin [7]. Believed to be formed by all cell types, MP formation has been observed in cells of the vasculature (endothelial cells, platelets, leukocytes and vascular smooth muscle cells, erythrocytes) and podocytes, as well as cancer and progenitor cell populations (Fig. 2). MPs may be distinguished from other common extracellular vesicles (such as exososomes or apoptotic bodies) on the basis of size, mechanism of formation, and content. Exososomes are smaller (approximately 40–100 nm) than MPs and are formed through a multi-step process [8]. Apoptotic bodies are much larger than exosomes or MPs with a size of 1–5 µm. They are formed exclusively during the late stages of apoptosis during cell shrinkage/collapse and after externalization of phosphatidylserine, increases in membrane permeability, and karyorrhexis (nuclear fragmentation).

MPs composition, formation, and release

In multicellular organisms, homeostasis results from a subtle balance between cell proliferation and degenerescence. Cells differentiate, expand, fulfill particular functions, then undergo programmed death, and are finally cleared by phagocytosis. At each stage of its life, the cell is subjected to a variety of stimulations leading to the

release of submicron fragments from the plasma membrane, usually termed microparticles or microvesicles. MPs hijack membrane constituents and cytoplasmic content and survive the cell. Membrane microparticles are shed from the plasma membrane of stimulated cells. They harbor membrane and carry cytoplasmic proteins as well as bioactive lipids implicated in a variety of fundamental processes. This representation does not intend to be exhaustive with respect to the different hijacked components [9]. MPs contain a wide range of biomolecules: proteins (signal proteins and receptors, cytoskeleton, and effector proteins), lipids, and nucleic acids (e.g., microRNA, mRNA, and even DNA). MP surface protein content may be different from that of the plasma. Membrane of the original cell, as the incorporation of protein molecules into MPs, can be selective and modulated by agonist activators and/or microenvironments of the parental cells. Depending on the stimulus, the protein content of MPs derived from the same cell lineage can vary [10]. Although the precise molecular determinants of MP are unknown, mechanisms of plasma membrane remodeling cause MP formation including cytoskeletal reorganization and externalization of phosphatidylserine (PS). Furthermore, lipid-rich microdomains including lipid rafts and caveolae have also been implicated in the formation of endothelial, monocyte, and platelet MPs.

In PS externalization (loss of membrane phospholipid asymmetry), under resting conditions, phospholipids are asymmetrically distributed in the membrane of eukaryotic cells. The outer leaflet is enriched in phosphatidylcholine and sphingomyelin, whereas the inner leaflet contains the aminophospholipids PS and phosphatidylethanolamine. The appearance of PS or phosphatidylethanolamine on the outer leaflet results in a back-transportation to the inner leaflet by an aminophospholipid translocase with "flippase" activity that maintains the normal resting phospholipid distribution. Because uncatalyzed transbilayer transport is slow, lipid asymmetry is stable in quiescent cells. This distribution is controlled by three proteins, namely a flippase (governing their inward translocation), a floppase (governing their outward translocation), and a lipid scramblase. The phospholipid transient mass imbalance between the two leaflets due to membrane randomization and the proteolysis of the cytoskeleton promoted by calcium-activated calpains promote the shedding of MPs. Importantly, PS exposure appears to be a nearly universal feature of cells undergoing activation or apoptosis and a common underlying feature of MP release by these cells [11].

In cytoskeletal reorganization, cytoskeleton integrity is believed to participate in the maintenance of membrane asymmetry and cell shape, its reorganization could

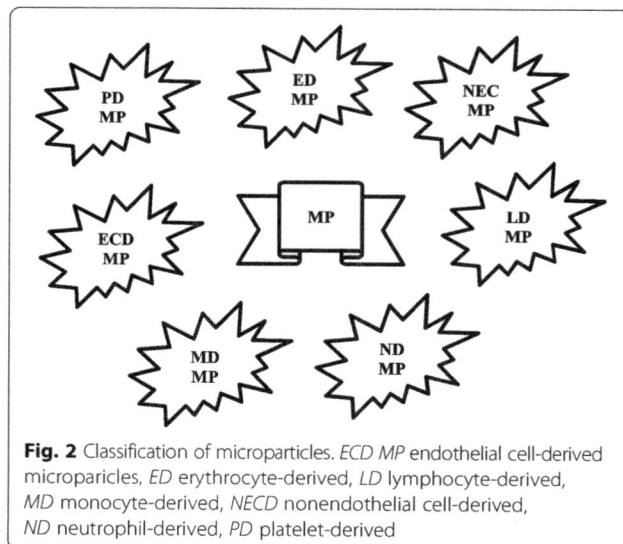

Fig. 2 Classification of microparticles. *ECD MP* endothelial cell-derived microparicles, *ED* erythrocyte-derived, *LD* lymphocyte-derived, *MD* monocyte-derived, *NECD* nonendothelial cell-derived, *ND* neutrophil-derived, *PD* platelet-derived

therefore favor membrane budding in stimulated cells. Unlike agonist-induced MP generation, this mechanism does not require either Ca^{2+} elevation or the activity of calpain, a Ca^{2+}-dependent thiol protease known to modify platelet cytoskeleton and some signal transduction enzymes. Although baseline calpain activity seems insufficient to degrade cytoskeleton components, agonist-induced Ca^{2+} influx is necessary to reach Ca^{2+} concentrations sufficiently high to induce maximum protease activity. Calpains have been known for more than a decade to play a crucial role in platelet shedding. Caspases are cytoplasm proteases from the apoptotic cascade involved in the reorganization of the cytoskeleton, possibly related to either membrane remodeling or cell differentiation. Caspases or calpain is responsible for the proteolytic cleavage of prominent cytoskeletal proteins such as filamin-1 (a marker of megakaryocyte derived MPs), gelosin, talin, and myosin. In the Jurkat T lymphocyte cell line, caspase-3 mediates the cleavage of Rho-associated coiled-coil containing protein kinases (ROCK I), a Rho-kinase acting by myosin light chain phosphorylation that induces cell membrane contraction and MP release during apoptosis. ROCK-I, the Rho-kinase isoform that is activated by caspase-3, was not modulated by thrombin. A group of genes are linked to the cytoskeleton reorganization and involved in MP release from endothelial cells. Of these, the Rho-kinase ROCK-II activated by caspase-$_2$ showed a high transcription rate [12–14].

The current knowledge on MP formation derives mainly from experiments on isolated or cultured cells showing that both cell activation and cell apoptosis can lead to MP release. However, in vivo mechanisms involved in MP formation and shedding remain mostly unknown. MPs are released from cell membranes by triggers such as cytokines, thrombin, endotoxins, hypoxia, and shear stress, capable of inducing activation or apoptosis. Phosphatidylserine exposure is not always followed by the release of MPs, which may be regulated by the level of intracellular calcium. Moreover, MP shedding necessitates modifications in cell structural architecture involving disruption of cytoskeleton protein organization. In platelets, MP release seems to be controlled by calcium-dependent activation of calpain, a cytosolic cysteine protease involved in rearrangement of cytoskeleton proteins and protein cleavage to activate various receptors and proenzymes. Platelets release MPs after activation by thrombin, adenosine diphosphate (ADP) plus collagen, the complement complex C5b-9, the calcium ionophore A23187, and by high shear stress. Endothelial cells, monocytes, vascular smooth muscle cells, and hepatocytes can also release MPs after activation by bacterial lipopolysaccharides, inflammatory cytokines including tumor necrosis factor or interleukin-1,

the complement complex C5b-9, aggregated low density lipoproteins, or reactive oxygen species. Increase in intracellular calcium, most likely at the site of membrane vesicle formation, seems to be a critical step for MP release, but the role of cytoskeleton is not yet fully elucidated. In apoptosis-induced MP release, apoptosis is characterized by cell contraction and DNA fragmentation. Blebbing of the cellular membrane occurs rapidly after cells enter the apoptotic process. Bleb formation depends on actin cytoskeleton and actin–myosin contraction, which is regulated by caspase 3-induced Rho-kinase I activation. Rho-kinase activation is required for relocalization of DNA fragments from the nuclear region to membrane blebs, suggesting that MPs from apoptotic cells may contain nuclear material. Interestingly, statins inhibit MP release from cultured endothelial cells by altering the Rho-kinase pathway [15]. Distler et al. in a study determined the effects of microparticles released from Jurkat T cells on RAW 264.7 cells for elucidating the interactions of microparticles with macrophages. Microparticles were isolated by differential centrifugation, using FACS analysis with annexin V and cell surface markers for identification. Various inducers of apoptosis increased the release of microparticles from Jurkat cells up to 5-fold. Furthermore, microparticles stimulated the release of microparticles from macrophages. These findings indicate that microparticles can induce macrophages to undergo apoptosis [16].

Stimuli for MP production

Membrane vesiculation occurs in vivo as a result of various stimuli and signaling mechanisms [17]. A number of cell activation and apoptosis triggers which induce MP formation have been identified including chemical stimuli such as cytokines, thrombin, and endotoxin or physical stimuli such as shear stress or hypoxia. In particular, high shear stress can initiate both platelet aggregation and shedding of procoagulant-containing platelet-derived microparticles (PDMPs) [18]. Higher shear stress-induced activation of platelets and the addition of platelet microparticles (PMPs) may also enhance the expression of cell adhesion of molecules and the production of the cytokines in the human monocytic leukemia cell line (THP-1) and ECs. Platelets release MPs after activation by thrombin, ADP plus collagen, the complement complex C5b-9, the calcium ionophore A23187, and by high shear stress. Endothelial cells, monocytes, vascular smooth muscle cells, and hepatocytes can also release MPs after activation by bacterial lipopolysaccharides, inflammatory cytokines including tumor necrosis factor or interleukin-1, the complement complex C5b-9, aggregated low density lipoproteins, or reactive oxygen species [19] (Fig. 3).

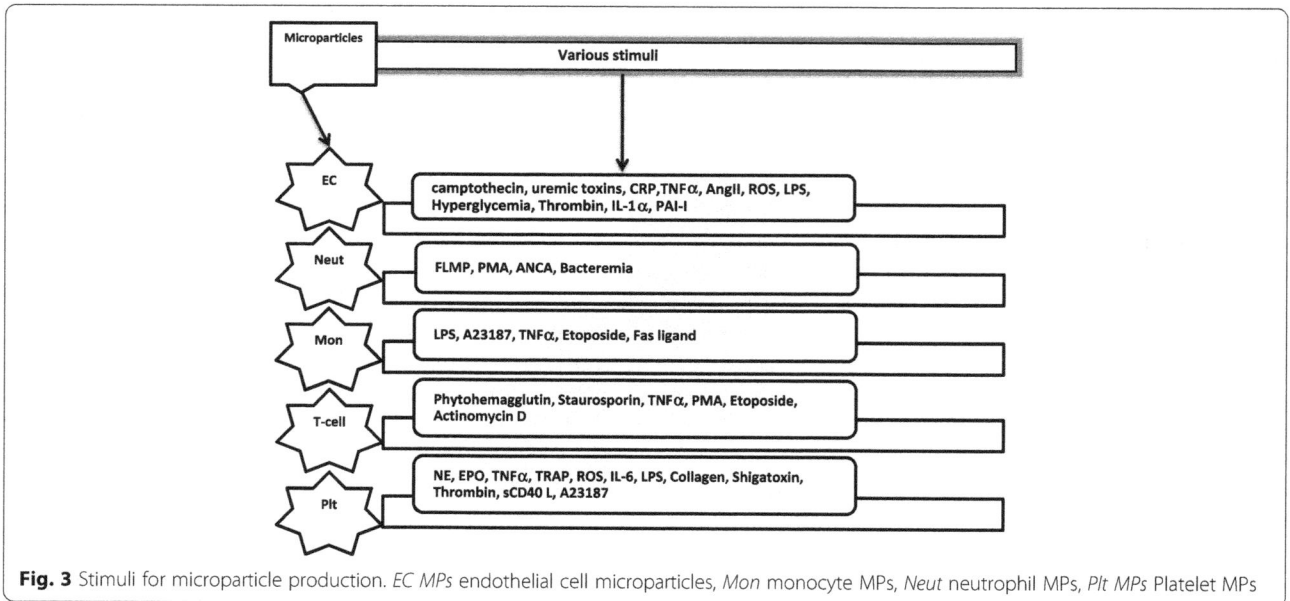

Fig. 3 Stimuli for microparticle production. *EC MPs* endothelial cell microparticles, *Mon* monocyte MPs, *Neut* neutrophil MPs, *Plt MPs* Platelet MPs

MP elimination

Cells become susceptible to complement-induced lysis when they lose key complement inhibitors such as CD46, CD55, and CD59. These inhibitors are sorted to microparticles and exosomes, most likely to prevent complement deposition and lysis of these vesicles, thereby increasing their chance of survival in the extracellular environment. Although exosomes can be internalized via phagocytosis by binding to the PS receptor T cell immunoglobulin and mucin-domain containing molecule (TIM-4), the extent to which exosomes and microvesicles expose PS in vivo remains unclear. Phagocytosis of PS-exposing cells and microparticles may be mediated by lactadherin, because lactadherin knockout mice have an increased concentration of (platelet-derived) microparticles, and splenic macrophages from these mice show a decreased capacity to phagocytose these microparticles, resulting in a hypercoagulable state. In most other studies, however, relatively fast (10–30 min) but also much slower (5–6 h) half-life times of vesicle disappearance were reported. The clearance of vesicles will undoubtedly depend on the organism studied, the clinical conditions, and whether artificial phospholipid vesicles or cell-derived vesicles were studied [3]. Clearance of MPs occurs through several main mechanisms. The major one is degradation due to the action of phospholipases and proteases. Other potential routes of MP clearance include opsonization with subsequent phagocytosis, uptake of MPs from the circulation by liver Kupffer cells in a PS-dependent manner, phagocytosis of MPs by splenocytes, and uptake of MPs by the lung macrophages [13, 20]. Jurkat T cell-derived apoptotic MPs have been shown to be engulfed by macrophages in vitro [16]. Moreover, study by Litvack et al. revealed that natural IgM is an important antibody to clear microbes and other bioparticles, and that shape is critical to particle uptake by macrophages as such there is an inverse relationship between IgM-mediated clearance by macrophages and the particle size [21].

MP measurement

The majority of studies investigate isolated-MPs from plasma samples, which typically contain endothelial-, leukocyte-, platelet- and erythrocyte-derived MPs. Under pathological conditions, MPs derived from non-circulating cells, for example, vascular smooth muscle cells or fibroblasts, might also be detectable, although there is a dearth of knowledge in this area. The main methods of MP detection include flow cytometry, enzyme-linked immunoassays, and functional coagulative assays. A recently developed new method for the detection of plasma MPs using a fluorescence-based antibody array system can rapidly identify the cell origin of MPs. MP counting, as currently performed by flow cytometry, certainly needs to be standardized [22]. Both methods of MP analysis rely on antibody detection of specific cellular markers and annexin V binding of phosphatidylserine. In addition to the above techniques, the antigenic characteristics and the membrane composition of blood MPs have been studied using electron microscopy, confocal microscopy, high performance liquid chromatography, capillary electrophoresis, and mass spectrometry with varying degrees of success [7]. Other methods include western blotting, flow imaging cytometry, and nanoparticle tracking analysis [1, 7, 9, 23]

(Table 1). Additionally, MPs of varying origins may be found in urine [24–29], bronchoalveolar lavage fluid [30], sputum [31], synovial fluid [32], ascites [33], and saliva [34]. There is presently no reliable approach for obtaining and/or characterizing MPs from tissue samples, and knowledge of MP biology in tissue is lacking.

Pathophysiological processes induced by MPs in kidney diseases

Increased levels of circulating microparticles, mainly originating from platelets and endothelial cells, have been proposed as causing vascular and endothelial dysfunction in renal diseases. Neutrophil MPs carry a large set of cell adhesion molecules and proteases such as proteinase 3 or elastase. During chronic renal failure progression, pro-inflammatory cytokines are increased and inflammation could explain in part the decline of renal function because of accerelated atherosclerosis. During acute vascular lesions such as wegener granulomatosis or micro-polyangitis, PMP and NMP are increased. Elevation of endothelial microparticles (EMP) has also been reported in antiphospholipid syndrome and uremic patients in the absence of a clinical history of vascular disease. High platelet MP levels are observed in micro-angiopathies and chronic renal failure patients (pre-dialyzed, under hemodialysis, and under continuous ambulatory peritoneal dialysis). In patients with ESRD, platelet, erythrocyte, and endothelial MPs are increased. EMP levels correlate with a loss of flow-mediated dilatation and increased aortic pulse wave velocity, suggesting that they are highly associated with arterial and endothelial dysfunction. A dramatic increase in PMP is observed at the end of dialysis session. This is probably due to membrane-induced complement activation and biological effects of extracorporeal dialyzers. Endotoxins of the dialysate fluid are another cause of MP release. MPs behave as effectors that play a deleterious role in renal diseases. They also represent novel biomarker that are useful to appreciate cardiovascular risk associated with chronic kidney disease and sometimes disease activity. In the following, pathophysiological processes induced by MPs in different renal diseases are discussed here.

MP in intercellular communication

There are many known ways in which cells communicate and exchange information. Cytokines, interleukins, growth factors, chemokines, and additional small molecules provide one mechanism for cell–cell interaction. Furthermore, via specialized adhesion molecules and nanotubules, cells are capable of connecting and exchanging information. Recently, the armamentarium was extended to MP which was identified as a valuable transport and information tool. At present, there is evidence that MPs use various mechanisms to transfer information. First, MPs function as signaling molecule; second, they are enabled to transfer entire receptors; third, MPs shift mRNA and proteins, and fourth, they are even capable of transporting whole cell organelles [35]. MPs may stimulate target cells directly by surface ligands. They are equipped with different signaling proteins and lipids on their surface. MPs are carrying

Table 1 Different methods for MPs measurement

Assay	Method	Advantages	Disadvantages
■ Flow cytometry ■ (fluorescence-activated cell sorting) ✓ MP counting	■ Utilization of fluorescence probes and light-scattering properties ■ MPs in suspension	■ Available to most research facilities ■ Rapid ■ Multiple antigens may be analyzed in a single sample ■ MPs analyzed on an individual basis ■ The gold standard of human cell-derived MPs	■ Antibody binding might not occur attributable to the small fraction of surface antigens available ■ Size limitations and not able to detect microvesicles with diameters less than 300–400 nm
■ Immunoassays	■ ELISA-based MP capture assays by annexin V as a means of capturing phospholipids or antibodies to specific blood MP membrane antigens or antibodies to nonspecific antigens (detection antibody)	■ Available at most research institutions ■ Alternative to flow cytometry approach ■ Less costly than flow cytometry ■ Not restricted by size	■ Analysis done in batches ■ No size determination possible ■ Quantifies based on a single antigen
■ Functional assays	■ Procoagulant or prothrombinase activity	■ Available at most research institutions ■ Provides an indication of biological activity	■ The inability to quantitate the MPs ■ Analysis done in batches, no size determination possible, measures procoagulant activity—not specific MP detection
■ Atomic force microscopy	■ Scanning of MPs utilizing specialized microscope	■ MP size detection very accurate ■ Allows for 3D structure of MP ■ Quantitation of MPs	■ Allows for very accurate sizing of MPs ■ Allows for 3D view of MP structure ■ May be used for quantification
■ Nanoparticle tracking	■ Light-scattering properties of MPs detected, video capture of MP motion	■ MP size detection, quantitation of MPs	■ Technology not readily available, long analysis times, costly

Elisa enzyme-linked immunosorbant assay, *MPs* microparticles

certain proteins like hedgehog proteins stemming from lymphocytes. They are also able to direct the differentiation of early hematopoietic cells towards a megakaryocytic differentiation. Platelet-derived MPs exert different surface molecules allowing attachment on endothelial cells. Proteins like CD41 (αII/βIII-integrins) and CD62P (P-selectin) as well as bioactive lipids like arachidonic acid and sphingosine-1-phosphate are involved in these various biological processes mediated by platelet-derived MP. It has been reported that MPs activate endothelial cells, polymorphonuclear leukocytes, and monocytes. Additionally, they may also induce apoptosis in leukocytes and promote secretion of cytokines and tissue factor expression in endothelial cells. MP represents a novel mechanism of intercellular communication mediating inflammation, immunity, and blood coagulation. Their effect on target cells was long accredited to their specific lipid composition, as well as to intravesicular chemokines. However, recent data indicate that MP can also affect protein expression of their target cells by delivering RNAs [36].

A prospective study by Bitzer et al. evaluated the protective effect to miR-126 and miR-296, which are detected in the microvesicles by real-time polymerase chain reaction (RT-PCR). MiR-126 and many of its targets are highly expressed in endothelial cells, and both miR-126 and miR-296 have been implicated in angiogenesis [37]. There are several potential ways for microparticles to interact with target cells: binding to the cell surface, fusion with the plasma membrane, and endocytic uptake and recycling to the membrane. In the immunoelectron microscopy of cell surface CD81, researchers observed that endocytosed gold particles were occasionally associated with small vesicles. This indicates endocytic uptake of CD81-positive microparticles and potential recycling to the membrane of target cells. It also shows that donor cells themselves are not resistant to binding and uptake of CD81-positive vesicles. CD81 on microparticles might therefore affect cells in an autocrine and paracrine way [38].

MP in blood coagulation and angiogenesis

With respect to activated platelets, circulating MPs provide an additional procoagulant phospholipid surface for the assembly of the characteristic enzyme complexes of the blood coagulation cascade. Their catalytic properties rely on a procoagulant anionic aminophospholipid, PhtdSer, translocated to the exoplasmic leaflet after membrane remodeling. Once accessible to circulating blood factors, PhtdSer enables local concentrations necessary to achieve the kinetics requisites for optimal thrombin generation and efficient hemostasis. Indeed, shielding PhtdSer-rich surfaces decreases the catalytic efficiency of both tenase and prothrombinase complexes

by 200- and 1000-fold respectively. Additionally, PhtdSer considerably enhances the procoagulant activity of tissue factor (TF), the main cellular initiator of blood coagulation. Apoptosis and vascular cell activation are main contributors to the release of procoagulant microparticles (MPs), deleterious partners in atherothrombosis. Elevated levels of circulating platelet, monocyte, or endothelial-derived MPs are associated with most of the cardiovascular risk factors and appear indicative of poor clinical outcome. In addition to being a valuable hallmark of vascular cell damage, MPs are at the crossroad of atherothrombosis processes by exerting direct effects on vascular or blood cells. Under pathological circumstances, circulating MPs would support cellular cross-talk leading to vascular inflammation and tissue remodeling, endothelial dysfunction, leukocyte adhesion, and stimulation. Exposed membrane phosphatidylserine and functional TF are two procoagulant entities conveyed by circulating MPs. At sites of vascular injury, P-selectin exposure by activated endothelial cells or platelets leads to the rapid recruitment of MPs bearing the P-selectin glycoprotein ligand-1 and blood-borne TF, thereby triggering coagulation. Within the atherosclerotic plaque, sequestered MPs constitute the main reservoir of TF activity, promoting coagulation after plaque erosion or rupture. Lesion-bound MPs, eventually harboring proteolytic and angiogenic effectors, are additional actors in plaque vulnerability [8]. Among the non-cell-bound TF present in blood, a variant form that results from alternative splicing of the primary RNA transcript was identified: alternatively spliced TF (asTF). asTF is soluble, circulates in plasma, and is biologically active. During thrombus formation, platelet deposition may separate catalytic enzyme complexes from circulating blood. Binding of asTF as well as TF-bearing monocyte-derived MPs to platelets provides a rationale for thrombus formation and growing [12, 39]. Elevated numbers of MPs have been reported in a variety of diseases, including patients with acute coronary syndromes, cancer, antiphospholipid antibody syndrome, sickle cell disease, sepsis, and diabetes. Although all MPs are procoagulant, those with the highest procoagulant activity are MPs derived from activated monocytes because of the presence of tissue factor. This transmembrane receptor is a potent activator of the coagulation cascade [4]. The procoagulant activity of MPs can be quantified using the thrombin generation test. In this system, MPs supply the procoagulant surface, while TF and plasma provide the necessary coagulation factors. By adding calcium ions, coagulation factors bind to MPs to initiate coagulation. In this assay, the generation of thrombin is dependent on the presence and activity of MPs, and in their absence, no coagulation would occur

[18]. MPs were shown to induce angiogenesis, in vitro and in vivo.

The controversial effects and the importance of direct stimulation of endothelial cells by MP was shown using MP generated from activated T cells harboring the morphogen sonic hedgehog. These MPs induced an inhibition of endothelial cell migration and proliferation. However, these same MP increased capillary-like formation through the upregulation of proteins such as intercellular adhesion molecule-1 and Rho A and the activation of focal adhesion kinase (FAK) and other proangiogenic factors, mainly vascular endothelial growth factor (VEGF), via the activation of the sonic hedgehog pathway [40]. A direct consequence of PS expression on EMP is that PS can bind to coagulation factors and promote their activation, consistent with a procoagulant potential for EMP. In addition to PS exposure, EMP harbor tissue factor (TF), the initiator of the extrinsic coagulation pathway, suggesting that EMP could promote the assembly of clotting enzymes leading to thrombin generation. Besides their procoagulant activity, EMP also behave as a surface supporting plasmin generation by expressing the urokinase-type plasminogen activator (uPA) and its receptor (uPAR), which could counteract the thrombin generated by EMP. In this context, EMP supports a link between hemostasis and angiogenesis. Indeed, the plasminogen activation system plays a pivotal role in maintaining vascular patency and facilitating cell migration and angiogenesis. This proteolytic potential affects the angiogenic potential of endothelial progenitor cells. By conveying plasmin, EMP activate matrix metalloproteases (MMP) which are involved in the extracellular matrix degradation and the release of growth factors that play a crucial role in tissue remodeling, angiogenesis, and cancer spreading. Endothelial-, platelet-, and tumor-cell-derived MPs appear to be able to angiogenesis, an effect mediated by reactive oxygen species, metalloproteinases, growth factors such as vascular endothelial growth factor, or sphingomyelin. Apoptotic bodies from endothelial cells could also contribute to tissue repair mechanisms by stimulating the differentiation of progenitor cells. The polypeptide VEGF is a potent regulator of normal and abnormal angiogenesis. Chuang et al. in a comparative study investigated three groups of patients: group I include 23 hemodialysis (HD) patients with recurrent vascular access failure (<2-year survival or synthetic arteriovenous graft <1-year survival), group II included 15 HD patients with longer vascular access survival (>5 year), and group III included 10 healthy volunteers as control. The expression of platelet activation markers (CD62P and fibrinogen receptor) and the numbers of platelet-derived MPs were measured. CD62P-positive platelets were significantly

higher in group I than in groups II and III. Fibrinogen receptor-positive platelets were also significantly higher in group I than in group II and group III. A higher level of circulating activated platelets is associated with shorter survival of vascular access in HD patients [41]. Andro et al. in an experimental study investigated 29 healthy subjects, 46 HD patients, 23 continuous ambulatory peritoneal dialysis (CAPD) patients, and 20 pre-dialyzed uremic patients. Analyses of platelet MPs were performed using a flow cytometer. Anexin V was used to probe procoagulant activity of PMPs. PMP counts at this study were significantly greater in each uremic groups than in controls. Platelet MP counts were significantly higher in uremic patients with thrombotic events than in those without thrombotic events. The HD procedure and existence of arteriovenous (AV) fistula did not affect PMP counts, but recombinant human erythropoietin (rHu EPO) treatment possibly enhanced the PMP release in these patients. Therefore, elevated PMP counts may trigger thrombosis in uremic patients [42].

MP in immunity and inflammation

It is now well established that MPs play a crucial role in inflammation. As a source of aminophospholipids and also a preferential substrate for phospholipase A_2, MPs are involved in the release of lysophosphatidic acid, which, in turn, triggers platelet aggregation and the inflammatory process. MPs are able to deliver arachidonic acid, leading to an increased expression of endothelial cyclooxygenase type 2. Cytokines also participate in the generation of MPs including PMPs with pro-inflammatory properties. It is documented that the released MPs contains interleukin-1, an important inflammatory factor. In addition, there is evidence showing that MPs shed by platelets can stimulate the production of pro-inflammatory cytokines such as IL-1, IL-6, IL-8, and TNF-a. These cytokines in turn activate inflammatory cells to generate more MPs, forming a positive feedback loop. MPs can also promote the expression of cell adhesion molecules in endothelial cells; MPs released by leukocytes have been demonstrated to contribute to the activated phenotype of rheumatoid arthritis synovial fibroblasts. MPs released by leukocytes may stimulate the expression of proangiogenic chemokines of CXCL1, CXCL2, CXCL3, CXCL5, CXCL6, and CXCL8. Taken together, MPs from certain cells may induce and intensify inflammatory response. This suggests that MPs can act as agonists of inflammation [5]. Neutrophil MPs are able to increase cytokine and chemokine release by endothelial cells by a nuclear factor-kB-independent pathway. Moreover, proteinase 3 (PR3) has been shown to be present on neutrophil MPs. Pro-inflammatory activities of PR3 include its ability to degrade matrix components, to enhance chemokine and tissue factor production by endothelial cells, and/or provoke endothelial cell apoptosis. The dissemination of highly adhesive MPs containing PR3 could thus greatly enhance inflammatory vascular lesions. On the contrary, neutrophil MPs could promote the resolution of inflammation, since they increase the release of transforming growth factor beta 1 by activated macrophages. Platelet MPs could participate to these modulations by adding new adhesion molecules to MPs aggregates (GPIIbIIIa, b1 integrins, GPIb, and P-selectin). Platelet MPs also contain bioactive lipids able to activate cyclooxygenase-2-dependent prostaglandin production in monocytes and endothelial cells. Finally, upon activation, platelets synthesize IL-1, which is released and processed on platelet MPs [43] (Fig. 4). In several studies, it has been shown that microparticles released by platelets, leukocytes, and endothelial cells can be found in conditions of endothelial dysfunction, acute and chronic vascular inflammation, and hypercoagulation. Endothelial microparticles can be found in several conditions that are associated with arterial hypertension. EMP are not only valuable surrogate markers reflecting the extent of endothelial dysfunction

but additionally might promote the progression of arterial hypertension and its complications [44].

MP in increasing cardiovascular disease

MVs secreted from platelets play an important role in both coagulation and development of atherosclerosis. Increased levels of MVs derived from platelets can be found in patients with acute coronary syndrome, stroke, and peripheral arterial disease. Microparticles behave as effectors that play a deleterious role in renal diseases. They also represent novel biomarkers that are useful to appreciate cardiovascular risk associated with chronic kidney disease and sometimes disease activity [45]. In a prospective pilot study by Amabile et al., 81 stable hemodialyzed end-stage renal disease (ESRD) patients were enrolled. Platelet-free plasma obtained 72 h after last dialysis was analyzed by flow cytometry, and MPs with cellular origin are identified as endothelial, platelets, or erythrocyte. They concluded that increased plasma levels of EMP is a robust independent predictor of severe cardiovascular (CV) outcome in ESRD patients [46]. Moreover, the role of coagulation, thrombosis, platelet activation, and microparticles in the pathology

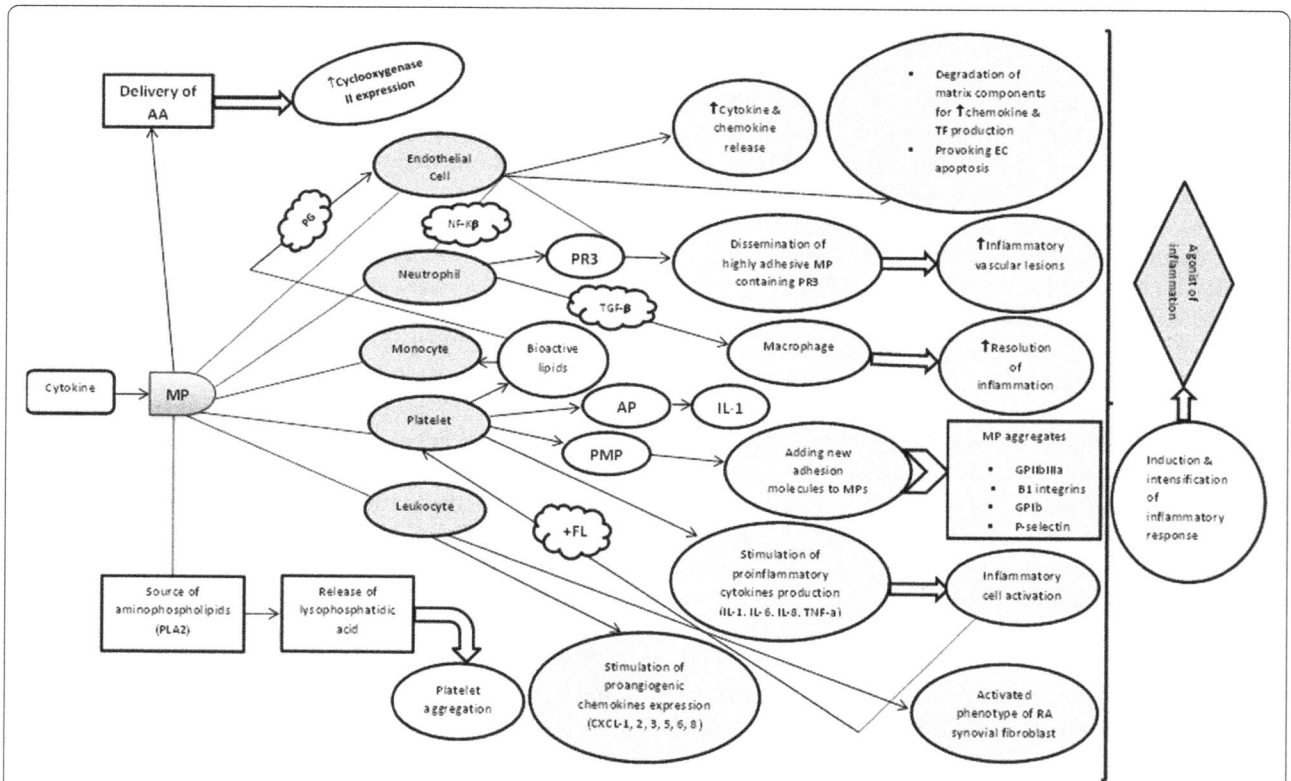

Fig. 4 Schematic actions of microparticles in immunity and inflammation. *AA* arachidonic acid, *AP* activated platelet, *EC* endothelial cells, *IL-1* interleukin-1, *MPs* microparticles, *NF-kB* nuclear factor-kapa B, *+FL* positive feedback loop, *PG* prostaglandin, *PLA2* phospholipase A2, *PMP* platelet microparticles, *PR3* proteinase 3, *RA* rheumatoid arthritis, *TGF-β* transforming growth factor of beta, *TF* tissue factor, *TNF-α* tumor necrosis factor-α

and progression of pulmonary arterial hypertension (PAH) is clearly characterized [47]. Endothelial microvesicles (eMVs) are considered to be markers of inflammation, endothelial injury, and endothelial dysfunction. As endothelial dysfunction is a well-known predictor of future cardiovascular diseases, endothelial MVs could be used to as biomarkers of vascular health. Similarly to eMVs in endothelial activation, platelet MVs (pMVs) are considered as platelet activation markers that contributes in cardiovascular diseases. pMVs possibly represent novel players in the network between inflammation and autoimmunity. Furthermore, circulating CD31$^+$/annexin V$^+$ apoptotic microparticles highly significantly predict the degree of endothelial dysfunction in humans with coronary artery disease [48]. Chronic renal failure patients are at high risk of cardiovascular events and display endothelial dysfunction, a critical element in the pathogenesis of atherosclerosis. Faure et al. in a cross-sectional study evaluated 45 chronic renal failure patients, 30 HD patients, and 36 healthy subjects. Circulating endothelial MPs were numerated by flow cytometry, and platelet MPs (CD41), leukocyte MPs (CD45) and annexin V MPs were also counted. CD144 EMP and CD146 EMP were significantly higher in chronic renal failure (CRF) and HD patients than in healthy subjects. Furthermore, annexin V MPs were elevated in both groups of uremic patients, and CD41PMPs and CD45 LMPs were increased in CRF and HD patients respectively. In vitro, para-cresol and indoxyl sulfate significantly increased both CD 146 and annexin-V EMP release. Increased levels of circulating EMP in CRF and HD patients represent a new marker of endothelial dysfunction in uremia [49].

MP in apoptosis

MPs derived from various origins, including monocytes, erythrocytes, endothelial cells, and platelets, have been reported to contain caspase 3. This process is believed to be a protective mechanism directed at removing pro-apoptotic machinery, since inhibition of MP-mediated caspase 3 release in endothelial cells is associated with increased apoptosis. It has been suggested that MPs may deliver caspase 3 to target cells, leading to the induction of apoptosis. However, as caspase 3 is involved in numerous cellular processes beyond cell death, the delivery of caspases may have an impact on several cellular processes [8].

Wang et al. in a prospective study investigated that starving stress endothelial progenitor MVs (sEPCs-MVs) and apoptotic stress endothelial progenitor MVs (aEPC-MVs) are functionally different on hypoxia/reoxygenation (H/R)-induced apoptosis and dysfunction. These functional roles might rely on the orchestrated mechanisms associated with MV-carried ribonucleic

acids (RNAs) in control of reactive oxygen species (ROS) production and phosphatidylinositol-3 kinase/endothelial nitric oxide synthase/nitric oxide (PI3K/eNOS/NO) pathway in the target cells. These findings indicate that EPC-MVs could be used as a novel vehicle for treating H/R injury [50].

MP in oxidative stress

MPs have been shown to regulate the production of reactive oxygen species (ROS). Interestingly, both the source of MPs and the manner in which they are formed appear to be a critical determinant of MP-mediated pro-oxidative effects. Thus, the majority of studies suggest that MPs (endothelial-, monocyte-, and lymphocyte-derived) are capable of promoting oxidative stress in the endothelium through processes which may involve several enzymatic systems [8]. Fontaine et al. in a prospective study investigated blood plasmas of 24 patients on-pump and 10 off-pump before, 1 h, and 24 h after cardiac surgery. Rings of rat thoracic aortas were incubated for 20 h with these different plasmas or saline. Then, superoxide anion production was assessed. Plasma isolated after on-pump, but not off-pump coronary bypass surgery can induce superoxide generation by the vascular wall which seems related to circulating microparticles remaining present at least 24 h after the procedure that might be of endothelial origin [51]. In patients with CRF, one could speculate that the initial stimuli that lead to MP generation could result from a release of lipopolysaccharide (LPS), advanced glycation end-products (AGEs), pro-inflammatory cytokines [TNFα (tumor necrosis factor-a and interleukin-1 (IL-1)], or oxidized low density lipoprotein (LDL), reflecting the oxidant stress.

Microparticles in kidney transplantation

In addition to their diagnostic role as markers of kidney and vascular damage, these microparticles have various functions, e.g., intercellular communication, anti-inflammation and anticoagulation, regulation of vascular tone, vascular wall permeability, and cell growth. MPs in kidney transplantation have dual effects, and, as such, some effects may cause pathologic conditions and sometimes they are considered as extracellular vesicles. For example, endothelial MPs may induce endothelial dysfunction, but at the same time, it has also been suggested that endothelial MPs are novel markers of endothelial dysfunction. Numerous studies indicate that MPs may trigger endothelial dysfunction by disrupting production of nitric oxide, promoting coagulation and inflammation, or altering angiogenesis and apoptosis (Fig. 5). MP are also implicated in the exchange of mRNA and proteins between cells. Circulating miRNAs are included into lipid or lipoprotein complexes such as

investigated the identified miRNA signature in kidney transplant recipients. Total RNA was extracted from trizol from biopsy tissue or urinary cell fractions. Real-time quantitative-PCR were used for quantifying the expression of miR-142-3p, miR-32, miR-107, miR-204, and miR-211 in paired urine sample using pre-designed TaqMan® miRNA expression assays. They confirmed the differential expression of these five miRNAs. Differential expression was detected for miR-142-3p, miR-204, miR-107, miR-211, and miR-32. Furthermore, differential expression of miR-142-3p, miR-204, and miR-211 was also observed between patient groups in urine samples. A characteristic miRNA signature for interstitial fibrosis/tubular atrophy (IF/TA) that correlates with paired urine samples was identified. These results support the potential use of miRNAs as noninvasive markers of IF/TA and for monitoring graft function [54].

VEGF is a mitogen for endothelial cells and is expressed widely by renal tissue and T cells. VEGF influences adhesion and migration of leukocytes across the endothelium. In a study, Shahbazi et al. investigated VEGF promoter polymorphisms by using sequence-specific primer-PCR in 173 renal transplant recipients. Acute rejection occurred in 38.7%. VEGF in vitro expression was investigated in stimulated leukocytes from 30 controls. The VEGF-1154*G and VEGF-2578*C alleles were associated with higher VEGF production. VEGF-1154 GG and GA genotypes were significantly associated with acute rejection risk at 3 months. VEGF-2578 CC and CA genotypes were associated with increased rejection risk. These data indicate that the VEGF-1154*G and VEGF-2578*C containing genotypes, encoding higher VEGF production, are strongly associated with acute rejection and may be useful markers of rejection risk [55]. A logical, but unstudied, extrapolation is that platelet-derived microparticles may also have an important function in transplant vasculopathy [56].

Ullal et al. in an experimental study investigated that particle binding to an antibody represents a useful serological assay to characterize autoantibody specificity as particles may represent an important antigenic form of deoxyribonucleic acid (DNA) that is exposed to the immune system in vivo. This DNA may have unique associations with other nuclear and cellular components on particles which may affect antigenicity as well as immunogenicity. Indeed, particles can display cytokines and serve as adjuvants. It is well known that the endothelium is the primary target of immunological attack in allograft rejection that could be detected early for effective patient care and management. Moreover, platelet microparticles suggest that they can migrate out of blood vessels by attaching to neutrophils thereby increasing their range of impact.

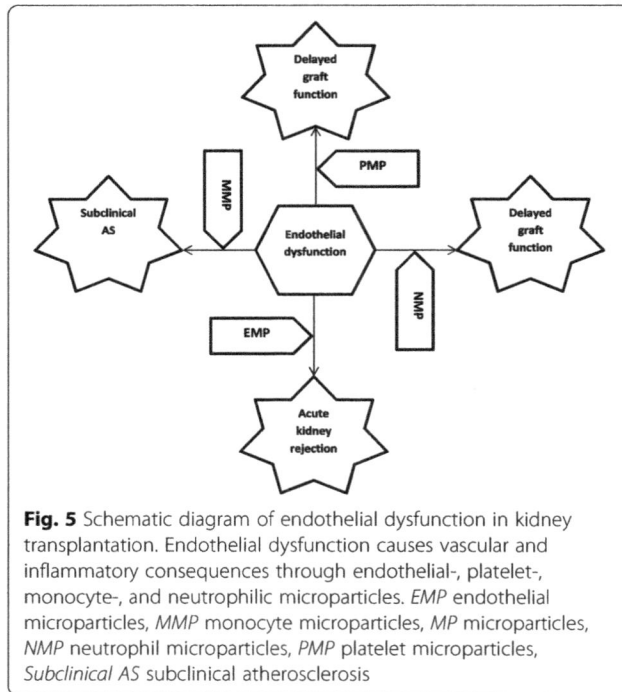

Fig. 5 Schematic diagram of endothelial dysfunction in kidney transplantation. Endothelial dysfunction causes vascular and inflammatory consequences through endothelial-, platelet-, monocyte-, and neutrophilic microparticles. *EMP* endothelial microparticles, *MMP* monocyte microparticles, *MP* microparticles, *NMP* neutrophil microparticles, *PMP* platelet microparticles, *Subclinical AS* subclinical atherosclerosis

microvesicles/microparticles or exosomes. Anglicheau et al. in a study investigated the miRNA profile in peripheral blood mononuclear cells (PBMCs) as well as kidney biopsies in patients with acute renal allograft rejection. These patients were shown to display a unique miRNA expression profile PBMCs and paired renal biopsy specimens. miRNAs overexpressed in renal biopsies (miR-142-5p, miR-155, and miR-223) followed the same pattern of expression in PBMCs, indicating that miRNA expression analysis might serve as a diagnostic test in this patient cohort [52]. Another study by Lorenzen et al. analyzed the miRNA expression profile in urine samples (quantitative real time PCR-based miRNA microarray) of patients with acute T cell-mediated renal allograft rejection. This approach was chosen to identify miRNAs deregulated in easily accessible urine to circumvent the potential risks associated with an invasive procedure such as kidney biopsy. Urine samples of patients were obtained at the time of biopsy. Patients with an acute rejection as diagnosed by a kidney biopsy showed reduced urinary levels of miR-210. In samples taken before and after the rejection period, miR-210 increased to levels of controls. In addition, a disease control group of transplant patients with urinary tract infection did not display altered miR-210 levels. These results underline a potential specificity of urinary miR-210 for the diagnosis of acute T cell-mediated rejection. Moreover, urinary miR-210 at the time of rejection predicted GFR decline at 1 year after transplantation [53]. Scian et al. in a prospective study

Considering the fact that the platelet microparticles express p-selectin and CD-154, extravascular distribution of microparticles could influence the responses of graft infiltrating cells [57].

As certain miRNAs are characteristic for tumors, their presence within tumor-derived exosomes and microvesicles may serve novel biomarkers of cancer [58]. Thus, the genetic content of circulating microvesicles may be of great use for diagnostic and prognostic purposes after organ transplantation. MPs contain membrane proteins and cytosolic material derived from the cell from which they originate. The circulating EMP could be used as a marker of vascular endothelial cell damage and to determine asymptomatic patients who might be at higher risk of developing cardiovascular disease in CKD and renal transplant.

In a study by Jarmo et al., chronic renal allograft rejection is characterized by gradual progression suggesting persistent low-grade injury. Apoptotic cell death may be initiated by low-grade injury secondary to external factors, making apoptosis a potential pathway of chronic rejection. Protocol kidney biopsies of 20 pediatric renal allograft recipients (12 with chronic rejection and 8 with normal histology), 9 pediatric liver allograft recipients, and 7 children with minimal change nephrotic syndrome were evaluated. The presence of apoptotic cell death was studied by determining apoptosis-induced oligonucleosomal DNA fragmentation in the biopsy specimens. Significant DNA fragmentation was found only in the specimens from patients with chronic rejection. In situ investigation revealed increased apoptosis of both proximal and distal tubular epithelial cells, but not in the glomeruli or interstitium. The mean number of apoptotic tubular epithelial cells was higher in the renal allografts than in kidneys of liver transplant recipients or patients with minimal change nephrotic syndrome. These data provide biochemical evidence of increased apoptotic cell death of renal tubular epithelial cells in patients undergoing chronic renal allograft rejection [59].

Simmons et al. in a prospective cohort study time-dependent changes in biomarkers of inflammation and oxidative stress before and after renal transplantation. Nineteen end-stage renal disease patients undergoing living-donor renal transplantation were enrolled. Pre-transplant levels of the pro-inflammatory proteins IL-6, TNF-α, and CRP, as well as the oxidative stress markers plasma protein carbonyls and F2-isoprostanes, were significantly elevated in ESRD patients compared with healthy control subjects. They observed rapid and significant declines in all of these biomarkers after transplantation that persisted for 2 months. These findings indicate that restoration of renal function by transplantation improves the chronic inflammation and increased oxidative stress associated with uremia, which

may contribute to the improved survival afforded to ESRD patients by renal transplantation [60].

A recent study defined the safety and clinical feasibility of autologous mesenchymal stem cell transplantation in two human recipients of kidneys from living-related donors. It has been shown that infusion of MSCs after kidney transplantation is feasible and restricts T memory cell expansion while enlarging the T regulatory population, even if graft dysfunction is induced. One possible alternative to the MSC infusion in organ transplantation might be MV treatment [61].

Circulating MVs may have a great potential to detect possible immune rejections, and MV modulation may emerge as a therapeutic approach in organ rejection therapy [62, 63]. Their actions in immunity, cardiovascular diseases, cancer, oxidative stress, blood coagulation, angiogenesis, apoptosis, rejection, and intercellular communication have been clearly demonstrated. Lactadherin, also known as milk fat globule–epidermal growth factor 8 (EGF-8), is a 45-kDa glycoprotein secreted by macrophages. Lactadherin contains EGF-like domains at the amino terminus and two C-domains at the carboxyl terminus that share homology to the phosphatidylserine-binding domains of blood coagulation factors V and VIII. Lactadherin binds to apoptotic cells, activated platelets, and phosphatidylserine expressing red blood cells via the C-domains and anchors them to macrophage integrins via its RGD sequence in the EGF domain. Dasgupta et al. examined the role of lactadherin in the clearance of phosphotidylserine-rich platelet-derived microvesicles. Investigators demonstrated that a defective clearance of platelet-derived MV can induce a hypercoagulable state [64]. Furthermore, investigations showed that attenuated platelet MV formation may be a sign of former activation of platelets that could influence graft function and survival. On the other hand, binding of PMP to cells can modify cell functional properties. For example, it has been elegantly demonstrated that PMP can bind hematopoietic progenitors and stimulate their engraftment [65]. An early decrease of circulating microparticle levels and procoagulant activity is observed after renal transplantation and persists during the 1 year of follow-up. Therefore, researchers suggest that MP could be associated to improvement of vascular dysfunction reported after transplant. Furthermore, endothelial dysfunction occurs in hemodialysis and kidney-transplanted patients and can be enhanced by immunosuppressive therapy. Circulating endothelial cells (CEC), endothelial microparticles (EMP), and soluble vascular cell adhesion molecule-1 (sVCAM-1) provide information on endothelium activation and damage. In study by Al-massarani et al., the impact of two immunosuppressive regimens [Cyclosporine A/ Azathioprine vs. Tacrolimus/Mycophenolate Mofetil

(CsA/Aza vs. Tac/MMF)] on the kinetics of CEC, EMP, and sVCAM-1 levels in 52 patients, both before graft and 3, 6, 9 and 12 months after graft, was evaluated. They reported the beneficial impact of renal transplantation on endothelial injury through circulating levels of endothelial markers and concluded that these effects are more pronounced in patients treated by CsA/Aza and are impaired in relation with cytomegalovirus (CMV) and cardiovascular diseases. These results are suggestive of the noninvasive endothelial evaluation as an early index of vascular injury [66].

Patients with chronic renal failure suffer from dysfunction in coagulation. Kidney transplantation induces inflammatory reactions and thus activation of platelets. Activated platelets, in turn, form microvesicles by shedding. These microvesicles have been shown to have coagulant activities. Activated platelets in prolonged cold ischemia were associated with delayed graft function and inferior survival. They concluded decreased platelet microvesicle formation after ex vivo stimulation with tartrate-resistant acid phosphatase (TRAP) was associated with longer graft ischemia time. This may be a sign of former activation of platelets which could influence graft function and survival (Table 2). Although it has been known that platelets modify vascular inflammation by secretion of soluble mediators and release of microparticles, new aspects of these mechanisms are being defined. New findings also demonstrate heterologous interactions of platelet microparticles with leukocytes that may increase their range of impact. By attaching to neutrophils, platelet microparticles appear to migrate out of blood vessels and into other compartments where they stimulate secretion of cytokines. Contact of platelets with extracellular matrix also can result in cleavage of hyaluronan into fragments that serve as an endogenous danger signal. Considering the fact that platelet microparticles express p-selectin and CD154, extravascular distribution of microparticles could influence the responses of graft-infiltrating cells [67]. Contrastly, Trappenburg et al., in a cross-sectional study, investigated blood samples of 27 patients with chronic kidney disease (8 CKD stage 4, 9 peritoneal disease, 10 hemodialysis patients) and 10 controls before and after hemodialysis. Degree and nature of endothelial activation were measured by von Willebrand factor (vWF) and vWF propeptide levels. Cellular MPs were characterized by flow cytometry, and MP-specific thrombin generation (TG) measurements showed renal failure is accompanied by endothelial activation of a different nature in CKD4 and peritoneal dialysis (PD) patients compared to hemodialysis (HD) patients, and results in all subgroups in an increase of mainly platelet-derived MPs that appear to be less procoagulant than in other disease states, possibly because of the uremic functional defect of their cellular source [68]. In organ transplantation, blood-borne cells and macromolecules (e.g., antibodies) of the host immune system are brought into direct contact with the endothelial cell (EC) lining of graft vessels. In this location, graft ECs play several roles in allograft rejection, including the initiation of rejection responses by presentation of alloantigen to circulating T cells, the development of inflammation and thrombosis, and as targets of injury and agents of repair [69]. The use of urinary extracellular vesicles (EVs) as a source of biomarkers for kidney injury after renal transplantation (RTx) was probed by Alvarez et al. In this study, the authors demonstrated the presence of neutrophil gelatinase-associated lipocalin (NGAL) in cellular fraction and in urinary EVs from patients. Urinary EVs NGAL detection differed between patients and controls. Interestingly, different quantities of NGAL were detected between deceased and living donors. Thus, various studies suggest that NGAL could be a biomarker of damage and delayed graft function [70, 71].

Concerning kidney function, experiments revealed that the beneficial effect of MSCs on recovery from acute kidney injury is in part mediated via MVs. MV function in this setting was CD-44 and beta-1 integrin dependent. Because miRNAs treatment of MSC-derived MVs abolished the beneficial effects, the authors concluded that this effect is most likely mediated via horizontal gene transfer [72]. MPs contain membrane proteins and cytosolic material that are derived from their original cells. EMP having CD144, CD 146, CD31+/CD41−, CD51, and CD105 may be used to evaluate the vascular endothelial cell damage and determine asymptomatic patients who might be at higher risk of developing cardiovascular disease in CKD and renal transplantation [73]. Urinary extracellular vesicles contain proteins from all sections of the nephron, whereas the most of studied circulating extracellular vesicles are derived from platelets, immune cells, and the endothelium. In addition to their diagnostic role as markers of kidney and vascular damage, extracellular vesicles may have functional significance in renal health and disease by facilitating communication between cells and protecting against kidney injury and bacterial infection in the urinary tract. It is crucial that researchers provide detailed information about their methodology and use several techniques to ensure that the particles that they are studying are truly EVs and not non-EV components, such as lipids or protein complexes. In addition, a standard and uniform language should be used among all scientific communications [74].

Conclusions

Elevated levels of MP have been detected throughout the entire process of vascular damage associated with

Table 2 Clinical studies of microparticles in renal transplantation

Author/year	Design of study	Patients	Main outcomes	Conclusion
Dimuccio V et al. 2014 [75]	prospective, randomized and monocentric trial	25 transplanted patients 20 age-matched control 5 ESRD patients with residual diuresis	Urinary CD133 EVs significantly increased	1. CD133 EVs may reflect activity of CD133 progenitor cells in renal homeostasis and may provide information on their regenerative potential after kidney injury
Al-Massarani et al. 2009 [76]	Open, prospective, randomized and mono-	52 patients 50 healthy control	At 12 months after Tx,↓ in MP and MP procoagulant was more pronounced in patients without CVD history	↓ MP and MP procoagulant activity in renal graft even in patients without CVD history
Quamri et al. 2014 [77]	Prospective, randomized and monocentric trial	213 patients with KTx, 14 KTx and 60 healthy donors	No difference in the quantity of circulating EMP in the pre-KTx or after KTx recipient sera and healthy donor sera	↓ in circulating EMP and Scr after kidney transplantation
Al-Massarani et al. 2008 [66]	Open, prospective, randomized and mono	52 patients 50 healthy control	Positive correlation between circulating endothelial cells (CEC) and history of CVD and between EMP and CMV infection at M_{12} (month of 12)	CEC usage in indexing vascular injury therapeutic options
Wu et al. 2014 [78]	Randomized, double blind, placebo-controlled crossover trial	84 patients with moderate risk of CVD (GG $n = 40$; GT/TT $n = 44$)	No significant effect of fish oil supplementation on BP plasma lipids or plasma glucose	GT/TT subjects tended to higher concentrations total cholesterol and LDL but vascular function not affected by Tx or eNOS genotype
Schuerholz et al. 2007 [79]	Clinical controlled trial	20 patients Group 1 with 10.4+/−6.1 h Group 2 with 23.7+/−3.8 h	Platelet-derived ex vivo microvesicle formation was higher in group 1 Platelet count was higher in short term ischemia	Lower platelet microvesicle formation after ex vivo stimulation with TRAP was associated with Cr that was lower in both groups longer graft ischemia
Renner et al. 2013 [80]	Animal and human experimental study	Animal Cyclosporine injection (subcutaneously) for 8–12 weeks to old-man C57BL/6 mice Human EDTA-plasma from five patients before renal Tx and 14 days after initiation of treatment with tacrolimus	Cyclosporine-induced microparticles caused injury to bystander endothelial cells and complement mediated injury of the kidneys and vasculature in cyclosporine-treated mice Number of endothelial MPs in plasma of renal transplant patients increases 2 weeks after initiation of tacrolimus and it was associated with increased C3 deposition on endothelial MPs in some of patients	Injury-associated release of endothelial MPs is a mechanism for systemic insults trigger intravascular complement activation and complement-dependent renal diseases
Kas-Deelen et al. 2000 [81]	Prospective clinical trial	54 patients before HCMV infection at ~15 days after Tx weekly (40, 50, 60 days) in first antigenemia test until negative antigenemia 32 patients high antigenemia 12 patients mild antigenemia (<5 pp 65-positive granulocytes/50000 cells) 10 patients without HCMV infection	1. Cytomegalic endothelial cells in moderate or high HCMV antigenemia 2. Uninfected endothelial cells in patients with or without HCMV antigenemia 3. Incidence of either CEC, EC or combination of both cells was with HCMV-related symptoms ($p < 0.01$)	Occurrence of rejection episodes before HCMV infection was an important risk for the occurrence of ECs in blood (ECs, CECs, or both) during HCMV infection ($p < 0.001$)
Werner et al. 2006 [48]	Prospective clinical trial			

Table 2 Clinical studies of microparticles in renal transplantation (*Continued*)

	50 patients with coronary artery disease underwent coronary angiography Circulating CD31+/annexin V+ apoptotic microparticles in peripheral blood was quantified by flow cytometry	Increased apoptotic microparticles counts positively correlated with impairment of coronary endothelial function	In patients with CAD endothelial-dependent vasodilatation closely relies on the degree of endothelial cell apoptosis. In patients with CAD, endothelial-dependent vasodilatation closely relies on the degree of endothelial cell apoptosis increased apoptotic MPs counts predict sever endothelial dysfunction independent of classical risk factors such as HTN, hypercholesterolemia, smoking, diabetes, age or sex
Shahbazian et al. 2002 [55]	Prospective clinical trial	173 renal transplant recipients were examined for VEGF promoter Polymorphism using sequence-specific primer-PCR	Acute rejection occurred in 38.7%; -1154*G and -2578*C alleles were associated with higher VEGF production VEGF-1154 GG and GA genotypes were significantly associated with acute rejection risk at 3 months VEGF-2578 CC and CA genotypes were associated with increased rejection risk	-1154*G and -2578*C containing genotypes, encoding higher VEGF production as strongly associated with acute rejection and may be a useful marker for acute rejection
Lorenzen et al. 2011 [53]	Prospective cohort study	62 patients with acute rejection 19 control transplant patients without rejection 13 stable transplant patients with UTI by quantitative RT-PCR	The miR-10b and miR-210 were downregulated and miR-10a upregulated in patients with acute rejection compared to controls. Only miR-210 differed between patients with acute rejection when compared with UTI or transplant patients before/after rejection	Low miR-210 levels were associated with higher decline in GFR 1 year after transplantation. Selected miRNA are strongly altered in urine of the patients with acute renal graft rejection. The miR-210 levels identify patients with acute rejection and predict long-term kidney function. Urinary miR-210 may thus serve as a novel biomarker of acute rejection
Scian et al. 2011 [54]	Prospective study	65 miRNA in samples with CAD with IF/TA vs. normal allografts by microarray Five miRNAs were selected and differential expression By RT-qPCR	Differential expression were detected for miR-142-3p, miR-204, miR-107, and miR-211	Differential expression of miR-142-3p, miR-204, and miR-211 were observed between patient groups in urine samples. A characteristic miRNA signature for IF/TA that correlates with paired urine samples was identified. This study support the potential use of miRNAs as noninvasive markers of IF/TA and for monitoring graft function.
Simmons et al. 2005 [60]	Prospective cohort study	19 patients of living-donor kidney Txs were enrolled. CRP, IL-1, IL-6, IL-10, TNF-a, protein-associated carbonyl content, and F-2 isoprostanes at 1 week pretransplant and 1 week and 2 months posttransplant	↑pretransplant levels of the pro-inflammatory proteins IL-6, TNF-a, CRP, oxidative markers (plasma protein carbonyls and F2-isoprostanes in ESRD patients vs. healthy control subjects ↓ posttransplant levels of pro-inflammatory proteins and oxidative markers on 2 months	Kidney Tx improves the chronic inflammation and ↑ oxidative stress due to uremia and may contribute to survival

Table 2 Clinical studies of microparticles in renal transplantation (Continued)

Jarmo et al. 1997 [59]	Prospective study	20 pediatric renal allograft recipients 12 patients with chronic rejection and 8 with normal histology 9 pediatric liver allograft recipients 7 children with minimal change nephrotic syndrome Apoptotic cell death by apoptosis-induced oligonucleosomal DNA fragmentation in the biopsy using 3′ end labeling with terminal transferase gel fractionation and southern blotting specific cell types with ↑ DNA fragmentation using 3′ end labeling were determined	Specific DNA fragmentation in chronic rejection ↑apoptosis of both the proximal and distal tubular epithelial cells Mean number of apoptotic tubular cells was higher in the renal allografts than liver allograft recipients and patients with minimal change nephrotic syndrome	Increased apoptotic cell death of renal tubular epithelial cells in patients undergoing chronic renal allograft rejection

AR acute rejection, BP blood pressure, CAD coronary artery disease, CECs circulating endothelial cells, CD cluster of differentiation, CRP C-reactive protein, CSA cyclosporine A, CVD cardiovascular disease, ECs endothelial cells, EDTA ethylene diamine tetra-acetate, eNOS endothelial nitric oxide synthase, ESRD end-stage renal disease, EVs extracellular vesicles, GFR glomerular filtration rate, HCMV human cytomegalovirus, HRECs human renal epithelial cells, HTN hypertension, IF/TA interstitial fibrosis/tubular atrophy, KTx kidney transplantation, LDL low density lipoprotein, MPs microparticles, mRNAs messenger RNAs, miRNAs microRNAs, PBMCs peripheral blood mononuclear cells, RT-qPCR real-time quantitative-polymerase chain reaction, Scr serum creatinine, TRAP tartrate-resistant acid phosphatase, VEGF vascular endothelial growth factor

renal diseases. Furthermore, MPs are key actors in cardiovascular diseases that are associated with renal diseases and are elevated in patients with hemodialysis. Furthermore, it recently has demonstrated that higher levels of endothelial MPs observed in hemodialyzed patients reach to normal values after graft. Circulating microvesicles may have a great potential to detect possible immune rejections, and microvesicle modulation may emerge as a therapeutic approach in organ rejection therapy. Because we are unaware from the other functional roles of microparticles, more key and original studies which be cost-effective are necessary to characterize functional roles of microparticles in renal diseases and clinical research.

Acknowledgements
None.

Funding
Not applicable.

Competing interests
The author declares that she has no competing interests.

References
1. Fang YD, King WH, Li YJ, Gleadle MJ. Exosomes and the kidney: blaming the messenger. Nephrology. 2013;18:1–10.
2. Lovren F, Verma S. Evolving role of microparticles in the pathophysiology of endothelial dysfunction. Clin Chem. 2013;59:1166–74.
3. Van der Pol E, Böing AN, Harrison P, Sturk A, Nieuwland R. Classification, functions, and clinical relevance of extracellular vesicles. Pharmacol Rev. 2012;64:676–705.
4. Mackman N. On the trail of microparticles. Circ Res. 2009;104:925–7.
5. ZH W, CL J, Li H, Qiu GX, Gao CJ, Weng XS. Membrane microparticles and diseases. Eur Rev Med Pharmacol Sci. 2013; 17:2420-7.
6. Rubin O, Canellini G, Delobel J, Lion N, Tissot JD. Red blood cell microparticles: clinical relevance. Transfus Med Hemother. 2012;39:342–7.
7. Shet AS. Characterizing blood microparticles: technical aspects and challenges. Vasc Health Risk Manag. 2008;4:769–74.
8. Burger D, Schock S, Thombson SC, Montezano CA, Hakim MA, Touyz MR. Microparticles:biomarkers and beyond. Clin Sci. 2013;124:423–41.
9. Hugel B, Martinez MC, Kunzelmann C, Freyssinet JM. Membrane microparticles: two sides of the coin. Physiology. 2005;20:22–7.
10. Barteneva NS, Fasler-Kan E, Bernimoulin M, Stern JN, Ponomarev ED, Duckett L, et al. Circulating microparticles: square the circle. BMC Cell Biol. 2013;14:1–21.
11. Morel O, Jesel L, Freyssinet JM, Toti F. Cellular mechanisms underlying the formation of circulating microparticles. Arterioscler Thromb Vasc Biol. 2011; 31:15–26.
12. Dignat-George F, Boulanger CM. The many faces of endothelial microparticles. Arterioscler Thromb Vasc Biol. 2011;31:27–33.
13. Sadallah S, Eken C, Schifferli JA. Ectosomes as modulators of inflammation and immunity. Clin Exp Immunol. 2010;163:26–32.
14. Puddu P, Puddu GM, Cravero E, Muscari S, Muscari A. The involvement of circulating microparticles in inflammation, coagulation and cardiovascular diseases. Can J Cardiol. 2010;26:140–5.
15. Boulanger CM, Amabile N, Tedgui A. Circulating microparticles: a potential prognostic marker for atherosclerotic vascular disease. Hypertension. 2006; 48:180–6.
16. Distler JH, Huber LC, Hueber AJ, Reich 3rd CF, Gay S, Distler O, et al. The release of microparticles by apoptotic cells and their effects on macrophages. Apoptosis. 2005;10:731–41.
17. Herring JM, McMichael MA, Smith SA. Microparticles in health and disease. Vet Intern Med. 2013;27:1020–33.
18. Nomura S, Ozaki Y, Ikeda Y. Function and role of microparticles in various clinical settings. Thromb Res. 2008;123:8–23.
19. Mesri M, Altieri DC. Endothelial cell activation by leukocyte microparticles. J Immunol. 1998;161:4382–7.
20. Zwaal RF, Comfurius P, Bevers EM. Surface exposure of phosphatidylserine in pathological cells. Cell Mol Life Sci. 2005;62:971–88.
21. Litvack ML, Post M, Palaniyar N. IgM promotes the clearance of small particles and apoptotic microparticles by macrophages. PLoS One. 2011;6: 17223.
22. Morel O, Toti F, Hugel B, Bakouboula B, Camoin-Jau L, Dignat-George F, et al. Procoagulant microparticles disrupting the vascular homeostasis equation? Arterioscler Thromb Vasc Biol. 2006;26:2594–604.
23. Burton JO, Hamali HA, Singh R, Abbasian N, Parsons R, Patel AK, et al. Elevated levels of procoagulant plasma microvesicles in dialysis patients. PLoS One. 2013;8:72663.
24. Burger D, Thibodeau JF, Holterman CE, Burns KD, Touyz RM, Kennedy CR, et al. Urinary podocyte microparticles identify prealbuminuric diabetic glomerular injury. J Am Soc Nephrol. 2014;25:1401–7.
25. Santucci L, Bruschi M, Candiano G, Lugani F, Petretto A, Bonanni A, et al. Urine proteome biomarkers in kidney diseases. I. Limits, perspectives, and first focus on normal urine. Biomark Insights. 2016;11:41–8.
26. Lorenzen JM, Thum T. Circulating and urinary microRNAs in kidney disease. Clin J Am Soc Nephrol. 2012;7:1528–33.
27. Salih M, Zietse R, Hoorn EJ. Urinary extracellular vesicles and the kidney: biomarkers and beyond. Am J Physiol Renal Physiol. 2014;306:1251–9.
28. Aatonen MT, Ohman T, Nyman TA, Laitinen S, Gronholm M, Siljander PR. Isolation and characterization of platelet-derived extracellular vesicles. J Extracell Vesicles. 2014;3:1–15.
29. Nolan S, Dixon R, Norman K, Hellewell P, Ridger V. Nitric oxide regulates neutrophil migration through microparticle formation. Am J Pathol. 2008; 172:265–73.
30. Mutschler DK, Larsson AO, Basu S, Nordgren A, Eriksson MB. Effects of mechanical ventilation on platelet microparticles in bronchoalveolar lavage fluid. Thromb Res. 2002;108:215–20.
31. Porro C, Lepore S, Trotta T, Castellani S, Ratclif L, Battaglino A, et al. Isolation and characterization of microparticles in sputum from cystic fibrosis patients. Respir Res. 2010;11:94.
32. Berckmans RJ, Nieuwland R, Tak PP, Böing AN, Romijn FP, Kraan MC, et al. Cell-derived microparticles in synovial fluid from inflamed arthritic joints support coagulation exclusively via a factor VII-dependent mechanism. Arthritis Rheum. 2012;46:2857–66.
33. Press JZ, Reyes M, Pitteri SJ, Pennil C, Garcia R, Goff BA, et al. Microparticles from ovarian carcinomas are shed into ascites and promote cell migration. Int J Gynecol Cancer. 2012;22:546–2.
34. Berckmans RJ, Sturk A, van Tienen LM, Schaap MC, Nieuwland R. Cell-derived vesicles exposing coagulant tissue factor in saliva. Blood. 2011;117:3172–73.
35. Hoyer FF, Nickenig G, Werner N. Microparticles—messengers of biological information. J Cell Mol Med. 2010;14:2250–6.
36. Diehl P, Fricke A, Sander L, Stamm J, Bassler N, Htun N, et al. Microparticles: major transport vehicles for distinct microRNAs in circulation. Cardiovasc Res. 2012;93:633–44.
37. Bitzer M, Ben-Dove IZ, Thum T. Microparticles and microRNAs of endothelial progenitor cells ameliorate acute kidney injury. Kidney Int. 2012;82:377–5.
38. Fritzsching B, Schwer B, Kartenbeck J, Pedal A, Horejsi V, Ott M. Release and intercellular transfer of cell surface CD81 via microparticles. Immunol. 2002; 169:5531–7.
39. Zwicker JI, Trenor III CC, Furie BC, Furie B. Tissue factor—bearing microparticles and thrombus formation. Arterioscler Thromb Vasc Biol. 2011; 31:728–33.
40. Shai E, Varon D. Development, cell differentiation, angiogenesis-microparticles and their roles in angiogenesis. Arterioscler Thromb Vasc Biol. 2011;31:10–4.
41. Chuang YC, Chen JB, Yang LC, Kuo CY. Significance of platelet activation in vascular access survival of haemodialysis patients. Nephrol Dial Transplant. 2003;18:947–54.
42. Ando M, Iwata A, Ozeki Y, Tsuchiya K, Akiba T, Nihei H. circulating platelet-

derived microparticles with procoagulant activity may be a potential cause of thrombosis in uremic patients. Kidney Int. 2002;62:1757–63.

43. Daniel L, Fakhouri F, Joly D, Lesavre P, Mecarelli-Halbwalchs L, Dignat-George F, et al. Increase of circulating neutrophil and platelet microparticles during acute vasculitis and hemodialysis. Kidney Int. 2006;69:1416–23.

44. Helbing T, Olivier C, Bode C, Moser M, Diehl P. Role of microparticles in endothelial dysfunction and arterial hypertension. World J Cardiol. 2014;6: 1135–39.

45. Daniel L, Die L, Berland Y, Lesavre P, Mecarelli-Halbwalchs L, Dignat-George F. Circulating microparticles in renal diseases. Nephrol Dial Transplant. 2008; 23:2129–32.

46. Amabile N, Guerin AP, Tedgui A, Boulanger CM, London GM. Predictive value of circulating endothelial microparticles for cardiovascular mortality in end-stage renal failure: a pilot study. Nephrol Dial Transplant. 2012;27:1873–80.

47. Lannan KL, Phipp RP, White RJ. Thrombosis, platelets, microparticles, and PAH: more than clot. Drug Discov Today. 2014;19:1230–5.

48. Werner N, Wassmann S, Ahlers P, Kosiol S, Nickenig G. Circulating CD31+/annexin V+ apoptotic microparticles correlate with coronary endothelial function in patients with coronary artery disease. Arterioscler Thromb Vasc Biol. 2006;26:112–6.

49. Faure V, Dou L, Sabatier F, Cerini C, Sampol J, Berland Y, Brunet P, Dignat-George F. Elevation of circulating endothelial microparticles in patients with chronic renal failure. J Thromb Haemost. 2006;4:566–73.

50. Wang J, Chen S, Ma X, Cheng C, Xiao X, Chen J, et al. Effects of endothelial progenitor cell-derived microvesicles on hypoxia/reoxygenation-induced endothelial dysfunction and apoptosis. Oxid Med Cell Longev. 2013;2013:572729.

51. Fontaine D, Pradier O, Haqcuabard M, Stefanidis C, Carpentier Y, de Canniere D, et al. Oxidative stress induced by circulating microparticles in on-pump but not in off-pump coronary surgery. Acta Cardiol. 2009;64:715–22.

52. Anglicheau D, Sharma VK, Ding R, Stamm J, Bassler N, Htun N, et al. MicroRNA expression profiles predictive of human renal allograft status. Proc Natl Acad Sci U S A. 2009;106:5330–35.

53. Lorenzen JM, Volkmann I, Fiedler J, et al. Urinary miR-210 as a mediator of acute T-cell mediated rejection in renal allograft recipients. Am J Transplant. 2011;11:2221–7.

54. Scian MJ, Maluf DG, David KG, Archer KJ, Suh JL, Wolen AR, et al. MicroRNA profiles in allograft tissues and paired urines associate with chronic allograft dysfunction with IF/TA. Am J Transplant. 2011;11:2110–22.

55. Shahbazian M, Fryer AA, Pravica V, Brogan IJ, Ramsay HM, Hutchinson IV, et al. Vascular endothelial growth factor gene polymorphisms are associated with acute renal allograft rejection. J Am Soc Nephrol. 2002;13:260–4.

56. Morrell CN, Sun H, Swaim AM, Baldwin III WM. Platelets an inflammatory force in transplantation. Am J Transplant. 2007;7:2447–54.

57. Ullal AJ, Marion TN, Pisetsky DS. The role of antigen specificity in the binding of murine monoclonal anti-DNA antibodies to microparticles from apoptotic cells. Clin Immunol. 2014;154:178–87.

58. Gyorgy B, Szabo TG, Pasztoi M, Pál Z, Misják P, Aradi B, et al. Membrane vesicles, current state-of-the-art: emerging role of extracellular vesicles. Cell Mol Life Sci. 2011;68:2667–88.

59. Jarmo L, Pauliina E, Christer H, Leo D. Apoptotic cell death in human chronic renal renal allograft rejection. Transplantation. 1997;63:101–5.

60. Simmons EM, Langone A, Sezer MT, Vella JP, Recupero J, Morrow JD, et al. Effect of renal transplantation on biomarkers of inflammation and oxidative stress in end-stage renal disease patients. Transplantation. 2005;79:914–9.

61. Tetta C, Bruno S, Fonsato V, Deregibus MC, Camussi G. The role of microvesicles in tissue repair. Organogenesis. 2011;7:105–15.

62. Fleissner F, Goerzig Y, Haverich A, Thum T. Microvesicles as novel biomarkers and therapeutic targets in transplantation medicine. Am J Transplant. 2012;12:289–97.

63. Cui J, Yang J, Cao W, Sun Y. Differential diagnosis of acute rejection and chronic cyclosporine nephropathy after rat renal transplantation by detection of endothelial microparticles (EMP). Med Hypotheses. 2010;75:666–8.

64. Dasgupta SK, Abdel-Monem H, Niravath P, Le A, Bellera RV, Langlois K, et al. Lactadherin and clearance of platelet-derived microvesicles. Blood. 2009;113: 1332–9.

65. Janowska-Wieczorek A, Majka M, Kijowski J, Baj-Krzyworzeka M, Reca R, Turner AR, et al. Platelet-derived microparticles bind to hematopoietic stem/progenitor cells and enhance their engraftment. Blood. 2001;98:3143–9.

66. Al-Massarani G, Vacher-Coponat H, Paul P, Widemann A, Arnaud L, Loundou A, et al. Impact of immunosuppressive treatment on endothelial biomarkers after kidney transplantation. Am J Transplant. 2008;8:2360–67.

67. Baldwin III WM, Kuo HH, Morrell CN. Platelets: versatile modifiers of innate and adaptive immune responses to transplants. Curr Opin Organ Transplant. 2011; 16:41–6.

68. Trappenburg MC, Van Schilfgaarde M, Frerichs FC, Spronk HM, ten Cate H, de Fijter CW, et al. Chronic renal failure is accompanied by endothelial activation and a large increase in microparticle numbers with reduced procoagulant capacity. Nephrol Dial Transplant. 2012;27:1446–53.

69. Al-Lamki RS, Bradley JR, Pober JS. Endothelial cells in allograft rejection. Transplantation. 2008;86:1340–48.

70. Alvarez S, Suazo C, Boltansky A, Ursu M, Carvajal D, Innocenti G, et al. Urinary exosomes as a source of kidney dysfunction biomarker in renal transplantation. Transplant Proc. 2013;45:3719–23.

71. Gamez-valero A, Lozano-Ramos SI, Bancu I, Lauzurica-Valdemoros R, Borràs FE. Urinary extracellular vesicles as source of biomarkers in kidney diseases. Front Immunol. 2015;6:6.

72. Bruno S, Grange C, Deregibus MC, Calogero RA, Saviozzi S, Collino F, et al. Mesenchymal stem cell derived microvesicles protect against acute tubular injury. J Am Soc Nephrol. 2009;20:1053–67.

73. Dursun I, Yel S, Unsur E. Dynamics of circulating microparticles in chronic kidney disease and transplantation: is it really reliable marker? World J Transplant. 2015;5:267–75.

74. Erdbrugger U, Le TH. Extracellular vesicles in renal diseases: more than novel biomarkers? J Am Soc Nephrol. 2016;27:12–26.

75. Dimuccio V, Ranghino A, Barbato LP, et al. Urinary CD133+ extracellular vesicles are decreased in kidney transplanted patients with slow graft function and vascular damage. PLoS One. 2014;9:104490.

76. Al-Massarani G, Vacher-Coponat H, Paul P, Arnaud L, Loundou A, Robert S, et al. Kidney transplantation decreases the level and procoagulant activity of circulating microparticles. Am J Transplant. 2009;9:550–7.

77. Quamri Z, Pelletier R, Foster J, Kumar S, Momani H, Ware K, et al. Early posttransplant changes in circulating endothelial microparticles in patients with kidney transplantation. Transplant Immunol. 2014;3:60–4.

78. Wu SY, Mayneris-Perxachs J, Lovegrove JA, Todd S, Yaqoob P. Fish-oil supplementation alters numbers of circulating endothelial progenitor cells and microparticles independently of eNOS genotype. Am J Clin Nutr. 2014; 100:1232–43.

79. Schuerholz T, Weissig A, Juettner B, Becker T, Scheinichen D. Ex vivo microvesicle formation after prolonged ischemia in renal transplantation. Thromb Res. 2007;120:231–6.

80. Renner B, Klawitter J, Goldberg R, McCullough JW, Ferreira VP, Cooper JE, et al. Cyclosporine induces endothelial cell release of complement-activating microparticles. J Am Soc Nephrol. 2013;24:1849–62.

81. Kas-Deelen AM, De Maar EF, Harmsen MC, Driessen C, Van Son WJ, The TH, et al. Uninfected and cytomegalic endothelial cells in blood during cytomegalovirus infection: effect of acute rejection. J Infect Dis. 2000;181:721–4.

9

Modified A-DROP score and mortality in hemodialysis patients with pneumonia

Makoto Harada[1,2*], Takeshi Masubuchi[3,4], Kazuaki Fujii[1,2], Yukifumi Kurasawa[1,2], Tohru Ichikawa[1] and Mamoru Kobayashi[1]

Abstract

Background: Pneumonia is common in hemodialysis (HD) patients and has a poor prognosis, but there is little information on an accurate method for evaluating the severity of pneumonia, which is closely associated with prognosis, in HD patients. This study examined a method for evaluating the severity of pneumonia that was closely associated with 30-day mortality in HD patients.

Methods: This was a retrospective observational study of 64 HD patients. We determined the relationship between the severity of pneumonia using a modified A-DROP (excluding the dehydration section) score and 30-day mortality.

Results: Nine patients (14.1%) died and 40% of patients with an A-DROP score of 3 or 4 died within 30 days. Logistic regression analysis showed that the A-DROP score was significantly associated with 30-day mortality. The discriminatory ability of the A-DROP score was assessed using area under the receiver operating characteristic curve analysis (0.810; 95% confidence interval 0.653–0.967; $p < 0.01$).

Conclusions: This modified A-DROP scoring system reflected the severity of pneumonia and was significantly associated with 30-day mortality. Patients with a modified A-DROP score of 3 or 4 had a poor prognosis.

Keywords: Pneumonia, Hemodialysis patients, A-DROP score

Background

Infectious diseases are one of the main causes of death among hemodialysis (HD) patients, and respiratory infectious diseases, especially pneumonia, are common and resulting in high mortality [1, 2]. HD patients who develop pneumonia are often difficult to treat because they are immune-compromised. They also tend to be elderly, and controlling the antibiotic dose is important [1, 2]. HD patients are also at high risk for blood stream-related infections [3] and methicillin-resistant *Staphylococcus aureus* or drug-resistant bacterial infections [4].

Pneumonia that develops in HD patients is included under the definitions of healthcare-associated pneumonia (HCAP) [5] and nursing and healthcare-associated pneumonia (NHCAP) [6]. Previous reports have suggested that the bacteria causing pneumonia are the same in HD and HCAP patients [4, 7]. However, when evaluating the severity of pneumonia, it is important to differentiate pneumonia in HD patients from HCAP.

There are several scoring systems used to evaluate the severity of community-acquired pneumonia, such as the pneumonia severity index (PSI), CURB65, and A-DROP [8–10]. PSI is a well-known but complex index that includes blood urea nitrogen and pleural effusion and is strongly influenced by dialysis. CURB65 and A-DROP also include blood urea nitrogen [8–10].

It is possible that pneumonia in patients with HD should be distinguished from non-HD patients with HCAP. The method for evaluating the severity of pneumonia in HD patients has not been fully investigated, and the relationship between the severity of pneumonia and prognosis in HD patients is not completely understood.

The Japanese Respiratory Society has recommended that the A-DROP score is used for evaluating the severity of community-acquired pneumonia (CAP) [10]. The A-DROP score is well-known and widely used in Japan. Although the A-DROP score is used for CAP and

* Correspondence: tokomadaraha@yahoo.co.jp
[1]Department of Nephrology, Nagano Red Cross Hospital, 5-22-1, Wakasato, Nagano 380-8582, Japan
[2]Department of Nephrology, Shinshu University School of Medicine, 3-1-1, Asahi, Matsumoto 390-8621, Japan
Full list of author information is available at the end of the article

pneumonia in HD patients categorized as NHCAP [6], a previous report suggests that a very high A-DROP score should be included as a prognostic factor for NHCAP [11]. In the current study, we adopted an A-DROP score based on a new scoring method, a "modified A-DROP score," to evaluate the severity of pneumonia. The modified A-DROP score did not include the dehydration section. We aimed to clarify the usefulness of the modified A-DROP score for evaluating the severity of pneumonia, which is significantly associated with prognosis in HD patients.

Methods

Study design

This was a retrospective observational study. Between January 2011 and December 2016, 64 maintenance HD patients with newly developed pneumonia were admitted to Nagano Red Cross Hospital and all of them were enrolled in the study. The study protocol was approved by the institutional review board of the ethical committee at Nagano Red Cross Hospital and was conducted in accordance with the principles contained within the Declaration of Helsinki as revised in 2013.

Definitions

Pneumonia was defined as the presence of newly developed infiltration on chest X-ray and/or computed tomography and an increase in serum markers of inflammation (C-reactive protein >0.3 mg/dL and/or white blood cell count >10,000/μL). History of cardiovascular disease included angina pectoris, acute myocardial infarction, cerebral hemorrhage, cerebral infarction, peripheral arterial disease, and aortic dissection. History of malignancy included solid tumors, such as colon cancer and gastric cancer, and hematological malignancies, such as lymphoma and myeloma. Chronic lung disease was defined as the presence of chronic obstructive pulmonary disease or interstitial pulmonary disease. Disorientation was evaluated as altered mentality. Altered mentality was defined as a decrease in Japan Coma Scale score. Hypoxia was defined as patients who could not maintain an oxygen saturation level greater than 90% without supplemental oxygen supply. The presence of infiltrates in two or more lobes on chest X-ray and/or computed tomography was defined as multi-lobar lesions. The severity of pneumonia was evaluated using A-DROP score (age [male >70, female >75], dehydration, respiratory failure, orientation disturbance, and low blood pressure) [10]. In general, the dehydration section of the A-DROP scoring system is defined by blood urea nitrogen and physiological findings. In the current study, because our participants were HD patients, we excluded the dehydration section. Briefly, we defined the A-DROP score without including the dehydration section as the

modified A-DROP score. The modified A-DROP score provided values of 0 to 4. Blood culture examinations were obtained within 24 h from admission and before the start of antibiotic therapy. Blood culture examinations were performed on either one or two sets. Clinical outcomes were defined as all-cause mortality within 30 days of hospital admission, clinical success of antibiotic therapy, duration of antibiotic therapy, and hospital mortality. Clinical success meant that pneumonia was successfully treated with the antibiotic selected at admission and that antibiotic was not changed except for the purpose of de-escalation. Failure of treatment was defined as death or a change in antibiotic from the initial therapy.

Statistical analysis

Continuous variables between the two groups were compared using the Mann–Whitney U test, and categorical variables were compared using Fisher's exact probability test. Continuous variables among three groups were compared using the Kruskal–Wallis test, and multiple comparisons between two groups were compared using the Mann–Whitney U test with Bonferroni correction. Factors associated with the clinical outcomes were analyzed using logistic regression analyses. The discriminatory ability of the factors was evaluated using the area under the receiver operating characteristic curve (AUC) analysis. A p value <0.05 was considered statistically significant. Analyses were performed using EZR (Saitama Medical Center, Jichi Medical University, Saitama, Japan), which is a graphical user interface for R (the R Foundation for Statistical Computing, Vienna, Austria) [12].

Results

Patient characteristics

The clinical characteristics of all 64 patients are shown in Table 1. The median age was 75 years. Forty-seven patients were male and 17 female. The main cause of HD was diabetic nephropathy (27 patients, 42.2%). Arteriovenous fistula or arteriovenous graft was the main type of vascular access. Thirty-four patients (53.1%) had cardiovascular disease complications, 21 (32.8%) had altered mentality, and 45 (70.3%) had hypoxia. Blood culture examinations were performed for 47 patients (73.4%), and three patients (6.4%) were positive. Forty-two patients (65.6%) had multi-lobar lung infiltration, and 43 patients (67.2%) had pleural effusion. The severities of pneumonia evaluated using the modified A-DROP score were eight patients (12.5%) scored 0, 19 (29.7%) scored 1, 22 (34.4%) scored 2, 13 (20.3%) scored 3, and two (3.1%) scored 4. Nine patients (14.1%) died within 30 days of hospitalization, and 11 patients (17.2%) died in the all hospitalization period.

Table 1 Background clinical data and characteristics of all patients

Clinical characteristics		
Age (years)	75	37–88
Male (n, %)	47	73.4
BMI (kg/m^2)	20.3	14.3–40.9
Duration of HD (months)	40	1–290
Cause of HD		
DMN (n, %)	27	42.2
Chronic GN (n, %)	21	32.8
Nephrosclerosis (n, %)	10	15.7
RPGN (n, %)	4	6.2
Other (n, %)	2	3.1
Vascular access		
AVF (n, %)	42	65.6
AVG (n, %)	15	23.5
Catheter (n, %)	7	10.9
Comorbidity		
CVD (n, %)	34	53.1
Malignancy (n, %)	12	18.8
CLD (n, %)	13	20.3
Vital signs		
Systolic BP (mmHg)	138	68–204
Diastolic BP (mmHg)	70	40–141
Heart rate (/min)	95	58–142
Altered mentality (n, %)	21	32.8
Fever (degree)	37.6	35.0–39.6
Hypoxia (n, %)	45	70.3
Blood examination		
Alb (g/dL)	3.1	2.0–4.3
BUN (mg/dL)	36.6	12.9–84.5
Cr (mg/dL)	5.49	1.48–13.32
Na (mEq/L)	139	129–147
K (mEq/L)	4.3	2.9–8.4
CRP (mg/dL)	8.2	0.9–43.1
WBC (/µL)	9590	3130–33520
Hb (g/dL)	10.7	4.1–16.5
Plt (×10^4/µL)	15.6	2.1–72.0
Bacterial cultures		
Sputum (n, %)	54	84.4
Blood (n, %)	47	73.4
Radiological findings		
Multi-lobar lesion (n, %)	42	65.6
Pleural effusion (n, %)	43	67.2

Table 1 Background clinical data and characteristics of all patients (Continued)

Severity of pneumonia		
Modified A-DROP		
0 (n, %)	8	12.5
1 (n, %)	19	29.7
2 (n, %)	22	34.4
3 (n, %)	13	20.3
4 (n, %)	2	3.1
Therapy and prognosis		
Success of initial therapy (n, %)	46	71.9
Duration of antibiotics (days)	11	1–43
30-day mortality (n, %)	9	14.1
Hospital mortality (n, %)	11	17.2

Data for continuous variables are expressed as median and range, and categorical variables are expressed as number and percentage
Alb albumin, AVF arteriovenous fistula, AVG arteriovenous graft, BMI body mass index, BP blood pressure, BUN blood urea nitrogen, CLD chronic lung diseases, Cr creatinine, CRP C-reactive protein, CVD cardiovascular disease, DMN diabetes mellitus nephropathy, K potassium, Na sodium, GN glomerulonephritis, HD hemodialysis, Hb hemoglobin, Plt platelet, RPGN rapid progressive glomerunephritis, WBC white blood cell count

Severity of pneumonia and clinical outcomes

One patient (3.7%) with a modified A-DROP score of 0 or 1 died, two patients (9.1%) with a modified A-DROP score of 2 died, and six patients (40.0%) with a modified A-DROP score of 3 or 4 died within 30 days of hospitalization (Fig. 1). Forty-six patients (71.9%) were successfully treated with initial antibiotic therapy. The median duration of antibiotic therapy was 11 days. The clinical characteristics among the three groups (modified A-DROP score 0 or 1, 2 or 3, or 4) is shown in Table 2.

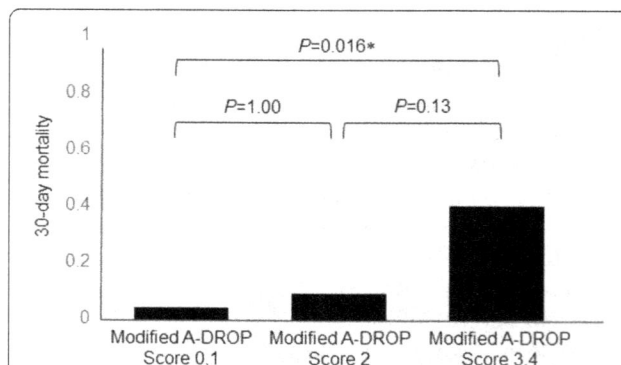

Fig. 1 Relationship between modified A-DROP score and 30-day mortality. Thirty-day mortality in patients with A-DROP score of 0 or 1 were 3.7%, with A-DROP score of 2 were 9.1%, and with A-DROP score of 3 or 4 were 40.0%. 30-day mortality in patients with A-DROP score of 3 or 4 were significantly higher than that in patients with A-DROP score of 0 or 1. A $p < 0.05$ was considered statistically significant and asterisk indicated $p < 0.05$

Table 2 Background clinical data and characteristics of each group

Severity of pneumonia	Modified A-DROP 0, 1 n = 27		Modified A-DROP 2 n = 22		Modified A-DROP 3, 4 n = 15		p value
Age (years)	65	37–81	76	59–88	81	74–88	<0.001***
Male (n, %)	16	59.3	19	86.4	12	80.0	0.09
BMI (kg/m^2)	20.7	16.1–40.9	19.4	14.3–26.3	20.4	14.8–23.9	0.66
Duration of HD (months)	47	3–231	37	2–290	48	1–154	0.97
Cause of HD							
DMN (n, %)	8	29.7	12	54.6	7	46.7	0.20
Chronic GN (n, %)	10	37.0	6	27.3	5	33.3	0.75
Nephrosclerosis (n, %)	5	18.5	2	9.1	3	20.0	0.62
RPGN (n, %)	3	11.1	1	4.5	0	0	0.54
Other (n, %)	1	3.7	1	4.5	0	0	1.00
Vascular access							
AVF (n, %)	21	77.8	13	59.1	8	53.3	0.21
AVG (n, %)	3	11.1	8	36.4	4	26.7	0.10
Catheter (n, %)	3	11.1	1	4.5	3	20.0	0.40
Comorbidity							
CVD (n, %)	13	48.1	10	45.5	11	73.3	0.23
Malignancy (n, %)	4	14.8	4	18.2	4	26.7	0.65
CLD (n, %)	6	22.2	5	22.7	2	13.3	0.85
Vital signs							
Systolic BP (mmHg)	129	88–204	150	97–170	120	68–203	0.18
Diastolic BP (mmHg)	74	53–103	72	47–141	64	40–99	0.24
Heart rate (/min)	98	68–142	96	68–136	94	58–130	0.49
Altered mentality (n, %)	0	0	7	31.8	14	93.3	<0.001***
Fever (degree)	37.1	35.5–39.6	37.7	35.0–39.3	37.8	36.1–39.3	0.38
Hypoxia (n, %)	11	40.7	19	86.4	15	100	<0.001***
Blood examination							
Alb (g/dL)	3.1	2.1–4.1	3.3	2.1–4.3	3.0	2.0–3.9	0.39
BUN (mg/dL)	35.2	13.2–80.7	39.4	12.9–84.5	34.2	13.6–74.3	0.48
Cr (mg/dL)	5.99	1.48–13.32	5.23	2.10–13.05	5.25	2.65–11.20	0.26
Na (mEq/L)	138	129–145	140	132–147	140	131–147	0.11
K (mEq/L)	4.2	3.2-5.9	4.5	3.5–8.2	4.1	2.9–8.4	0.25
CRP (mg/dL)	7.91	1.21–30.80	9.16	0.85–43.12	9.54	1.37–13.99	0.98
WBC (/μL)	9600	4220–23100	9910	3130–33520	9580	3600–28910	0.99
Hb (g/dL)	10.6	4.1–16.5	10.9	7.6–14.4	10.5	7.1–13.5	0.98
Plt (x 10^4/μL)	16.2	2.7–50.0	17.6	2.1–31.3	14.4	6.8–72.0	0.88
Bacterial cultures							
Sputum (n, %)	20	74.1	20	90.9	14	93.3	0.22
Blood (n, %)	17	63.0	20	90.9	10	66.7	0.07
Radiological findings							
Multi-lobar lesion (n, %)	15	55.6	15	68.2	12	80.0	0.26
Pleural effusion (n, %)	14	51.9	15	68.2	14	93.3	0.012*

Table 2 Background clinical data and characteristics of each group *(Continued)*

Therapy and prognosis							
Success of initial therapy							
(n, %)	21	77.8	17	77.3	8	53.3	0.22
Duration of antibiotics							
(days)	8	1–43	12	3–36	13	3–36	0.023*
30-day mortality (n, %)	1	3.7	2	9.1	6	40.0	0.004**
Hospital mortality (n, %)	1	3.7	3	13.6	7	46.7	0.003**

Data for continuous variables are expressed as median and range, and categorical variables are expressed as number and percentages. Categorical variables were compared using Fisher's exact probability test, and continuous variables among three groups were compared using the Kruskal–Wallis test. Significant difference are indicated with asterisks (***$p < 0.001$, **$p < 0.01$, *$p < 0.05$)

Alb albumin, *AVF* arteriovenous fistula, *AVG* arteriovenous graft, *BMI* body mass index, *BP* blood pressure, *BUN* blood urea nitrogen, *CLD* chronic lung diseases, *Cr* creatinine, *CRP* C-reactive protein, *CVD* cardiovascular diseases, *DMN* diabetes mellitus nephropathy, *K* potassium, *Na* sodium, *GN* glomerulonephritis, *HD* hemodialysis, *Hb* hemoglobin, *Plt* platelet, *RPGN* rapid progressive glomerulonephritis, *WBC* white blood cell count

Age, altered mentality, hypoxia, pleural effusion, duration of antibiotic therapy, 30-day mortality, and hospital mortality were significantly different among the three groups. Logistic regression analysis showed that the modified A-DROP score was significantly associated with 30-day mortality (Table 3). The discriminatory ability of the modified A-DROP score was assessed using AUC analysis (AUC 0.810; 95%CI 0.653–0.967; $p < 0.01$) (Fig. 2).

Bacteria and antibiotic therapy

α-Streptococcus, *Candida*, *Neisseria*, and *S. aureus* were the main pathogens detected in sputum cultures, while *Streptococcus pneumoniae* and *Branhamella catarrhalis* were detected in a few cases only (Table 4). *Klebsiella pneumoniae* was detected in two patients and *S. pneumoniae* was detected in one patient from blood cultures. Ampicillin/sulbactam, tazobactam/piperacillin, and meropenem were the main initial antibiotic therapies (Table 5).

Discussion

Previous studies have reported hospital mortality from pneumonia in HD patients as 12.4% and 30-day mortality as 11.6% [1, 13]. In the current study, 30-day mortality was 14.1% and prognosis was similar as the previous studies. A previous study compared the prognosis between HD patients with pneumonia and patients with HCAP and did not find a significant difference [7]. In addition, the bacteria causing pneumonia in HD patients

and HCAP are similar. Thus, the clinical characteristics between the two groups are similar.

When predicting the prognosis of pneumonia or evaluating the severity of pneumonia, either the PSI, CURB65, or A-DROP scoring systems are used. However, these scoring systems include blood urea nitrogen, dehydration, or pleural effusion [8–10], which are strongly influenced by renal impairment and dialysis. This means that it is difficult to accurately evaluate the severity of pneumonia in dialysis patients. In such patients, the severity of pneumonia should be evaluated using a scoring system that excludes those factors associated with kidney function or dialysis.

Table 3 Association between 30-day mortality and modified A-DROP score

	OR	CI	p value
Modified A-DROP	4.67	1.63–13.3	0.004**

Logistic regression analysis reveals the association between 30-day mortality and modified A-DROP score. Significant difference are indicated with asterisks (**$p < 0.01$)

CI confidence interval, *OR* odds ratio

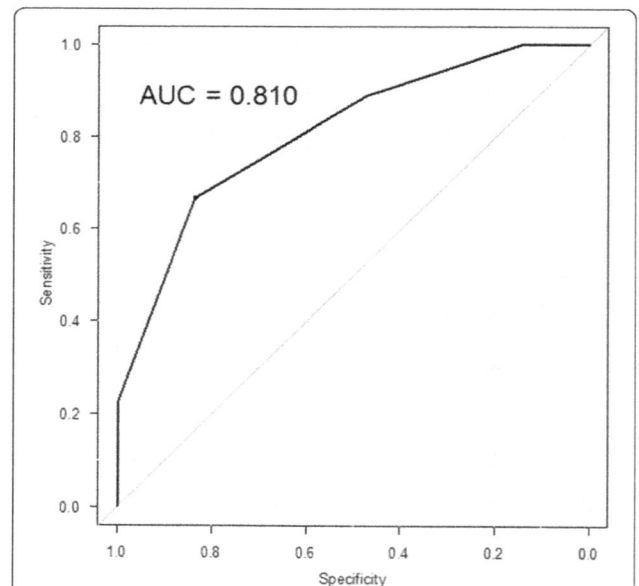

Fig. 2 Area under the receiver operating characteristic curve analysis between the death within 30 days of hospital admission and modified A-DROP score. The discriminatory ability of the modified A-DROP score evaluated by using AUC analysis (AUC 0.810; 95%CI 0.653–0.967; $p < 0.01$)

Table 4 Type of bacteria isolated from sputum cultures

Type of bacteria	n
α-Streptococcus spp.	35
Candida spp.	35
Neisseria spp.	20
Staphylococcus aureus (including MRSA)	17
Haemophilus parainfluenzae	8
Corynebacterium spp.	7
Klebsiella oxytoca	6
Escherichia coli (including ESBL-producing E. coli)	6
Staphylococcus epidermidis	5
Klebsiella pneumoniae	3
Pseudomonas aeruginosa	3
Branhamella catarrhalis	2
Serratia marcescens	1
Streptococcus pneumoniae	1
Streptococcus agalactiae	1
Acinetobacter baumannii	1
Enterobacter	1
Citrobacter spp.	1

ESBL extended spectrum beta-lactamase, MRSA methicillin-resistant Staphylococcus aureus, Spp species

Table 5 Details of initial antibiotic therapy

Initial antibiotic therapy	n
ABPC/SBT	16
ABPC/SBT + CPFX	4
ABPC/SBT + LVFX	1
TAZ/PIPC	8
TAZ/PIPC + LZD	1
CMZ	1
CTRX	4
CTRX + CLDM	3
CPZ/SBT	1
CPZ/SBT + AZM	1
CFPM	1
CFPM + CLDM	1
BIPM	1
MEPM	10
MEPM + CPFX	1
MEPM + PZFX	1
MEPM + LZD	1
DRPM + TEIC	1
AZM	1
AZT + VCM	1
PZFX	4
LVFX	1

ABPC/SBT ampicillin/sulbactam, AZM azithromycin, AZT aztreonam, BIPM biapenem, CFPM cefepime, CLDM clindamycin, CMZ cefmetazole, CPFX ciprofloxacin, CPZ/SBT cefoperazone/sulbactam, CTRX ceftriaxone, DRPM doripenem, LVFX levofloxacin, LZD linezolid, MEPM meropenem, PZFX pazufloxacin, TAZ/PIPC tazobactam/piperacillin, TEIC teicoplanin, VCM vancomycin

In the current study, we used the A-DROP scoring system but excluded the dehydration section to evaluate the severity of pneumonia in HD patients. The modified A-DROP score was found to be significantly associated with prognosis in HD patients with pneumonia. It is suggested that the modified A-DROP score is useful for evaluating the severity of pneumonia in HD patients. A benefit of this system is that clinical data (age, blood pressure, orientation, and hypoxia) are easy to obtain and do not require blood examinations. In short, the modified A-DROP score is a good and convenient option not only in hospitals but also in HD clinics.

With regard to the bacteria isolated from sputum cultures, gram-positive coccus such as α-Streptococcus and S. aureus were the main species detected. S. pneumoniae and B. catarrhalis are often detected in non-HD patients presenting with pneumonia [14, 15]. A previous study by Kawasaki et al. reported that S. pneumonia is the second most frequently detected pathogen in HD patients with pneumonia [13]. However, S. pneumonia and B. catarrhalis were detected in only a few cases. Most patients were elderly and some presented with dysphagia and might develop aspiration pneumonia. Therefore, the detected bacteria were not S. pneumonia or B. catarrhalis but indigenous bacterium of the oral cavity such as α-Streptococcus.

This study examined HD patients, who have an increased risk for blood stream infections; however, there were only three patients (6.4%) with positive blood cultures. A previous study of non-HD patients with pneumonia reported a positive blood culture rate of 5.7%, and it was not associated with the severity of pneumonia evaluated using PSI [16]. These results suggest that blood culture examination is not useful for detecting the causative microorganism in patients with bacterial pneumonia. Recently, routine blood culture examinations have been not recommended for patients presenting with pneumonia [17].

This study had some limitations. We could not fully evaluate the severity of pneumonia using CURB65 or PSI. Because we could not obtain data for respiration rates, we evaluated the severity of pneumonia using the modified A-DROP score. Although smoking is a risk factor for community-acquired pneumonia [18], we were unable to obtain patient smoking histories. Bedridden patients or patients with dysphagia often have repeated aspiration pneumonia and have a poor prognosis, and activities of daily living and cognitive impairment are important for the prognosis of pneumonia [19]. However, we could not obtain data about patients' activities of daily living or cognitive function. Although this study had a small sample size, we collected and analyzed clinical data such as the severity of pneumonia and prognosis, duration of antibiotic therapy, and success of initial therapy in details. We could not diagnose whether a patient had aspiration pneumonia as it is difficult to correctly diagnose if a patient presenting with pneumonia has aspiration pneumonia. Because information of the quality of sputum could not be obtained, some sputum samples mainly contained salivary contents, resulting detecting indigenous bacterium of the oral cavity.

We could not unify the timing of evaluation of the modified A-DROP score in the current study. Therefore, we examined when the modified A-DROP score was evaluated. According to the timing of HD sessions, we divided the timing of the modified A-DROP score evaluation into three groups: (1) before HD sessions, (2) between HD sessions, and (3) after HD sessions. Eighteen patients were evaluated for the modified A-DROP score before HD sessions, 25 were evaluated between HD sessions, and 21 were evaluated after HD sessions. Because it is possible that blood pressure, fluid volume, and hypoxia can change depending on the timing of a HD session, and this can influence the evaluation of the A-DROP score (as well as the modified A-DROP score being influenced by when the modified A-DROP score was evaluated), we compared the frequency of the modified A-DROP score among the three groups (before HD sessions, between HD sessions, and after HD sessions). As a result, the frequency of the modified A-DROP score was not significantly different among the groups (Additional file 1: Table S1). However, not unifying the timing of evaluation of the modified A-DROP score is a limitation of the current study.

Conclusions

In conclusion, the modified A-DROP score reflected the severity of pneumonia and was significantly associated with 30-day mortality in this population of HD patients. Patients with a modified A-DROP score of 3 or 4 had a poor prognosis.

Abbreviations
AUC: Area under the receiver operating characteristic curve; HCAP: Healthcare-associated pneumonia; HD: Hemodialysis; PSI: Pneumonia severity index

Acknowledgements
None.

Funding
Not applicable.

Authors' contributions
MH, KF, and YK designed the study and collected the data. MH and TI wrote the manuscript. TM and MK corrected the manuscript, tables, and figures. All authors read and approved the final manuscript.

Competing interests
The authors declare that they have no competing interests.

Author details
[1]Department of Nephrology, Nagano Red Cross Hospital, 5-22-1, Wakasato, Nagano 380-8582, Japan. [2]Department of Nephrology, Shinshu University School of Medicine, 3-1-1, Asahi, Matsumoto 390-8621, Japan. [3]Department of Infection and Host Defense, Nagano Red Cross Hospital, 5-22-1, Wakasato, Nagano 380-8582, Japan. [4]Department of Respiratory Medicine, Nagano Red Cross Hospital, 5-22-1, Wakasato, Nagano 380-8582, Japan.

References
1. Slinin Y, Foley RN, Collins AJ. Clinical epidemiology of pneumonia in hemodialysis patients: the USRDS waves 1, 3, and 4 study. Kidney Int. 2006; 70:1135–41.
2. Sarnak MJ, Jaber BL. Pulmonary infectious mortality among patients with end-stage renal disease. Chest. 2001;120:1883–7.
3. Patel PR, Yi SH, Booth S, Bren V, Downham G, Hess S, et al. Bloodstream infection rates in outpatient hemodialysis facilities participating in a collaborative prevention effort: a quality improvement report. Am J Kidney Dis. 2013;62:322–30.
4. Wang PH, Wang HC. Risk factors to predict drug-resistant pathogens in hemodialysis-associated pneumonia. BMC Infect Dis. 2016;16:377.
5. Kollef MH, Morrow LE, Baughman RP, Craven DE, McGowan Jr JE, Micek ST, et al. Health care-associated pneumonia (HCAP): a critical appraisal to improve identification, management, and outcomes—proceedings of the HCAP Summit. Clin Infect Dis. 2008;46 Suppl 4:S296–334.
6. Kohno S, Imamura Y, Shindo Y, Seki M, Ishida T, Teramoto S, et al. Clinical practice guidelines for nursing- and healthcare-associated pneumonia (NHCAP). Respir Investig. 2013;51:103–26 [complete translation].
7. Lee JH, Moon JC. Clinical characteristics of patients with hemodialysis-associated pneumonia compared to patients with non-hemodialysis community-onset pneumonia. Respir Med. 2016;111:84–90.
8. Arnold FW, Ramirez JA, McDonald LC, Xia EL. Hospitalization for community-acquired pneumonia: the pneumonia severity index vs clinical judgment. Chest. 2003;124:121–4.
9. Barlow G, Nathwani D, Davey P. The CURB65 pneumonia severity score outperforms generic sepsis and early warning scores in predicting mortality in community-acquired pneumonia. Thorax. 2007;62:253–9.
10. Shindo Y, Sato S, Maruyama E, Ohashi T, Ogawa M, Imaizumi K, et al. Comparison of severity scoring systems A-DROP and CURB-65 for community-acquired pneumonia. Respirology. 2008;13:731–5.
11. Oshitani Y, Nagai H, Matsui H, Aoshima M. Reevaluation of the Japanese guideline for healthcare-associated pneumonia in a medium-sized community hospital in Japan. J Infect Chemother. 2013;19:579–87.
12. Kanda Y. Investigation of the freely available easy-to-use software 'EZR' for medical statistics. Bone Marrow Transplant. 2013;48:452–8.
13. Kawasaki S, Aoki N, Kikuchi H, Nakayama H, Saito N, Shimada H, et al. Clinical and microbiological evaluation of hemodialysis-associated pneumonia (HDAP): should HDAP be included in healthcare-associated pneumonia? J Infect Chemother. 2011;17:640–5.
14. Saito A, Kohno S, Matsushima T, Watanabe A, Oizumi K, Yamaguchi K, et al. Prospective multicenter study of the causative organisms of community-acquired pneumonia in adults in Japan. J Infect Chemother. 2006;12:63–9.
15. Ishida T, Hashimoto T, Arita M, Tojo Y, Tachibana H, Jinnai M. A 3-year prospective study of a urinary antigen-detection test for Streptococcus pneumoniae in community-acquired pneumonia: utility and clinical impact on the reported etiology. J Infect Chemother. 2004;10:359–63.

16. Campbell SG, Marrie TJ, Anstey R, Dickinson G, Ackroyd-Stolarz S. The contribution of blood cultures to the clinical management of adult patients admitted to the hospital with community-acquired pneumonia: a prospective observational study. Chest. 2003;123:1142–50.

17. Wunderink RG, Waterer GW. Clinical practice. Community-acquired pneumonia. N Engl J Med. 2014;370:543–51.

18. Baik I, Curhan GC, Rimm EB, Bendich A, Willett WC, Fawzi WW. A prospective study of age and lifestyle factors in relation to community-acquired pneumonia in US men and women. Arch Intern Med. 2000;160:3082–8.

19. Salive ME, Satterfield S, Ostfeld AM, Wallace RB, Havlik RJ. Disability and cognitive impairment are risk factors for pneumonia-related mortality in older adults. Public Health Rep. 1993;108:314–22.

10

Association between B-lines detected during lung ultrasound and various factors in hemodialysis patients

Shinzo Kuzuhara[1,2], Shigeru Otsubo[1,3*], Katsuya Kajimoto[4], Takashi Akiba[2] and Kosaku Nitta[1]

Abstract

Background: In recent years, the use of chest ultrasonography to detect lung water has received growing attention in clinical research. Estimation of the number of B-lines using lung ultrasound is now a standard method for the evaluation of pulmonary congestion. In the present study, we examined the relation between the number of B-lines and clinical parameters in hemodialysis patients.

Methods: A total of 49 consecutive patients receiving maintenance hemodialysis were enrolled in this study. Lung ultrasound was performed using Vscan® (GE Healthcare, Japan). Bilateral scanning of the anterior and lateral chest walls was performed with the patient in a supine position just after the start of the hemodialysis therapy. The total number of B-lines was estimated. We investigated the relationships between the number of B-lines and other clinical parameters.

Results: Patient heart rate and the serum log [NT-proBNP] level were positively correlated ($P = 0.009$ and 0.003, respectively), and body weight and the serum albumin and creatinine level were negatively correlated with the number of B-lines ($P = 0.023$, 0.001, and 0.011, respectively).

Conclusions: The number of B-lines was positively correlated with the serum N-terminal pro-brain natriuretic peptide level. Lung ultrasound can quantify lung edema. Body weight and the serum albumin and creatinine level were negatively correlated with the number of B-lines. Careful attention to the presence of pulmonary edema is needed in patients with a low body weight and a low serum albumin and creatinine level.

Keywords: B-lines, Hemodialysis, Lung ultrasound, N-terminal pro-brain natriuretic peptide

Background

Chronic fluid overloading frequently occurs in hemodialysis patients, so one of the major targets of hemodialysis therapy is to maintain a normal extracellular volume status. Preventing volume overload is a central recommendation when it comes to nephrology best-practice guidelines for dialysis patients [1], as this goal is directly associated with hypertension, increased arterial stiffness, left ventricular hypertrophy, heart failure, and ultimately higher rates of mortality and morbidity [2].

To estimate the volume status, several methods have been proposed, such as evaluating the natriuretic peptide levels [3, 4], the dimensions and collapsibility of the inferior vena cava [5], chest X-ray signs, and bioelectrical impedance analysis techniques [6, 7]. However, each of these methods has significant theoretical and practical limitations.

In recent years, the use of chest ultrasonography to detect lung water has received growing attention in clinical research focused on intensive care patients [8] and patients with heart failure [9]. The most commonly observed finding was a comet tail artifact fanning out from the lung-wall interface and spreading upwards to the edge of the screen, previously named a "B-line" (Fig. 1) [10]. In patients with heart failure, the number of B-lines was correlated with the degree of extravascular lung water [11], and

---
* Correspondence: sotsubo@hb.tp1.jp
[1]Department of Medicine, Kidney Center, Tokyo Women's Medical University, Tokyo, Japan
[3]Department of Blood Purification, Tohto Sangenjaya Clinic, 2-13-2 Taishido, Setagaya-ku, Tokyo 154-0004, Japan
Full list of author information is available at the end of the article

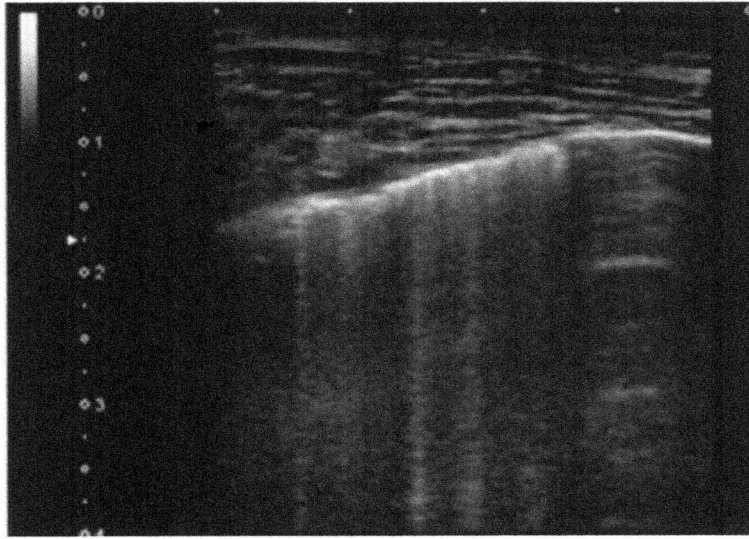

Fig. 1 B-lines: comet tail artifacts fanning out from the lung-wall interface and spreading upwards to the edge of the screen

a reduction in the number of B-lines reflected the efficacy of treatment [1]. Previous studies have also shown that lung ultrasound can detect extravascular lung water and can be used to show a significant reduction after a dialytic session (both hemodialysis and peritoneal dialysis) [12–15]. Existing data suggest that lung ultrasound characteristics might be suitable for assessing the ideal body weight in hemodialysis patients, since this technique is simple, inexpensive, nonionizing, and can easily be performed at the patient's bedside [16, 17].

Consequently, estimation of the number of B-lines using lung ultrasound is now a standard method for the evaluation of pulmonary congestion [18]. In the present study, we examined the relation between the number of B-lines and clinical parameters in hemodialysis patients.

Methods

The proportion of hospitalization for acute heart failure in hemodialysis patients was significantly higher on Monday (approximately 1/3) compared with other days [19]. So we selected patients who underwent hemodialysis therapy on Monday (the first day after weekend interval). A total of 49 consecutive patients receiving maintenance hemodialysis at Sekikawa Hospital on Monday were enrolled in this study. Informed consents were obtained in all patients.

Clinical data including age, sex, duration of hemodialysis therapy, presence of diabetes mellitus and/or hypertension and/or dyslipidemia complications, use of antihypertensive drug, history of coronary artery disease, and the results of biological examinations were collected from the patient's clinical records. Hypertension was defined as a systolic

blood pressure of 140 mmHg or higher, a diastolic blood pressure of 90 mmHg or higher, and/or the current use of antihypertensive drugs. Diabetes mellitus was defined as a fasting glucose level $\geq$126 mg/dL, a nonfasting glucose level $\geq$200 mg/dL, or the use of medication. Dyslipidemia was defined as a low-density lipoprotein-cholesterol level $\geq$140 mg/dL, a high-density lipoprotein-cholesterol level <40 mg/dL, a triglyceride level $\geq$150 mg/dL, or the use of medication.

A peripheral blood sample was obtained before hemodialysis during the first session of the week. The serum N-terminal pro-brain natriuretic peptide (NT-proBNP) level in the pre-dialysis blood sample was measured using an electrochemiluminescence immunoassay on an Elecsys platform (Roche, Basel, Switzerland).

Lung ultrasound was performed at the first session of the week, the same time of peripheral blood sample preparation, using Vscan® (GE Healthcare, Japan), a hand-held ultrasound device with a wide-bandwidth phased-array probe (1.7–3.5 MHz) [20, 21]. Bilateral scanning of the anterior and lateral chest walls was performed with the patient in a supine position just after the start of the hemodialysis therapy. An intercostal scan with maximum extension of the visual pleural line was performed. The chest wall was divided into eight areas (two anterior and two lateral areas per side), and two scan was obtained for each area [22–26]. The anterior zone of the chest wall was designated from the sternum to the anterior axillary line and was then divided into upper and lower halves (from the clavicle to the third intercostal spaces and from the third space to the diaphragm). The lateral zone was positioned from the anterior axillary line to the posterior axillary line and was also divided into the upper and lower halves. Cardiologist, who is blind to the result of blood peripheral blood sample, attempted to detect comet tail artifacts fanning out from the lung-wall interface and spreading to the edge of the screen, which were previously named B-lines (Additional file 1: Movie S1) [23, 24]. The total number of B-lines was estimated. Echocardiographic measurements were obtained at the same time and left ventricular ejection fraction (LVEF) was estimated.

We investigated the relationships between the number of B-lines and other clinical parameters. This study was conducted in accordance with the principles of the Declaration of Helsinki and was permitted by the research ethics committee of Sekikawa Hospital (Approved No. H2705). The data were expressed as the means ± SD or median (interquartile range, IQR). A simple and multivariate regression analysis was used to examine the relationship between two continuous variables. Because of the skewed distribution of the NT-proBNP levels, the data were normalized using a logarithmic transformation for further statistical analysis. All the statistical calculations were performed using JMP 5.1 software. P values less than 0.05 were considered statistically significant.

Results

The patient background characteristics are shown in Table 1. The mean age was 74.5 ± 11.2 years. Elderly patients were common in this study. Diabetic nephropathy was the major cause of end-stage kidney disease. Hypertension, diabetes mellitus, and dyslipidemia were present in 83.7, 42.9, and 20.4% of the study participants, respectively. The mean number of B-lines was 10.8 ± 4.6. The results of the biochemistry analyses, including the NT-proBNP level, are shown in Table 2. The serum albumin level was relatively low (3.2 ± 0.5 g/dL), and the serum NT-proBNP level was relatively high (13,404 (4355–28,011) pg/mL) among the study participants.

Table 3 shows the relationships between the number of B-lines and other clinical parameters. Heart rate and the serum log [NT-proBNP] level were positively correlated (P = 0.009 and 0.003, respectively), and body weight and the serum albumin and creatinine levels were negatively correlated with the number of B-lines (P = 0.023, 0.001 and 0.011, respectively). Patient age tended to be positively associate with the number of B-lines (P = 0.055). LVEF tended to negatively relate to the number of B-lines (P = 0.056). In multivariate analysis including body weight and heart rate and the serum albumin, creatinine, and log [NT-proBNP] levels, only the serum log [NT-proBNP] level remained significant relation to the number of B-lines (P = 0.014).

Discussion

We showed that the number of B-lines was positively correlated with heart rate and the serum NT-proBNP

Table 1 Background characteristics of the study participants

Characteristic	Quantity
Gender (M/F)	24/25
Age (year)	74.5 ± 11.2
Duration of HD (year)	3.4 (2.1–7.2)
Primary cause of ESKD, n (%)	
Chronic glomerulonephritis	8 (16.3)
Diabetic nephropathy	22 (44.9)
Nephrosclerosis	10 (20.4)
Unknown and others	9 (18.4)
Hypertension, n (%)	41 (83.7)
Diabetes mellitus, n (%)	21 (42.9)
Dyslipidemia, n (%)	10 (20.4)
Atrial fibrillation, n (%)	6 (12.2)
Use of antihypertensive drug, n (%)	38 (77.6)
History of coronary artery disease, n (%)	
PCI	4 (8.2)
CABG	3 (6.1)
Vascular access	
Arteriovenous fistula	43 (87.8)
Arteriovenous graft	2 (4.1)
Subcutaneously fixed superficial artery	2 (4.1)
Venous catheter	2 (4.1)
Body weight (kg)	52.7 ± 11.5
Systolic blood pressure (mmHg)	141 ± 26
Diastolic blood pressure (mmHg)	73 ± 16
Heart rate (beat/minute)	75 ± 13
Ejection fraction (%)	60 ± 12
B-lines (number)	10.8 ± 4.6

Mean ± SD, median (interquartile range: IQR)
HD hemodialysis, *ESKD* end-stage kidney disease, *PCI* percutaneous coronary intervention, *CABG* coronary artery bypass grafting

Table 2 Background characteristics of laboratory data

Characteristic	Quantity
Albumin (g/dL)	3.2 ± 0.5
Urea nitrogen (mg/dL)	51.8 ± 19.0
Creatinine (mg/dL)	7.57 ± 2.41
Sodium (mEq/L)	137 ± 4
C-reactive protein (mg/dL)	0.26 (0.10–0.91)
Hemoglobin (g/dL)	10.4 ± 1.2
NT-proBNP (pg/mL)	13,650 (4355–28,011)
log [NT-ProBNP (pg/mL)]	9.26 ± 1.33

Mean ± SD, median (interquartile range: IQR)
NT-proBNP N-terminal pro-brain natriuretic peptide

Table 3 The relationship between the number of B-lines and other clinical parameters

	r	P value
Age (years)	0.276	0.055
Duration of HD (year)	0.026	0.576
Body weight (kg)	−0.325	0.023
Systolic blood pressure (mmHg)	−0.103	0.479
Diastolic blood pressure (mmHg)	0.013	0.928
Heart rate (beat/minute)	0.371	0.009
Ejection fraction (%)	−0.275	0.056
Albumin (g/dL)	−0.444	0.001
Urea nitrogen (mg/dL)	−0.159	0.276
Creatinine (mg/dL)	−0.360	0.011
Sodium (mEq/L)	−0.248	0.085
C-reactive protein (mg/dL)	0.063	0.666
Hemoglobin (g/dL)	−0.197	0.175
NT-ProBNP	0.523	<0.001
log [NT-ProBNP]	0.447	0.002

HD hemodialysis, *NT-proBNP* N-terminal pro-brain natriuretic peptide

level, while it was negatively correlated with the body weight and the serum albumin and creatinine level.

Lung ultrasound assessments of extravascular lung water based on the number of B-lines provide an excellent diagnostic alternative, expanding the already established role of transthoracic echocardiography for patients with heart failure [2, 27–29]. Bedetti et al. compared lung ultrasound information obtained by experienced echocardiologists and by inexperienced echocardiographer with very limited (30') dedicated training on B-lines assessment and reveal, there was a significant, tight correlation ($r = 0.958$, $p < 0.001$) between the two observations in the same patient [30]. B-lines can be evaluated anywhere (including extreme environmental conditions using pocket-sized instruments to detect high-altitude pulmonary edema), anytime (during dialysis), by anyone (even a novice sonographer after 1 h of training), and on anybody (since the chest acoustic window usually remains patent even when an echocardiography is not feasible) [18]. The pre-dialysis number of B-lines significantly correlated with a whole body bioimpedance spectroscopy device-derived extracellular water in hemodialysis patients [31]. Vitturi et al. investigated lung and bioimpedance spectroscopy results immediately before and after dialysis and reported that a reduction in the number of B-lines was correlated with fluid loss as a result of hemodialysis, conforming that lung ultrasound can identify extravascular lung water. The number of post-dialysis B-lines is correlated with the residual weight assessed using bioimpedance, suggesting a role for ultrasound in the management of

hemodialysis patients [32]. The serum NT-proBNP level is influenced not only by heart function but also by the volume status. Among nondialysis patients, lung congestion was correlated with the NT-proBNP level [22]. Natriuretic peptides may directly enhance capillary permeability, an effect that may explain the association in addition to filling pressure alone [33]. In this study, we also showed a positive and independent relationship between the number of B-lines and the serum NT-proBNP level in hemodialysis patients.

We also showed that the number of B-lines was positively correlated with heart rate and negatively correlated with body weight and the serum albumin and creatinine level. Volume overload results in lung congestion and also activates the sympathetic nervous system which increases the heart rate. Hypoalbuminemia is common in heart failure patients [34, 35]. Two mechanisms have been proposed to explain the relationship between hypoalbuminemia and congestion. On the one hand, an increase in vascular permeability mediated by an increase in hydrostatic venous pressure may increase the transcapillary escape rate of albumin from the intravascular to the extravascular space [36]; on the other hand, it is possible that intestinal congestion favors albumin enteric losses [37]. It is well documented that a decrease in the body mass index is correlated with an increased mortality rate in patients with heart failure [38, 39]. Serum level of albumin was positively related to body weight in our study participants ($r = 0.332$, $P = 0.020$, data not shown). Both hypoalbuminemia and body weight loss are result of malnutrition. That may be the reason of the relationship between B-lines and body weight. Giuseppe et al. previously reported that physical functioning was inversely associated with the number of B-lines and patient age and was positively associated with the serum albumin level [40]. In our study, patient age tended to be positively associate with the number of B-lines ($P = 0.055$). In elderly patients, hypoalbuminemia, body weight loss (which results in reduction of serum creatinine level), and a low level of physical functioning are known to affect each other. Under such conditions, lung congestion, which can be detected by lung ultrasound as B-lines, should be considered.

Left ventricular systolic dysfunction may cause overhydration which result in lung congestion. On the other hand, overhydration may cause lung congestion and increase venous return volume and ventricular filling, thereby increase the stroke volume by the Frank-Starling mechanism when LVEF is preserved. There are conflicting result about the relationship between the number of B-lines and LVEF. Mallamaci et al. [12] used this technique in a population of 75 hemodialysis patients and showed the number of B-lines was negatively associated with an LVEF. But in other study, Siriopol et al. reported the number of B-lines was not related to LVEF [31]. The differences are most certainly the result of differences in study populations. In Siriopol et al.'s study, the patients (being younger and possibly with less comorbidities) had a preserved left ventricular systolic function (only 6.3% of the patients had an LVEF of <50%) [31]. In our study, 11 (22.4%) of the patients had an LVEF of <50%. In hemodialysis patients, the relationship between hydration status, B-lines, and left ventricular systolic function is complex. Accordingly, additional investigation will be needed to clarify the mechanism underlying the association between overhydration and B-lines in hemodialysis patients with a preserved or reduced LVEF.

Our study had some limitations. The sample size was relatively small, and the study was performed at a single institution. B-lines represent the volume status of extravascular lung water. There are some markers of intravascular volume such as cardiothoracic ratio, inferior vena cava, and serum level of atrial natriuretic peptide. Bioimpedance spectroscopy device enables to derive the extracellular water and intracellular water. But we did not have such data, so we could not discuss the relation between these markers. Another limitation of this study was that the investigator who performed lung ultrasound was not blind for the clinical information of the patients such as age, gender, or clinical diagnosis. In addition, the limitations of lung ultrasound are essentially patient-dependent. Obese patients may be more difficult to examine because of the thickness of their ribcages and soft tissues. Furthermore, the cross-sectional design prevented us from making any conclusions regarding the effects of treatment. The study participants were also relatively old, their serum albumin levels were relatively low, and their serum NT-proBNP levels were relatively high because of the specificity of our institution.

Conclusions

The number of B-lines was positively correlated with the serum NT-proBNP level. Lung ultrasound can quantify lung edema noninvasively in real time and in a radiation-free manner, enabling the direct imaging of extravascular lung water. Patient age tended to be positively correlated and the body weight and the serum albumin and creatinine levels were negatively correlated with the number of B-lines. Careful attention to the presence of pulmonary edema is needed in elderly patients with a low body weight and a low serum albumin and creatinine level.

Abbreviations

CABG: Coronary artery bypass grafting; ESKD: End-stage kidney disease; HD: Hemodialysis; LVEF: Left ventricular ejection fraction; NT-proBNP: N-terminal pro-brain natriuretic peptide; PCI: Percutaneous coronary intervention

Acknowledgements
The authors are very grateful to dialysis staff who understood the clinical importance of this study and who provided high-quality data in Sekikawa Hospital.

Funding
This study was not supported by any grants or funding.

Authors' contributions
SK planned the study, searched the literature, assessed the studies, extracted the data, analyzed the data, and prepared the article. SO and KK searched the literature, assessed the studies, and assisted in the article preparation. KK performed the lung echo. KN and TA assisted in the article preparation. All authors read and approved the final manuscript.

Competing interests
The authors declare that they have no competing interests.

Author details
[1]Department of Medicine, Kidney Center, Tokyo Women's Medical University, Tokyo, Japan. [2]Department of Nephrology, Sekikawa Hospital, Tokyo, Japan. [3]Department of Blood Purification, Tohto Sangenjaya Clinic, 2-13-2 Taishido, Setagaya-ku, Tokyo 154-0004, Japan. [4]Department of Cardiology, Sekikawa Hospital, Tokyo, Japan.

References
1. DOQI. Clinical practice guidelines and clinical practice recommendations for 2006 updates: hemodialysis adequacy, peritoneal dialysis adequacy and vascular access. Am J Kidney Dis. 2006;48(1):S1–322.
2. Tonelli M, Wiebe N, Culleton B, Tonelli M, Wiebe N, Culleton B, et al. Chronic kidney disease and mortality risk: a systematic review. J Am Soc Nephrol. 2006;17:2034–47.
3. Wang AY. Clinical utility of natriuretic peptides in dialysis patients. Semin Dial. 2012;25:326–33.
4. David S, Kumpers P, Seidler V, Biertz F, Haller H, Fliser D. Diagnostic value of N-terminal pro-B-type natriuretic peptide (NT-proBNP) for left ventricular dysfunction in patients with chronic kidney disease stage 5 on hemodialysis. Nephrol Dial Transplant. 2008;23:1370–7.
5. Ando Y, Yanagiba S, Asano Y. The inferior vena cava diameter as a marker of dry weight in chronic hemodialyzed patients. Artif Organs. 1995;9:1237–42.
6. Jaeger JQ, Mehta RL. Assessment of dry weight in hemodialysis: an overview. J Am Soc Nephrol. 1999;10:392–403.
7. Donadio C, Consani C, Ardini M, Bernabini G, Caprio F, Grassi G, et al. Estimate of body water compartments and of body composition in maintenance hemodialysis patients: comparison of single and multifrequency bioimpedance analysis. J Ren Nutr. 2005;15:332–44.
8. Jambrik Z, Monti S, Coppola V, Agricola E, Mottola G, Miniati M, et al. Usefulness of ultrasound lung comets as a nonradiologic sign of extravascular lung water. Am J Cardiol. 2004;93:1265–70.
9. Kajimoto K, Madeen K, Nakayama T, Tsudo H, Kuroda T, Abe T. Rapid evaluation by lung-cardiac-inferior vena cava (LCI) integrated ultrasound for differentiating heart failure from pulmonary disease as the cause of acute dyspnea in the emergency setting. Cardiovasc Ultrasound. 2012;10:49–51.
10. Lichtenstein D. Pneumothorax and introduction to ultrasound signs in the lung. In: Heilmann U, Wilbertz H, Gosling A, editors. General ultrasound in the critically ill. 1st ed. Heidelberg: Springer-Verlag; 2005. p. 105–15.
11. Agricola E, Bove T, Oppizzi M, Marino G, Zangrillo A, Margonato A, et al. "Ultrasound comet-tail images": a marker of pulmonary edema: a comparative study with wedge pressure and extravascular lung water. Chest. 2005;127:1690–5.
12. Mallamaci F, Benedetto FA, Tripepi R, Rastelli S, Castellino P, Tripepi G, et al.

Detection of pulmonary congestion by chest ultrasound in dialysis patients. JACC Cardiovasc Imaging. 2010;3:586–94.

13. Noble VE, Murray AF, Capp R, Sylvia-Reardon MH, Steele DJ, Liteplo A. Ultrasound assessment for extravascular lung water in patients undergoing hemodialysis. Chest. 2009;135:1433–9.

14. Trezzi M, Torzillo D, Ceriani E, Costantino G, Caruso S, Damavandi PT, et al. Lung ultrasonography for the assessment of rapid extravascular water variation: evidence from hemodialysis patients. Intern Emerg Med. 2013;8:409–15.

15. Panuccio V, Enia G, Tripepi R, Torino C, Garozzo M, Battaglia GG, et al. Chest ultrasound and hidden lung congestion in peritoneal dialysis patients. Nephrol Dial Transplant. 2012;27:3601–5.

16. Gargani L. Lung ultrasound: a new tool for the cardiologist. Cardiovasc Ultrasound. 2011; 27. doi:10.1186/1476-7120-9-6.

17. Bedetti G, Gargani L, Corbisiero A, Frassi F, Poggianti E, Mottola G. Evaluation of ultrasound lung comets by hand held echocardiography. Cardiovasc Ultrasound. 2006;31:4–34.

18. Picano E, Pellikka PA. Ultrasound of extravascular lung water: a new standard for pulmonary congestion. Eur Heart J. 2016;37:2097–104.

19. Minami Y, Kajimoto K, Sato N, Hagiwara N, Takano T. End-stage renal disease patients on chronic maintenance hemodialysis in a hospitalized acute heart failure cohort: Prevalence, clinical characteristics, therapeutic options, and mortality. Int J Cardiol. 2016;224:267–70.

20. Cardim N, Fernandez Golfin C, Ferreira D, Aubele A, Toste J, Cobos MA, et al. Usefulness of a new miniaturized echocardiographic system in outpatient cardiology consultations as an extension of physical examination. J Am Soc Echocardiogr. 2011;24:117–24.

21. Liebo MJ, Israel RL, Lillie EO, Smith MR, Rubenson DS, Topol EJ. Is pocket mobile echocardiography the next-generation stethoscope? A cross-sectional comparison of rapidly acquired images with standard transthoracic echocardiography. Ann Intern Med. 2011;155:33–8.

22. Liteplo AS, Marill KA, Villen T, Miller RM, Murray AF, Croft PE, et al. Emergency thoracic ultrasound in the differentiation of the etiology of shortness of breath (ETUDES): sonographic B-lines and N-terminal pro-brain-type natriuretic peptide in diagnosing congestive heart failure. Acad Emerg Med. 2009;16:201–10.

23. Volpicelli G, Elbarbary M, Blaivas M, Lichtenstein DA, Mathis G, Kirkpatrick AW, et al. International Liaison Committee on Lung Ultrasound (ILC-LUS) for International Consensus Conference on Lung Ultrasound (ICC-LUS). International evidence-based recommendations for point-of-care lung ultrasound. Intensive Care Med. 2012;38:577–91.

24. Volpicelli G, Mussa A, Garofalo G, Cardinale L, Casoli G, Perotto F, et al. Bedside lung ultrasound in the assessment of alveolar-interstitial syndrome. Am J Emerg Med. 2006;24:689–96.

25. Cardinale L, Volpicelli G, Binello F, Garofalo G, Priola SM, Veltri A, et al. Clinical application of lung ultrasound in patients with acute dyspnea: differential diagnosis between cardiogenic and pulmonary causes. Radiol Med. 2009;114:1053–64.

26. Prosen G, Klemen P, Strnad M, Grmec S. Combination of lung ultrasound (a comet-tail sign) and N-terminal pro-brain natriuretic peptide in differentiating acute heart failure from chronic obstructive pulmonary disease and asthma as cause of acute dyspnea in prehospital emergency setting. Crit Care. 2011;15:114–22.

27. Volpicelli G, Caramello V, Cardinale L, Mussa A, Bar F, Frascisco MF. Bedside ultrasound of the lung for the monitoring of acute decompensated heart failure. Am J Emerg Med. 2008;26:585–91.

28. Lichtenstein D, Mézière G, Biderman P, Gepner A, Barré O. The comet-tail artifact. An ultrasound sign of alveolar-interstitial syndrome. Am J Respir Crit Care Med. 1997;156:1640–6.

29. Picano E, Frassi F, Agricola E, Gligorova S, Gargani L, Mottola G. Ultrasound lung comets: a clinically useful sign of extravascular lung water. J Am Soc Echocardiogr. 2006;19:356–63.

30. Bedetti G, Gargani L, Corbisiero A, Frassi F, Poggianti E, Mottola G. Evaluation of ultrasound lung comets by hand-held echocardiography. Cardiovasc Ultrasound. 2006;4:34.

31. Siriopol D, Hogas S, Voroneanu L, Onofriescu M, Apetrii M, Oleniuc M, et al. Predicting mortality in haemodialysis patients: a comparison between lung ultrasonography, bioimpedance data and echocardiography parameters. Nephrol Dial Transplant. 2013;28:2851–9.

32. Vitturi N, Dugo M, Soattin M, Simoni F, Maresca L, Zagatti R, et al. Lung ultrasound during hemodialysis: the role in the assessment of volume status. Int Urol Nephrol. 2014;46:169–74.

33. Chen W, Gassner B, Borner S, Nikolaev VO, Schlegel N, Waschke J, et al. Atrial natriuretic peptide enhances microvascular albumin permeability by the caveolae-mediated transcellular pathway. Cardiovasc Res. 2012;93:141–51.

34. Horwich TB, Kalantar-Zadeh K, MacLellan RW, Fonarow GC. Albumin levels predict survival in patients with systolic heart failure. Am Heart J. 2008;155:883–9.

35. Liu M, Chan CP, Yan BP, Zhang Q, Lam YY, Li RJ, et al. Albumin levels predict survival in patients with heart failure and preserved ejection fraction. Eur J Heart Fail. 2012;14:39–44.

36. Hesse B, Parving HH, Lund-Jacobsen H, Noer I. Transcapillary escape rate of albumin and right atrial pressure in chronic congestive heart failure before and after treatment. Circ Res. 1976;39:358–62.

37. Battin DL, Ali S, Shahbaz AU, Massie JD, Munir A, Davis Jr RC. Hypoalbuminemia and lymphocytopenia in patients with decompensated biventricular failure. Am J Med Sci. 2010;339:31–5.

38. Shah R, Gayat E, Januzzi Jr JL, Sato N, Cohen-Solal A, diSomma S, et al. Body mass index and mortality in acutely decompensated heart failure across the world: a global obesity paradox. J Am Coll Cardiol. 2014;63:778–85.

39. Kenchaiah S, Pocock SJ, Wang D, Finn PV, Zornoff LA, Skali H, et al. Body mass index and prognosis in patients with chronic heart failure: insights from the Candesartan in Heart failure: Assessment of Reduction in Mortality and morbidity (CHARM) program. Circulation. 2007;116:627–36.

40. Enia G, Torino C, Panuccio V, Tripepi R, Postorino M, Aliotta R, et al. Asymptomatic pulmonary congestion and physical functioning in hemodialysis patients. Clin J Am Soc Nephrol. 2013;8:1343–8.

11

Higher reticulocyte counts are associated with higher mortality rates in hemodialysis patients: a retrospective single-center cohort study

Chieko Takagi[1,4*], Kumeo Ono[2], Hidenori Matsuo[1], Nobuo Nagano[1] and Yoshihisa Nojima[3]

Abstract

Background: We assessed laboratory data related to mortality in hemodialysis (HD) patients. In our preliminary study, we examined all of the data for HD outpatients in our facility according to whether the patient had survived. A statistically significant difference was observed for the reticulocyte count, which has not previously been considered a prognostic factor. We subsequently verified the relationship between all-cause and cardiovascular mortality and reticulocyte count.

Methods: We retrospectively analyzed the data of 358 hemodialysis outpatients who were followed up for an average of 41.4 months. The patients were divided into quartiles according to the reticulocyte count levels.

Results: Higher reticulocyte counts were associated with female gender, an increase in interdialytic body weight gain, serum erythropoietin level, white blood cell count, and increased levels of lactate dehydrogenase, inorganic phosphorus, non-high-density lipoprotein, and glucose. As compared with patients in the lowest quartile, those in the highest quartile showed significantly higher adjusted hazard ratios (HRs) for all-cause (HR 3.12; 95% confidence interval (CI) 1.26 to 7.74) and cardiovascular (HR 4.93; 95% CI 1.24 to 19.56) mortality. For every 10^4 cells/µL increment in the reticulocyte count, the adjusted HRs for all-cause and cardiovascular mortality were 1.33 (95% CI 1.17 to 1.51) and 1.38 (95% CI 1.17 to 1.63), respectively. The association of reticulocyte count with all-cause and cardiovascular mortality was independent of other prognostic factors. Stepwise multivariable Cox analysis indicated that only age showed stronger association with all-cause mortality than reticulocyte count. Regarding cardiovascular mortality, reticulocyte count was found as the strongest progenitor. We also examined the relationship between the reticulocyte count and the temporal hemoglobin trend (a slope of changes in hemoglobin levels over time). A statistically significant negative correlation was found.

Conclusions: Higher reticulocyte counts were associated with higher mortality. We speculate that this result reflects tissue hypoxia, which results in a higher erythropoietin level, or a compensatory erythropoietic response due to the accelerated clearance of erythrocytes. Prospective studies are warranted to confirm our findings.

Keywords: Reticulocyte, Mortality, Hemodialysis, Anemia, Erythropoietin, Microvascular dysfunction

* Correspondence: chiekot@cj8.so-net.ne.jp
[1]Hidaka Hospital, Takasaki, Gunma, Japan
[4]Present address: Dialysis Center, Ogo Clinic, 245-7, Motogi-machi, Maebashi-shi, Gunma 371-0232, Japan
Full list of author information is available at the end of the article

Background

To improve the prognosis of chronic maintenance hemodialysis (HD) patients, it is important to identify simple and inexpensive prognostic factors. In our preliminary analysis, we examined data from a total of 1,814,698 HD outpatients. These data were obtained from January 4, 1999 to December 26, 2003. We divided patients into two groups depending on whether they had survived until the end of 2003. Student's t tests were performed for each comparison. In addition to the established prognostic factors, we found that the mean reticulocyte count was significantly higher in the non-survivor group. The means +/− standard deviations (SDs) of the reticulocyte count were 46.4×10^3 +/− 0.2×10^3 cells (sample count 8732) in the survivor group and 52.4×10^3 +/− 0.2×10^3 cells in the non-survivor group (sample count 1111) $p = 6.09$ E−15.

Reticulocytes are young red blood cells that develop from erythroblasts and circulate in the bloodstream for approximately 1–4 days before maturing into erythrocytes [1]. These cells provide a real-time assessment of the functional state of erythropoiesis [2] and are thus useful in both diagnosing anemias and monitoring the bone marrow response to therapy [3]. While reticulocyte count is widely measured in routine laboratory work, the clinical significance of the reticulocyte count in patients on chronic maintenance HD has yet to be clearly delineated [4].

In this study, we conducted a retrospective single-center analysis of the data of 358 patients under chronic maintenance HD to examine the association of reticulocyte counts with all-cause/cardiovascular mortality and hemoglobin trends (Hb trend).

Methods

Study design and patients

This is a retrospective observational study of 358 patients under regular maintenance hemodialysis at Hidaka Hospital. Patients were excluded from the study, when they had required hospitalization during 3 months prior to enrollment due to hematologic disorder, active bleeding, acute cardiovascular events, infectious diseases, or other comorbid conditions such as blood access troubles or traffic accidents. No patient had received chemotherapy for malignancy during the 3 months prior to enrollment. In addition, we did not include patients who had obvious inflammatory symptoms at the beginning of the enrollment period. The observation period was from January 2000 to July 2005, which was 5 years before darbepoetin therapy was introduced in our facility. The mean ± SD of the age of the cohort was 60.2 ± 12.6 years (range, 29 to 89 years), and the patients had been on maintenance hemodialysis for 8.5 ± 7.0 years, on average (range, 0.3 to 27.9 years). During the follow-up period,

52 patients were censored at departure to another dialysis unit. The mean follow-up period was 41.4 ± 16.6 months (range, 0.5 to 53.3 months).

The demographic and medical data were obtained from the medical records and interviews with the patients. The demographic data included age, gender, duration of dialysis, primary cause of renal failure, interdialysis weight gain, body mass index (BMI), dry weight, systolic blood pressure, diastolic blood pressure, vascular disease history, and smoking history (ever versus never). Vascular disease history was defined as a history of hospitalization due to coronary heart disease, heart failure, arrhythmia, valvular disease, aortic aneurysm, peripheral arterial disease, atrial septal defect, deep vein thrombosis, or cerebrovascular accident, including cerebral bleeding or infarction. The medication exposure data included the use of angiotensin-converting enzyme inhibitors (ACE-Is) or angiotensin receptor blockers (ARBs), the use of intravenous iron injections during the week prior to enrollment, and the average weekly dose of recombinant human erythropoietin (rHuEPO) at 1, 2, or 4 weeks prior to the observation period. None of the patients was receiving darbepoetin or continuous erythropoietin receptor activator (CERA) during the observation period in our cohort. Medical data were obtained from the records for the week prior to the enrollment. The doses of rHuEPO and iron were adjusted to maintain the hemoglobin level at approximately 10.0 g/dl, according to the dosage column of the Insurance Price List [5].

Blood samples were obtained on the first day of the week before the start of the dialysis sessions undertaken at 2-day intervals and were subjected to determination for Hb, reticulocyte count, white blood cell count (WBC), platelet count (Plt), transferrin saturation (TSAT), ferritin, albumin (Alb), lactate dehydrogenase (LDH), blood urea nitrogen (BUN), creatinine (Cr), phosphorus inorganic (iP), total cholesterol, triglyceride, high-density-lipoprotein, blood sugar, C reactive protein (CRP), and erythropoietin (EPO). Determination for most of these parameters was undertaken as a part of the routine clinical work. The data obtained at a single time point within a week before enrollment were used for subsequent entire analysis. Concentrations of BUN were measured before and after a single dialysis session at enrollment to determine KT/V according to the procedure of Shinzato et al. [6]. The reticulocyte count was measured according to the method of Brecher [7].

Hb trend was obtained to determine the slope of the changes in the Hb levels over time, a best-fit (ordinary least squares) line of Hb over time until 2 weeks or 6 months after the start of the observation period was plotted for each subject; the temporal trend in Hb was represented by the slope of this line [8].

Statistical analyses

Data are expressed as mean ± SD. We used χ^2 or ANOVA to test for differences in the categorical or continuous factors, respectively, among the four quartiles of patients divided according to the reticulocyte count. The primary outcome was all-cause and cardiovascular mortality. Cardiovascular death was defined as death from coronary heart disease, heart failure, peripheral artery disease, cardiomyopathy, arrhythmia, cardiac arrest, valvular disease, infective endocarditis, rupture of aortic aneurysm, mesenteric artery occlusion, or cerebral bleeding. Survival curves were estimated by the Kaplan-Meier method, followed by a log-rank test. Univariate and multivariate analyses were conducted using the Cox proportional hazards model. Statistical significance was defined as $p < 0.05$. The models of association for all-cause mortality and death due to cardiovascular disease were built using a forward stepwise multivariate Cox modeling with $p < 0.05$ set as the inclusion criterion. The 20 candidate parameters were evaluated to identify associations between variables and outcome. The parameters tested were age, sex, diabetic nephropathy (DMN), duration of dialysis, interdialysis body weight gain, vascular disease history, use of ACE-I or ARB, systolic blood pressure, diastolic blood pressure, weekly dose of rHuEPO for a week before the enrollment (1w rHuEPO), Hb, WBC, Plt, iP, Cr, Alb, CRP, ferritin, TSAT, and reticulocyte count. The statistical contribution of each variable to the association of the outcome was assessed by the χ^2 statistic. Pearson correlations were used to test the relationships among the reticulocyte count, temporal trend of Hb, and dose of rHuEPO.

Results

Patient characteristics

We retrospectively analyzed the data of a total of 358 patients undergoing regular hemodialysis at Hidaka Hospital. The observation period extended from January 2000 to July 2005. During a mean follow-up of 41.4 months (0.5 to 53.3 months), 82 deaths were documented (heart failure $n = 19$, coronary heart disease $n = 14$, infection $n = 12$, malignant disease $n = 9$, peripheral artery disease $n = 3$, cardiomyopathy $n = 4$, gastrointestinal tract bleeding $n = 4$, cerebral bleeding $n = 3$, infective endocarditis $n = 2$, valvular disease $n = 2$, arrhythmia $n = 2$, cardiac arrest $n = 2$, rupture of aortic aneurysm $n = 1$, mesenteric artery occlusion $n = 1$, and miscellaneous $n = 4$), among which 53 were cardiovascular-related deaths.

Patients were divided into quartiles according to the reticulocyte counts. Table 1 shows the baseline characteristics of all the patients and of the patients in each reticulocyte count quartile. Higher reticulocyte counts were associated with female gender ($p = 0.01$), interdialysis

body weight gain ($p = 0.02$), and a lower frequency of the use of ACE-I or ARB ($p < 0.01$). Meanwhile, age, duration of dialysis, blood pressure, history of smoking, weekly dose of rHuEPO, and use of iron injections were not correlated with the reticulocyte count.

As for the laboratory parameters, the serum Hb values were not significantly correlated with the reticulocyte counts. Patients with higher reticulocyte counts were more likely to have decreased TSAT, Hb trend (2 weeks and 6 months) and increase of such parameters as the serum EPO, WBC, LDH, BUN, iP, total cholesterol, triglyceride, non-high-density lipoprotein (non-HDL), and glucose.

Association of the reticulocyte count with all-cause and cardiovascular mortality

Crude survival was determined using Kaplan-Meier analysis with the log-rank test. The risk for all-cause death differed significantly among the reticulocyte count quartiles (log-rank test $\chi^2 = 28.34$, $p < 0.001$; Fig. 1a). In univariate Cox proportional hazard model, the all-cause mortality rate was highest in the highest quartile, and there was a survival gradient across quartiles (Table 2). After adjustments for background covariates, the hazard ratio (HR) for all-cause mortality in the highest versus the lowest quartile of reticulocyte count remained significantly high at 4.37 (95% confidence interval (CI) 1.94 to 9.84) (model 1 in Table 2). Additional adjustment for background and other prognostic factors Hb, WBC, Plt, TSAT, ferritin, iP, Cr, Alb, and CRP partially attenuated this estimate (HR 3.12; 95% CI 1.26 to 7.74), but the difference remained significant. The increase in mortality was in a relatively linear fashion. In the univariate analysis, the HR was significantly high for reticulocyte count increments of $1 \times 10^4/\mu L$ (HR 1.29; 95% CI 1.18 to 1.42; $p < 0.001$). The effect of reticulocyte count on the survival remained statistically significant after adjustments (model 1, HR 1.37, 95% CI 1.23 to 1.53; model 2, HR 1.33, 95% CI 1.17 to 1.51).

Significant increase of the cardiovascular death rates was also observed from the lowest to the highest reticulocyte count quartiles (log-rank test, $\chi^2 = 20.36$, $p < 0.001$) (Fig. 1b). The HR for cardiovascular death in the highest quartiles of reticulocyte count was significantly higher as compared with that in the lowest quartile at 5.67 (95% CI 1.94 to 16.59) (Table 2). The highest quartile of reticulocyte count, compared with the lowest, was significantly associated with the risk of cardiovascular death after adjustments (models 1 and 2). The effect of every 10^4 cells/μL increment in the reticulocyte count on the cardiovascular death also remained statistically significant after adjustments (models 1 and 2 in Table 2)

Table 1 Baseline patient characteristics

| Characteristics | All Patients | Reticulocyte count | | | | p |
		Q1	Q2	Q3	Q4	ANOVA or χ^2
No. of patients	358	89	90	89	90	
Range of reticulocyte count (10^3/μL)	9.3 to 147.9	≤30.1	30.2 to 39.4	39.6 to 53.6	≤53.7	
Demographics						
Age (year)	60.2 (12.6)	60.4 (13.8)	60.4 (12.7)	61.0 (12.6)	59.1 (11.4)	0.78
Male gender (%)	67.3	78.7	70.0	64.0	56.7	0.01
Duration of dialysis (year)	8.5 (7.0)	7.9 (6.2)	8.8 (6.6)	8.8 (7.6)	8.7 (7.4)	0.80
Cause of renal failure						
Diabetes mellitus (%)	29.9	23.6	27.8	33.7	34.4	0.34
BMI	20.6 (3.0)	20.0 (2.4)	20.6 (3.0)	20.6 (2.8)	21.1 (3.5)	0.09
Dry weight (kg)	53.1 (10.3)	53.0 (9.0)	53.3 (12.1)	52.2 (9.1)	53.7 (10.7)	0.80
Interdialysis weight gain (%)	5.6 (1.9)	5.1 (1.9)	5.6 (1.9)	5.4 (2.0)	6.0 (1.7)	0.02
Smoking history (%)	44.9	48.8	42.9	45.3	42.5	0.84
Vascular disease history (%)	47.8	41.6	42.2	53.9	53.3	0.18
Medication						
ACE or ARB (%)	30.7	40.4	38.1	25.6	18.9	<0.01
Injection of Fe (%)	25.1	22.5	30.0	25.8	22.2	0.60
1w rHuEPO/week (IU/w)	3694 (3077)	3396 (2874)	4321 (2949)	3584 (3281)	3508 (3154)	0.19
2w rHuEPO/week (IU/w)	3727 (3079)	3459 (2906)	4415 (2971)	3576 (3255)	3496 (3079)	0.13
4w rHuEPO/week (IU/w)	3752 (3063)	3550 (2912)	4339 (2900)	3628 (3259)	3521 (3142)	0.25
Systolic blood pressure (mmHg)	151.9 (23.6)	154.8 (20.9)	155.5 (22.4)	146.8 (25.6)	150.33 (24.5)	0.05
Diastolic blood pressure (mmHg)	78.4 (11.6)	79.4 (12.1)	80.4 (11.1)	76.8 (10.0)	76.9 (13.0)	0.11
Laboratory parameters						
Reticulocyte count (10^3/μL)	43.4 (19.4)	22.5 (5.1)	35.1 (2.7)	45.8 (4.0)	69.6 (16.1)	<0.001
Hemoglobin (g/dL)	9.9 (1.1)	9.8 (1.2)	9.9 (1.0)	9.8 (1.0)	10.1 (1.2)	0.20
Mean corpuscular volume (fL)	97.8 (6.8)	97.2 (6.3)	98.9 (6.2)	97.9 (7.0)	97.0 (7.7)	0.22
White cell count (10^3/μL)	6.1 (2.1)	5.4 (1.5)	6.0 (1.8)	6.2 (2.2)	6.9 (2.5)	<0.001
Platelet count (10^3/μL)	185 (67)	172 (53)	182 (58)	187 (65)	199 (87)	0.06
Iron (μg/dL)	57.2 (23.3)	58.9 (25.9)	60.3 (25.0)	57.2 (20.0)	52.6 (21.4)	0.13
TSAT (%)	21.9 (10.1)	24.1 (11.8)	23.0 (10.1)	21.8 (9.1)	18.9 (8.5)	<0.01
Ferritin (ng/mL)	101 (135)	116 (167)	94 (107)	108 (160)	85 (92)	0.43
AST (U/L)	15.9 (8.8)	15.5 (6.4)	14.8 (6.0)	17.2 (12.6)	16.1 (8.5)	0.32
ALT (U/L)	14.2 (10.3)	13.6 (7.3)	13.7 (8.0)	15.4 (15.9)	14.0 (7.7)	0.62
Alkaline phosphatase (U/L)	251 (101)	253 (115)	249 (78)	246 (96)	255 (114)	0.94
Total bilirubin (mg/dL)	0.20 (0.09)	0.21 (0.10)	0.19 (0.06)	0.20 (0.10)	0.20 (0.09)	0.60
Lactate dehydrogenase (U/L)	335 (81)	323 (70)	322 (66)	342 (83)	353 (98)	0.03
Blood urea nitrogen (mg/dL)	77.4 (17.4)	70.1 (14.5)	80.3 (18.1)	79.1 (18.2)	80.1 (16.7)	<0.001
Creatinine (mg/dL)	11.7 (2.8)	11.5 (3.1)	12.0 (2.6)	11.5 (2.7)	11.8 (2.7)	0.63
Corrected calcium (mg/dL)	9.30 (0.88)	9.25 (0.84)	9.19 (0.92)	9.28 (0.88)	9.48 (0.87)	0.14
Phosphorus inorganic (mg/dL)	5.95 (1.50)	5.49 (1.42)	5.90 (1.33)	5.91 (1.56)	6.43 (1.53)	<0.001
Parathyroid hormone intact (pg/mL)	212 (191)	212 (206)	229 (172)	198 (292)	210 (184)	0.75
Albumin (g/dL)	3.72 (0.36)	3.71 (0.35)	3.80 (0.36)	3.68 (0.76)	3.68 (0.35)	0.07
Total protein (g/dL)	6.46 (0.51)	6.43 (0.49)	6.49 (0.50)	6.43 (0.58)	6.49 (0.50)	0.71
Glucose (mg/dL)	135 (62)	122 (40)	128 (47)	141 (72)	149 (78)	0.01

Table 1 Baseline patient characteristics *(Continued)*

Total cholesterol (mg/dL)	157 (34)	147 (31)	154 (33)	162 (31)	165 (36)	<0.01
High-density lipoprotein (mg/dL)	45 (14)	43 (12)	46 (14)	46 (15)	45 (15)	0.43
Triglyceride (mg/dL)	117 (68)	97 (48)	107 (62)	120 (62)	143 (87)	<0.001
Non-HDL (mg/dL)	112.1 (32.3)	104.2 (29.8)	108.1 (31.1)	116.4 (31.3)	119.9 (34.9)	<0.01
C-reactive protein (mg/dL)	0.57 (1.33)	0.41 (0.76)	0.45 (1.16)	0.56 (1.23)	0.86 (1.88)	0.11
Serum erythropoietin (U/L)	16.2 (22.8)	11.0 (9.0)	12.0 (8.0)	14.7 (12.0)	26.6 (40.4)	<0.001
Kt/V	1.23 (0.25)	1.19 (0.24)	1.26 (0.27)	1.24 (0.23)	1.23 (0.24)	0.41
Hb trend 0.5 mo (g/dL/week) $n = 353$	−0.02 (0.39)	0.01 (0.06)	0.08 (0.37)	−0.03 (0.31)	−0.12 (0.44)	0.01
Hb trend 6 mo (g/dL/week) $n = 338$	0.01 (0.07)	0.03 (0.06)	0.01 (0.06)	0.00 (0.05)	−0.01 (0.09)	<0.01

Results are displayed as mean (standard deviation). Patients were quartiled according to reticulocyte count. Q1, $\leq 30.1 \times 10^3$ cells/μL; Q2, 30.2 to 39.4×10^3 cells/μL; Q3, 39.6 to 53.6×10^3 cells/μL; and Q4, $\geq 53.7 \times 10^3$ cells/μL

Note: *BMI* body mass index, *ACE* angiotensin-converting enzyme, *ARB* angiotensin receptor blocker, *rHuEPO* recombinant human erythropoietin, *1w rHuEPO/week* the dose of rHuEPO per week for 1 week prior to enrollment, *2w rHuEPO/week* the average dose of rHuEPO per week for 2 weeks prior to enrollment, *4w rHuEPO/week* the average dose of rHuEPO per week for 4 weeks prior to enrollment, *TSAT* transferrin saturation, *AST* aspartate aminotransferase, *ALT* alanine aminotransferase, *non-HDL* non-high-density lipoprotein, *Hb trend 0.5 mo* hemoglobin trend untill 0.5 month, *Hb tred 6 mo* hemoglobin trend untill 6 months

Table 3 shows the association models for all-cause and cardiovascular mortality. For each outcome, Cox proportional hazards models were built using a forward stepwise procedure. The variables are listed in order of their statistical strength of association with outcome, as represented by the χ^2 statistic. Reticulocyte count showed the second most powerful association with death from any cause, with χ^2 of 29.85. In this model, increased reticulocyte count showed among the most significant overall correlations of outcome, showing stronger statistical association than presence/absence of DMN, CRP, iP, and vascular disease history. Only age showed stronger independent association with outcomes. In our model for cardiovascular death, reticulocyte count showed the strongest association ($\chi^2 = 25.38$).

Correlation between the reticulocyte count and temporal trend of Hb

We next examined whether higher reticulocyte counts translated into a rise of the Hb levels during the following period. To determine the slope of the change in the Hb levels over time, we evaluated Hb trend until 2 weeks and 6 months after the start of the observation period. Among the 358 subjects, 8 died within the first 6 months of enrollment, before the trend in Hb levels could be determined. Hb concentrations were distributed in a very narrow range; the mean Hb trend was −0.02 +/− 0.39 g/dL/week at 2 weeks and 0.01 +/− 0.07 g/dL/week at 6 months. As shown in Fig. 2a, b, the reticulocyte count was negatively correlated with the temporal trend of Hb at 2 weeks ($r = -0.20$, $p < 0.001$, $n = 358$) as well as 6 months ($r = -0.21$, $p < 0.001$, $n = 338$).

Dose of rHuEPO and mortality

We examined all subjects in the cohort, including those who had received ($n = 281$) and those who had not

received ($n = 73$) 1 week of treatment with rHuEPO (four patients' data were not available). We re-examined the prognostic impact of the reticulocyte count by separately analyzing subgroups of patients according to whether they had received rHuEPO. The prognostic impact of a high reticulocyte count with respect to the all-cause mortality remained significant not only in patients who had been treated with rHuEPO (HR per 10^4 cells/μL 1.33; 95% CI 1.20 to 1.47) but also in those who had not been treated with rHuEPO (HR per 10^4 cells/μL 1.28; 95% CI 1.03 to 1.59). Furthermore, the HR for all-cause mortality in the subgroup that had been treated with rHuEPO was not attenuated by an adjustment for the rHuEPO dose (HR 1.34; 95% CI 1.20 to 1.48). These data suggested that the association of the reticulocyte count with mortality was not dependent on the dose of rHuEPO.

Reproducibility of the association between reticulocyte count and all-cause and cardiovascular mortality

We also evaluated the association between the reticulocyte count and mortality at different time points. A total of 203 patients whose reticulocyte count data were available at 1 year prior to enrollment were divided into quartiles according to the reticulocyte count. A total of 32 deaths were documented, among which 25 were due to a cardiovascular cause. The range of each group was as follows: pQ1 $\leq 31.5 \times 10^3$ cells/μL, pQ2 (31.5×10^{33} cells/μL to 42.1×10^3 cells/μL), pQ3 (42.2×10^3 cells/μL to 54.2×10^3 cells/μL), and pQ4 $\geq 54.4 \times 10^3$ cells/μL. Survival curves were estimated via the Kaplan-Meier method, followed by the log-rank test. The risk for all-cause and cardiovascular death differed significantly among the reticulocyte count quartiles (all-cause death log-rank test $\chi^2 = 9.479$, $p = 0.02$; Fig. 3a/cardiovascular death log-rank test $\chi^2 = 9.914$, $p = 0.02$; Fig. 3b). In the

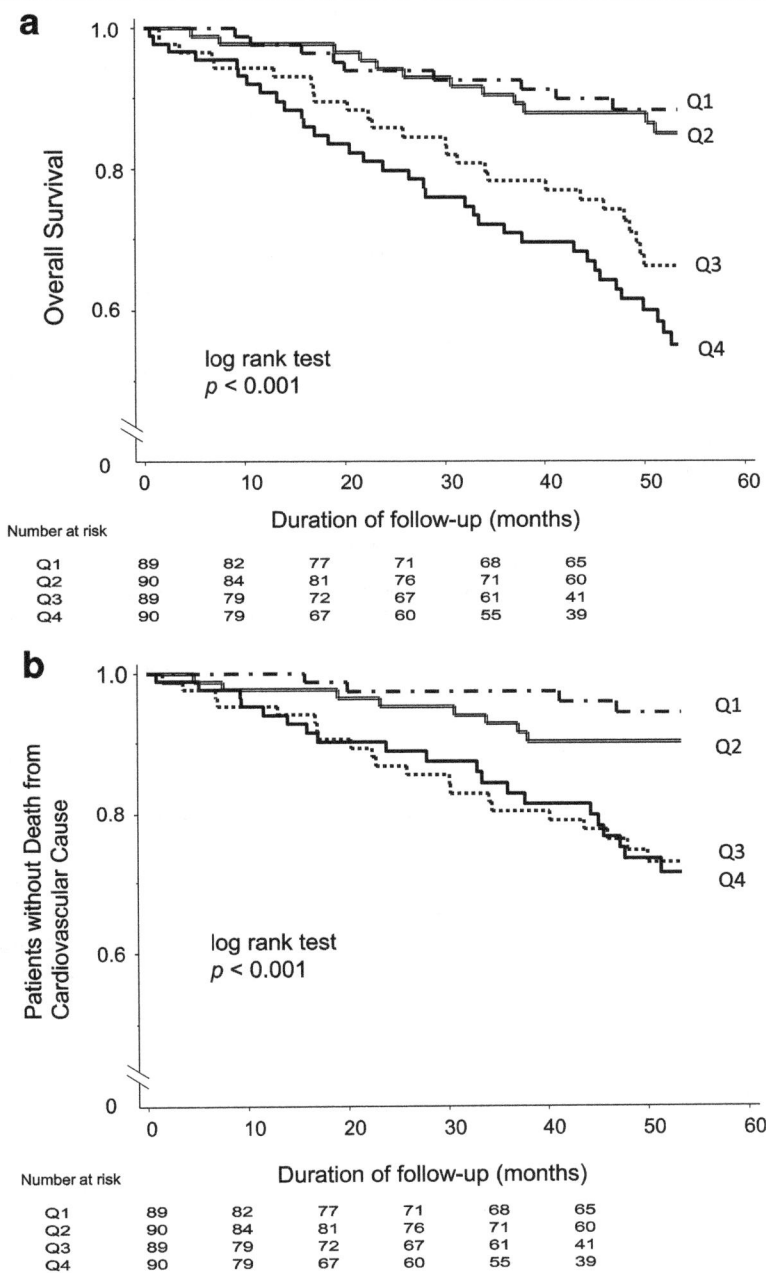

Fig. 1 Kaplan-Meier survival curves according to reticulocyte count quartiles. Patients were divided into quartiles according to the reticulocyte count. Q1, ≤30.1 × 10^3 cells/μL; Q2, 30.2 to 39.4 × 10^3 cells/μL; Q3, 39.6 to 53.6 × 10^3 cells/μL; and Q4, ≥53.7 × 10^3 cells/μL. **a** Overall survival; $p < 0.001$ as determined by a log-rank test conducted to compare the four groups. **b** Patients who had not died from cardiovascular causes; $p < 0.001$ according to a log-rank test conducted to compare the four groups

univariate Cox proportional hazard model, the HR was significantly higher for reticulocyte count increments of 1×10^4/μL for both all-cause mortality (HR 1.35; 95% CI 1.14 to 1.60; $p < 0.001$) and cardiovascular mortality (HR 1.41; 95% I 1.14 to 1.73; $p < 0.001$). Thus, our findings revealed that the reticulocyte count was related to mortality at 1 year prior to enrollment.

Discussion

One striking finding of this retrospective study was that the reticulocyte count showed very strong correlation with the all-cause and cardiovascular mortality in patients on maintenance HD. Multivariate analysis revealed that reticulocyte count was associated with all-cause and cardiovascular mortality, even after adjusting

Table 2 Adjusted association between quartile of reticulocyte count and mortality

	Unadjusted		Model 1		Model 2	
	HR (95% CI)	p	HR (95% CI)	p	HR (95% CI)	p
All-cause mortality						
Q1	1 (Reference)	<0.001[†]	1 (Reference)	<0.001[†]	1 (Reference)	0.003[†]
Q2	1.23 (0.52 to 2.93)		0.95 (0.37 to 2.49)		0.71 (0.26 to 1.96)	
Q3	3.06 (1.43 to 6.52)		2.24 (0.98 to 5.16)		1.94 (0.83 to 4.58)	
Q4	4.37 (2.10 to 9.10)		4.37 (1.94 to 9.84)		3.12 (1.26 to 7.74)	
per 10^4 cells/µL	1.29 (1.18 to 1.42)	<0.001	1.37 (1.23 to 1.53)	<0.001	1.33 (1.17 to 1.51)	<0.001
Cardiovascular mortality						
Q1	1 (Reference)	<0.001[†]	1 (Reference)	0.005[†]	1 (Reference)	0.03[†]
Q2	1.86 (0.56 to 6.19)		1.91 (0.47 to 7.62)		1.59 (0.37 to 6.79)	
Q3	5.59 (1.92 to 16.27)		4.97 (1.41 to 17.46)		4.18 (1.14 to 15.25)	
Q4	5.67 (1.94 to 16.59)		6.57 (1.85 to 23.34)		4.93 (1.24 to 19.56)	
per 10^4 cells/µL	1.28 (1.14 to 1.43)	<0.001	1.37 (1.19 to 1.56)	<0.001	1.38 (1.17 to 1.63)	<0.001

Patients were quartiled according to reticulocyte count. Q1, ≤30.1 × 10^3 cells/µL; Q2, 30.2 to 39.4 × 10^3 cells/µL; Q3, 39.6 to 53.6 × 10^3 cells/µL; Q4, ≥53.7 × 10^3 cells. Model 1 is adjusted for age, sex, diabetic nephropathy, duration of dialysis, interdialysis weight gain, smoking status, vascular disease history, use of angiotensin-converting enzyme inhibitors or angiotensin receptor blockers, systolic blood pressure, diastolic blood pressure, and weekly dose of recombinant human erythropoietin. Model 2 is adjusted for model 1 covariates and hemoglobin, white blood cell, platelet count, transferrin saturation, ferritin, phosphorus inorganic, creatinine, albumin, and C-reactive protein
Note: *HR* hazard ratio, *CI* confidence interval
[†]*p* for linear trend

for other risk factors known to affect mortality in HD patients, such as age, history of DMN, preexisting vascular disease, weekly dose of rHuEPO, Hb, WBC count, serum Alb, Cr, iP, or CRP. The correlation between all-cause mortality and reticulocyte count showed stronger statistical relation than the presence/absence of DMN, CRP, iP, and vascular disease history. Only age showed stronger independent association with outcomes. In

addition, the strongest correlation was observed between cardiovascular mortality and reticulocyte count. There is only one previously reported study in the literature, by Cantaro et al., in which the prognostic value of the reticulocyte count was investigated [9]. This study, in which the data of 117 HD patients were analyzed for a period of 12 months and the reticulocyte count tended to be higher in the deceased group, however, failed to

Table 3 Correlation models for all-cause and cardiovascular mortality based on forward stepwise Cox proportional hazard regression

Variables	HR	95% CI	χ2	p
All-cause mortality				
Age (per 1 year)	1.08	1.06 to 1.11	40.00	<0.001
Reticulocyte count (per 10^4 cells/µL)	1.36	1.22 to 1.51	29.85	<0.001
Diabetic nephropathy yes vs no	3.19	1.98 to 5.13	22.65	<0.001
C-reactive protein (per 1 mg/dL)	1.28	1.14 to 1.44	16.21	<0.001
Phosphorus inorganic (per 1 mg/dL)	1.24	1.03 to 1.46	5.18	0.02
Vascular disease yes vs no	1.77	1.06 to 2.95	4.84	0.03
Cardiovascular mortality				
Reticulocyte count (per 10^4 cells/µL)	1.40	1.23 to 1.60	25.38	<0.001
Diabetic nephropathy yes vs no	4.62	2.51 to 8.50	24.20	<0.001
C-reactive protein (per 1 mg/dL)	1.38	1.21 to 1.58	22.87	<0.001
Age (per 1 year)	1.08	1.04 to 1.10	21.15	<0.001
Diastolic blood presure (per 1 mmHg)	0.97	0.95 to 0.99	6.56	0.01

Stepwise, multivariate Cox proportional regression models were developed using candidate variables to predict all-cause and cardiovascular mortality. Candidate variables are age, sex, diabetic nephropathy, duration of dialysis, interdialysis weight gain, vascular disease history, use of angiotensin-converting enzyme inhibitors or angiotensin receptor blockers, systolic blood pressure, diastolic blood pressure, weekly dose of recombinant human erythropoietin, hemoglobin, white blood cell, platelet count, transferrin saturation, ferritin, phosphorus inorganic, creatinine, albumin, C-reactive protein, and reticulocyte count. Inclusion criterion is *p* < 0.05
Note: *HR* hazard ratio, *CI* confidence interval

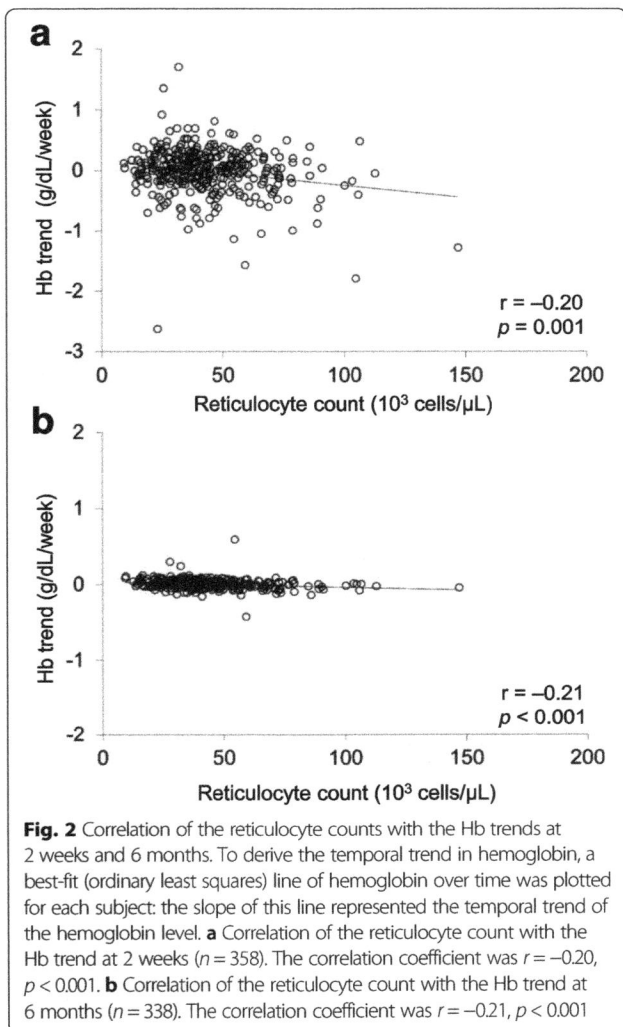

Fig. 2 Correlation of the reticulocyte counts with the Hb trends at 2 weeks and 6 months. To derive the temporal trend in hemoglobin, a best-fit (ordinary least squares) line of hemoglobin over time was plotted for each subject: the slope of this line represented the temporal trend of the hemoglobin level. **a** Correlation of the reticulocyte count with the Hb trend at 2 weeks ($n = 358$). The correlation coefficient was $r = -0.20$, $p < 0.001$. **b** Correlation of the reticulocyte count with the Hb trend at 6 months ($n = 338$). The correlation coefficient was $r = -0.21$, $p < 0.001$

show any significant correlation between the reticulocyte count and mortality. This discrepant result from our present study may be attributable to differences in the sample size, observation period, and/or methodology between the two studies.

The second important finding of this study was that reticulocyte counts showed a strong positive association with female gender, interdialytic body weight gain, and levels of serum EPO, WBC, LDH, iP, non-HDL, and glucose. EPO levels were assessed at intervals of more than 72 h from the last injection of rHuEPO; therefore, the impact of rHuEPO might have been small. Several studies have reported an increased level of plasma EPO in patients with heart failure, which was correlated to a more severe outcome [10–13]. Meanwhile, female gender, inflammation, hyperphosphatemia, hyperglycemia, and dyslipidemia were identified as potential risk factors of microvascular dysfunction [14–16]. In postmenopausal women, microvascular dysfunction has been

linked with adverse outcomes, such as Syndrome X [14]. Recently, Shah et al. reported that global coronary flow reserve, which is defined as the ratio of stress to rest for absolute myocardial blood flow and is a reliable indicator of coronary microvascular function, may provide independent and incremental risk stratification for all-cause and cardiovascular mortality in patients with dialysis-dependent end-stage renal disease (ESRD) [17].

The third finding is that high reticulocyte counts were associated with negative Hb trends. The mean value of Hb at the time of enrollment was not significantly different among the four groups, and the slope of the change in Hb level over half of 1 year was very gentle (0.01 +/– 0.07 g/dL/w); however, the reticulocyte count was wide-ranging ($9.27 \times 10^3/\mu L$ to $146.9 \times 10^3/\mu L$). We theorize that those patients who need a high reticulocyte count to maintain the target Hb level may experience a poorer prognosis.

Given these findings, we would like to present two hypotheses for the relationship between high reticulocyte count and poor outcome. The first is that the reticulocyte count could be a sensitive marker of tissue hypoxia. Reductions in tissue oxygen tension due to microvascular dysfunction would be expected to lead to the activation of hypoxia-inducible transcription factors [15], which in turn might initiate the production of EPO. EPO increases reticulocyte release from the bone marrow and therefore prolongs the maturation time of circulating reticulocytes; this is likely the reason for findings showing a high reticulocyte count [18]. Even HD patients might produce EPO in response to chronic hypoxia. Indeed, Brookhart et al. suspected that ESRD patients who lived at high altitudes could increase endogenous EPO production [19].

The second hypothesis is that reticulocytosis is a result of the accelerated clearance of red blood cells (RBCs). A study showed that the RBC lifespan was significantly and negatively correlated with the erythropoiesis-stimulating agent (ESA) requirement of the patients [20]. Our findings imply that the reticulocytosis found in patients with a poorer prognosis may reflect the compensatory increase of erythropoiesis against the accelerated clearance of circulating RBCs as result of occult bleeding or impairment of RBC survival, including hemolysis [21], or increased eryptosis (apoptotic erythrocyte death) [22, 23]. Oxidative stress [24] and mechanical pressure [25] might play some roles.

There were some limitations to our study; first, it was a retrospective study without a pre-specified hypothesis; therefore, data on some important parameters were lacking. Although we speculated that hemolysis or eryptosis might have been the reason for the increased reticulocyte counts, we did not measure either the serum haptoglobin, phosphatidylserine-positive erythrocyte counts,

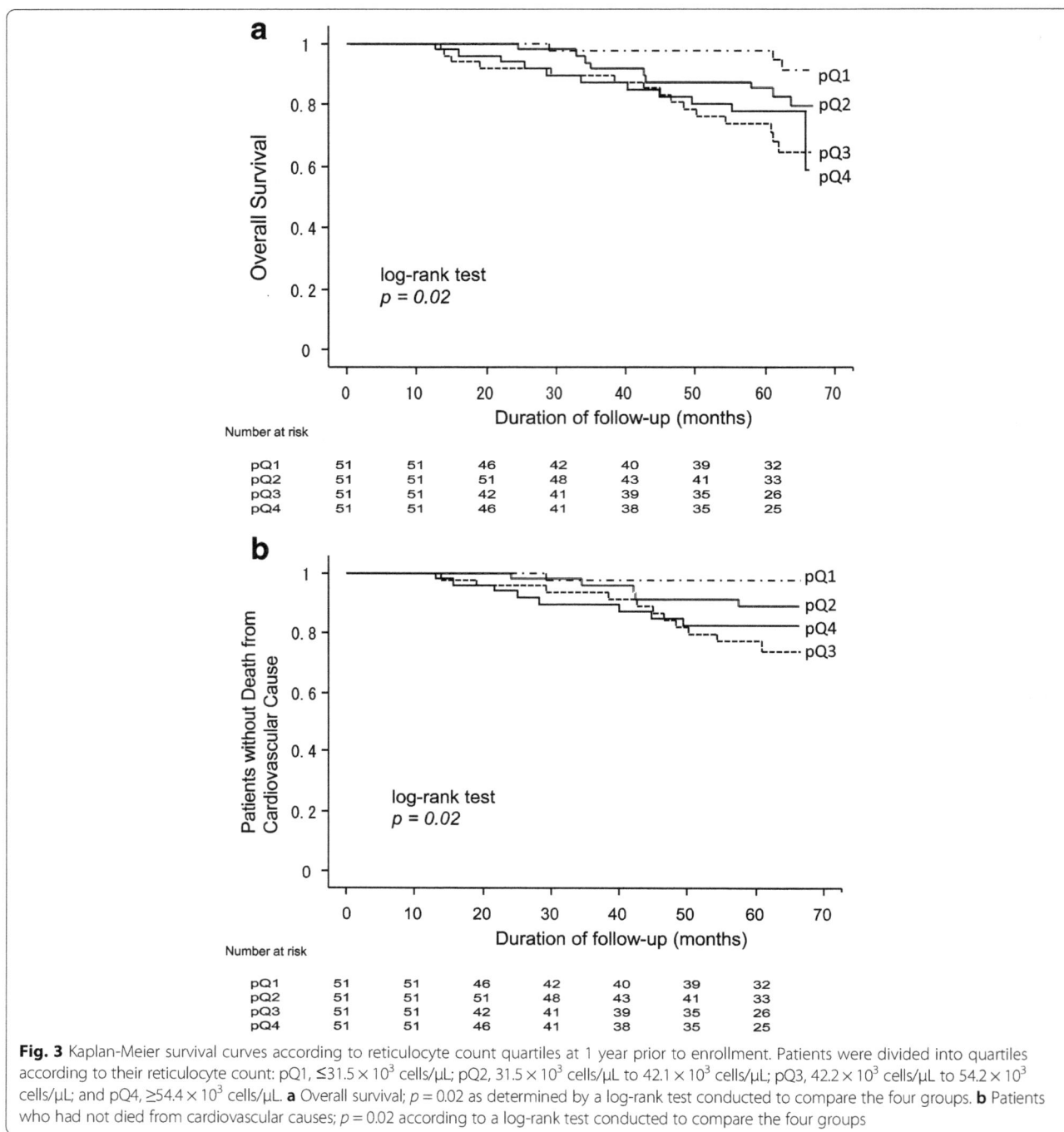

Fig. 3 Kaplan-Meier survival curves according to reticulocyte count quartiles at 1 year prior to enrollment. Patients were divided into quartiles according to their reticulocyte count: pQ1, $\leq$31.5 $\times$ 10^3 cells/μL; pQ2, 31.5 $\times$ 10^3 cells/μL to 42.1 $\times$ 10^3 cells/μL; pQ3, 42.2 $\times$ 10^3 cells/μL to 54.2 $\times$ 10^3 cells/μL; and pQ4, $\geq$54.4 $\times$ 10^3 cells/μL. **a** Overall survival; p = 0.02 as determined by a log-rank test conducted to compare the four groups. **b** Patients who had not died from cardiovascular causes; p = 0.02 according to a log-rank test conducted to compare the four groups

or spleen size. Second, our patients were treated with short-acting ESAs, and it would be unreasonable to extrapolate our findings to patients treated with darbepoetin or CERA. Finally, the average Hb level in our study subjects was lower than the target Hb level recommended in the guidelines published in Europe and the USA [26, 27], although this level was within the average range in Japan [28].

Conclusions

In summary, our findings demonstrated that higher reticulocyte counts in hemodialysis patients are associated with a higher mortality rate. The exact mechanisms underlying the association of the reticulocyte count with the mortality are still unknown. We propose that the increased reticulocyte count is a result of tissue hypoxia or is a compensatory mechanism to maintain the target Hb concentration. Further studies are necessary to explore the mechanisms underlying the close association between the reticulocyte count and mortality in HD patients.

Abbreviations
ACE-I: Angiotensin-converting enzyme inhibitors; Alb: Albumin; ARB: Angiotensin receptor blockers; BMI: Body mass index; BUN: Blood urea nitrogen; CERA: Continuous erythropoietin receptor activator; CI: Confidence interval; Cr: Creatinine; CRP: C-reactive protein; DMN: Diabetic nephropathy; EPO: Erythropoietin; ESAs: Erythropoiesis-stimulating agents; ESRD: End-stage renal disease; Hb: Hemoglobin; HD: Hemodialysis; HR: Hazard ratio; iP: Phosphorus inorganic; LDH: Lactate dehydrogenase; non-HDL: Non-high-density lipoprotein; PLT: Platelet count; RBC: Red blood cell; rHuEPO: Recombinant human erythropoietin; SD: Standard deviation; TSAT: Transferrin saturation; WBC: White blood cell count

Acknowledgements
We thank Dr. Takaaki Tsutsui, Dr. Kyoko Ito, Dr. Tetsuo Ando, Mr. Hideki Ishida, and Mr. Shinsuke Moki for the help in the study operation and data collection. We also express appreciation to the staff of Hidaka Hospital.

Funding
We have no financial support.

Authors' contributions
CT conceived of the study. CT and KO participated in the design of the study, performed the statistical analysis, and drafted the manuscript. HM took the lead in the data collection. NN and YN participated in its design and edited the manuscript. All authors read and approved the final manuscript.

Competing interests
N.N. is a member of the speaker's bureau for Kyowa Hakko Kirin Co., Ltd. The authors declare that they have no competing interests.

Author details
[1]Hidaka Hospital, Takasaki, Gunma, Japan. [2]Ono Naika Clinic, Maebashi, Gunma, Japan. [3]Department of Medicine and Clinical Science, Gunma University Graduate School of Medicine, Maebashi, Gunma, Japan. [4]Present address: Dialysis Center, Ogo Clinic, 245-7, Motogi-machi, Maebashi-shi, Gunma 371-0232, Japan.

References
1. Lombardi G, Colombini A, Lanteri P, Banfi G. Reticulocytes in sports medicine: an update. Adv Clin Chem. 2013;59:125–53. PubMed https://www.ncbi.nlm.nih.gov/pubmed/23461135.
2. Lawrence T, Goodnough, Barry S, Carlo B. Erythropoietin, iron, and erythropoiesis. Blood. 2000;96:823–33. View Article http://www.bloodjournal.org/content/96/3/823?sso-checked=true. PubMed https://www.ncbi.nlm.nih.gov/pubmed/10910892.
3. Piva E, Brugnara C, Spolaore F, Plebani M. Clinical utility of reticulocyte parameters. Clin Lab Med. 2015;35:133–63. PubMedhttps://www.ncbi.nlm.nih.gov/pubmed/25676377.
4. KDOQI, National Kidney Foundation. KDOQI clinical practice guidelines and clinical practice recommendations for anemia in chronic kidney disease. Am J Kidney Dis. 2006;47 suppl 3:S11–145. View Article http://www.ajkd.org/article/S0272-6386(06)00454-9/abstract.
5. Gejyo F, Saito A, Akizawa T, Akiba T, Sakai T, Suzuki M, et al. 2004 Japanese Society for Dialysis Therapy guidelines for renal anemia in chronic hemodialysis patients. Ther Apher Dial. 2004;8:443–59. View Article http://onlinelibrary.wiley.com/doi/10.1111/j.1774-9987.2004.00199.x/abstract;jsessionid=EA4D4497AEF539F2058AA16608445DB9.f04t01. PubMed http://www.ncbi.nlm.nih.gov/pubmed/15663544.
6. Shinzato T, Nakai S, Fujita Y, Takai I, Morita H, Nakane K, et al. Determination of Kt/V and protein catabolic rate using pre and postdialysis blood urea nitrogen concentrations. Nephron. 1994;67:280–90. https://www.ncbi.nlm.nih.gov/pubmed/7936017.
7. Brecher G. New methylene blue as a reticulocyte stain. Am J Clin Pathol. 1949;19:895. PubMedhttp://www.ncbi.nlm.nih.gov/pubmed/18137789.
8. Yang W, Israni RK, Brunelli SM, Joffe MM, Fishbane S, Feldman HI. Hemoglobin variability and mortality in ESRD. J Am Soc Nephrol. 2007;18:3164–70. View Article http://jasn.asnjournals.org/content/18/12/3164.long. PubMed http://www.ncbi.nlm.nih.gov/pubmed/18003781.
9. Cantaro S, Piva E. Hematological and iron parameters to predict mortality in ESRD. G Ital Nefrol. 2005;22 suppl 31:S135–9. PubMed https://www.ncbi.nlm.nih.gov/pubmed/15786388.
10. van der Meer P, Voors AA, Lipsic E, Smilde TD, van Gilst WH, van Veldhuisen DJ. Prognostic value of plasma erythropoietin on mortality in patients with chronic heart failure. J Am Coll Cardiol. 2004;44:63–7. View Article http://www.sciencedirect.com/science/article/pii/S0735109704007764. PubMed https://www.ncbi.nlm.nih.gov/pubmed/15234408.
11. Volpe M, Tritto C, Testa U, Rao MA, Martucci R, Mirante A, et al. Blood levels of erythropoietin in congestive heart failure and correlation with clinical, hemodynamic, and hormonal profiles. Am J Cardiol. 1994;74:468–73. PubMedhttps://www.ncbi.nlm.nih.gov/pubmed/8059727/.
12. George J, Patal S, Wexler D, Abashidze A, Shmilovich H, Barak T, et al. Circulating erythropoietin levels and prognosis in patients with congestive heart failure: comparison with neurohormonal and inflammatory markers. Arch Intern Med. 2005;165:1304–9. View Articles http://jamanetwork.com/journals/jamainternalmedicine/fullarticle/486589. PubMed https://www.ncbi.nlm.nih.gov/pubmed/15956012.
13. Nagai T, Nishimura K, Honma T, Higashiyama A, Sugano Y, Nakai M, Honda S et al, NaDEF investigators. Prognostic significance of endogenous erythropoietin in long-term outcome of patients with acute decompensated heart failure. View Article http://onlinelibrary.wiley.com/doi/10.1002/ejhf.537/abstract;jsessionid=3A8BA63C63C85535B54855201BE0DB75.f01t02. PubMed https://www.ncbi.nlm.nih.gov/pubmed/27126377
14. Pepine CJ, Kerensky RA, Lambert CR, Smith KM, von Mering GO, Sopko G, et al. Some thoughts on the vasculopathy of women with ischemic heart disease. J Am Coll Cardiol. 2006;47(3 Suppl):S30–5. View Article http://www.sciencedirect.com/science/article/pii/S0735109705025088. PubMed https://www.ncbi.nlm.nih.gov/pubmed/16458168.
15. Ostergaard L, Kristiansen SB, Angleys H, Frøkiær J, Michael Hasenkam J, Jespersen SN, et al. The role of capillary transit time heterogeneity in myocardial oxygenation and ischemic heart disease. Basic Res Cardiol. 2014;109:409. View Article https://www.ncbi.nlm.nih.gov/pmc/articles/PMC4013440/. PubMed https://www.ncbi.nlm.nih.gov/pubmed/24743925.
16. Thang OH, Serné EH, Grooteman MP, Smulders YM, ter Wee PM, Tangelder GJ, et al. Capillary rarefaction in advanced chronic kidney disease is associated with high phosphorus and bicarbonate levels. Nephrol Dial Transplant. 2011;26:3529–36. View Article http://ndt.oxfordjournals.org/content/26/11/3529.long. PubMed https://www.ncbi.nlm.nih.gov/pubmed/21414968.
17. Shah NR, Charytan DM, Murthy VL, Skali Lami H, Veeranna V, Cheezum MK, et al. Prognostic value of coronary flow reserve in patients with dialysis-dependent ESRD. J Am Soc Nephrol. 2016;27:1823–9. View Article http://jasn.asnjournals.org/content/27/6/1823.long. PubMed https://www.ncbi.nlm.nih.gov/pubmed/26459635.
18. Krzyzanski W, Perez-Ruixo JJ. An assessment of recombinant human erythropoietin effect on reticulocyte production rate and lifespan

distribution in healthy subjects. Pharm Res. 2007;24:758–72. View Article http://link.springer.com/article/10.1007%2Fs11095-006-9195-y. PubMed https://www.ncbi.nlm.nih.gov/pubmed/17318417.

19. Brookhart MA, Schneeweiss S, Avorn J, Bradbury BD, Rothman KJ, Fischer M, Mehta J, et al. The effect of altitude on dosing and response to erythropoietin in ESRD. J Am Soc Nephrol. 2008;19:1389–95. View Article http://jasn.asnjournals.org/content/19/7/1389.long. PubMed https://www.ncbi.nlm.nih.gov/pubmed/18385423.

20. Sato Y, Mizuguchi T, Shigenaga S, Yoshikawa E, Chujo K, Minakuchi J, Kawashima S. Shortened red blood cell lifespan is related to the dose of erythropoiesis-stimulating agents requirement in patients on hemodialysis. Ther Apher Dial. 2012;16:522–8. View Article http://onlinelibrary.wiley.com/doi/10.1111/j.1744-9987.2012.01089.x/abstract. PubMed https://www.ncbi.nlm.nih.gov/pubmed/23190511.

21. Gallucci MT, Lubrano R, Meloni C, Morosetti M, Manca di Villahermosa S, Scoppi P, et al. Red blood cell membrane lipid peroxidation and resistance to erythropoietin therapy in hemodialysis patients. Clin Nephrol. 1999;52:239–45. PubMedhttp://www.ncbi.nlm.nih.gov/pubmed/10543326.

22. Mahmud H, Ruifrok WP, Westenbrink BD, Cannon MV, Vreeswijk-Baudoin I, van Gilst WH, et al. Suicidal erythrocyte death, eryptosis, as a novel mechanism in heart failure-associated anaemia. Cardiovasc Res. 2013;98:37–46. View Article http://cardiovascres.oxfordjournals.org/content/98/1/37.long. PubMed https://www.ncbi.nlm.nih.gov/pubmed/23341574.

23. Bonomini M, Sirolli V, Settefrati N, Dottori S, Di Liberato L, Arduini A. Increased erythrocyte phosphatidylserine exposure in chronic renal failure. J Am Soc Nephrol. 1999;10:1982–90. View Article http://jasn.asnjournals.org/content/10/9/1982.long. PubMed http://www.ncbi.nlm.nih.gov/pubmed/10477151.

24. Huang KC, Yang CC, Hsu SP, Lee KT, Liu HW, Morisawa S, Otsubo K, Chien CT. Electrolyzed-reduced water reduced hemodialysis-induced erythrocyte impairment in end-stage renal disease patients. Kidney Int. 2006;70:391–8. PubMed https://www.ncbi.nlm.nih.gov/pubmed/16760903.

25. Yang MC, Lin CC. In vitro characterization of the occurrence of hemolysis during extracorporeal blood circulation using a mini hemodialyzer. ASAIO J. 2000;46:293–7. View Article http://journals.lww.com/asaiojournal/pages/articleviewer.aspx?year=2000&issue=05000&article=00010&type=abstract. PubMed https://www.ncbi.nlm.nih.gov/pubmed/10826739.

26. Kidney Disease: Improving Global Outcomes (KDIGO) Anemia Work Group. KDIGO clinical practice guideline for anemia in chronic kidney disease. Kidney Int Suppl. 2012;2:279–335. View Article http://www.kdigo.org/clinical_practice_guidelines/pdf/KDIGO-Anemia%20GL.pdf.

27. KDOQI, et al. KDOQI clinical practice guideline and clinical practice recommendations for anemia in chronic kidney disease: 2007 update of hemoglobin target. Am J Kidney Dis. 2007;50:471–530. View Article http://www.ajkd.org/article/S0272-6386(07)00934-1/pdf.

28. Pisoni RL, Bragg-Gresham JL, Young EW, Akizawa T, Asano Y, Locatelli F, et al. Anemia management and outcomes from 12 countries in the dialysis outcomes and practice patterns study (DOPPS). Am J Kidney Dis. 2004;44:94–111. View Article http://www.ajkd.org/article/S0272-6386(04)00506-2/abstract. PubMed http://www.ncbi.nlm.nih.gov/pubmed/15211443.

12

Frailty and mortality among dialysis patients

Kosaku Nitta[1*], Norio Hanafusa[2] and Ken Tsuchiya[2]

Abstract

Frailty is a clinical state in which there is an increase in the individual's vulnerability to developing increased dependency and/or mortality when exposed to a stressor. Since the mean age of dialysis patients is increasing worldwide, frailty has recently come to be considered one of the risk factors for mortality in the older dialysis population. The prevalence of frailty among dialysis patients has ranged from 3.0- to 10-fold higher than that among community-dwelling elderly, depending on the method of assessing frailty and patient characteristics. Since frailty has been found to be associated with higher mortality, independent of clinical characteristics and comorbidity, interventions to improve frailty have the potential to contribute to better quality of life and lower mortality among dialysis patients. In addition, greater attention should be focused on the possibility that early rehabilitation of dialysis patients might improve poor outcomes. Clinical research should aim to devise an adequate strategy to address frailty, including identifying the optimal timing for intervention.

Keywords: Frailty, Chronic kidney disease, Dialysis, Mortality, Intervention

Background

Because Japan has the world's highest life expectancy and a persistently low birth rate, Japan's population is aging more rapidly than any other country [1]. A systematic review and meta-analysis [2] identified five studies incorporating 11,940 Japanese people aged 65 years or older living in the community and demonstrated that the pooled prevalences of frailty, prefrailty, and robustness based on the Fried criteria were 7.4, 48.1, and 44.4%, respectively. Stratified analyses showed that women were frailer than men and that prevalence of frailty increased with age.

The age of the dialysis patient population in Japan is also increasing yearly. The number of prevalent dialysis patients in Japan was 320,448 in 2014 [3], and the mean age of prevalent dialysis patients was 67.5 years and are likely the older dialysis populations of most other countries in the world. Since 65% of Japanese dialysis patients in 2014 are 65 years of age or more, and 32% are 75 years of age or above (Fig. 1), it is becoming important for dialysis staff members to understand frailty, which is common in elderly dialysis populations.

Frailty has been described as a loss of functional, cognitive, and physiologic reserves that leads to a vulnerable condition [4]. Frailty is a state of increased vulnerability to poor recovery of homeostasis following a stress, and it increases the risk of adverse outcomes, including falls, delirium, and disability [5]. An important perspective for therapeutic approach to frailty is to consider how the complex mechanism of aging promotes the cumulative decline of multiple physiological systems, consequent disturbance of homeostatic reserves, and vulnerability to disproportionate changes in health status in response to relatively minor stressor events.

Chronic kidney disease (CKD) accelerates the aging process via protein energy wasting, uremic toxins, inflammation, and oxidative stresses [6]. These combined effects of chronological and pathological aging may explain why the frailty phenotype is much more common in the CKD population irrespective of dialysis therapy. This article reviews focus on the recent frailty consensus in older adults and how to apply it to the dialysis population.

Definition of frailty

Operational definitions of frailty have incorporated the concepts of multiple contributing causes and multiple manifestations in the form of a syndrome. Fried et al. [4]

* Correspondence: knitta@twmu.ac.jp
[1]Department of Medicine, Kidney Center, Tokyo Women's Medical University, 8-1 Kawada-cho, Shinjuku-ku, Tokyo 162-8666, Japan
Full list of author information is available at the end of the article

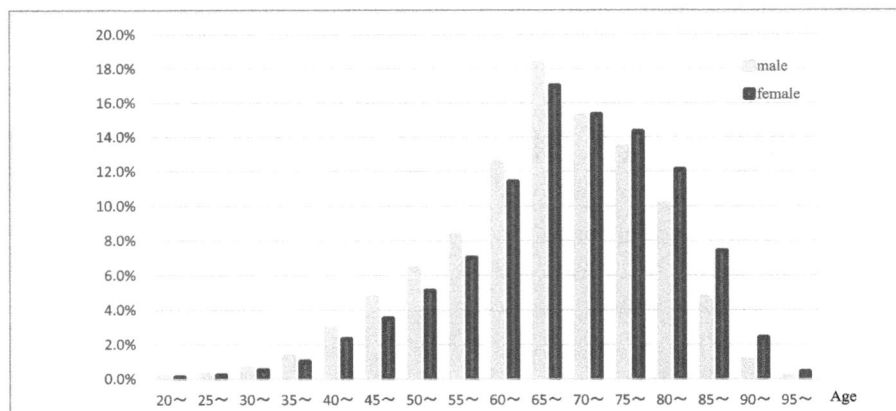

Fig. 1 Distribution of dialysis patients according to age in the Annual Report of the Japanese Society for Dialysis Therapy as of 31 December 2014

have defined a frailty phenotype consisting of at least three of the following unintentional weight loss, exhaustion, physical inactivity, slow gait speed, and weak grip strength. According to this definition, approximately 7% of community-dwelling elderly in a large US cohort study were frail, and frailty was significantly associated with female sex, older age, and higher comorbidity burden. In order to apply the concept of frailty to patients with CKD or end-stage renal disease (ESRD), the frailty phenotype has been adapted in numerous ways, the most common of which is to substitute patients' self-report of physical functioning for direct measures of physical performance [7, 8].

Two approaches to define physical frailty have become popular. The first deficit model consists of adding together an individual's number of impairments and conditions to create a frailty index [9]. The second model was originally defined as a specific physical phenotype consisting of a constellation of five possible components: weight loss, exhaustion, weakness, slowness, and reduced physical activity, which marked an underlying physiologic state of multisystem and energy dysregulation [10]. Both of these definitions are currently used to define a frail state and a prefrail state, a condition between the frail state and nonfrail state. Many other definitions of frailty have been proposed, but the heterogeneity of definitions may have contributed to the inability to agree on a single operational definition of frailty that satisfies all experts.

A recent consensus conference of European and American frailty experts defined frailty as a medical syndrome with multiple causes and contributors that is characterized by diminished strength, endurance, and reduced physiologic function that increases an individual's vulnerability to developing increased dependency and/or to death [11]. The consensus conference showed four recommendations: (1) physical frailty is an important medical syndrome, (2) simple screening tests are available to be used by physicians to recognize frail persons and identify persons with physical frailty or at risk of frailty, (3) physical frailty is a manageable condition, and (4) all persons older than 70 years should be screened for frailty. Since aging and chronic diseases likely contribute to the development of frailty through mechanisms that include oxidative stress, inflammation, and reductions in serum anabolic hormone levels [10], it is not surprising that CKD, which itself can lead to all of the above, is associated with a higher prevalence of frailty in community-dwelling elderly [12]. However, the definition or the diagnostic criteria of 'frailty' have not gained the broad consensus.

Prevalence of frailty in the predialysis and dialysis population

CKD represents a formidable cause of biochemical changes and is also a physiological stressor, causing premature occurrence of age-related changes. The combined effect of aging and CKD may represent a higher dose of physiological changes that lead to unsuccessful aging [12]. An association between frailty and predialysis CKD has recently recognized. A systematic review of frailty in CKD found that multiple studies have demonstrated a strong and consistent relationship between worsening kidney function and poor performance on physical function tests [13]. In a large study of predialysis CKD patients enrolled in the third National Health and Nutrition Evaluation Survey, increasing severity of predialysis CKD patients was strongly associated with occurrence of frailty [14], suggesting that more severe metabolic abnormalities carried by worsening kidney function lead to more significant levels of frailty.

Johansen et al. used a self-report-based definition of frailty to assess the prevalence and significance of frailty among the 2275 dialysis patients participating in the Dialysis Morbidity and Mortality Wave 2 study [8]. The results revealed that two thirds of the patients were frail, including those who were under the age of 65 years. A multivariable logistic regression analysis suggested that older age, female sex, and hemodialysis were independently associated with frailty. A Cox proportional hazards model indicated that frailty was independently associated with higher risk of death (adjusted hazard ratio (HR) 2.24, 95% confidence interval (CI) 1.60–3.15) and with a combined outcome of death and hospitalization (adjusted HR 1.63, 95% CI 1.41–1.87). Since then, the Fried frailty phenotype has been applied to prevalent dialysis populations in the USA [15, 16]. The prevalence was lower when measured by this method, 30–42%, but was still four to six times that of healthy elderly persons despite inclusion of all adults in these studies rather than only those above 65 years of age. The prevalence of frailty among ESRD patients has varied with the cohorts, probably as a result of differences between the methods used to assess frailty [17]. Differences in patient characteristics, such as dialysis vintage and severity of co-morbidities, probably contribute to the variation. Nevertheless, all studies have shown a substantially higher prevalence of frailty among ESRD patients than among community-dwelling elderly.

Because of the high burden of comorbid illness in dialysis patients and the high overall mortality, it is important to consider whether frailty provides prognostic information in this population. If comorbidity and inflammatory exist already in the dialysis population, the presence of frailty may not improve prediction of adverse outcomes. However, frailty has been found to be independently associated with higher mortality in all studies that have examined the association between frailty and mortality to date. Frailty has also been found to be associated with higher risk of falls and fractures [18, 19]. There is an ongoing debate about the value of frailty assessment in dialysis populations and the methods by which frailty should be assessed [20, 21], and longitudinal studies are needed to provide the answers.

Screening and management of frailty

Sufficient evidence exists for the implementation of frailty screening of persons 70 years of age and older by health care providers. Simple rapid screening tests that allow physicians to rapidly identify frail persons have been developed and validated. Examples of some commonly used and validated frailty tools are the FRAIL (Table 1) [22] and the Clinical Frailty Scale (Table 2) [23]. A screening approach is also being carried out widely in Japan, and interventions suggested by the consensus group have been provided successfully [24]. They

Table 1 The simple "FRAIL" questionnaire screening tool

3 or greater = frailty; 1 or 2 = prefrail
Fatigue: are you fatigued?
Resistance: cannot walk up 1 flight of stairs?
Aerobic: cannot walk 1 block?
Illnesses: do you have more than 5 illnesses?
Loss of weight: have you lost more than 5% of your weight in the past 6 months?

compared the comprehensive geriatric assessment (CGA) between specified elderly individuals at risk of requiring long-term care insurance and uncertified elderly people, and also compared CGA between the risk group and non-risk group, in subcategories of the "Kihon Checklist," including the physical strength, nutrition/oral function, overall low score on questions 1–20, houseboundness, cognitive function, and depression risk (Fig. 2). They concluded that the assessments of physical strength and cognitive function were more useful as means of identifying frail elderly.

We are aware of a few published studies that were specifically designed to examine frailty in the dialysis population. Unfortunately, the results of recent studies suggest that the functional status in the absence of intervention declines further after initiating dialysis among very elderly patients [25, 26], making it imperative to consider treatments or interventions that reverse their downward trajectory. Since physical inactivity is part of the definition of frailty, interventions that increase activity may reverse frailty directly or indirectly if they also improve physical performance or symptoms of fatigue and exhaustion. Some studies have shown that hemodialysis patients are extremely inactive [27–29] and that their low physical activity is associated with poorer physical performance [30] and lower survival rates [31, 32]. Few studies have focused on increasing the habitual physical activity of the dialysis population [33, 34], but such a strategy seems promising and should be investigated. Even in the absence of solid evidence for a benefit in the dialysis population, dialysis patients should be encouraged to follow physical activity guidelines for older patients.

There have been numerous studies of more vigorous exercise training programs designed to increase the exercise capacity or physical performance of dialysis patients [35], and although many of the studies have been small and/or of low quality, since the majority have shown improvements and patients with lower baseline functioning have been found to derive greater benefit in one of the largest exercise intervention studies [36], aerobic exercise training would seem to have the potential to improve frailty. However, the vigorous nature of such training programs has led to the exclusion of large numbers of hemodialysis patients as ineligible, and frail patients

Table 2 The clinical frailty scale (CFS)

CFS score	Interpretation
1	Very fit: robust, active, energetic, motivated, and fit; fittest in their age group
2	Well: without active disease but not as fit as those in category 1
3	Well: with treated comorbid disease
4	Apparently vulnerable: not dependent but has symptoms from comorbid disease (such as being slowed up)
5	Mildly frail: limited dependence on others for instrumental activities of daily living
6	Moderately frail: help is needed for instrumental activities of daily living and activities of daily living
7	Severely frail: completely dependent on others for instrumental activities of daily living and activities of daily living or terminally ill
8	Very severely frail: completely dependent, approaching the end of life. Typically, they could not recover even from a minor illness.
9	Terminally ill: approaching the end of life. This category applies to people with a life expectancy <6 months, who are not otherwise evidently frail.

would be more likely have factors that lead to exclusion. Moreover, there has been a high rate of patient refusal to participate in such programs when offered, suggesting that fear or reluctance to engage in vigorous activity is a barrier to patients' adoption of exercise programs. Thus, the extent to which aerobic exercise training during dialysis or at some other time can reverse frailty remains to be determined.

Because weakness is part of frailty, and muscle atrophy is a key underlying mechanism [37], resistance exercises or other anabolic interventions might be logical choices to ameliorate frailty in the dialysis population [38]. Indeed, resistance training has been shown to increase muscle strength in both hemodialysis patients [38] and institutionalized nonagenarians [39], thereby demonstrating that such programs are possible, even among patients with extremely low functioning, and that they can be beneficial. Thus, referral of frail individuals for physical therapy and strength training should be considered when weakness or frailty is detected.

Interventions for frail older adults

The development of strategies, such as community-based interventions, to reduce the risk of disability, including physical frailty, is required worldwide. Physical frailty is bidirectional and potentially reversible. Therefore, interventions have been developed for the condition, and exercise has been shown to exert a positive functional effect on physical frailty [40]. Although interventions, including exercise, nutrition, and education, for older adults at high risk of disability may improve their quality of life, there is little evidence available to show whether interventions reduce the onset of disability with physical frailty [41]. Makizato et al. [42] has recently reported the effects of a community disability prevention program for frail older adults. A total of 514 community-dwelling older adults aged 65 years or older with physical frailty who had undergone baseline assessment and participated in community-based intervention studies (participants) or did not (non-participants) were included in the study. They conclude that participation in community-based

1	Do you use public transportation (bus or train) to go out on your own?	
2	Do you shop for daily necessities?	
3	Do you manage financial matters such as savings or deposits by yourself?	
4	Do you visit the homes of friends?	
5	Do you give advice to friends or family members who confide in you?	
6	Are you able to go up stairs without using handrails or the wall for support?	
7	Are you able to stand up from a sitting position without support?	Physical strength
8	Are you able to walk continuously for 15 minutes?	
9	Have you experienced a fall in the past year?	
10	Do you feel anxious about falling when you walk?	
11	Has your weight declined by 2-3 kg in the past 6 months?	Nutritional status
12	Height: cm Weight: kg BMI	
13	Have you experienced more difficulty chewing tough foods than you did 6 months ago?	
14	Do you ever experience choking or coughing when drinking tea or soup?	Oral function
15	Are you bothered by feelings of thirst or dry mouth?	
16	Do you go out at least one time a week?	Houseboundness
17	Do you go out less often than you did last year?	
18	Do others point out your forgetfulness or tell you "You always ask the same thing."	
19	When you want to make a call, do you usually search for the telephone number and call on your own?	
20	Do you sometimes not know what the date is?	Cognitive function
21	(in the past 2 weeks) You feel no sense of fulfillment in your life.	
22	(in the past 2 weeks) You cannot enjoy things that you enjoyed before.	Depression risk
23	(in the past 2 weeks) Things that you could do easily before are now difficult.	
24	(in the past 2 weeks) You do not feel that you are a useful person.	
25	(in the past 2 weeks) You feel exhausted for no apparent reason.	

Overall low score on questions 1–20

Fig. 2 Kihon Checklist of 25 items and seven categories for screening "specified elderly" individuals for frailty

intervention studies could reduce the incidence of disability in older adults with physical frailty.

A systematic review has shown that exercise interventions are beneficial and feasible and can be implemented safely in the ESRD population [43]. Both aerobic and resistance exercise interventions, administered in the dialysis facility or outside of dialysis, have resulted in improvements in physical function [44]. However, there are several limitations of the methodologic issues with studies of exercise in dialysis patients, including uncertainty about the optimal modality and dose of exercise, the best time for intervention, safety and health concerns, and frequent hospitalizations and clinical status changes in the dialysis population that can interrupt training. Conclusions were limited by the heterogeneity of the ESRD population, the presence of multiple comorbid conditions, and difficulty in implementing long-term interventions given the high rate of drop-out in the studies to date and the high mortality in the patient population.

Conclusion

Frailty is common in the older dialysis population and is associated with adverse outcomes, including death, hospitalization, falls, and fractures. Studies are required to determine whether interventions can improve frailty. The potential association between frailty of predialysis patients and higher risk of ESRD would suggest that early intervention may be effective, but it is also important to consider the dialysis population whose current functioning is extremely impaired.

Acknowledgements
The authors would like to thank all dialysis staffs who gave us the chance to write this review.

Funding
None.

Authors' contributions
KN planned the review, searched the literature, and prepared the article. NH searched the literature and assisted in writing the article. KT planned the context of this article and assisted in writing the article. All authors read and approved the final manuscript.

Competing interests
The authors declare that they have no competing interests.

Author details
[1]Department of Medicine, Kidney Center, Tokyo Women's Medical University, 8-1 Kawada-cho, Shinjuku-ku, Tokyo 162-8666, Japan. [2]Department of Blood Purification, Kidney Center, Tokyo Women's Medical University, Tokyo, Japan.

References

1. Arai H, Ouchi Y, Toba K, Endo T, Shimokado K, Tsubota K, et al. Japan as the front-runner of super-aged societies: perspectives from medicine and medical care in Japan. Geriatr Gerontol Int. 2015;15:673–87.
2. Kojima G, Iliffe S, Taniguchi Y, Shimada H, Rakugi H, Walters K. Prevalence of frailty in Japan: a systematic review and meta-analysis. J Epidemiol. 2016.
3. Masakane I, Nakai S, Ogata S, Kimata N, Hanafusa N, Hamano T, et al. Annual dialysis data report 2014, JSDT renal data registry (JRDR). Ren Replace Ther. 2017;3:18.
4. Fried LP, Tangen CM, Walston J, Newman AB, Hirsch C, Gottdiener J, et al. Frailty in older adults: evidence for a phenotype. J Gerontol A Viol Sci Med Sci. 2001;56:M146–56.
5. Walston J, Hadley EC, Ferrucci L, Guralnik JM, Newman AB, Studenski SA, et al. Research agenda for frailty in doler sdults: toward a better understanding of physiology and etiology: summary from the American Geriatrics Society/National Institute on Aging Research Conference on Frailty in Older Adults. J Am Geriatr Soc. 2006;54:991–1001.
6. Nitta K, Hanafusa N, Tsuchiya K. Recent advances in the pathophysiology and management of protein-energy wasting in chronic kidney disease. Ren Replace Ther. 2016;2:4.
7. Woods N, LaCroix A, Gray S, Aragaki A, Cochrane B, Brunner R, et al. Frailty: emergence and consequences in women aged 65 and older in the Women's Health Initiative Observational Study. J Am Geriatr Soc. 2005;53:1321–30.
8. Johansen KL, Chertow GM, Jin C, Kutner NG. Significance of frailty among dialysis patients. J Am Soc Nephrol. 2007;18:2960–7.
9. Rockwood K, Mitnitski A. Frailty defined by deficit accumulation and geriatric medicine defined by frailty. Clin Geriatr Med. 2011;27:17–26.
10. Fried LP, Ferrucci L, Darer J, Williamson JD, Anderson G. Untangling the concepts of disability, frailty, and comorbidity: implications for improved targeting and care. J Gerontol A Biol Sci Med Sci. 2004;59:255–63.
11. Morley JE, Vellas B, van Kan GA, Anker SD, Bauer JM, Bernabei R, et al. Frailty consensus: a call to action. J Am Med Dir Assoc. 2013;14:392–7.
12. Shlipak M, Stehman-Breen C, Fried L, Song X, Siscovick D, Fried L, et al. The presence of frailty in elderly persons with chronic renal insufficiency. Am J Kidney Dis. 2004;43:861–7.
13. Kalantar-Zadeh K, Ikizler TA, Block G, Avram MM, Kopple JD. Malnutrition-inflammation complex syndrome in dialysis patients: causes and consequences. Am J Kidney Dis. 2003;42:864–81.
14. Wilhelm-Leen ER, Hall YN, Tamura MK, Chertow GM. Frailty and chronic kidney disease: the Third National Health and Nutrition Evaluation Survey. Am J Med. 2009;122:664–71.
15. McAdams-Demarco MA, Law A, Salter ML, Boyarsky B, Gimenez L, Jaar BG, et al. Frailty as a novel predictor of mortality and hospitalization in individuals of all ages undergoing hemodialysis. J Am Geriatr Soc. 2013;61:896–901.
16. Johansen KL, Dalrymple LS, Delgado C, Kaysen GA, Kornak J, Grimes B, et al. Association between body composition and frailty among prevalent hemodialysis patients: a USRDS special study. J Am Soc Nephrol. 2014;25:381–9.
17. Johansen KL. The frail dialysis population: a growing burden for the dialysis community. Blood Purif. 2015;40:288–92.
18. McAdams-DeMarco MA, Suresh S, Law A, Salter ML, Gimenez LF, Jaar BG, et al. Frailty and falls among adult patients undergoing chronic hemodialysis: a prospective cohort study. BMC Nephrol. 2013;14:224.
19. Delgado C, Shieh S, Grimes B, Chertow GM, Dalrymple LS, Kaysen GA, et al. Association of self-reported frailty with falls and fractures among patients new to dialysis. Am J Nephrol. 2015;42:134–40. Epub ahead of print.
20. Painter P, Kuskowski M. A closer look at frailty in ESRD: getting the measure right. Hemodialysis Int. 2013;17:41–9.
21. Johansen KL, Dalrymple LS, Delgado C, Kaysen GA, Kornak J, Grimes B, et al. Comparison of self-report-based and physical performance-based frailty definitions among patients receiving maintenance hemodialysis. Am J Kidney Dis. 2014;64:600–7.

22. Morley JE, Malmstrom TK, Miller DK. A simple frailty questionnaire (FRAIL) predicts outcomes in middle aged African Americans. J Nutr Health Aging. 2012;16:601–8.

23. Rockwood K, Song X, MacKnight C, Bergman H, Hogan DB, McDowell I, et al. A global clinical measure of fitness and frailty in elderly people. CMAJ. 2005;173:489–95.

24. Fukutomi E, Okumiya K, Wada T, Sakamoto R, Ishimoto Y, Kimura Y, et al. Importance of cognitive assessment as part of the "Kihon Checklist" developed by the Japanese Ministry of Health, Labor and Welfare for prediction of frailty at a 2-year follow up. Geriatr Gerontol Int. 2013;13:654–62.

25. Kurella Tamura M, Covinsky KE, Chertow GM, Yaffe K, Landefeld CS, McCulloch CE. Functional status of elderly adults before and after initiation of dialysis. N Engl J Med. 2009;361:1539–47.

26. Jassal SV, Chiu E, Hladunewich M. Loss of independence in patients starting dialysis at 80 years of age or older. N Engl J Med. 2009;361:1612–3.

27. Johansen KL, Chertow GM, Kutner NG, Dalrymple LS, Grimes BA, Kaysen GA. Low level of self-reported physical activity in ambulatory patients new to dialysis. Kidney Int. 2010;78:1164–70.

28. Avesani C, Trolonge S, Deleaval P, Baria F, Mafra D, Faxen-Irving G, et al. Physical activity and energy expenditure in haemodialysis patients: an international study. Nephrol Dial Transplant. 2012;27:2430–4.

29. Matsuzawa R, Matsunaga A, Wang G, Kutsuna T, Ishii A, Abe Y, et al. Habitual physical activity measured by accelerometer and survival in maintenance hemodialysis patients. Clin J Am Soc Nephrol. 2012;7:2010–6.

30. Johansen KL, Painter P, Kent-Braun JA, Ng AV, Carey S, Da Silva M, et al. Validation of questionnaires to estimate physical activity and functioning in end-stage renal disease. Kidney Int. 2001;59:1121–7.

31. O'Hare AM, Tawney K, Bacchetti P, Johansen KL. Decreased survival among sedentary patients undergoing dialysis: results from the dialysis morbidity and mortality study wave 2. Am J Kidney Dis. 2003;41:447–54.

32. Johansen KL, Kaysen GA, Dalrymple LS, Grimes BA, Glidden DV, Anand S, et al. Association of physical activity with survival among ambulatory patients on dialysis: the comprehensive dialysis study. Clin J Am Soc Nephrol. 2013;8: 248–53.

33. Bulckaen M, Capitanini A, Lange S, Caciula A, Giuntoli F, Cupisti A. Implementation of exercise training programs in a hemodialysis unit: effects on physical performance. J Nephrol. 2011;24:790–7.

34. Nowicki M, Murlikiewicz K, Jagodzińska M. Pedometers as a means to increase spontaneous physical activity in chronic hemodialysis patients. J Nephrol. 2010;23:297–305.

35. Johansen KL. Exercise in the end-stage renal disease population. J Am Soc Nephrol. 2007;18:1845–54.

36. Painter P, Carlson L, Carey S, Paul SM, Myll J. Low-functioning hemodialysis patients improve with exercise training. Am J Kidney Dis. 2000;36:600–8.

37. Delgado C, Doyle JW, Johansen KL. Association of frailty with body composition among patients on hemodialysis. J Ren Nutr. 2013;23:356–62.

38. Johansen KL, Painter PL, Sakkas GK, Gordon P, Doyle J, Shubert T. Effects of resistance exercise training and nandrolone decanoate on body composition and muscle function among patients who receive hemodialysis: a randomized, controlled trial. J Am Soc Nephrol. 2006;17:2307–14.

39. Fiatarone MA, Marks EC, Ryan ND, Meredith CN, Lipsitz LA, Evans WJ. High-intensity strength training in nonagenarians. Effects on skeletal muscle. JAMA. 1990;263:3029–34.

40. Theou O, Stathokostas L, Roland KP, Jakobi JM, Patterson C, Vandervoort AA, et al. The effectiveness of exercise interventions for the management of frailty: a systematic review. J Aging Res. 2011;2011:569194.

41. Michel JP, Cruz-Jentoft AJ, Cederholm T. Frailty, exercise and nutrition. Clin Geriatr Med. 2015;31:375–87.

42. Makizato H, Shimada H, Doi T, Tsutumimoto K, Yoshida D, Suzuki T. Effects of a community disability prevention program for frail older adults at 48-month follow up. Geriatr Gerontol Int 2017. in press

43. Barcellos FC, Santos IS, Umpierre D, Bohlke M, Hallal PC. Effects of exercise in the whole spectrum of chronic kidney disease: a systematic review. Clin Kidney J. 2015;8:753–65.

44. Sheshadri A, Johansen KL. Prehabitation for the frail patients approaching ESRD. Semin Nephrol. 2017;37:159–72.

13

Annual peritoneal dialysis report 2014, the peritoneal dialysis registry

Ikuto Masakane[1,4*], Takeshi Hasegawa[2], Satoshi Ogata[1], Naoki Kimata[1], Shigeru Nakai[1], Norio Hanafusa[1], Takayuki Hamano[1], Kenji Wakai[1], Atsushi Wada[1], Kosaku Nitta[3], on behalf of the Committee of Renal Data Registry (CRDR), the Japanese Society for Dialysis Therapy (JSDT)

Abstract

Background: Since 2009, the peritoneal dialysis (PD) registry has been carried out as part of Japanese Society for Dialysis Therapy (JSDT) Renal Data Registry with the cooperation of Japanese Society for Peritoneal Dialysis. In this study, the current status of PD patients is reported on the basis of the results of the survey conducted at the end of 2014.

Methods: The subjects were PD patients who lived in Japan and participated in the 2014 survey. Descriptive analysis was performed for various items including the current status of the combined use of PD and another dialysis modalities such as hemodialysis or hemodiafiltration, the method of exchanging PD fluid, the use of an automated peritoneal dialysis machine, and the incidences of peritonitis and catheter exit-site infection.

Results: From the results of the facility survey in 2014, the number of PD patients was 9255, a decrease of 137 from that in 2013. Among the entire dialysis patient population, 2.9% were PD patients, a decrease of 0.1%. One thousand thirteen (21%) among them were on the combination therapy of PD and hemodialysis or hemodiafiltration. The mean incidence of peritonitis was 0.21 per patient per year in another expression as once per 57.1 patients per month. The mean incidence of catheter exit-site infection was 0.40 per patient per year in the other expression as once per 30.0 patients per month.

Conclusions: The number of PD patients has been stable around 9000~10,000 in these 10 years. High percentage of the combination therapy of PD and other dialysis modality and the lower PD dialysis dose was a unique point of the current PD in Japan. The patient's and center's peritonitis rates were very low as around 0.2 per patient-year. PD registry clearly showed the current trends in PD in Japan which were a little different from those in other many countries.

Keywords: PD registry, Dialysis fluid exchange maneuver, Peritonitis, Catheter exit-site infection

Introduction

Japanese Society for Dialysis Therapy (JSDT) has been conducting an annual survey on the current status of regular dialysis treatment in Japan (JSDT Renal Data Registry (JRDR)) at the end of each year since 1968. Since 1983, survey items relating to all dialysis patients

* Correspondence: imasakan.aipod@seieig.or.jp
[1]Committee of Renal Data Registry (CRDR), Japanese Society for Dialysis Therapy (JSDT), Aramido Building 2F, 2-38-21 Hongo, Bunkyo-ku, Tokyo 113-0033, Japan
[4]Department Nephrology, Yabuki Hospital, 4-4-5 Shima Kita, Yamagata City, Yamagata 990-0885, Japan
Full list of author information is available at the end of the article

treated in dialysis facilities that participated in the surveys have been included and the obtained data have been registered in an electronic database [1]. In the 2009 survey, JSDT started the peritoneal dialysis (PD) registry survey of patients who underwent PD, in cooperation with Japanese Society for Peritoneal Dialysis (JSPD) [2]. The targets of the PD registry survey include facilities that offer PD alone, which were not targeted in the conventional surveys conducted at the end of each year. The results of the PD registry survey have been reported annually in the sections "Current status of PD treatment" and "Items associated with PD" of the "An

Overview of Regular Dialysis Treatment in Japan" compiled by Committee of Renal Data Registry (CRDR) in JSDT. In 2012, the results of the PD registry survey were separated from the above overview and independently summarized in the PD registry survey report as an academic paper. The current manuscript is the second publication of "Peritoneal dialysis (PD) registry with 2014 survey report. J Jpn Soc Dial Ther 49(1):35–40, 2016," written in Japanese.

Here, the data obtained from the 2014 PD registry survey are summarized in the following six topics:

I. Current status of PD patients
II. Urine output and volume of water removed by PD
III. Dialysate/plasma creatinine (D/P Cr) ratio in a peritoneal equilibration test (PET)
IV. Kt/V for residual renal function (residual renal Kt/V) and Kt/V for PD (PD Kt/V)
V. Peritonitis and catheter exit-site infections
VI. Encapsulating peritoneal sclerosis (EPS)

Outline of the PD registry in 2014
Survey methods
This survey was conducted by sending questionnaires to individual dialysis facilities. A total of 4367 facilities participating in this survey were either member facilities of JSDT, nonmember facilities offering regular hemodialysis (HD), or nonmember facilities offering PD but not HD, as of December 31, 2014. The number of participating facilities increased by 42 (1.0%) from the previous year (4325 facilities) [3]. Among the 4367 facilities, 986 treated PD patients.

Universal serial bus (USB) memory devices that stored electronic spreadsheets in Microsoft Excel® or paper questionnaires were sent to and collected from the individual dialysis facilities, mainly by postal mail; for some facilities, the questionnaires were sent and collected by fax. In the 2014 survey, two sets of questionnaires were used. One was for the facility survey, which included items on individual dialysis facilities, such as the numbers of patients and staff members. The other was for the patient survey, which included items on individual dialysis patients, such as their demographical background, treatment conditions, and outcomes of treatment. The deadline for acceptance of responses was the end of January 2015. The acceptance of responses submitted after this deadline, including those of the additional surveys, ended on August 7, 2015.

Before 2014, the results from JRDR had been reported in the following three types of report. First, quick analyses of the data obtained by April in the following year were reported at the annual meeting of the JSDT held in June and compiled in "The Atlas, Overview of Regular Dialysis Treatment in Japan," Second, the responses to

the survey had been continuously collected until September, and the obtained data were screened to determine the definite survey results, which were published in the "An Overview of Regular Dialysis Treatment in Japan, the CD-ROM Report." Third, the tabulated results based on the definite values in the CD-ROM Report were published as an annual dialysis data report in the Journal of Japanese Society for Dialysis Therapy. Therefore, the values in the atlas were different from the definite values in the CD-ROM. The quick estimations were prepared only for the atlas in the annual meeting of JSDT. However, the values in the atlas had been occasionally cited as if they were officially approved values because they were expressed by attractive graphs. To avoid these mal-citations, we decided to publish all the official reports from the 2014 survey based on the definite database.

For the CD-ROM Report, the number of facilities that responded to the facility survey was 4330 (99.2%) and the number of those that responded to both the facility and patient surveys was 4191 (96.0%) [4]. Moreover, the number of facilities that completed the questionnaires using the electronic medium was 3764 (86.9%), which was higher than that in the 2013 survey (3698 facilities, 86.6%). This increase contributed to the accurate and simplified analysis of survey data.

Survey items
The 2014 survey included the following survey items. For the items included in the previous surveys, refer to the members-only pages of the JSDT website (http://member.jsdt.or.jp/member/contents/data/research_list_2000-2015.pdf).

Facility survey items

- Name of facility, contact numbers (telephone and fax), name of representative (doctor), and name of respondent
- Year and month when the facility started offering dialysis treatment

Table 1 Number of prevalent PD patients

	Number of patients
Prevalent PD patients	9255
Patients with a catheter for PD such as those who underwent only peritoneal lavage	278
New patients who started on PD in 2014 but switched to other methods in the same year	193
Patients who underwent PD + HD(F)	1913

These data were obtained by the facility survey

Table 2 Distribution of prevalent PD patients, by PD vintage and combination frequency

PD vintage	<1 year	1–<2 years	2–<4 years	4–<6 years	6–<8 years	8–<10 years	≥10 years	Subtotal	No information available	Total	Mean	SD
PD only (%)	1252 (96.7)	948 (89.9)	1269 (83.7)	640 (73.1)	269 (59.1)	101 (46.5)	109 (41.3)	4588 (80.8)	2600 (77.8)	7188 (79.7)	2.80	2.72
PD + HD(F) once a week (%)	35 (2.7)	93 (8.8)	219 (14.4)	205 (23.4)	151 (33.2)	86 (39.6)	113 (42.8)	902 (15.9)	642 (19.2)	1544 (17.1)	5.69	3.92
PD + HD(F) twice a week (%)	4 (0.3)	7 (0.7)	12 (0.8)	20 (2.3)	27 (5.9)	26 (12.0)	26 (9.8)	122 (2.1)	55 (1.6)	177 (2.0)	7.53	4.15
PD + HD(F) three times a week (%)	–	3 (0.3)	3 (0.2)	2 (0.2)	2 (0.4)	–	5 (1.9)	15 (0.3)	25 (0.7)	40 (0.4)	6.58	5.05
PD + HD(F) at other frequencies (%)	4 (0.3)	4 (0.4)	14 (0.9)	8 (0.9)	6 (1.3)	4 (1.8)	11 (4.2)	51 (0.9)	22 (0.7)	73 (0.8)	6.47	4.99
Total (%)	1295 (100.0)	1055 (100.0)	1517 (100.0)	875 (100.0)	455 (100.0)	217 (100.0)	264 (100.0)	5678 (100.0)	3344 (100.0)	9022 (100.0)	3.40	3.27

These data were obtained by the patient survey

Table 3 Changing maneuver of PD fluids

Method of PD solution exchange	Completely manual exchange	Double-bag system with ultraviolet light irradiation	Double-bag system with sterile connecting device	Double-bag system (methods other than those on the left columns, including semimanual methods)	Subtotal	Unspecified	No information available	Total
Number of patients (%)	1422 (32.2)	2322 (52.6)	607 (13.7)	66 (1.5)	4417 (100.0)	76	2695	7188

These data were obtained from the PD-only patients in the patient survey

- Number of bedside consoles, total number of patients who can simultaneously receive dialysis, and maximum number of admissible patients
- Number of full-time and part-time workers engaged in dialysis treatment (e.g., doctors, nurses, clinical engineers, nutritionists, case workers)
- Number of dialysis doctors
- Number of outpatients and inpatients who underwent dialysis (daytime dialysis, nighttime dialysis, home HD, and PD)
- Number of prevalent dialysis patients at the end of 2014
- Number of new patients who were started incident dialysis patients in 2014
- Number of dialysis patients who died during 2014
- Number of patients who underwent HD or hemodiafiltration (HDF) and did not undergo PD despite having a catheter for PD (underwent only peritoneal lavage), number of patients who underwent both PD and HD or HDF, and number of new patients who were started on PD in 2014 but introduced to another blood purification method in the same year
- Current status of dialysate quality control (details not shown)

Patient survey items

The following are the basic survey items that have been annually surveyed since 1983.

- Anonymized name
- Gender and date of birth
- Year and month of start of dialysis and year and month of transfer from another hospital
- Primary disease
- Prefecture where the patient lives
- Dialysis method
- Outcome, year, and month (transfer, death, change in dialysis method, or transplantation) (code of facility to which the patient is transferred)
- Cause of death

The following were added to the basic survey items and were surveyed using both paper and electronic media.

- Dialysis modality, current status of combined use of PD, and HD or HDF
- History of PD
- Number of renal transplantations

Table 4 Use or nonuse of APD machine, by PD vintage

PD vintage	Use	Nonuse	Subtotal	Unspecified	No information available	Total
<1 year (%)	627 (52.8)	561 (47.2)	1188 (100.0)	3	61	1252
1–<2 years (%)	451 (50.0)	451 (50.0)	902 (100.0)	2	44	948
2–<4 years (%)	672 (55.8)	532 (44.2)	1204 (100.0)	16	49	1269
4–<6 years (%)	340 (55.6)	272 (44.4)	612 (100.0)	7	21	640
6–<8 years (%)	163 (63.7)	93 (36.3)	256 (100.0)	–	13	269
8–<10 years (%)	66 (70.2)	28 (29.8)	94 (100.0)	2	5	101
≥10 years (%)	71 (68.3)	33 (31.7)	104 (100.0)	–	5	109
Subtotal (%)	2390 (54.8)	1970 (45.2)	4360 (100.0)	30	198	4588
No information available (%)	48 (55.8)	38 (44.2)	86 (100.0)	–	2514	2600
Total (%)	2438 (54.8)	2008 (45.2)	4446 (100.0)	30	2712	7188
Mean	2.99	2.56	2.80	3.41	2.67	2.80
SD	2.91	2.42	2.71	2.02	3.02	2.72

These data were obtained from the PD-only patients in the patient survey
Values in parentheses under each figure represent the percentage relative to the total in each row
APD automated peritoneal dialysis

Table 5 PD treatment time, by PD vintage

PD vintage	1–<5 h	5–<9 h	9–<13 h	13–<18 h	18–<24 h	24 h	Subtotal	No information available	Total	Mean	SD
<1 year (%)	21 (1.8)	294 (25.5)	221 (19.2)	91 (7.9)	33 (2.9)	493 (42.8)	1153 (100.0)	99	1252	15.97	7.46
1–<2 years (%)	13 (1.5)	181 (20.5)	135 (15.3)	73 (8.3)	32 (3.6)	450 (50.9)	884 (100.0)	64	948	17.38	7.27
2–<4 years (%)	23 (2.0)	157 (13.4)	159 (13.6)	108 (9.2)	48 (4.1)	678 (57.8)	1173 (100.0)	96	1269	18.54	6.98
4–<6 years (%)	5 (0.8)	67 (11.2)	62 (10.3)	43 (7.2)	20 (3.3)	403 (67.2)	600 (100.0)	40	640	19.81	6.46
6–<8 years (%)	6 (2.4)	19 (7.8)	16 (6.5)	14 (5.7)	7 (2.9)	183 (74.7)	245 (100.0)	24	269	20.65	6.20
8–<10 years (%)	2 (2.2)	5 (5.4)	4 (4.3)	5 (5.4)	3 (3.2)	74 (79.6)	93 (100.0)	8	101	21.42	5.55
≥10 years (%)	1 (1.0)	5 (5.2)	10 (10.4)	3 (3.1)	4 (4.2)	73 (76.0)	96 (100.0)	13	109	20.97	5.89
Subtotal (%)	71 (1.7)	728 (17.2)	607 (14.3)	337 (7.9)	147 (3.5)	2354 (55.5)	4244 (100.0)	344	4588	18.02	7.19
No information available (%)	8 (20.5)	5 (12.8)	6 (15.4)	3 (7.7)	1 (2.6)	16 (41.0)	39 (100.0)	2561	2600	14.67	8.62
Total (%)	79 (1.8)	733 (17.1)	613 (14.3)	340 (7.9)	148 (3.5)	2370 (55.3)	4283 (100.0)	2905	7188	17.99	7.21
Mean	2.61	1.88	2.13	2.51	2.86	3.27	2.78	2.95	2.80	–	–
SD	2.37	1.92	2.18	2.16	2.76	2.92	2.67	3.28	2.72	–	–

These data were obtained from the PD-only patients in the patient survey

Table 6 Urine output, by PD vintage

PD vintage	<100 mL/day	100–<400 mL/day	400–<800 mL/day	800–1200 mL/day	1200–<1600 mL/day	≥1600 mL/d	Subtotal	No information available	Total	Mean	SD
<1 year (%)	36 (3.6)	99 (10.0)	231 (23.3)	284 (28.6)	227 (22.9)	116 (11.7)	993 (100.0)	259	1252	970.04	552.21
1–<2 years (%)	51 (6.7)	112 (14.8)	215 (28.3)	193 (25.4)	108 (14.2)	80 (10.5)	759 (100.0)	189	948	826.58	554.06
2–<4 years (%)	102 (9.7)	211 (20.1)	304 (28.9)	241 (22.9)	127 (12.1)	66 (6.3)	1051 (100.0)	218	1269	711.19	539.97
4–<6 years (%)	107 (20.5)	124 (23.8)	133 (25.5)	86 (16.5)	47 (9.0)	25 (4.8)	522 (100.0)	118	640	564.16	528.89
6–<8 years (%)	83 (40.1)	44 (21.3)	40 (19.3)	24 (11.6)	10 (4.8)	6 (2.9)	207 (100.0)	62	269	385.73	480.29
8–<10 years (%)	37 (45.1)	11 (13.4)	13 (15.9)	9 (11.0)	7 (8.5)	5 (6.1)	82 (100.0)	19	101	473.66	659.63
≥10 years (%)	54 (61.4)	15 (17.0)	6 (6.8)	10 (11.4)	1 (1.1)	2 (2.3)	88 (100.0)	21	109	239.49	403.43
Subtotal (%)	470 (12.7)	616 (16.6)	942 (25.4)	847 (22.9)	527 (14.2)	300 (8.1)	3702 (100.0)	886	4588	748.87	572.45
No information available (%)	15 (40.5)	4 (10.8)	6 (16.2)	8 (21.6)	3 (8.1)	1 (2.7)	37 (100.0)	2563	2600	472.97	529.49
Total (%)	485 (13.0)	620 (16.6)	948 (25.4)	855 (22.9)	530 (14.2)	301 (8.1)	3739 (100.0)	3449	7188	746.14	572.62
Mean	5.48	3.25	2.51	2.19	1.85	1.96	2.80	2.77	2.80	–	–
SD	4.05	2.55	2.01	2.24	1.82	1.92	2.71	2.76	2.72	–	–

These data were obtained from the PD-only patients in the patient survey

Table 7 Ultrafiltration volume by PD, by PD vintage

PD vintage	<−1000 mL/day	−1000–<0 mL/day	0–<1000 mL/day	1000–<2000 mL/day	2000–<3000 mL/day	3000–<4000 mL/day	≥4000 mL/day	Subtotal	No information available	Total	Mean	SD
<1 year (%)	1 (0.1)	78 (7.5)	836 (79.9)	123 (11.8)	8 (0.8)	–	–	1046 (100.0)	206	1252	450.31	453.10
1–<2 years (%)	–	54 (6.5)	618 (74.9)	146 (17.7)	6 (0.7)	1 (0.1)	–	825 (100.0)	123	948	554.78	478.10
2–<4 years (%)	1 (0.1)	46 (4.2)	755 (69.3)	274 (25.1)	11 (1.0)	2 (0.2)	1 (0.1)	1090 (100.0)	179	1269	676.10	502.64
4–<6 years (%)	–	15 (2.7)	358 (64.0)	179 (32.0)	6 (1.1)	–	1 (0.2)	559 (100.0)	81	640	753.31	494.71
6–<8 years (%)	–	4 (1.8)	138 (60.8)	81 (35.7)	3 (1.3)	1 (0.4)	–	227 (100.0)	42	269	806.98	507.14
8–<10 years (%)	–	–	47 (56.6)	35 (42.2)	1 (1.2)	–	–	83 (100.0)	18	101	843.47	458.93
≥10 years (%)	–	1 (1.2)	51 (60.7)	31 (36.9)	1 (1.2)	–	–	84 (100.0)	25	109	838.49	474.98
Subtotal (%)	2 (0.1)	198 (5.1)	2803 (71.6)	869 (22.2)	36 (0.9)	4 (0.1)	2 (0.1)	3914 (100.0)	674	4588	615.84	498.33
No information available (%)	–	–	27 (77.1)	7 (20.0)	1 (2.9)	–	–	35 (100.0)	2565	2600	727.29	515.26
Total (%)	2 (0.1)	198 (5.0)	2830 (71.7)	876 (22.2)	37 (0.9)	4 (0.1)	2 (0.1)	3949 (100.0)	3239	7188	616.83	498.52
Mean	1.50	1.80	2.56	3.70	3.22	3.15	3.71	2.78	2.89	2.80	–	–
SD	1.89	1.67	2.56	2.88	3.21	2.40	0.41	2.65	3.06	2.72	–	–

These data were obtained from the PD-only patients in the patient survey

Table 8 History of PET

Performance or nonperformance of PET	Not performed	PET performed	Fast PET only	Subtotal	Unspecified	No information available	Total
Number of patients (%)	1513 (34.5)	1885 (42.9)	992 (22.6)	4390 (100.0)	90	2708	7188

These data were obtained from the PD-only patients in the patient survey

- Frequency of dialysis per week, duration of one session of dialysis (min/session), and blood flow rate (mL/min) (for patients who underwent blood purification by extracorporeal circulation)
- Method of diluting HDF solution and volume of substitution fluid per HDF session (L) (for patients who underwent HDF)
- Height and predialysis and postdialysis body weights
- Predialysis and postdialysis serum blood urea nitrogen (BUN) (mg/dL) and creatinine (mg/dL) levels
- Predialysis albumin (g/dL), C-reactive protein (CRP) (mg/dL), calcium (mg/dL), phosphorus (mg/dL), and blood hemoglobin (g/dL) levels and parathyroid hormone (PTH) (pg/mL) levels and the measurement method of PTH

- Use or nonuse of antihypertensive drugs and smoking habit
- History of comorbidity (diabetes, myocardial infarction, cerebral hemorrhage, cerebral infarction, quadruple amputation, femoral neck fracture, and EPS)

USB-only survey items

Details of PD were surveyed as USB-only survey items separately from the abovementioned questionnaires for the facility and patient surveys. The following are the USB-only survey items associated with PD.

- PD vintage (months)
- Number of months when PD was performed in 2014
- Performance or nonperformance of PET

Table 9 Type of PD fluid, by PET D/P Cr ratio

Type of PD fluid	<0.5	0.5–<0.65	0.65–<0.81	≥0.81	Subtotal	No information available	Total	Mean	SD
1.5% dextrose only (%)	143 (61.9)	485 (55.6)	402 (39.7)	103 (31.2)	1133 (46.3)	958 (46.5)	2091 (46.4)	0.63	0.13
1.5 and 2.5% dextrose (%)	26 (11.3)	110 (12.6)	128 (12.6)	29 (8.8)	293 (12.0)	272 (13.2)	565 (12.5)	0.65	0.14
2.5% dextrose only (%)	1 (0.4)	11 (1.3)	22 (2.2)	11 (3.3)	45 (1.8)	81 (3.9)	126 (2.8)	0.71	0.12
4.25% dextrose only (without icodextrin) (%)	1 (0.4)	1 (0.1)	–	–	2 (0.1)	5 (0.2)	7 (0.2)	0.44	0.21
Icodextrin only (without dextrose) (%)	2 (0.9)	7 (0.8)	7 (0.7)	4 (1.2)	20 (0.8)	31 (1.5)	51 (1.1)	0.70	0.16
1.5% dextrose + icodextrin (%)	37 (16.0)	146 (16.7)	275 (27.1)	108 (32.7)	566 (23.1)	439 (21.3)	1005 (22.3)	0.69	0.13
1.5 and 2.5% dextrose + icodextrin (%)	10 (4.3)	68 (7.8)	111 (11.0)	42 (12.7)	231 (9.4)	135 (6.6)	366 (8.1)	0.69	0.13
2.5% dextrose + icodextrin (%)	11 (4.8)	44 (5.0)	66 (6.5)	33 (10.0)	154 (6.3)	140 (6.8)	294 (6.5)	0.68	0.16
4.25% dextrose + icodextrin (%)	–	1 (0.1)	2 (0.2)	–	3 (0.1)	–	3 (0.1)	0.67	0.12
Subtotal (%)	231 (100.0)	873 (100.0)	1013 (100.0)	330 (100.0)	2447 (100.0)	2061 (100.0)	4508 (100.0)	0.66	0.14
Unspecified	5	19	9	2	35	13	48	0.59	0.15
No information available	3	8	17	3	31	2601	2632	0.67	0.11
Total	239	900	1039	335	2513	4675	7188	0.66	0.14

These data were obtained from the PD-only patients in the patient survey
PET peritoneal equilibration test, *D/P Cr* dialysate/plasma creatinine

Table 10 Residual renal Kt/V, by PD vintage

PD vintage	<0.1	0.1-<0.4	0.4-<0.8	0.8-<1.2	1.2-<1.7	1.7-<2.0	2.0-<2.4	≥2.4	Subtotal	Unspecified	Total	Mean	SD
<1 year (%)	16 (4.0)	49 (12.2)	126 (31.3)	121 (30.0)	56 (13.9)	18 (4.5)	14 (3.5)	3 (0.7)	403 (100.0)	849	1252	0.84	0.54
1-<2 years (%)	22 (5.7)	64 (16.7)	116 (30.3)	94 (24.5)	62 (16.2)	11 (2.9)	9 (2.3)	5 (1.3)	383 (100.0)	565	948	0.79	0.56
2-<4 years (%)	58 (10.9)	162 (30.4)	158 (29.6)	76 (14.3)	41 (7.7)	18 (3.4)	8 (1.5)	12 (2.3)	533 (100.0)	736	1269	0.65	0.81
4-<6 years (%)	74 (27.3)	79 (29.2)	64 (23.6)	29 (10.7)	14 (5.2)	2 (0.7)	6 (2.2)	3 (1.1)	271 (100.0)	369	640	0.45	0.57
6-<8 years (%)	49 (45.0)	30 (27.5)	15 (13.8)	9 (8.3)	5 (4.6)	–	–	1 (0.9)	109 (100.0)	160	269	0.29	0.46
8-<10 years (%)	16 (48.5)	6 (18.2)	4 (12.1)	3 (9.1)	1 (3.0)	1 (3.0)	–	2 (6.1)	33 (100.0)	68	101	0.5	0.94
≥10 years (%)	22 (68.8)	4 (12.5)	3 (9.4)	2 (6.3)	1 (3.1)	–	–	–	32 (100.0)	77	109	0.19	0.39
Subtotal (%)	257 (14.6)	394 (22.3)	486 (27.6)	334 (18.9)	180 (10.2)	50 (2.8)	37 (2.1)	26 (1.5)	1764 (100.0)	2824	4588	0.66	0.67
No information available (%)	2 (50.0)	1 (25.0)	–	–	1 (25.0)	–	(0.0)	–	4 (100.0)	2596	2600	0.38	0.57
Total (%)	259 (14.6)	395 (22.3)	486 (27.5)	334 (18.9)	181 (10.2)	50 (2.8)	37 (2.1)	26 (1.5)	1768 (100.0)	5420	7188	0.66	0.67
Mean	5.29	3.22	2.42	1.94	1.94	1.88	1.94	3.09	2.86	2.75	2.80	–	–
SD	3.51	2.09	1.98	1.88	1.73	1.67	1.55	2.48	2.50	2.85	2.72	–	–

These data were obtained from the PD-only patients in the patient survey

Kt/V index for standardized dialysis dose defined as; K: urea clearance, t dialysis time, V: body fluid volume

Table 11 PD Kt/V, by PD vintage

PD vintage	<0.1	0.1–<0.4	0.4–<0.8	0.8–<1.2	1.2–<1.7	1.7–<2.0	2.0–<2.4	≥2.4	Subtotal	Unspecified	Total	Mean	SD
<1 year (%)	5 (1.1)	30 (6.8)	82 (18.7)	144 (32.8)	118 (26.9)	31 (7.1)	15 (3.4)	14 (3.2)	439 (100.0)	813	1252	1.10	0.62
1–<2 years (%)	1 (0.2)	21 (5.0)	58 (13.8)	104 (24.7)	153 (36.3)	40 (9.5)	28 (6.7)	16 (3.8)	421 (100.0)	527	948	1.25	0.56
2–<4 years (%)	3 (0.5)	33 (5.8)	43 (7.5)	120 (21.1)	232 (40.7)	76 (13.3)	37 (6.5)	26 (4.6)	570 (100.0)	699	1269	1.38	0.89
4–<6 years (%)	–	15 (4.9)	28 (9.2)	46 (15.0)	118 (38.6)	53 (17.3)	29 (9.5)	17 (5.6)	306 (100.0)	334	640	1.47	0.94
6–<8 years (%)	–	11 (8.6)	7 (5.5)	8 (6.3)	48 (37.5)	34 (26.6)	17 (13.3)	3 (2.3)	128 (100.0)	141	269	1.47	0.56
8–<10 years (%)	–	2 (5.3)	5 (13.2)	5 (13.2)	11 (28.9)	8 (21.1)	4 (10.5)	3 (7.9)	38 (100.0)	63	101	1.54	1.03
≥10 years (%)	1 (2.9)	2 (5.7)	3 (8.6)	–	12 (34.3)	7 (20.0)	9 (25.7)	1 (2.9)	35 (100.0)	74	109	1.51	0.64
Subtotal (%)	10 (0.5)	114 (5.9)	226 (11.7)	427 (22.0)	692 (35.7)	249 (12.9)	139 (7.2)	80 (4.1)	1937 (100.0)	2651	4588	1.31	0.77
No information available (%)	–	2 (33.3)	–	2 (33.3)	1 (16.7)	–	1 (16.7)	–	6 (100.0)	2594	2600	0.95	0.69
Total (%)	10 (0.5)	116 (6.0)	226 (11.6)	429 (22.1)	693 (35.7)	249 (12.8)	140 (7.2)	80 (4.1)	1943 (100.0)	5245	7188	1.31	0.77
Mean	2.39	2.89	2.25	2.04	3.02	3.99	3.90	3.11	2.89	2.72	2.80	–	–
SD	2.10	2.45	2.24	1.71	2.37	3.24	2.92	2.55	2.51	2.86	2.72	–	–

These data were obtained from the PD-only patients in the patient survey

Table 12 Patient's peritonitis rate

Peritonitis episodes per patient-year	0	1.0–<2.0	2.0–<3.0	3.0–<4.0	4.0–<5.0	≥5.0	Subtotal	Unspecified/no information available	Total	Mean
Number of patients (%)	3758 (86.7)	400 (9.5)	82 (2.3)	25 (0.8)	13 (0.3)	23 (0.4)	4301 (100.0)	2887	7188	0.21

These data were obtained from the PD-only patients in the patient survey
Patient's peritonitis rate per patient-year = (Peritonitis episodes in 2014 in all subjects ÷ Total months on PD in 2014 in all subjects) × 12

- PET-derived 4-h dialysate/plasma creatinine ratio (PET D/P Cr ratio)
- Type of PD fluid
- Volume of PD fluid per day
- Remaining renal function (daily urine output)
- Mean ultrafiltration (UF) volume per day (UF volume)
- Residual renal Kt/V and PD Kt/V
- Changing maneuver of PD fluids
- Use or nonuse of automated peritoneal dialysis (APD) machine
- PD treatment time per day
- Past history of peritonitis during 2014
- At history of catheter exit-site infections (ESI) in 2014

Results and discussion
Current status of PD patients
Number of patients
According to the facility survey, the number of PD patients was 9255 at the end of 2014, a decrease of 137 from the previous year. The percentage of PD patients among the entire dialysis patient population was 2.9%, a decrease of 0.1% from the previous year. The number of patients who underwent a nonPD modality but despite having a PD catheter, most of whom are considered to have undergone only peritoneal lavage, was 278 and it was a decrease of 14 from the previous year. The number of new patients who were started PD in 2014 but switched to another method in the same year was 193, an increase of 19 from the previous year. The number of patients on the combination therapy of PD and HD or HDF was 1913, a decrease of 7 from the previous year (Table 1).

Current status of the combination therapy of PD + HD(F) with respect to PD vintage
To the questions regarding PD vintage and current status of PD + HD(F), 5678 patients responded. The percentage of patients who underwent PD + HD(F) increased with PD vintage (<1 year, 3.3%; 1–<2 years, 10.1%; 2–<4 years, 16.3%; 4–<6 years, 26.9%; 6–<8 years, 40.9%; 8–<10 years, 53.5%; and ≥10 years, 58.7%). Regarding the frequency of HD(F), the majority of the PD patients underwent HD(F) once a week (nearly 82.8%) (Table 2).

Changing maneuver of PD fluids
To the questions regarding the method of PD solution exchange, 4417 of the PD-only patients responded. The number of PD patients who performed completely manual PD fluid exchanges was 1422 (32.2%). The number of PD patients who used a double-bag system with ultraviolet light irradiation was 2322 (52.6%), and the number of those who used the same system but with a sterile connecting device was 607 (13.7%) (Table 3).

Use or nonuse of APD machine with respect to PD vintage
Among the PD-only patients, 4446 responded to the questions regarding their PD vintage and use or nonuse of an APD machine. The percentage of PD-only patients who used an APD machine was 45.2%. The percentages of PD-only patients who used an APD machine were ≥40% for PD vintages of <6 years (<1 year, 47.2%; 1–<2 years, 50.0%; 2–<4 years, 44.2%; and 4–<6 years, 44.4%). However, the percentage of PD-only patients who used an APD machine decreased to around 30% for PD vintages of ≥6 years (≥10 years, 31.7%) (Table 4).

Number of hours of PD session per day with respect to PD vintage
Among the PD-only patients, 4244 responded to the questions regarding their PD vintage and PD treatment time per day. The percentage of patients who underwent PD for the whole day (24 h) was 55.5%. The percentages of patients who underwent PD for the whole day tended to increase with PD vintage (<1 year, 42.8%; 8–<10 years, 79.6%; and ≥10 years, 76.0%) (Table 5).

Table 13 Center's peritonitis rate

Peritonitis rate (episodes per year per facility)	0~	1.0~	2.0~	3.0~	4.0~	5.0~	Subtotal	No information available	Total	Mean
Number of facilities (%)	195 (85.9)	25 (11.0)	5 (2.2)	1 (0.4)	0 (0.0)	1 (0.4)	227 (100.0)	263	490	0.21

These data were obtained from the PD-only patients in the patient survey
Center's peritonitis rate per patient-year = (Peritonitis episodes in 2014 in all patients in the facility ÷ Total months on PD in 2014 in all patients in the facility) × 12

Table 14 Patient's ESI rate

ESI episodes per patient-year	0	1.0–<2.0	2.0–<3.0	3.0–<4.0	4.0–<5.0	≥5.0	Subtotal	Unspecified/no information available	Total	Mean
Number of patients (%)	3465 (80.8)	495 (11.5)	159 (3.7)	58 (1.4)	40 (0.9)	72 (1.7)	4289 (100.0)	2899	7188	0.40

These data were obtained from the PD-only patients in the patient survey
The patient's ESI rate per patient-year = (ESI episodes in 2014 in all subjects ÷ Total months on PD in 2014 in all subjects) × 12

Urine output and ultrafiltration volume by PD
Urine output by PD vintage
To the questions regarding urine output and PD vintage, 3702 of the PD-only patients responded. The mean urine output of the PD patients was 748.9 mL/day. The urine output tended to decrease with increasing PD vintage (<1 year, 970.0 mL/day and ≥10 years, 239.5 mL/day) (Table 6).

Ultrafiltration volume by PD by PD vintage
To the questions regarding the ultrafiltration volume by PD and PD vintage, 3914 of the PD-only patients responded. The mean ultrafiltration volume by PD was 615.8 mL/day. The mean ultrafiltration volume by PD tended to increase with PD vintage (<1 year, 450.3 mL/day and ≥10 years, 838.5 mL/day) (Table 7).

Peritoneal equilibration test (PET)
History of PET
To the questions regarding the history of PET, 4390 of the PD-only patients responded. Among these patients, 1885 (42.9%) underwent a standard PET and 992 (22.6%) underwent a fast PET; that is, a total of 2877 (65.5%) underwent PET (Table 8).

PET D/P Cr ratio and type of PD fluid
To the questions regarding the type of PD fluid, 4508 of the PD-only patients responded. Among these patients, 2782 (61.7%) used 1.5 or 2.5% dextrose and only 10 (0.2%) used 4.25% dextrose. The number of patients who used icodextrin was 1719 (38.1%). The percentage of patients who used icodextrin increased with PET D/P Cr ratio (<0.5, 26.0%; 0.5–<0.65, 30.5%; 0.65–<0.81, 45.5%; and ≥0.81, 56.7%) (Table 9).

Residual renal Kt/V and PD Kt/V
Residual renal Kt/V by PD vintage
To the questions regarding the residual renal Kt/V and PD vintage, 1764 of the PD-only patients responded. The mean residual renal Kt/V was 0.66. The mean residual renal Kt/V decreased with increasing PD vintage of <8. For patients with PD vintage of ≥8, the residual renal Kt/V was considered to be varied significantly among patients (Table 10).

PD Kt/V by PD vintage
To the questions regarding PD Kt/V and PD vintage, 1937 of the PD-only patients responded. The mean PD Kt/V was 1.31. The mean PD Kt/V tended to increase with increasing PD vintage (<1 year, 1.10 and ≥10 years, 1.51) (Table 11).

Peritonitis and catheter exit-site infections
Peritonitis is defined as a white blood cell count of ≥100/μL (neutrophil, ≥50%) in waste PD fluid. A catheter exit-site infection is defined by the presence of purulent drainage from the exit site. The rates of peritonitis and catheter exit-site infections were calculated in the PD-only patients using the following formulae.

Patient's peritonitis rate
The patient's peritonitis rate per patient-year was calculated as follows,

The patient's peritonitis rate per patient-year
= (Peritonitis episodes in 2014 in all subjects
÷ Total months on PD in 2014 in all subjects) × 12

According to the International Society for Peritoneal Dialysis (ISPD) guidelines (Peritoneal Dialysis-Related Infection Recommendations: 2010 Update) [5], "the center's peritonitis rate should be no more than 1 episode every 18 months (0.67 per patient-year)."

To the questions regarding peritonitis, 4301 of the PD-only patients responded. The mean peritonitis rate was 0.21 per patient-year (1 episode every 57.1 patient-months). This was much lower than the recommendation in the ISPD guidelines. The number of patients who did not develop peritonitis in 2014 was 3758 (87.4%). The number of patients with a peritonitis rate

Table 15 Center's ESI rate

Episodes of ESI per patient-year	0~	1.0~	2.0~	3.0~	4.0~	5.0~	Subtotal	No information available	Total	Mean
Number of facilities (%)	191 (75.9)	51 (15.2)	11 (5.2)	1 (1.1)	3 (0.7)	4 (1.9)	261 (100.0)	229	490	0.40

These data were obtained from the PD-only patients in the patient survey
The center's ESI rate per patient-year = (ESI episodes in 2014 in all patients in the center ÷ Total months on PD in 2014 in all patients in the center) × 12

of 1.0–<2.0 was 400 (9.3%) and that with a peritonitis rate of ≥2.0 was 143 (3.3%) (Table 12).

Center's peritonitis rate

The center's peritonitis rate was calculated as follows,

> The center's peritonitis rate per patient-year
> = (Peritonitis episodes in 2014 in all patients in the center
> ÷ Total months on PD in 2014 in all patients in the center) × 12

On the basis of the valid responses obtained from 227 centers, the mean center's peritonitis rate was 0.21 per patient-year (1 episode each 57.1 patient-months) (Table 13).

Patient's catheter exit-site infection (ESI) rates

The patient's ESI rate was calculated as follows,

> The patient's ESI rate per patient-year
> = (ESI episodes in 2014 in all subjects
> ÷ Total months on PD in 2014 in all subjects) × 12

To the questions regarding ESI, 4289 of the PD-only patients responded. The mean patient's ESI rate in the PD-only dialysis patients was 0.40 per patient-year (1 episode every 30.0 patient-months). The number of patients who did not develop ESI in 2014 was 3465 (80.8%). The number of patients with ESI rate of 1.0–<2.0 was 495 (11.5%) and that with ESI rate of ≥2.0 was 329 (7.7%) (Table 14).

Center's ESI rate

The center's ESI rate was calculated as follows.

> The center's ESI rate per patient-year
> = (ESI episodes in 2014 in all patients in the center
> ÷ Total months on PD in 2014 in all patients in the center) × 12

On the basis of the valid responses obtained from 261 centers, the mean center's ESI rate was 0.40 per patient-year (1 episode each 30.0 patient-months) (Table 15).

Encapsulating peritoneal sclerosis (EPS)
History of EPS in the patients with PD history

The history of EPS and the treatments for EPS, surgical treatment and/or steroids, were surveyed on the patients on PD and the patients with past PD history currently on another dialysis modality. Among the 12,865 patients who responded to the questions regarding their history of EPS, 676 (5.3%) had a history of EPS. Among these 676 patients, 541 (80.0%) had received surgical treatments (Table 16).

History of EPS by PD vintage

Responses to the questions regarding PD vintage and EPS history were obtained from 4917 patients. The percentages of patients with a history of EPS who had undergone PD for <6 years were low (<1 year, 0.4%; 1–<2 years, 0.7%; 2–<4 years, 0.5%; and 4–<6 years, 0.3%). However, the percentages of such patients who had undergone PD for a longer duration increased to around 1% (6–<8 years, 1.6%; 8–<10 years, 1.1%; and ≥10 years, 0.9%) (Table 17).

Table 16 PD patient distribution, by treatment for EPS and dialysis modality

Treatment for EPS	EPS (−)	EPS (+)				Subtotal	Unspecified	No information available	Total
		Surgery (+) steroids (+)	Surgery (+) steroids (−)	Surgery (−) steroids (+)	Surgery (−) steroids (−)				
In-center HD (%)	5051 (91.2)	376 (6.8)	12 (0.2)	56 (1.0)	46 (0.8)	5541 (100.0)	198	730	6469
HDF (%)	1250 (90.5)	104 (7.5)	3 (0.2)	9 (0.7)	15 (1.1)	1381 (100.0)	35	161	1577
Hemofiltration (%)	1 (100.0)	–	–	–	–	1 (100.0)	–	–	1
Hemoadsorption (%)	46 (79.3)	8 (13.8)	1 (1.7)	–	3 (5.2)	58 (100.0)	4	3	65
Home HD (%)	72 (98.6)	1 (1.4)	–	–	–	73 (100.0)	–	4	77
PD (%)	5769 (99.3)	36 (0.6)	–	3 (0.1)	3 (0.1)	5811 (100.0)	67	3063	8941
Subtotal (%)	12,189 (94.7)	525 (4.1)	16 (0.1)	68 (0.5)	67 (0.5)	12,865 (100.0)	304	3961	17,130
No information available (%)	–	–	–	–	–	–	–	–	–
Total (%)	12,189 (94.7)	525 (4.2)	16 (0.2)	68 (0.6)	67 (0.4)	12,865 (100.0)	304	3961	17,130

These data were obtained from the patients on PD and the patients with past PD history currently on another dialysis modality
EPS encapsulating peritoneal sclerosis

Table 17 PD patient distribution, by PD vintage and treatment for EPS

PD vintage	<1 year	1–<2 years	2–<4 years	4–<6 years	6–<8 years	8–<10 years	≥10 years	Subtotal	No information available	Total	Mean	SD
EPS (−) (%)	1130 (99.6)	909 (99.3)	1326 (99.5)	764 (99.7)	371 (98.4)	172 (98.9)	215 (99.1)	4887 (99.4)	7302 (91.9)	12,189 (94.7)	3.34	3.19
EPS (+) surgery (+), steroids (+) EPS (+) surgery (+), steroids (+) (%)	4 (0.4)	6 (0.7)	6 (0.5)	1 (0.1)	5 (1.3)	2 (1.1)	1 (0.5)	25 (0.5)	500 (6.3)	525 (4.1)	4.15	3.89
EPS (+) surgery (+), steroids (−) EPS (+) surgery (+), steroids (−) (%)	–	–	–	–	–	–	–	–	16 (0.2)	16 (0.1)	–	–
EPS (+) surgery (−), steroids (+) EPS (+) surgery (−), steroids (+) (%)	1 (0.1)	–	1 (0.1)	–	1 (0.3)	–	–	3 (0.1)	65 (0.8)	68 (0.5)	3.89	3.29
EPS (+) surgery (−), steroids (−) EPS (+) surgery (−), steroids (−) (%)	–	–	–	1 (0.1)	–	–	1 (0.5)	2 (0.0)	65 (0.8)	67 (0.5)	8.38	4.89
Subtotal (%)	1135 (100.0)	915 (100.0)	1333 (100.0)	766 (100.0)	377 (100.0)	174 (100.0)	217 (100.0)	4917 (100.0)	7948 (100.0)	12,865 (100.0)	3.35	3.20
Unspecified	8	1	12	9	6	5	5	46	258	304	5.26	4.37
No information available	152	140	173	100	71	38	42	716	3245	3961	3.65	3.60
Total	1295	1056	1518	875	454	217	264	5679	11,451	17,130	3.40	3.27

These data were obtained from the patients on PD and the patients with past PD history currently on another dialysis modality

Conclusions

The number of PD patients has been stable around 9000~10,000 in these 10 years, and the penetration rate of PD among all dialysis patients was just 2.9%, which is one of the lowest numbers in the world. There were several unique points in the current status of PD therapy in Japan compared with other many countries. One of them was the combination therapy of PD and other dialysis modality and 21% of the PD patients were on the combination therapy. The second is lower PD dialysis dose as the mean PD Kt/V was 1.31, and it was supposed to be smaller than that from the world reports. The third is the lower risk of PD-related infections as the patient's peritonitis rate was 0.21 per patient-year and it was smaller than that of ISPD guideline. The final is about EPS. The percentage of the patients with the history of EPS among the patients with current and past PD treatment was 5.3%, and 80% of them had received the surgical treatment. The PD registry in Japan has clarified unique points in the current status of PD therapy in Japan and the differences from the trends in the other countries in the world. Based on the further analysis of the PD registry data, we would like to improve the quality of PD therapy in Japan and send messages about the merits of our therapeutic policy to the world.

Abbreviations
APD: Automated peritoneal dialysis; BUN: Blood urea nitrogen; CRDR: The committee of renal data registry; CRP: C-reactive protein; D/P Cr: Dialysate/plasma creatinine; EPS: Encapsulating peritoneal sclerosis; ESI: Exit-site infection; HDF: Hemodiafiltration; ISPD: The International Society for Peritoneal Dialysis; JRDR: JSDT renal data registry; JSDT: Japanese Society for Dialysis Therapy; Kt/V: Index for standardized dialysis dose defined as; K: urea clearance; PD: Peritoneal dialysis; PET: Peritoneal equilibration test; PTH: Parathyroid hormone; t: Dialysis time, V: body fluid volume; USB: Universal serial bus

Acknowledgements
We owe the completion of this survey to the efforts of the members of the subcommittee of local cooperation mentioned as follows and the staff members of dialysis facilities who participated in the survey and responded to the questionnaires. We would like to express our deepest gratitude to all these people.
District Cooperative Committee in JRDR
Noritomo Itami, Tetsuya Kawata, Chikara Oyama, Koji Seino, Toshinobu Sato, Shigeru Sato, Minoru Ito, Masaaki Nakayama, Atsushi Ueda, Takashi Yagisawa, Tetsuo Ando, Tomonari Ogawa, Hiroo Kumagai, Makoto Ogura, Takahiro Mochizuki, Ryoichi Ando, Kazuyoshi Okada, Tetsuya Kashiwagi, Chieko Hamada, Yugo Shibagaki, Nobuhito Hirawa, Junichiro Kazama, Yoichi Ishida, Hitoshi Yokoyama, Ryoichi Miyazaki, Mizuya Fukasawa, Masaki Nagasawa, Teppei Matsuoka, Akihiko Kato, Noriko Mori, Yasuhiko Ito, Hirotake Kasuga, Sukenari Koyabu, Takashi Udu, Tetsuya Hashimoto, Masaaki Inaba, Terumasa Hayashi, Tomoyuki Yamakawa, Shinichi Nishi, Akira Fujimori, Tatsuo Yoneda, Shigeo Negi, Akihisa Nakaoka, Takafumi Ito, Hitoshi Sugiyama, Takao Masaki, Yutaka Nitta, Hirofumi Hashimoto, Masato Yamanaka, Masaharu Kan, Kazumichi Ota, Masahito Tamura, Koji Mitsuiki, Yuji Ikeda, Masaharu Nishikido, Akira Miyata, Tadashi Tomo, Shoichi Fujimoto, Tsuyoshi Nosaki, Yoshinori Oshiro

Funding
There are no funding for the current study.
All efforts and costs for the 2014 JRDR survey and making the report were totally given by JSDT.

Authors' contributions
IM was the director of CRDR in 2014 and directed all of the 2014 JRDR survey. IM and TH finalized the results of the survey and made this manuscript. SO and AW designed the survey sheets and made a special program mounted in MS Excel worksheet for the convenience of self-assessment for the dialysis quality of each dialysis facility. SN, NK, and TH had the responsibilities on the data analysis. KW had the responsibility on the ethical aspect of the JRDR survey. KN was the president of the JSDT in 2014 and checked all the results from the 2014 JRDR survey and approved them to be published. All authors read and approved the final manuscript.

Competing interests
The authors declare that they have no competing interests.

Author details
[1]Committee of Renal Data Registry (CRDR), Japanese Society for Dialysis Therapy (JSDT), Aramido Building 2F, 2-38-21 Hongo, Bunkyo-ku, Tokyo 113-0033, Japan. [2]Subcommittee of Statical Analysis of CRDR, Japanese Society for Dialysis Therapy, Tokyo, Japan. [3]Japanese Society for Dialysis Therapy, Tokyo, Japan. [4]Department Nephrology, Yabuki Hospital, 4-4-5 Shima Kita, Yamagata City, Yamagata 990-0885, Japan.

References
1. Nakai S. History of statistical survey of the Japanese Society for Dialysis Therapy. J Jpn Soc Dial Ther. 2010;43:119–52 (in Japanese).
2. Nakai S, Iseki K, Itami N, Ogata S, Kazama JJ, Kimata N, et al. Overview of regular dialysis treatment in Japan (as of 31 December 2009). Ther Apher Dial. 2012;16:11–53.
3. Masakane I, Nakai S, Ogata S, Kimata N, Hanafusa N, Hamano T, et al. An overview of regular dialysis treatment in Japan (as of 31 December 2013). Ther Apher Dial. 2015;19:540–74.
4. Masakane I, Nakai S, Ogata S, Kimata N, Hanafusa N, Hamano T, et al. Overview of regular dialysis treatment in Japan (as of 31 December 2014). J Jpn Soc Dial Ther. 2016;49:1–34.
5. Li PK, Szeto CC, Piraino B, Bernardini J, Figueiredo AE, Gupta A, et al. Peritoneal dialysis-related infections recommendations: 2010 update. Perit Dial Int. 2010;30:393–423.

14

Effect of cardiovascular risk factors and time of hospital presentation on mortality of maintenance hemodialysis patients presenting with acute pulmonary edema

Saki Hasegawa[1], Shintaro Nakano[1*], Jun Tanno[1], Shiro Iwanaga[1], Ritsushi Kato[1], Toshihiro Muramatsu[1], Yusuke Watanabe[2], Hirokazu Okada[2], Takaaki Senbonmatsu[1], Hidetomo Nakamoto[3] and Shigeyuki Nishimura[1]

Abstract

Background: Acute pulmonary edema (APE) has a poor prognosis in the general population. Mortality associated with APE in patients with end-stage renal disease (ESRD) is especially high, although specific predictors are not well understood. This study aimed to determine the potential predictive factors of outcome in patients with ESRD presenting with APE.

Methods: Sixty-eight patients with ESRD (mean age, 68.9 ± 9.9 years; males, 66.2%; median duration of maintenance hemodialysis, 55.5 months) presenting with APE to a single tertiary medical center were retrospectively evaluated. The effects of patients' characteristics, cardiovascular risk factors, variables at hospital presentation, and clinical presentation patterns on all-cause mortality were evaluated.

Results: Throughout the observational period (median follow-up period, 575 days; range, 10–2546 days), 32 (47%) patients died. In univariate analysis, older age, diabetes mellitus, peripheral artery or aortic disease, hypotension, atrial fibrillation rhythm, anemia, and hypoalbuminemia were associated with higher mortality, whereas hospital presentation from midnight to 8 am was associated with lower mortality. In multivariate analysis, age (hazard ratio (HR) = 1.05, 95% confidential interval (CI) 1.01–1.09, $p = 0.018$), presence of peripheral artery or aortic disease (HR = 3.36, 95% CI 1.52–7.42, $p = 0.003$), time of presentation from midnight to 8 am (HR = 0.40, 95% CI 0.15–0.99, $p = 0.047$), and atrial fibrillation rhythm at presentation (HR = 3.12, 95% CI 1.04–9.13, $p = 0.044$) were significantly independently associated with mortality.

Conclusions: Our findings indicate important predictive roles of the clinical presentation pattern specific to ESRD patients, as well as their characteristics, including cardiovascular risk factors.

Keywords: Pulmonary edema, End-stage renal disease, Dialysis, Clinical presentation

Background

The number of patients on maintenance hemodialysis suffering from end-stage renal disease (ESRD) is approximately 400,000 in the USA [1] and approximately 300,000 in Japan [2]. Cardiovascular disease accounts for 50% of death among these patients [3], with congestive heart failure comprising approximately 25% of death in Japan [2].

Acute pulmonary edema (APE), which is a common symptom of acute heart failure requiring hospital admission, is associated with considerable mortality [4, 5]. This condition is accompanied by severe respiratory distress, audible crackles, and orthopnea and is verified by chest X-ray [6]. In addition to respiratory support, initial treatment of APE aims to ameliorate preload and afterload [7]. In the general population, factors such as older age, hypotension, hyponatremia, and anemia at presentation are predictors of poor outcome in patients presenting with acute heart

* Correspondence: snakano@saitama-med.ac.jp
[1]Department of Cardiovascular Medicine, Saitama Medical University International Medical Center, 1397-1 Yamane, 350-1298 Hidaka, Saitama, Japan
Full list of author information is available at the end of the article

failure [8–11]. In patients with APE only, older age and hypotension predict mortality [5].

Despite high mortality (approximately 80% mortality at 5 years) and morbidity of APE [12, 13], evidence regarding APE in patients undergoing maintenance hemodialysis is lacking. Patients with ESRD on maintenance hemodialysis should be considered as different from the general population because they have different cardiovascular disease characteristics and responses to therapy [1, 3]. Moreover, periodic hemodialysis therapy jeopardizes their preload to fluctuate non-physiologically. Therefore, risk stratification and therapeutic guidelines according to clinical presentation described in acute heart failure in the general population, such as the clinical scenario [9, 14], may not be applicable to this cohort.

Considering the distinct patho-physiology and high mortality, specific predictors in patients with ESRD on maintenance hemodialysis presenting with APE need to be investigated. This study aimed to determine the effects of demographics, non-cardiovascular and cardiovascular factors, and clinical presentation on all-cause mortality in patients on maintenance hemodialysis presenting with APE.

Methods

Study design and population

The medical records of 132 patients with ESRD on maintenance hemodialysis presenting with APE who required emergent admission were retrospectively reviewed. Patients were admitted to the Intensive Care Unit or Cardiac Care Unit in Saitama Medical University International Medical Center because of APE between April 2007 and October 2015. Maintenance hemodialysis was defined as performance of maintenance hemodialysis for 3 months or longer before admission. Patients were included if they showed pulmonary edema on an initial chest X-ray as determined by two observers (S.N. and S.H.). Patients who showed marginal X-ray findings with their clinical course that were inconsistent with APE were excluded after discussion with a third observer using clinical information. Figure 1 shows representative X-rays of the included and excluded patients. Other exclusion criteria are shown in Fig. 2. Patients who required immediate invasive therapy for acute cardiovascular collapse (such as acute coronary syndrome) were excluded because the impact of sudden cardiac dysfunction and procedure-related outcomes may cancel the effects of the factors specifically related to maintenance hemodialysis or ESRD.

Data collection

Baseline demographics of patients, maintenance hemodialysis data, and coexisting or previous conditions were recorded. Hypertension was defined as current or previous treatment with anti-hypertensive medication. Diabetes mellitus was defined as treatment with anti-diabetic medication or hemoglobin A1c concentration of $\geq 6.5\%$ [15]. Dyslipidemia was defined as treatment with anti-dyslipidemic medication or fasting serum concentration of low-density lipoprotein cholesterol ≥ 160 mg/dl, high-density lipoprotein cholesterol ≤ 40 mg/dl, or total cholesterol ≥ 240 mg/dl [16].

Malignancy, peripheral artery and aortic disease (e.g., aortic dissection and aortic aneurysm, either treated or untreated), previous myocardial infarction, and previous cerebral infarction and hemorrhage were recorded. Previous cardiovascular interventions, such as percutaneous coronary intervention, coronary artery bypass grafting,

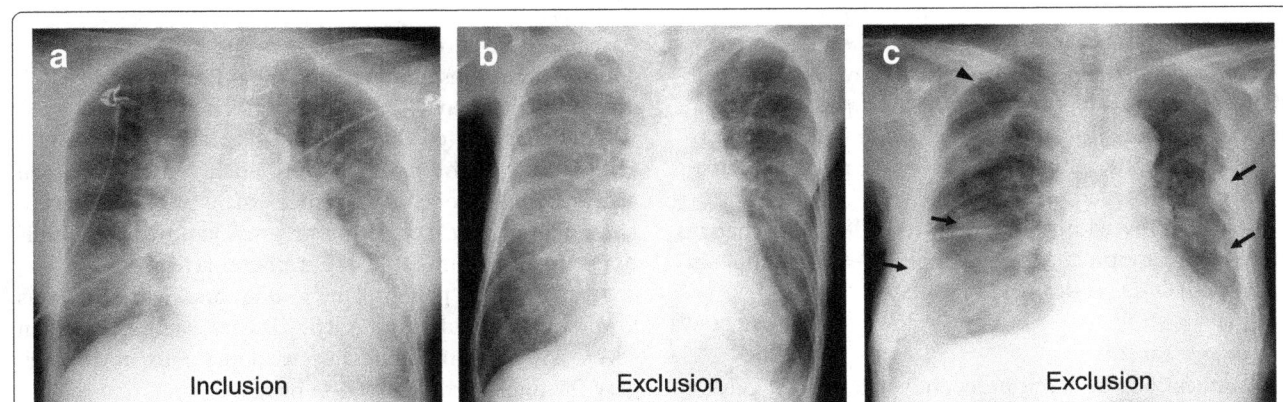

Fig. 1 Chest X-rays of included and excluded patients. **a** Included patient: A 58-year-old woman with X-ray findings typical of pulmonary edema. **b** Excluded patient: A 58-year-old woman with marginal X-ray findings showing right-side-dominant infiltration and modest cardiomegaly. Upon admission, this patient had hypotension (systolic blood pressure 70 mmHg), fever (>38°), and elevated levels of acute inflammatory biomarkers (white blood cell count 23,140/μl, serum C-reactive protein 20.0 mg/dl). A systemic inflammatory response due to infection was suspected, and these abnormal parameters and X-ray findings were subsequently resolved with antibiotic therapy. **c** (excluded patient) An 81-year-old man with marginal X-ray findings showing abnormal pleural and pulmonary shadows (*arrows*) and pneumothorax (*arrowhead*). The patient had pleural and pulmonary metastases secondary to renal cancer

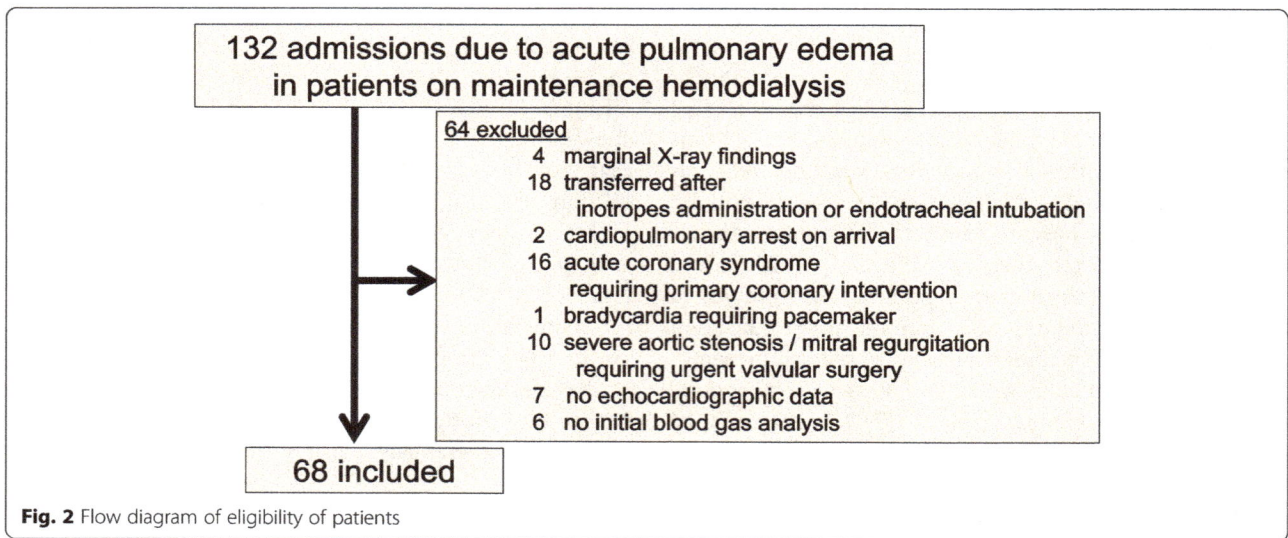

Fig. 2 Flow diagram of eligibility of patients

aortic surgery, percutaneous transluminal angioplasty or surgery for peripheral artery disease, valvular surgery, and pacemaker/cardio-defibrillator implantation, were recorded. Coronary artery anatomy collected from coronary angiography during the index or previous hospitalization was recorded. Medications that were administered prior to presentation were recorded.

For the prehospital course, the time elapsed from symptom (defined as dyspnea on exertion, paroxysmal nocturnal dyspnea, or orthopnea) onset to arrival was recorded, and the patients were divided into two groups (>72 and ≤72 h); in the >72-h group, their symptoms started before the last dialysis session. Hospital presentation time was recorded and divided into the following three groups: 8 am to 4 pm, 4 pm to midnight, and midnight to 8 am [17]. The 2-day interdialytic gap, body weight gain, and body weight gain rate were recorded.

Vital signs, arterial blood gases (before initiating specific respiratory support other than oxygen supplement alone), and laboratory findings at presentation were recorded. Echocardiographic and electrocardiographic variables were recorded.

Initial therapy within 48 h was recorded, and changes in subjective dyspnea and vital signs after the initial single hemodialysis session were evaluated.

Outcome measures
The associations between independent factors at presentation and all-cause death throughout the observation period were evaluated.

Statistical analysis
Continuous variables are expressed as the mean ± standard deviation or median (first to third quartile) and categorical variables as number (%). The Shapiro–Wilk test

was performed for testing normal distribution. Univariate Cox proportional regression analyses were performed to identify the association between independent variables and all-cause death. Subsequently, multivariate Cox proportional regression analyses were performed to identify potential predictors of all-cause death. Because there are no established predictors of mortality in patients on maintenance hemodialysis presenting with APE, a multivariate model was constructed with independent variables using $p < 0.05$ in univariate analysis. Kaplan–Meier analyses were performed to test the predictive value of independent variables for mortality with the log-rank test. All statistical analyses were performed using JMP Pro.11.2.0 (SAS Institute, Inc., Cary, USA).

Results
Baseline characteristics, variables of the prehospital course and at presentation, and initial therapy and response of patients
A flow diagram of the patients' eligibility is shown in Fig. 2. Sixty-eight patients were included in the final analysis. Baseline characteristics, data on maintenance hemodialysis, and coexisting or previous medical conditions are shown in Table 1. Peripheral artery disease was observed in 20 patients, including one with previous lower limb amputation. Aortic disease was observed in seven patients, including five with previous aortic surgery for their aortic dissection or aneurysm.

Coronary artery anatomy was only evaluated in 50 (73.5%) patients. Medications and previous cardiovascular interventions are shown in Additional file 1: Tables S1 and S2.

Variables of the prehospital course and at presentation are shown in Table 2. Most patients were hypertensive at presentation. Their initial therapy within 48 h after

Table 1 Baseline characteristics of patients and univariate Cox proportional analysis for all-cause death

	Total (n = 68)	Hazard ratio	p
Demographics			
Age (years)	68.9 ± 9.9	1.06	0.003*
Male, n (%)	45 (66.2)	2.03	0.08
Body mass index (kg/m²)	21.1 (19.1–24.3)	0.95	0.30
Maintenance hemodialysis data			
Etiology of kidney disease			
Diabetic nephropathy, n (%)	44 (64.7)	1.16	0.70
Nephrosclerosis, n (%)	6 (8.8)	1.74	0.33
Others, n (%)	18 (26.5)	0.65	0.30
Duration of maintenance hemodialysis (months)	55.5 (27.3–85.5)	1.00	0.95
Frequency (times/week)	3 (3–3)	NA	NA
Each hemodialysis time (hours/day)	4.0 (4.0–4.0)	1.05	0.88
Coexisting/previous conditions, n (%)			
Previous acute pulmonary edema	24 (35.3)	1.09	0.82
Hypertension	60 (88.2)	0.64	0.44
Diabetes mellitus	52 (76.5)	2.47	0.04*
Dyslipidemia	34 (50.0)	0.97	0.94
Current smoking	10 (14.7)	0.98	0.97
Malignancy	11 (16.2)	1.12	0.82
Peripheral artery or aortic disease	21 (30.9)	2.98	0.005*
Previous myocardial infarction	21 (30.9)	1.00	0.99
Previous cerebral infarction	9 (13.2)	2.17	0.12
Previous cerebral hemorrhage	4 (5.9)	1.08	0.91
Coronary anatomy (n = 50)			
Normal coronary artery, n (%)	10 (20.0)	0.87	0.80
Left main trunk disease, n (%)	3 (6.0)	0.95	0.96
Triple vessel disease, n (%)	10 (20.0)	1.54	0.38

Continuous variables are shown as the mean ± SD or median (first to third quartile) and categorical variables as number (%)
NA not analyzed
*p<0.05

presentation and their responses are shown in Additional file 1: Table S3; 56 (82.4%) patients required emergent hemodialysis, including continuous hemodialysis for expected hemodynamic instability. Most patients (86.4%) demonstrated relief of subjective dyspnea and hypertension after initial renal replacement therapy.

Univariate Cox proportional analyses for all-cause mortality

The median follow-up period was 575 days (174–966: range 10–2546 days), and the total follow-up time was 135.4 years. Throughout the observational period, 32 (47%) patients died from the following causes: myocardial infarction (n = 7), low-output circulatory failure (n = 6), acute pulmonary edema (n = 6), sudden death (n = 3), and other non-cardiovascular causes, such as malignancy (n = 3), liver failure (n = 3), pneumonia (n = 2), sepsis (n = 1), and an

unknown cause (n = 1). Index in-hospital death was observed in six (8.8%) patients. The potential cause of in-hospital death was cardiovascular events in all six patients, including low-output circulatory failure (n = 5) and acute myocardial infarction with shock (n = 1). However, most of these patients were complicated by sepsis or lower airway infection.

In univariate analysis, older age, the presence of diabetes mellitus, and peripheral artery disease or aortic disease were associated with higher all-cause mortality in the whole observational period. Lower systolic blood pressure, hematocrit, serum albumin levels, and AF rhythm at presentation were also significantly associated with higher mortality. The time of hospital presentation from midnight to 8 am was significantly associated with lower mortality (Tables 1 and 2).

Table 2 Variables of the prehospital course and at hospital presentation, and univariate Cox proportional analysis for all-cause death

	Total (n = 68)	Hazard ratio	p
Prehospital course			
>72 h from onset to arrival, n (%)	13 (19.1)	0.90	0.83
Time of hospital presentation, n (%)			
- 8 am to 4 pm	10 (14.7)	1.88	0.17
- 4 pm to midnight	22 (32.4)	1.96	0.07
- Midnight to 8 am	36 (52.9)	0.38	0.007[†]
2-day interdialytic gap, n (%)	37 (54.4)	1.09	0.81
Body weight gain (kg)	2.0 (1.0–4.0)	1.00	0.95
Body weight gain rate (%)	4.1 (1.4–6.0)	1.01	0.84
Vital signs			
Systolic blood pressure (mmHg)	182 (159–205)	0.99	0.04[†]
Diastolic blood pressure (mmHg)	94 (72–115)	0.99	0.13
Heart rate (bpm)	102 (90–116)	0.98	0.15
Respiratory rate (/minute)	26 (21–30)	0.97	0.35
Saturation of peripheral oxygen (%)	97 (92–99)	0.98	0.42
Arterial blood gases			
pH	7.37 (7.26–7.44)	6.98	0.19
pCO_2 (mmHg)	38.8 (34.5–50.6)	0.99	0.26
pO_2 (mmHg)	83.4 (61.4–97.5)	1.00	0.72
$HCO_3{-}$ (mmol/l)	22.1 (19.6–24.6)	1.03	0.60
Echocardiographic variables (Teichholz method)			
LVEDVI (ml/m^2)	77.6 (62.8–97.8)	1.00	0.53
LVESVI (ml/m^2)	36.9 (25.9–50.1)	1.00	0.73
Left ventricular ejection fraction (%)	53 (41.3–61)	0.99	0.61
Left ventricular mass index (g/m^2)	158 (133–190.5)	1.00	0.47
Electrocardiographic variables			
Atrial fibrillation rhythm, n (%)	10 (14.7)	3.34	0.01*
Artificially paced, n (%)	0 (0)	NA	NA
Left ventricular hypertrophy, n (%)	12 (17.6)	1.22	0.65
QRS duration (ms)	112 (101.5–120)	1.01	0.41
Laboratory findings			
White blood cell count (×10^3/µl)	10.2 (7.7–12.4)	0.97	0.56
Hematocrit (%)	34.4 ± 5.3	0.92	0.03[†]
Platelet count (×10^3/µl)	213.2 ± 69.2	0.99	0.07
Blood urea nitrogen (mg/dl)	47.0 ± 16.1	1.00	0.66

Table 2 Variables of the prehospital course and at hospital presentation, and univariate Cox proportional analysis for all-cause death *(Continued)*

Creatinine (mg/dl)	8.1 ± 2.3	0.88	0.08
Aspartate aminotransferase (U/l)	20 (15–30)	1.01	0.16
Alanine aminotransferase (U/l)	14 (8–17)	1.01	0.10
Albumin (g/dl)	3.7 ± 0.4	0.28	0.007[†]
Blood glucose (mg/dl)	161 (120.3–217.3)	1.00	0.31
Sodium (mmol/l)	139.1 ± 3.1	0.93	0.17
Potassium (mmol/l)	4.8 (4.3–5.4)	1.04	0.84
Chloride (mmol/l)	102.0 ± 3.2	0.95	0.31
Calcium (mg/dl), n = 61	8.9 ± 0.7	0.98	0.96
Phosphate (mg/dl), n = 56	5.0 (3.6–5.8)	1.06	0.61
C-reactive protein (mg/dl)	0.53 (0.15–1.85)	1.01	0.89

Continuous variables are shown as the mean ± SD or median (first to third quartile) and categorical variables as number (%)
LVEDVI left ventricular end-diastolic volume index, *LVESVI* left ventricular end-systolic volume index, *NA* not analyzed
*p<0.05 with a positive association, †p<0.05 with a negative association

Potential predictors of all-cause mortality using multivariate Cox regression analysis

Variables that were significantly associated with all-cause mortality were included in the multivariate regression model. Age (p = 0.018), presence of peripheral artery or aortic disease (p = 0.003), time of presentation from midnight to 8 am (p = 0.047), and AF rhythm at presentation (p = 0.044) were significantly independently associated with mortality (Table 3).

Kaplan–Meier analyses using potential predictors (Fig. 3) showed significantly higher all-cause mortality in patients with peripheral artery or aortic disease (p = 0.002) and with AF (p = 0.003). Lower mortality was found in patients presenting from midnight to 8 am than in those presenting during the rest of the day (p = 0.007).

Discussion

The current study aimed to determine the potential predictors of mortality in patients with ESRD presenting with APE. We found that older age, the presence of peripheral or aortic disease, and AF rhythm at hospital presentation were independently associated with higher mortality, whereas the time of hospital presentation from midnight to 8 am was associated with lower mortality. These findings suggest an important role of the specific clinical presentation pattern in predicting mortality, as well as the importance of readily accessible acute data, including cardiovascular parameters.

Table 3 Factors associated with all-cause death

	HR	95% CI	p
Age	1.05	1.01–1.09	0.018*
Diabetes mellitus	1.70	0.65–5.45	0.298
Peripheral artery or aortic disease	3.36	1.52–7.42	0.003*
Presentation from midnight to 8 am	0.40	0.15–0.99	0.047[†]
Systolic blood pressure	1.00	0.99–1.01	0.956
Atrial fibrillation rhythm	3.12	1.04–9.13	0.044*
Hematocrit	0.96	0.88–1.05	0.414
Albumin	0.30	0.08–1.02	0.053

Cox proportional regression analyses were performed

HR hazard ratio, *CI* confidence interval

*$p < 0.05$ with a positive association, [†]$p < 0.05$ with a negative association

Cardiac or non-cardiac APE in patients on maintenance hemodialysis

Acute pulmonary edema may be caused by cardiac or non-cardiac etiology. Distinguishing cardiac from non-cardiac APE using a single parameter, such as left ventricular contractility, is often difficult [18–20], especially in patients with ESRD whose fluid status is susceptible to excessive sodium and water intake. In these patients, underlying abnormal cardiac function is common because of volume overload (e.g., anemia, arteriovenous fistulas, and dialysis therapy per se), leading to left ventricular dilatation, or pressure overload (e.g., hypertension and atherosclerosis), leading to left ventricular hypertrophy and potential relative myocardial ischemia [3]. We speculate that their potential cardiovascular pathology may directly or indirectly lead to the development of APE. Therefore, comprehensive assessment of cardiovascular information, including previous or coexisting cardiovascular disease, and echocardiographic and electrocardiographic findings as candidate contributors

of APE may be reasonable, rather than distinguishing cardiac from non-cardiac etiology.

Effect of comorbidities and cardiac function

Some studies focused on acute heart failure or pulmonary edema in patients with ESRD. We found that older age was significantly associated with mortality, which is consistent with previous studies [12, 21].

In our study, some conventional cardiovascular risk factors in the general population, such as coexisting dyslipidemia, hypertension, or obesity, were not associated with mortality. This finding may be partly explained by the reverse epidemiology in which these factors may play protective roles in under-nutrition [22]. In contrast, in our study, diabetes mellitus was associated with mortality in univariate analysis. Diabetes mellitus and coexisting macro- and microvascular diseases are associated with a poor prognosis in patients on maintenance hemodialysis [12, 23–25]. We also found that the presence of peripheral artery or aortic disease was a strong predictor of mortality.

We found that AF rhythm at presentation was associated with mortality. Previous studies have reported an association between AF and all-cause mortality in patients with ESRD [21, 26]. Interestingly, as demonstrated in our study, the association of AF with poor outcome was reported to be superior to that of left ventricular ejection fraction in patients with ESRD [21]. In our study, the median heart rate and duration of maintenance hemodialysis were comparable between patients with and without AF. Although the exact mechanism of a worse outcome associated with AF is unclear, potential acceleration of atrial remodeling caused by hemodialytic therapy and a high prevalence of embolic or bleeding events [21, 27] have been reported to be involved in high mortality.

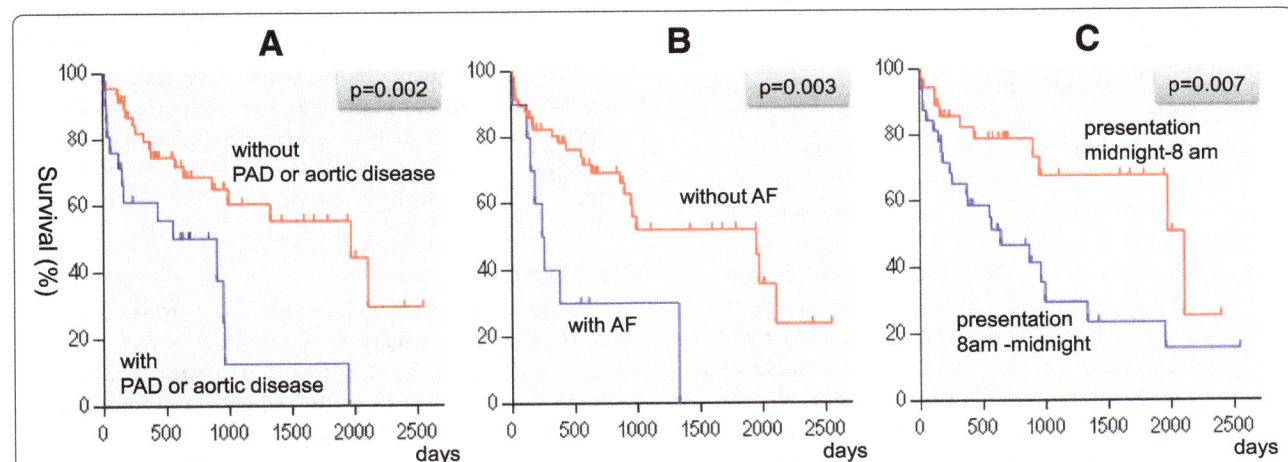

Fig. 3 Kaplan–Meier analyses. Kaplan–Meier analyses using the potential predictors showed significantly higher all-cause mortality in patients with peripheral artery disease (*PAD*) or aortic disease (**a**) and in those with atrial fibrillation (*AF*, **b**). Lower mortality was found in patients presenting from midnight to 8 am (**c**)

We also found that none of the acid–base parameters was associated with mortality. The acid–base imbalance observed in our cohort was mild (median pH, 7.37) and had little effect on outcome in patients with ESRD who are commonly exposed to mild acidosis [28].

Effect of the clinical presentation pattern

In patients undergoing maintenance hemodialysis, a substantial amount of fluid is retained in interdialytic period and quickly removed at hemodialysis treatment. This leads to non-physiological fluctuation of preload. Fluid retention is the main cause of emergent hospitalization in patients undergoing maintenance hemodialysis and is associated with mortality [13, 18]. However, greater weight gain or a 2-day gap after the last hemodialysis session was not associated with mortality in our study.

We found that hospital presentation from midnight to 8 am was significantly associated with lower mortality. The association between nighttime presentation and outcomes in general populations of patients with acute heart failure has not been determined [29, 30]. The definition of nighttime presentation varies among studies; in the current study, we recognized nighttime as the time from midnight to 8 am to eliminate the evening time when many patients were still awake. The concept of circadian fluid shift may partly explain this finding. Upon lying down at night, fluid that is accumulated during the daytime redistributes rostrally by gravity, resulting in fluid shift to the lungs, as well as the upper airway [31]. We speculate that APE developing at night may simply result from a fluid shift due to volume overload, whereas APE developing during the daytime might be attributable to underlying factors other than simple volume overload, such as an altered cardiovascular condition. Additionally, the potential presence of obstructive sleep apnea, which is a prevalent condition in patients with ESRD (50–70%) [32], should be considered as a contributing factor to the better prognosis in patients who presented at night, although our study lacks polysomnographic data. In patients with concurrent ESRD and obstructive sleep apnea, rostral overnight fluid shift is associated with the severity of obstructive sleep apnea [33], possibly via an increase in the jugular vein volume and pharyngeal water content [34]. Hence, nighttime rostral fluid shift, which may lead to acute pulmonary edema, may be enhanced by obstructive sleep apnea. From a therapeutic viewpoint, rostral fluid shift resulting from fluid overload can be corrected by a single emergent hemodialysis session. Moreover, positive airway pressure, which was performed as initial respiratory management in some of our patients (Additional file 1: Table S3), might have helped to alleviate symptoms in patients with obstructive sleep apnea by unloading the inspiratory muscles and left ventricular afterload [35].

Interestingly, patients presenting at night had a higher median systolic blood pressure than did those presenting during the rest of the day. Elevated systolic blood pressure at presentation, possibly related to increased filling pressure and sympathetic hyperactivity, may favorably respond to pharmacological therapy, such as vasodilators, and is associated with lower mortality [9, 11]. In the majority of our patients who presented at night, relief of dyspnea and hypertension was observed after a single emergent hemodialysis session. We speculate that these characteristic initial therapeutic strategies and their responses may be a reflection of the hemodynamics and neurohormonal responses that are specific to patients with ESRD.

The effect of delay from symptom onset to presentation has been discussed for general heart failure [36–40]. In our study, a delay in presenting to the hospital (>72 h after initial symptoms) was not associated with mortality. We consider that because of the meticulous titration of the fluid balance at regular clinic visits, prolonged symptoms may be less common in patients with ESRD than in the general population. This situation indicates that the role of a delay in presentation is less meaningful in patients with ESRD than in the general population.

Limitations

This study has some limitations. First, it was an observational study conducted at a single tertiary center and included relatively small number of patients. A center-specific bias involving medical transfer systems should be considered as a potential social and infrastructural factor that contributed to the better prognosis of patients who presented at night. However, we included objective variables accessible at presentation and the clinical presentation pattern and found potential predictors of mortality from our longitudinal observation. Second, coronary artery anatomy, which may be an important predictor of mortality, was evaluated in only 73.5% of patients; therefore, we might have underestimated the implication of coronary artery anatomy. Clinically accessible parameters, such as echocardiographic or electrocardiographic variables, might have partially compensated for the insufficient coronary information.

Conclusions

In patients on maintenance hemodialysis presenting with APE, older age, the presence of peripheral artery or aortic disease, and AF rhythm at presentation were significantly associated with higher mortality, whereas the time of hospital presentation from midnight to 8 am was significantly associated with lower mortality. Our findings indicate important predictive roles of the clinical presentation pattern specific to patients with ESRD, as well as their characteristics, including cardiovascular risk factors.

Acknowledgements
Not applicable

Funding
None to declare

Authors' contributions
SH and SNa designed the study and drafted the manuscript. SH, YW, and HO collected the data. SH, SNa, JT, YW, HO, TS, and SNi analyzed and interpreted the data. SI, RK, TM, and HN revised the manuscript for intellectual content. SNi approved the final manuscript. All authors read and approved the final manuscript.

Competing interests
The authors declare that they have no competing interests.

Author details
[1]Department of Cardiovascular Medicine, Saitama Medical University International Medical Center, 1397-1 Yamane, 350-1298 Hidaka, Saitama, Japan. [2]Department of Nephrology, Saitama Medical University, Saitama, Japan. [3]Department of General Internal Medicine, Saitama Medical University Hospital, Saitama, Japan.

References
1. Allon M. Evidence-based cardiology in hemodialysis patients. J Am Soc Nephrol. 2013;24(12):1934–43.
2. Masakane I, Nakai S, Ogata S, Kimata N, Hanafusa N, Hamano T, Wakai K, Wada A, Nitta K. An overview of regular dialysis treatment in Japan (as of 31 December 2013). Ther Apher Dial. 2015;19(6):540–74.
3. Fort J. Chronic renal failure: a cardiovascular risk factor. Kidney Int Suppl. 2005;99:S25–29.
4. Gheorghiade M, Zannad F, Sopko G, Klein L, Pina IL, Konstam MA, Massie BM, Roland E, Targum S, Collins SP, et al. Acute heart failure syndromes: current state and framework for future research. Circulation. 2005;112(25): 3958–68.
5. Gray A, Goodacre S, Nicholl J, Masson M, Sampson F, Elliott M, Crane S, Newby DE. The development of a simple risk score to predict early outcome in severe acute acidotic cardiogenic pulmonary edema: the 3CPO score. Circ Heart Fail. 2010;3(1):111–7.
6. Nieminen MS, Bohm M, Cowie MR, Drexler H, Filippatos GS, Jondeau G, Hasin Y, Lopez-Sendon J, Mebazaa A, Metra M, et al. Executive summary of the guidelines on the diagnosis and treatment of acute heart failure: the Task Force on Acute Heart Failure of the European Society of Cardiology. Eur Heart J. 2005;26(4):384–416.
7. Ellingsrud C, Agewall S. Morphine in the treatment of acute pulmonary oedema—why? Int J Cardiol. 2016;202:870–3.
8. Fonarow GC, Adams Jr KF, Abraham WT, Yancy CW, Boscardin WJ. Risk stratification for in-hospital mortality in acutely decompensated heart failure: classification and regression tree analysis. JAMA. 2005;293(5):572–80.
9. Gheorghiade M, Abraham WT, Albert NM, Greenberg BH, O'Connor CM, She L, Stough WG, Yancy CW, Young JB, Fonarow GC. Systolic blood pressure at admission, clinical characteristics, and outcomes in patients hospitalized with acute heart failure. JAMA. 2006;296(18):2217–26.
10. Klein L, O'Connor CM, Leimberger JD, Gattis-Stough W, Pina IL, Felker GM, Adams Jr KF, Califf RM, Gheorghiade M. Lower serum sodium is associated with increased short-term mortality in hospitalized patients with worsening heart failure: results from the Outcomes of a Prospective Trial of Intravenous Milrinone for Exacerbations of Chronic Heart Failure (OPTIME-CHF) study. Circulation. 2005;111(19):2454–60.
11. Felker GM, Leimberger JD, Califf RM, Cuffe MS, Massie BM, Adams Jr KF, Gheorghiade M, O'Connor CM. Risk stratification after hospitalization for decompensated heart failure. J Card Fail. 2004;10(6):460–6.
12. Banerjee D, Ma JZ, Collins AJ, Herzog CA. Long-term survival of incident hemodialysis patients who are hospitalized for congestive heart failure, pulmonary edema, or fluid overload. Clin J Am Soc Nephrol. 2007;2(6):1186–90.
13. Halle MP, Hertig A, Kengne AP, Ashuntantang G, Rondeau E, Ridel C. Acute pulmonary oedema in chronic dialysis patients admitted into an intensive care unit. Nephrol Dial Transplant. 2012;27(2):603–7.
14. Mebazaa A, Gheorghiade M, Pina IL, Harjola VP, Hollenberg SM, Follath F, Rhodes A, Plaisance P, Roland E, Nieminen M, et al. Practical recommendations for prehospital and early in-hospital management of patients presenting with acute heart failure syndromes. Crit Care Med. 2008; 36(1 Suppl):S129–139.
15. Gillett MJ. International Expert Committee report on the role of the A1c assay in the diagnosis of diabetes: diabetes care 2009; 32(7): 1327-1334. Clin Biochem Rev. 2009;30(4):197–200.
16. Executive Summary of The Third Report of The National Cholesterol Education Program (NCEP) expert panel on detection, evaluation, and treatment of high blood cholesterol in adults (adult treatment panel III). JAMA. 2001;285(19):2486-2497.
17. Herzog CA, Littrell K, Arko C, Frederick PD, Blaney M. Clinical characteristics of dialysis patients with acute myocardial infarction in the United States: a collaborative project of the United States Renal Data System and the National Registry of Myocardial Infarction. Circulation. 2007;116(13):1465–72.
18. Kalantar-Zadeh K, Regidor DL, Kovesdy CP, Van Wyck D, Bunnapradist S, Horwich TB, Fonarow GC. Fluid retention is associated with cardiovascular mortality in patients undergoing long-term hemodialysis. Circulation. 2009; 119(5):671–9.
19. Fonarow GC, Stough WG, Abraham WT, Albert NM, Gheorghiade M, Greenberg BH, O'Connor CM, Sun JL, Yancy CW, Young JB. Characteristics, treatments, and outcomes of patients with preserved systolic function hospitalized for heart failure: a report from the OPTIMIZE-HF Registry. J Am Coll Cardiol. 2007;50(8):768–77.
20. McIntyre CW, Goldsmith DJ. Ischemic brain injury in hemodialysis patients: which is more dangerous, hypertension or intradialytic hypotension? Kidney Int. 2015;87(6):1109–15.
21. Genovesi S, Vincenti A, Rossi E, Pogliani D, Acquistapace I, Stella A, Valsecchi MG. Atrial fibrillation and morbidity and mortality in a cohort of long-term hemodialysis patients. Am J Kidney Dis. 2008;51(2):255–62.
22. Kalantar-Zadeh K, Block G, Humphreys MH, Kopple JD. Reverse epidemiology of cardiovascular risk factors in maintenance dialysis patients. Kidney Int. 2003;63(3):793–808.
23. Chen SC, Chang JM, Hwang SJ, Tsai JC, Liu WC, Wang CS, Lin TH, Su HM, Chen HC. Ankle brachial index as a predictor for mortality in patients with chronic kidney disease and undergoing haemodialysis. Nephrology (Carlton). 2010;15(3):294–9.
24. Di Eusanio M, Schepens MA, Morshuis WJ, Dossche KM, Kazui T, Ohkura K, Washiyama N, Di Bartolomeo R, Pacini D, Pierangeli A. Separate grafts or en bloc anastomosis for arch vessels reimplantation to the aortic arch. Ann Thorac Surg. 2004;77(6):2021–8.
25. Kimmel PL, Varela MP, Peterson RA, Weihs KL, Simmens SJ, Alleyne S, Amarashinge A, Mishkin GJ, Cruz I, Veis JH. Interdialytic weight gain and survival in hemodialysis patients: effects of duration of ESRD and diabetes mellitus. Kidney Int. 2000;57(3):1141–51.
26. Mitsuma W, Matsubara T, Hatada K, Imai S, Saito N, Shimada H, Miyazaki S. Clinical characteristics of hemodialysis patients with atrial fibrillation: The RAKUEN (Registry of atrial fibrillation in chronic kidney disease under hemodialysis from Niigata) study. J Cardiol. 2016;68(2):148–55.
27. Genovesi S, Rossi E, Gallieni M, Stella A, Badiali F, Conte F, Pasquali S, Bertoli S, Ondei P, Bonforte G, et al. Warfarin use, mortality, bleeding and stroke in haemodialysis patients with atrial fibrillation. Nephrol Dial Transplant. 2015; 30(3):491–8.
28. Oh MS, Uribarri J, Weinstein J, Schreiber M, Kamel KS, Kraut JA, Madias NE, Laski ME. What unique acid-base considerations exist in dialysis patients? Semin Dial. 2004;17(5):351–64.
29. Minami Y, Kajimoto K, Sato N, Yumino D, Mizuno M, Aokage T, Murai K, Munakata R, Asai K, Sakata Y, et al. Admission time, variability in clinical characteristics, and in-hospital outcomes in acute heart failure syndromes: findings from the ATTEND registry. Int J Cardiol. 2011;153(1):102–5.
30. Matsushita M, Shirakabe A, Hata N, Shinada T, Kobayashi N, Tomita K, Tsurumi M, Shimura T, Okazaki H, Yamamoto Y, et al. Association between

the admission time and the clinical findings in patients with acute heart failure. J Cardiol. 2013;61(3):210–5.

31. Kalantar-Zadeh K, Abbott KC, Salahudeen AK, Kilpatrick RD, Horwich TB. Survival advantages of obesity in dialysis patients. Am J Clin Nutr. 2005; 81(3):543–54.

32. Roumelioti ME, Brown LK, Unruh ML. The relationship between volume overload in end-stage renal disease and obstructive sleep apnea. Semin Dial. 2015;28(5):508–13.

33. Elias RM, Bradley TD, Kasai T, Motwani SS, Chan CT. Rostral overnight fluid shift in end-stage renal disease: relationship with obstructive sleep apnea. Nephrol Dial Transplant. 2012;27(4):1569–73.

34. Elias RM, Chan CT, Paul N, Motwani SS, Kasai T, Gabriel JM, Spiller N, Bradley TD. Relationship of pharyngeal water content and jugular volume with severity of obstructive sleep apnea in renal failure. Nephrol Dial Transplant. 2013;28(4):937–44.

35. Naughton MT, Rahman MA, Hara K, Floras JS, Bradley TD. Effect of continuous positive airway pressure on intrathoracic and left ventricular transmural pressures in patients with congestive heart failure. Circulation. 1995;91(6):1725–31.

36. Gravely-Witte S, Jurgens CY, Tamim H, Grace SL. Length of delay in seeking medical care by patients with heart failure symptoms and the role of symptom-related factors: a narrative review. Eur J Heart Fail. 2010;12(10):1122–9.

37. Goldberg RJ, Goldberg JH, Pruell S, Yarzebski J, Lessard D, Spencer FA, Gore JM. Delays in seeking medical care in hospitalized patients with decompensated heart failure. Am J Med. 2008;121(3):212–8.

38. Shiraishi Y, Kohsaka S, Harada K, Sakai T, Takagi A, Miyamoto T, Iida K, Tanimoto S, Fukuda K, Nagao K, et al. Time interval from symptom onset to hospital care in patients with acute heart failure: a report from the Tokyo Cardiac Care Unit Network Emergency Medical Service Database. PLoS One. 2015;10(11):e0142017.

39. De Luca L, Abraham WT, Fonarow GC, Gheorghiade M. Congestion in acute heart failure syndromes: importance of early recognition and treatment. Rev Cardiovasc Med. 2006;7(2):69–74.

40. Sethares KA, Chin E, Jurgens CY. Predictors of delay in heart failure patients and consequences for outcomes. Curr Heart Fail Rep. 2015;12(1):94–105.

15

Presepsin is a potent biomarker for diagnosing skin wound infection in hemodialysis patients compared to white blood cell count, high-sensitivity C-reactive protein, procalcitonin, and soluble CD14

Jun Shiota[1,2]*, Hitoshi Tagawa[2], Norihiko Ohura[3] and Hitoshi Kasahara[2]

Abstract

Background: The production of presepsin has been shown to be strongly related to bacterial phagocytosis. The purpose of the present study is to compare the usefulness of presepsin for diagnosing localized skin wound infection with that of conventional infection biomarkers.

Methods: We enrolled 29 hemodialysis (HD) patients with skin wound infections of foot gangrene or decubitus ("localized infection group") and 20 HD patients without infection ("no infection group"). The white blood cell (WBC) count and high-sensitivity C-reactive protein (hsCRP) and presepsin levels were measured using blood samples collected before HD, 2 days after the previous dialysis session. Soluble CD14 (sCD14) and procalcitonin (PCT) levels were also measured in 12 patients with localized infection and 8 patients without infection.

Results: The levels of hsCRP and presepsin were significantly higher in the localized infection group ($N = 29$) than in the no infection group ($N = 20$) ($P = 0.0209$ and 0.0000, respectively). In receiver operating characteristics (ROC) analyses, when the cut-off values of hsCRP and presepsin were set at 1.07 mg/dL and 2080 pg/mL, respectively, the sensitivity was 0.69 and 0.86, and the specificity was 0.70 and 0.80, respectively. The area under the curve (AUC) was calculated as 0.696 for hsCRP and 0.874 for presepsin. The AUC for presepsin was significantly higher than that for hsCRP ($P = 0.0348$). No marked differences were found in the age, gender, WBC, or sCD14 or PCT levels between groups.

Conclusions: Presepsin is a potent, useful biomarker for diagnosing skin wound infection in HD patients compared to conventional infection biomarkers.

Keywords: Presepsin, Localized infection, Skin wound infection, Hemodialysis, hsCRP, Procalcitonin, Soluble CD 14

Background

Complex wounds develop rapidly and are refractory to healing in hemodialysis (HD) patients because of persistent bacterial infection due to immune deficiency and ischemic limbs due to peripheral arterial disease [1]. Bacterial phagocytosis by monocytes is required to overcome bacterial proliferation in order to localize the infection focus [2].

Although bacterial infection of skin wound can be diagnosed by physical signs [3], the bacterial burden is occasionally hard to evaluate in the presence of deep localized lesions or myelitis despite apparently mild skin lesions, resulting in overlooking indications for antibiotics therapy and surgical or vascular intervention.

Presepsin is an N-terminal fragment of CD14 on monocytes with a molecular weight of 13 kDa that was discovered in Japan in 2002 as a biomarker for diagnosing sepsis [4, 5]. In contrast to conventional infection biomarkers which are induced by endotoxins or cytokines, the novel production mechanism of presepsin has

* Correspondence: jun.siota@grp.zenjinkai.or.jp
[1]Department of Internal Medicine, Tsunashima Kidney Clinic, 1-10-4 Tsunashima-Higashi, Kohoku-ku, Yokohama 223-0052, Japan
[2]Department of Internal Medicine, Kichijoji Asahi Hospital, Tokyo, Japan
Full list of author information is available at the end of the article

been reported to be closely related to phagocytosis by monocytes [6, 7]. We previously reported the usefulness of presepsin for predicting the prognosis of foot gangrene in HD patients (cut-off plasma value 2083 pg/mL) [8]. In the present study, we hypothesized that presepsin might be useful for diagnosing localized infection, and we compared the diagnosing ability of presepsin for skin wound infection in HD patients with that of conventional infection biomarkers: white blood cell count (WBC) and levels of high-sensitivity C-reactive protein (hsCRP), soluble CD14 (sCD14), and procalcitonin (PCT).

Methods

Participants

We enrolled 29 HD patients (male, 48.3%) complicated with skin wound infections of foot gangrene or decubitus ("localized infection group") and 20 HD patients (male, 55.0%) without skin wound ("no infection group") who had been admitted to Kichijoji Asahi Hospital between 2014/1/1 and 2015/3/31. All patients were thoroughly examined to confirm the absence of infection of other organs. Patients who had received immunosuppressants were excluded. Patients with chronic hepatitis and liver cirrhosis were excluded because higher presepsin levels have been observed due to the bacterial translocation [9]. The skin wounds were all examined and evaluated by the same plastic surgeon (who is one of the authors). The localized infection group was defined by skin wounds with exudate/pus, friable tissue, or debris, suggesting critical colonization with ongoing bacterial proliferation [3]. A photograph of a localized skin wound infection is shown in Fig. 1.

Blood was collected with heparin as an anticoagulant using an endotoxin-free tube (TERUMO, Tokyo, Japan) before HD, 2 days after the previous dialysis session, and the blood samples were immediately measured or frozen prior to the analysis of the WBC and levels of hsCRP and presepsin (Table 1; shown as "all patients"). sCD14 and PCT levels were measured additionally in the 20 HD patients ($N = 12$, localized infection group; $N = 8$, no infection group) enrolled after 2015/1/1 (Table 1; shown as "patients examined for all biomarkers including sCD14 and PCT").

All of the patients received 4-h dialysis three times per week with a blood flow rate of 180–200 mL/min and a dialysate flow rate of 400 mL/min. We used high-flux membrane dialyzers that were not reused and standard bicarbonate dialysate diluted with ultrapure water. All dialysate samples were negative for bacteria measured in colony-forming units in bacterial culture and had an endotoxin (ET) level ≤0.001 EU/mL as measured by a chromogenic assay (Endospecy ES-24S; Seikagaku Corporation, Tokyo, Japan).

Measurement of biomarkers

The WBC was measured using an automated analyzer, LH780 (Beckman Coulter, Tokyo, Japan). The hsCRP levels were measured using an automated analyzer, JCA-BM8060 (JEOL, Tokyo, Japan) based on a turbidometeric immunoassay (CRP-latex X2 "Seiken"; Denka Seiken, Tokyo, Japan). The upper reference limit in healthy volunteers was 0.30 mg/dL. The presepsin levels were measured using an automated immunoanalyzer, PATHFAST, based on a non-competitive chemiluminescent enzyme immunoassay (CLEIA), which contained Magtration technology (LSI Medience Corporation, Tokyo, Japan) [10], modified from an enzyme-linked immunosorbent assay (ELISA) [11]. The method was calibrated using heparinized plasma samples that contained a recombinant human presepsin antigen. The reference range in healthy volunteers has not been established yet [12]. The sCD14 levels were measured using a commercially available ELISA kit (sCD14 Quantikine ELISA Kit; R&D Systems, Minneapolis, USA). The levels were measured in duplicate, and the mean value was used. The median value in healthy volunteers without infection has been reported as 1660 ng/mL [13]. The PCT levels were measured using an automated electrochemiluminescence immunoanalyzer based on Elecsys reagent (BRAHMS PCT; Roche Diagnostics, Tokyo, Japan). The median PCT level in healthy volunteers without infection has been reported as 0.034 ng/mL [14].

Statistical analyses

The data were presented as the median (interquartile range, IQR). The data were compared between the

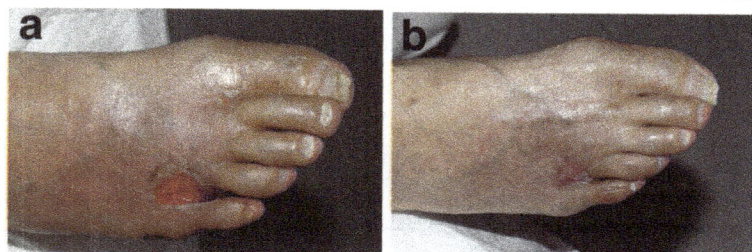

Fig. 1 a An exudative skin wound indicating a bacterial burden. Presepsin level 4480 pg/mL; b healed skin wound (the same case)

Table 1 Comparison of characteristics and infection biomarkers between the localized infection group and the no infection group

Group	All patients		Patients examined for all biomarkers including sCD14 and PCT	
	Localized infection	No infection	Localized infection	No infection
Number	29	20	12	8
Age, years	72 (66–77)	78 (74–83)	73 (65–78)	78 (72–84)
Male, %	48.3	55.0	66.7	62.5
WBC, μL	5700 (4333–7100)	5250 (4475–6000)	5800 (4675–6735)	5450 (4475–5750)
hsCRP, mg/dL	1.26 (0.71–2.24)*	0.23 (0.10–1.22)	1.30 (0.50–2.16)	0.17 (0.11–0.74)
Presepsin, pg/mL	3370 (2240–4480)**	1510 (1205–1810)	3330 (2515–3990)*	1560 (1488–1973)
sCD14, ng/mL			2278 (1969–2906)	2417 (2226–2732)
PCT, ng/mL			0.23 (0.20–0.27)	0.25 (0.21–0.28)

Data were presented as the median (interquartile range, IQR). Statistics were analyzed using the Mann-Whitney U test. A blood analysis was performed to determine the WBC count, and the hsCRP and presepsin levels of 49 HD patients who were enrolled in 2014/1/1–2015/3/31 (shown as "all patients"). sCD14 and PCT were also measured in the 20 HD patients enrolled after 2015/1/1 (shown as "patients examined for all biomarkers including sCD14 and PCT")
*$P < 0.05$, **$P < 0.01$ vs. the no infection group

localized infection group and the no infection group using Fisher's exact test or the Mann-Whitney U test. A receiver operating characteristic (ROC) analysis was performed to determine the area under the curve (AUC), sensitivity and specificity. Diagnostic AUCs were compared using DeLong's test [15]. The calculations were performed using R 3.3.1, which is open to the public. All analyses set a P value of 0.05 (two-tailed) to indicate significance.

Results

Comparison between two groups for all patients ($N = 49$)

The levels of hsCRP and presepsin were significantly higher in the localized infection group ($N = 29$) than in the no infection group ($N = 20$) ($P = 0.0209$ and 0.0000, respectively), although no marked differences were found in the age, gender, or WBC (Table 1). In ROC analyses (Fig. 2), when the cut-off values of hsCRP and presepsin were set at 1.07 mg/dL and 2080 pg/mL, respectively, the sensitivity was 0.69 and 0.86, and the specificity was 0.70 and 0.80, respectively. The AUC was calculated as 0.696 for hsCRP and 0.874 for presepsin. The AUC for presepsin was significantly higher than that for hsCRP ($P = 0.0348$) (Fig. 2).

Comparison between two groups for the patients examined additionally for sCD14 and PCT ($N = 20$)

The levels of presepsin were significantly higher in the localized infection group ($N = 12$) than in the no infection group ($N = 8$) ($P = 0.0206$), although no marked differences were found in the age, gender, WBC, hsCRP, sCD14, or PCT levels (Table 1, Fig. 3).

Discussion

Chronic wound infection is categorized into four stages: "contamination," "colonization," "critical colonization," and "infection". In the "critical colonization" stage,

bacterial proliferation has exceeded the phagocytosis potential of macrophages [2]. Sibbald et al. [16] created an assessment model using the mnemonic NERDS (exudate/pus, friable tissue, debris, nonhealing and smell) to predict critical colonization. Woo et al. [3] devised a semiquantitative bacterial culture system using wound swabs, in which the bacterial burden of the wound is classified as "scant," "light," "moderate," or "heavy" for bacterial growth; scant to light bacterial growth was considered to reflect critical colonization. The odds ratios for individual

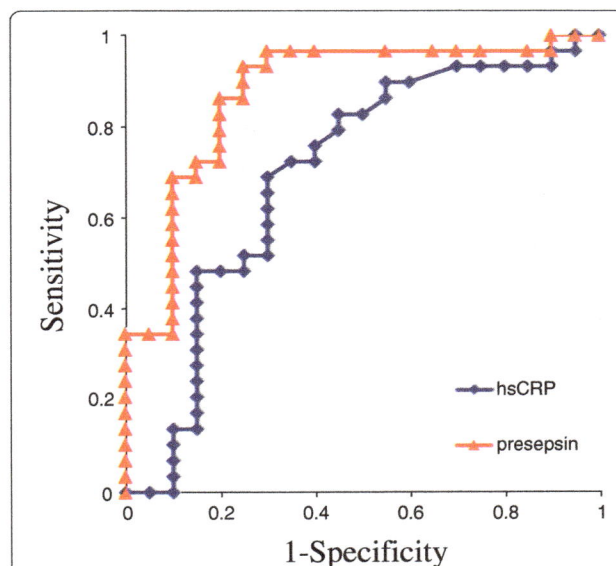

Fig. 2 Receiver operating characteristic (ROC) curves of presepsin and hsCRP for discriminating the localized infection group ($N = 29$) and the no infection group ($N = 20$). When the cut-off value of presepsin and hsCRP were set at 2080 pg/mL and 1.07 mg/dL, respectively, the sensitivity was 0.86 and 0.69, and the specificity was 0.80 and 0.70, respectively. The AUC was calculated as 0.874 for presepsin and 0.696 for hsCRP, and the AUC for presepsin was significantly higher than that for hsCRP ($P = 0.0348$)

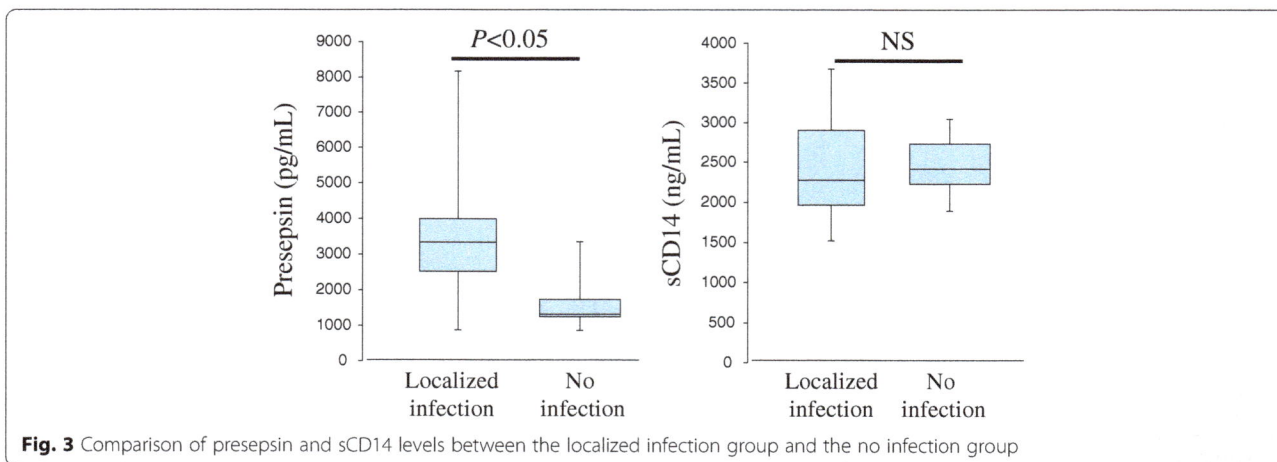

Fig. 3 Comparison of presepsin and sCD14 levels between the localized infection group and the no infection group

NERDS variables and scant/light bacterial growth were calculated and wounds were found to be five times more likely to have a scant/light bacterial growth in the presence of exudate/pus, friable tissue, or debris. In the present study, localized infection was defined as a state of critical colonization, which was diagnosed based on the presence of exudate/pus, friable tissue, or debris.

Presepsin and hsCRP were recognized as useful biomarkers in the present study but the WBC and the sCD14 and PCT levels were not useful for diagnosing localized skin wound infection. ROC analyses showed that the AUC of presepsin was significantly higher than that of hsCRP (0.874 vs. 0.696, $P = 0.0348$) and the sensitivity and specificity of presepsin were 0.86 and 0.80 respectively when the cut-off value was set at 2080 pg/mL. The AUC of presepsin was higher than the evaluation criterion of 0.75 required for the diagnostic ability of biomarkers [17]. The AUC, sensitivity, and specificity for localized infection in the present study were comparable to those for sepsis in meta-analyses (0.874, 0.86, 0.80 vs. 0.89, 0.83, 0.81) [18]. Therefore, presepsin may have the most reliable diagnostic ability among infection biomarkers for diagnosing localized infection.

An in vitro study showed that the stimulation of whole blood (including monocytes) from healthy volunteers by lipopolysaccharide (LPS) induced a significant increase in the plasma IL-6 levels, with no significant increase in presepsin levels [19]. CRP seemed to be stimulated by IL-6 released from monocytes in a localized infection group [20], but presepsin might be produced by different mechanisms. The relationship between presepsin production and bacterial phagocytosis by monocytes has been previously demonstrated. It has been shown that presepsin levels increased in a rabbit model of cecal ligation and puncture sepsis but not in a rabbit ET shock model and that presepsin production from peritoneal granulocyte was stimulated by *Escherichia coli* and suppressed by the inhibition of phagocytosis [7]. In vitro

presepsin production by peripheral mononuclear cells was increased by *Escherichia coli*, *Staphylococcus epidermidis*, and sterile monosodium urate crystals and suppressed by an inhibitor of phagocytosis, whereas presepsin production was not induced by peptidoglycan or LPS [6]. Taking into account a report that presepsin levels were not markedly different between systemic bacterial infection patients (positive blood culture) and localized bacterial infection patients (positive culture except blood) [21], presepsin produced by bacterial phagocytosis at a localized infection site might increase the presepsin levels in circulating blood.

CD14 is a pattern-recognition receptor that plays an immunomodulatory role in secreting pro-inflammatory humoral factors in response to not only ET but also lipoteichoic acid (LTA), which is a major constituent of Gram-positive bacteria [22]. sCD14 is a fragment of CD14, and its levels are increased by ET (LPS) stimulation in vitro [23]. In HD patients, sCD14 levels are increased compared with healthy volunteers, probably because of inevitable exposure to ET (LPS) due to contaminated dialysate, intestinal bacterial translocation, and an impaired liver macrophage function [24, 25]. As no marked differences in the sCD14 levels were observed between the localized infection group and the no infection group in the present study, a significant ET (LPS) load from skin wound infection site is unlikely to be observed. Therefore, sCD14 is not appropriate as a biomarker for diagnosing localized skin wound infection, in contrast to presepsin, which is also a fragment of CD14 (Fig. 3). Although both sCD14 and presepsin are released by proteolysis with protease from monocytes, the mechanism is likely to be different. In contrast to sCD14, which was reported to be produced from cell-surface CD14 of activated monocytes [26, 27], presepsin is reported to be produced from monocytes that are activated in the event of phagocytosis [6].

PCT is a polypeptide with a molecular weight of 13 kDa that was first described in 1993 as a biomarker for the diagnosis of sepsis. PCT is mainly produced by monocytes in circulating blood [28], and iatrogenic ET (LPS) load into circulating blood was reported to increase the PCT levels [29]. PCT is ubiquitously produced in response to ET (LPS) in HD patients. The PCT levels in HD patients without infection were reported to be about eight times as high as those in healthy volunteers without infection (median 0.260 vs. 0.034 ng/mL) [14]. In the present study, PCT was not useful for detecting localized skin wound infection, because the PCT levels were not elevated in the localized infection group compared with the no infection group (median 0.23 vs 0.25 ng/mL). The PCT values within a range of 0.13–0.30 ng/mL in the localized infection group of the present study were obviously lower than the cut-off value of 0.5 ng/mL reported in the HD patients with pneumonia and sepsis [30], suggesting that the bacterial load into the circulating blood from the skin wound infection was unlikely.

The presepsin levels of HD patients are higher than those of healthy volunteers [31], and the reference range of presepsin levels, even in healthy volunteers, has not been established yet [32]. It has been reported that the presepsin levels are inversely correlated with the glomerular filtration rate (GFR) and that they significantly decrease after an HD session [31]. As presepsin (a 13-kDa protein) is freely filtered through the glomeruli and is almost completely reabsorbed and catabolized within the proximal tubular cells [33], the increased levels in the patients with a decreased GFR might be caused by the decreased filtration and catabolism in the kidney. In addition, the increased presepsin levels in HD patients might also be caused by inevitable exposure to ET (LPS), due to the contamination of the dialysate, intestinal bacterial translocation, and an impaired liver macrophage function [24, 25].

Our results showed that the usefulness of presepsin in HD patients for diagnosing skin wound infection was comparable to that for sepsis and superior to the conventional infection biomarkers (WBC, hsCRP, sCD14, and PCT). The cut-off value (2080 pg/mL) for diagnosing skin wound infection was close to that (2083 pg/mL) for predicting the prognosis of foot gangrene [8].

To our knowledge, the present study is the first to address the potential value of presepsin for diagnosing localized infection in HD patients; however, further verification of the usefulness of presepsin for diagnosing localized infection using a larger number of HD patients is necessary before application in clinical practice. In addition, the usefulness of presepsin for diagnosing infection of various organs must also be verified.

Conclusions

Presepsin is a potent, useful infection biomarker for diagnosing skin wound infection in HD patients compared to conventional infection biomarkers.

Abbreviations
AUC: Area under the curve; ET: Endotoxin; hsCRP: High-sensitivity C-reactive protein; PCT: Procalcitonin; ROC: Receiver operating characteristic; WBC: White blood cell

Acknowledgements
The authors thank all the staff members working at Kichijoji Asahi Hospital.

Funding
Not applicable.

Author's contributions
JS was involved in the statistical analysis. All authors read and approved the final manuscript.

Competing interests
The authors declare that they have no competing interests.

Author details
[1]Department of Internal Medicine, Tsunashima Kidney Clinic, 1-10-4 Tsunashima-Higashi, Kohoku-ku, Yokohama 223-0052, Japan. [2]Department of Internal Medicine, Kichijoji Asahi Hospital, Tokyo, Japan. [3]Department of Plastic, Reconstructive and Aesthetic Surgery, Kyorin University School of Medicine, Tokyo, Japan.

References
1. Fujioka M, Oka K, Kitamura R, Yakabe A. Complex wounds tend to develop more rapidly in patients receiving hemodialysis because of diabetes mellitus. Hemodial Int. 2009;13:168–71.
2. Kingsley A. The wound infection continuum and its application to clinical practice. Ostomy Wound Manag. 2003;49(7A Suppl):1–7.
3. Woo KY, Sibbald RG. A cross-sectional validation study of using NERDS and STONEES to assess bacterial burden. Ostomy Wound Manag. 2009;55:40–8.
4. Yaegashi Y, Shirakawa K, Sato N, et al. Evaluation of a newly identified soluble CD14 subtype as a marker for sepsis. J Infect Chemother. 2005;11:234–8.
5. Shozushima T, Takahashi G, Matsumoto N, Kojika M, Okamura Y, Endo S. Usefulness of presepsin (sCD14-ST) measurements as a marker for the diagnosis and severity of sepsis that satisfied diagnostic criteria of systemic inflammatory response syndrome. J Infect Chemother. 2011;17:764–9.
6. Arai Y, Mizugishi K, Nonomura K, Naitoh K, Takaori-Kondo A, Yamashita K. Phagocytosis by human monocytes is required for the secretion of presepsin. J Infect Chemother. 2015;21:564–9.
7. Naitoh K, Shirakawa K, Hirose J, Nakamura M, et al. The new sepsis marker, sCD14-ST (PRESEPSIN), induction mechanism in the rabbit sepsis models. Crit Care. 2010;14 Suppl 2:19.
8. Shiota J, Ohura N, Higashikawa S, et al. Presepsin as a predictor of critical colonization in CLI hemodialysis patients. Wound Rep Reg. 2016;24:189–94.
9. Papp M, Tornai T, Vitalis Z, Tornai I, Dinya T, et al. Presepsin teardown-pitfalls of biomarkers in the diagnosis and prognosis of bacterial infection in cirrhosis. World J Gastroenterol. 2016;22:9172–85.
10. Okamura Y, Yokoi H. Development of a point-of-care assay system for measurement of presepsin (sCD14-ST). Clin Chim Acta. 2011;412:2157–61.
11. Shirakawa K, Naitoh K, Hirose J, Takahashi T, Furusako S. Presepsin (sCD14-ST): development and evaluation of one-step ELISA with a new standard that is similar to the form of presepsin in septic patients. Clin Chem Lab Med. 2011;49:937–9.
12. Chenevier-Gobeaux C, Borderie D, Weiss N, Mallet-Coste T, Claessens YE. Presepsin (sCD14-ST), an innate immune response marker in sepsis. Clin Chim Acta. 2015;450:97–103.

13. Sandler NG, Koh C, Roque A, et al. Host response to translocated microbial products predicts outcomes of patients with HBV or HCV infection. Gastroenterology. 2011;141:1220–30.
14. Trimarchi H, Dicugno M, Muryan A, et al. Pro-calcitonin and inflammation in chronic hemodialysis. Medicina. 2013;73:411–6.
15. DeLong ER, DeLong DM, Clarke-Peason DL. Comparing the areas under two or more correlated receiver operating characteristic curves: A nonparametric approach. Biometrics. 1988;44:837–45.
16. Sibbald RG, Woo K, Ayello EA. Increased bacterial burden and infection: the story of NERDS and STONES. Adv Skin Wound Care. 2006;19:447–61.
17. Behnes M, Bertsch T, Lepiorz D, et al. Diagnostic and prognostic utility of soluble CD14 subtype (presepsin) for severe sepsis and septic shock during the first week of intensive care treatment. Crit Care. 2014;18:507.
18. Tong X, Cao Y, Yu M, Han C. Presepsin as a diagnostic marker for sepsis: evidence from a bivariate meta-analysis. Ther Clin Risk Manag. 2015;11:1027–33.
19. Chenvier-Gobeaux C, Bardet V, Poupet H, Poyart C, Borderie D, Claessens YE. Presepsin (sCD14-ST) secretion and kinetics by peripheral blood mononuclear cells and monocytic THP-1 cell line. Ann Biol Clin. 2016;74:93–7.
20. Pepys MB, Hirschfield GM. C-reactive protein: a critical update. J Clin Invest. 2003;111:1805–12.
21. Endo S, Suzuki Y, Takahashi G, et al. Usefulness of presepsin in the diagnosis of sepsis in a multicenter prospective study. J Infect Chemothr. 2012;18:891–7.
22. Miyake K. Innate recognition of lipopolysaccharide by Toll-like receptor 4-MD-2. Trends Microbiol. 2004;12:186–92.
23. Marcos V, Latzin P, Hector A, et al. Expression, regulation and clinical significance of soluble and membrane CD14 receptors in pediatric inflammatory lung diseases. Respir Res. 2010;11:32.
24. Navarro-Gonzalez JF, Mora-Femandez C, Muros de Fuentes M, Donate-Correa J, Cazana-Perez V, Garcia-Perez J. Effect of phosphate binders on serum inflammatory profile, soluble CD14, and endotoxin levels in hemodialysis patients. Clin J Am Soc Nephrol. 2011;6:2272–9.
25. Seabra VF, Thomas G, Jaber BL. Soluble CD14 and endotoxin levels in hemodialysis patients: A tale of 2 molecules. Am J Kidney Dis. 2009;54:990–2.
26. Nockher WA, Scherberich JE. Monocyte cell-surface CD14 expression and soluble CD14 antigen in hemodialysis: evidence for chronic exposure to LPS. Kidney Int. 1995;48:1469–76.
27. Bazil V, Strominger JL. Shedding as a mechanism of down-modulation of CD14 on stimulated human monocytes. J Immunol. 1991;147:1567–74.
28. Oberhoffer M, Stonans I, Russwurm S, et al. Procalcitonin expression in human peripheral blood mononuclear cells and its modulation by lipopolysaccharides and sepsis-related cytokines in vitro. J Lab Clin Med. 1999;134:49–55.
29. Brunkhorst FM, Heinz U, Forycki ZF. Kinetics of procalcitonin in iatrogenic sepsis. Intensive Care Med. 1998;24:888–9.
30. Grace E, Tutner RM. Use of procalcitonin in patients with various degrees of chronic kidney disease including renal replacement therapy. Clin Infect Dis. 2014;59:1761–7.
31. Nagata T, Yasuda Y, Ando M, et al. Clinical impact of kidney function on presepsin levels. PloS one. 2015;10:e0129159. doi:10.1371/journal.pone.0129159.
32. Giavarina D, Carta M. Determination of reference interval for presepsin, an early marker for sepsis. Biochem Med. 2015;25:64–8.
33. Chenevier-Gobeaux C, Trabattoni E, Roelens M, Borderie D, Claessens Y-E. Presepsin (sCD14-ST) in emergency department: The need for adapted threshold values? Clin Chim Acta. 2014;427:34–6.

16

The importance of nutritional intervention by dietitians for hyperphosphatemia in maintained hemodialysis patients

Yuka Kawate[1] and Hitomi Miyata[2*]

Abstract

Hyperphosphatemia is a risk factor for cardiovascular disease and mortality in individuals with end-stage kidney disease (ESKD). Thus, it represents a potential target for interventions to improve clinical outcomes in ESKD. Phosphorus reduction therapy for maintained hemodialysis (MHD) patients encompasses phosphate binder medication, adequate dialysis, and also dietary phosphorus control. The main strategy in achieving dietary phosphorus reduction involves intensive education by a dietitian. The purposes of this patient education process are: (a) to obtain patient background information, (b) to assess patient knowledge, (c) to evaluate patient nutritional status, (d) to educate the patient using various approaches, and (e) to optimize the patient's nutritional state. Here, we review the management of dietary phosphorus by dietitians and summarize our strategy and the activities we use in diet counseling for MHD patients.

Keywords: Nutritional intervention, Hyperphosphatemia, MHD patients

Background

The occurrence of kidney disease and subsequent kidney failure continues to increase throughout Japan. By the end of 2012, the number of patients on dialysis reached as high as 300,000 [1]. It is currently estimated that more than 13,300,000 people suffer from chronic kidney disease (CKD) [2]. In CKD, progressive impairment of kidney function leads to the retention of many substances, including potassium and phosphorus. Thus, hyperphosphatemia is a common secondary complication in patients with end-stage kidney disease (ESKD). This complication is a consequence of the reduction in filtered phosphate load, which subsequently plays an important role in the development of renal osteodystrophy and in the increased risk of mortality and cardiovascular diseases [3–6].

Phosphate homeostasis is maintained through the concerted action of various hormones and factors in the intestine, kidney, and skeleton [7, 8]. Following further impairment of residual renal function in people with CKD, the reduction in phosphate excretion breaks down this complex balance and induces hyperphosphatemia. The management of serum phosphate is therefore vital for reducing the risk of mortality and cardiovascular events. Such management requires a multi-factorial approach, including appropriate use of phosphate-binding agents, delivery of an adequate dose of renal replacement therapy, and dietary restriction of phosphate [9–13]. Medical staff caring for maintained hemodialysis (MHD) patients often face difficulties in successfully implementing phosphate management.

Previous studies suggested that patient education may improve phosphate control, patient knowledge about dietary phosphorus, and patient compliance to an adequate diet regimen—variables essential to maintaining phosphorus at acceptable levels [14, 15]. Herein, we review the management of dietary phosphorus intake for MHD patients and introduce our approach for improving dietitians' skills at educating MHD patients.

The physiological role of dietary phosphorus

Phosphorus is an essential mineral used for growth and repair of the body's cells and tissues [8] and serves as a vital component of an array of biologically active molecules

* Correspondence: himiyata@katsura.com; himiyata@kuhp.kyoto-u.ac.jp
[2]Department of Nephrology, Kyoto Katsura Hospital, 17 Yamadahirao-cho Nishikyo-ku, Kyoto 615-8157, Japan
Full list of author information is available at the end of the article

such as nucleic acids, signaling proteins, phosphorylated enzymes, and cell membranes. While some phosphorus is stored in tissues throughout the body, most (85%) is present in the body as phosphate within bones and teeth. However, phosphorus is continuously in flux between the bone and extracellular fluid, and all tissues can absorb and secrete phosphate to meet physiological demands.

Phosphate homeostasis is a complex, highly regulated process. In individuals with CKD, the serum phosphorus concentration is usually maintained within the normal range (2.5 to 4.5 mg/dl) by a variety of compensatory mechanisms until CKD has progressed to stage 5 or become ESKD [16]. In ESKD patients who lose the ability to excrete excess phosphorus, the extent of phosphorus retention depends on the patient's intake of phosphorus-containing food [17]. Therefore, the management of dietary phosphorus is critical throughout the progressive course of kidney disease, up to dialysis-dependent end-stage renal failure.

Dietary sources of phosphorus

Because phosphorus is found in a wide variety of foods, complying with a dietary phosphorus restriction is very challenging for MHD patients. Kalantar-Zadeh et al. demonstrated a strong linear correlation ($R^2 = 0.83$) between dietary protein and phosphorus content (Fig. 1). This correlation yields a regression equation that can be used to estimate daily phosphorus intake from daily protein intake in MHD patients. On average, the ratio of

phosphorus to protein is 15 mg of phosphorus per gram of protein [11]. The Japanese Society for Dialysis Therapy recommendation for MHD patients is a phosphorus intake of (1.2–1.4 mg/day/kg) × 15 mg/day.

Information reporting the phosphorus content as milligram per gram of protein (mg/g protein) is especially useful to identify which foods supply less phosphorus for the same amount of protein. Dietitians recommend foods and supplements with an inorganic phosphorus-protein ratio of less than 10 mg/g. Analyses of phosphorus content (mg/100 g edible portion) in various natural food groups have shown that the highest phosphorus load comes from nuts, hard cheeses, egg yolks, meat, poultry, and fish [17–21]. Rather than compelling patients to give up their favorite foods, dietitians aim to provide appropriate recommendations and practical information. For example, rather than eliminating eggs entirely, patients can be advised to instead consume fresh, non-processed egg white (which has a phosphorus-protein ratio less than 2 mg/g), because egg white contains a high amount of essential amino acids and low amounts of fat, cholesterol, and phosphorus [22].

In addition to assessing food based on its phosphorus content as milligram per gram of protein, the protein digestibility-corrected amino acid score (PDCAAS) can also be used for the management of dietary phosphorus. PDCAAS is a method for evaluating protein quality based on both human requirements for, and the ability to digest, amino acids. Because the formula for calculating

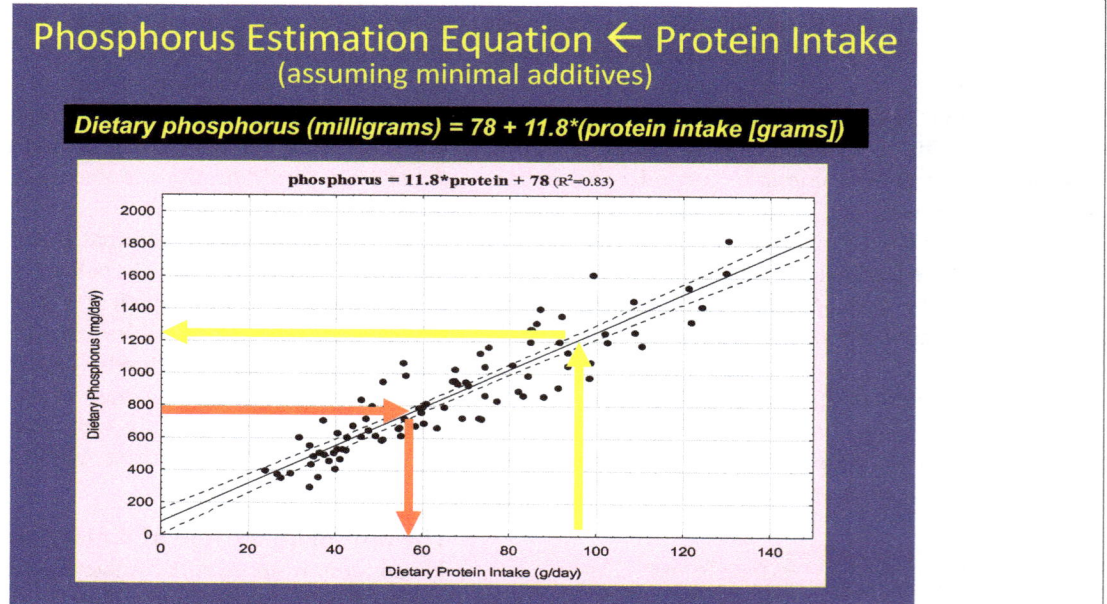

Phosphorus Estimation Equation ← Protein Intake
(assuming minimal additives)

Dietary phosphorus (milligrams) = 78 + 11.8*(protein intake [grams])

phosphorus = 11.8*protein + 78 (R²=0.83)

Fig. 1 Estimated phosphorus intake (in mg/dl) calculated from daily protein intake (in g/d) in 107 MHD patients from the NIED study. This figure was kindly provided by Prof. Kalantar-Zadeh. Regression equation: phosphorus = 11.8 protein + 78 ($r = 0.91$, $P = 0.001$)

the PDCAAS is very complicated, dietitians perform the calculations and use the assessment for educating patients [23].

Almost all foods contain phosphorus, although the actual intake of phosphorus depends upon the total amount of phosphorus in the diet and its bioavailability. In healthy individuals, the recommended dietary intake for phosphorus is 1000 mg/day for men and 800 mg/day for women (for further information, see Overview of Dietary intakes for Japanese 2015 [2]). In fact, total dietary phosphorus comes from three different sources which are thought to have different bioavailability and physiologic roles: (1) naturally occurring organic phosphorus, which serves as a component of cell membranes, tissue structures, and phosphoprotein; (2) inorganic phosphorus, which is added during food processing and is present to a lesser extent in naturally occurring phosphorus salts; and (3) inorganic phosphorus present as an active or inactive ingredient in over-the-counter medications, common prescription medications, dietary supplements, and food enrichment/fortification substances (Table 1) [20].

1. Dietary organic phosphorus
(a) Phosphorus from animal protein

The main dietary sources of phosphorus are members of the protein food group: meat, poultry, fish, eggs, and dairy products. Animal- and plant-based foods both each have high organic phosphorus content. However, different sources of animal protein contain different proportions of phosphorus. For example, Noori et al. showed that the amount of phosphorus in egg white is much less than in egg yolk or poultry (e.g., chicken, turkey) and that fish contain less phosphorus than the equivalent amount of red meat (e.g., beef, veal). Following ingestion, between 40 and 60% of animal-based phosphorus is absorbed; this varies by the degree of gastrointestinal vitamin receptor activation [24]. However, meat and dairy products are frequently supplemented with phosphate additives, which may markedly increase the total phosphorus content. Ando et al. recently reported that boiling food in soft water and cooking sliced food in a pressure cooker are

preferable cooking procedures for MHD patients as these procedures reduce phosphorus content while preserving protein content [25].

(b) Phosphorus from plants

Many fruits and vegetables contain only small amounts of organic phosphate, but some seeds and beans such as cacaos and soy possess a high phosphorus content. In plants—especially beans, peas, and nuts—phosphorus is present mostly in the storage form of phytic acid or phytate. Because humans lack the digestive enzymes to degrade phytate, plant phosphorus in its predominant phytate form is less absorbable. In contrast to animal-based foods, phosphorus absorption from plant-based foods by the human gastrointestinal tract is usually less than 40%. Therefore, a diet relying on plant protein rather than animal protein would presumably lead to better management of a patient's phosphorus burden [22, 26]. However, Noori et al. noted that there are three important caveats to this plant-based diet. First, the yeast-based phytate in whole grains makes the phosphorus content of leavened breads more effectively absorbed than the phosphorus content of cereals or flat breads. Second, the effects of probiotics on enhancing phytate-associated phosphorus release and absorption are currently unknown. Third, the biological value (quality) of plant proteins tends to be lower than that of animal proteins, and for people with marginal protein intakes, this could leads to inadequate protein nutrition [24].

(c) Rice as a major Japanese food

Rice is a staple food for Japanese people. In Japan, the average daily consumption per person reaches 155 g/day and, in the form of steamed rice, becomes 330 g/day [2]. Kanno et al. [27] and Watanabe et al. [28] reported that phosphorus intake is reduced by using wash-free rice. Uehara et al. [29] demonstrated that five rounds of washing polished rice for 20 s each could reduce its amount of phosphorus. Given that special protein-controlled rice for CKD patients is very expensive (usually 2.5 to 4.5 times the expense of ordinary steamed rice), it is

Table 1 Dietary phosphorus

Type	Source	Examples	GI absorption	Phos/protein ratio	Advantage
Organic plants	Plant proteins	Nuts, beans, chocolate	20–40%	5–15 mg/g	Protein gain
Organic animals	Animal proteins	Fish, meat, chicken	40–60%	10–20 mg/g Egg whites <5 Egg yolk >20	High value protein and amino acids
Inorganic	Additives	Soft drink, fast food	~100%	Very high (>>50 mg/g)	No gain (teenagers?)

economically better for patients to instead eat polished rice and/or well-washed rice.

2. Inorganic phosphorus from food additives

Phosphorus is the main component of many preservatives and additive salts found in processed foods (e.g., as an acidifier emulsifier or adhesive agent in foods such as processed cheese and some carbonated drinks) (Fig. 2). Additives are used in food processing for a variety of purposes such as extending shelf life, improving color, enhancing flavor, and retaining moisture [20, 30]. The presence of inorganic phosphorus in foods is often obscured by the use of complex names or ingredients on food labels (Fig. 3). Importantly, almost all the inorganic phosphorus in processed foods can be absorbed. In the USA and other Western countries, the phosphorus added during processing contributes an average of 500 mg/day per capita. Depending on food preferences, these compounds can contribute from 300 mg to as much as a gram of phosphorus towards an individual's daily intake. In Japan, both lifestyle and food preferences have changed and become more similar to those of Western cultures. Phosphate additives are a serious concern for kidney patients at all stages of CKD. Specific preparation methods for processed foods can reduce the food's amount of phosphorus [20, 25, 31, 32], Table 1. Recently, Takemasa et al. demonstrated that the phosphorus content in sausages could be reduced

by chopping and boiling [30]. Similarly, Ando et al. [25] reported that boiling food in soft water and cooking sliced food in a pressure cooker could reduce phosphorus content while preserving protein content.

Nutritional counseling

Serum phosphate concentrations reflect the dynamic balance between dietary phosphorus absorption, urinary phosphorus excretion, and internal exchange with the bone, soft tissue, and intracellular stores [33]. In MHD patients—who possess severely limited urinary phosphorus excretion and still-efficient gut phosphorus absorption—dietary absorption is a critical determinant of serum phosphate concentration. The importance of dietary phosphate intake is further boosted by the widespread use of activated vitamin D analogs, which increase gut absorption of phosphorus [34], and by the relatively poor phosphate clearance provided by standard hemodialysis three times per week. Preventing gut absorption of dietary phosphorus either by restricting intake or prescribing oral phosphorus binders is currently the cornerstone of managing hyperphosphatemia in MHD patients.

Compared to phosphate binders, dietary phosphorus restriction is underutilized in MHD patients. This is likely due to fear of exacerbating protein energy wasting (PEW), the assumption that patients will be poorly compliant with yet another layer of dietary restriction in

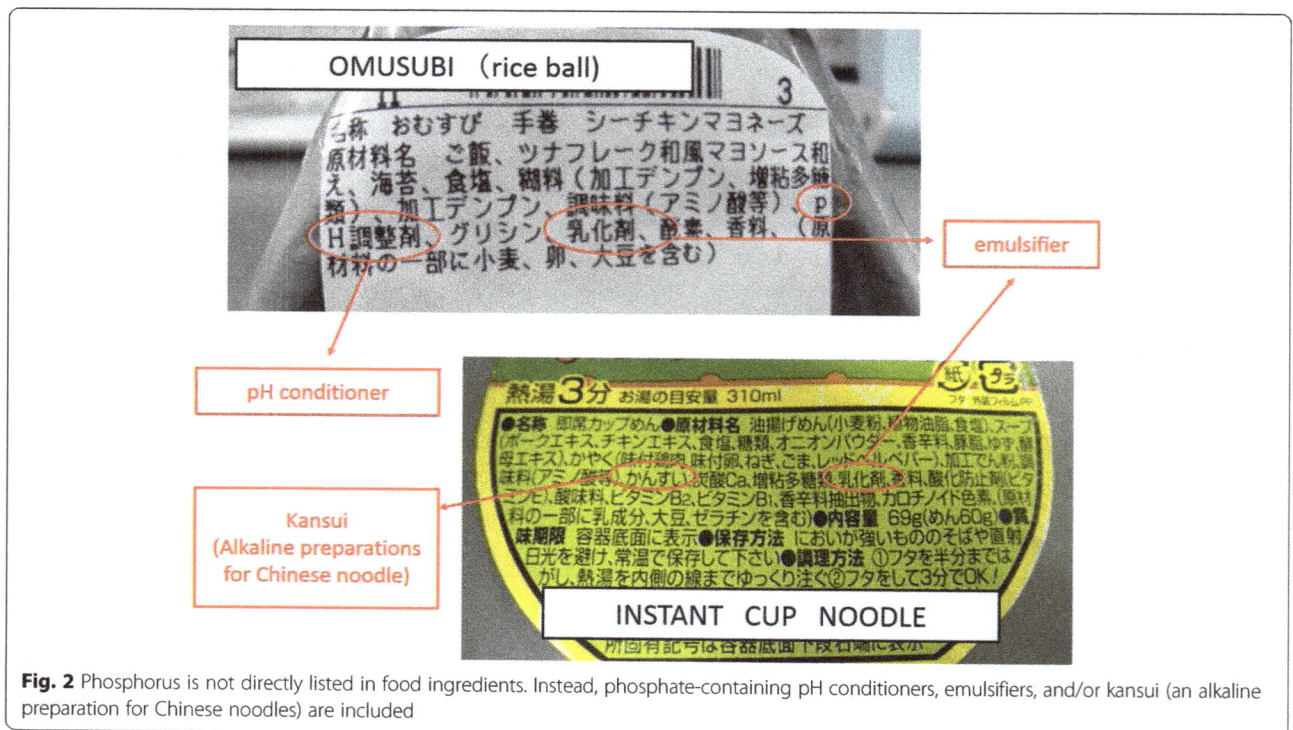

Fig. 2 Phosphorus is not directly listed in food ingredients. Instead, phosphate-containing pH conditioners, emulsifiers, and/or kansui (an alkaline preparation for Chinese noodles) are included

THE NUTRITION CARE PROCESS MODEL

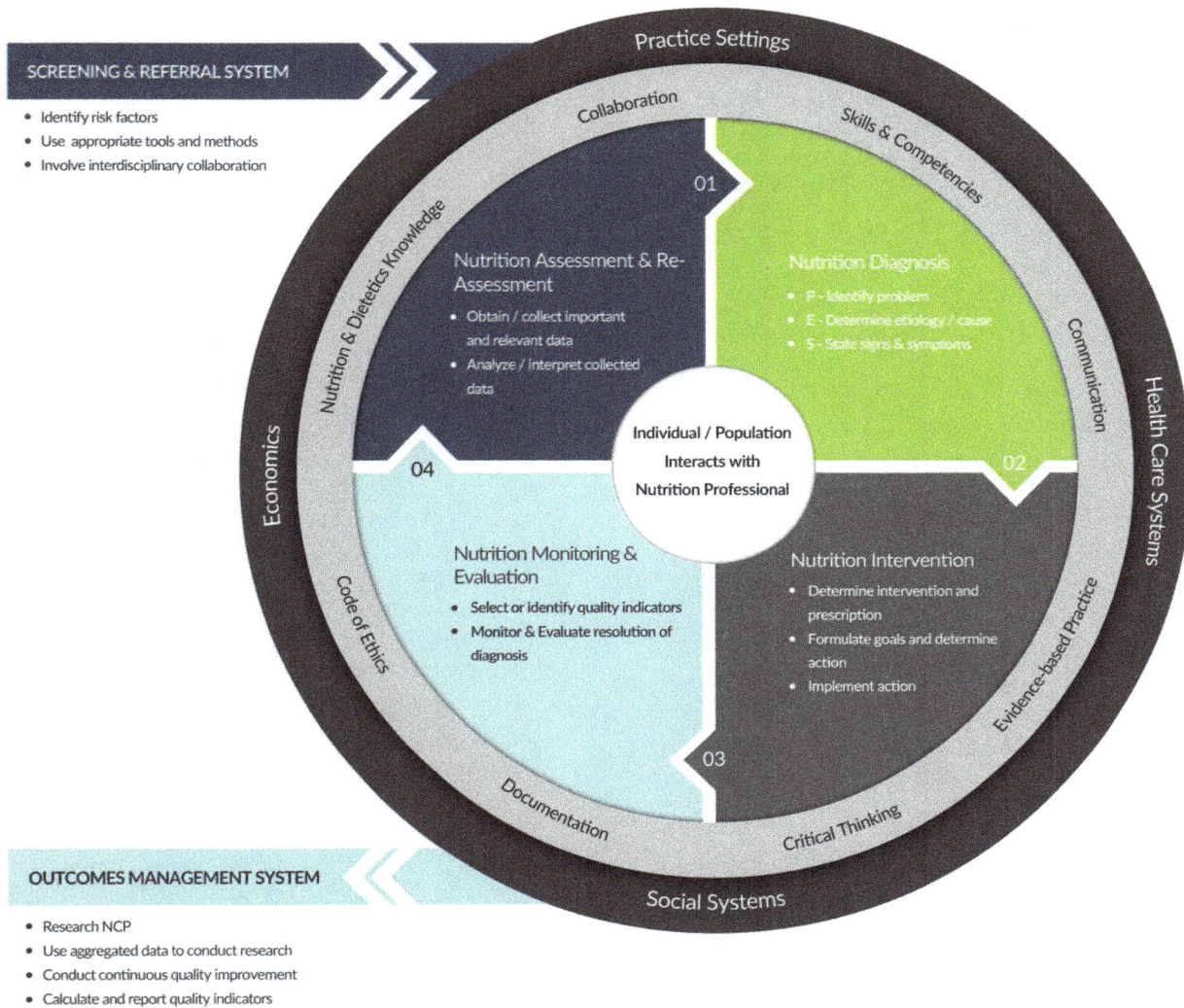

Fig. 3 The Nutrition Care Process (NCP) model. Permission to use this figure has been obtained from the Academy of Nutrition and Diabetes (USA). This model is a graphic visualization that illustrates the steps of the NCP as well as internal and external factors that impact application of the NCP. The central component of the model is the relationship of the target patients or group and the registered dietitian and nutritionist (RDN). One of the two outer rings represents the skill and abilities of the RDN along with application of evidenced-based practice, application of the Code of Ethics, and knowledge of the RDN. The second of the outer rings represents environmental factors such as healthcare system, socioeconomics, and practice setting that impacts the ability of the target patient or group to benefit from RDN services

addition to those already in place (e.g., for fluid, salt) and the logistical challenges of continuous dietary counseling. In support of these concerns, some previous reports suggest that hemodialysis patients are less likely to adhere to a phosphate dietary restriction than to potassium, sodium, or fluid restriction [14, 35].

To help a patient successfully follow phosphate dietary restrictions, dietitians must listen attentively to patients' concerns and actively identify issues to be solved in order to adequately manage serum phosphorus concentrations. Individual counseling, based on learning needs and preferences, is offered by dietitians to MHD patients with hyperphosphatemia [36–38]. This counseling includes advice on avoiding phosphate-rich foods and phosphate additives as shown in Tables 2 and 3. The dietary modification can be achieved through ongoing education from dietitians and other medical team members and through support from family and friends [39]. Towards this end, the

Table 2 Questionnaires about dietary phosphorus for dialysis patients

No.	Questions
1	Do you pay attention to your intake of phosphorus?
2	Approximately how many times do you eat fish or meat in a week?
3	What kind of dairy products do you eat? (e.g., yogurt, cheese, milk, etc.?) How many times in a week?
4	Approximately how many times a week do you eat processed foods? (e.g., ham, sausages, chikuwa etc.)
5	Do you go to restaurants, eat bento boxes, or instant meals? If you answered yes, how many times? (everyday/once a every few days/once a week/once a month/twice a month)
6	Who cooks at home? (you/partner/your child/your parents/others)
7	Do you pay attention to what's in your food? (e.g., Intake salt, use scale, restrict water, no attention, other)
8	Are you prescribed phosphate binders? If you answer yes, tell me their names.
9	If you take Fosrenol, tell me how do you take it? (crushed/ uncrushed)
10	Do you sometimes forget to take phosphate binders?
11	If you do forget to to take it, what do you then do? (e.g., nothing/take next meal time/when you remember/or other)
12	Do you take phosphate binders on an empty stomach?
13	Do you take laxatives? If you answer yes, how many, what kind? When do you take them? (the morning before HD/ Before sleeping/a non-dialysis morning) How many times do you defecate?
14	Do you know your blood level of phosphate?
15	Do you check your blood data? (Regularly/Sometimes/Never) If you do check, what do you see? (Phosphorus/potassium/neutral fat/bloodless data/blood sugar/others)
16	If you are told that your phosphorus levels are high, do you do something to combat it?(meals/take phosphate binders regularly/Do nothing/ Have never been told its high)
17	After paying attention to high phosphorus levels and trying to combat it, have your phosphorus levels declined?

Table 3 Self-management survey about dietary phosphorus for patients

No.	Questions	Yes	No
1	To prevent hyperphosphatemia, you should control your intake of phosphorus.		
2	A hypophosphate meal is defined as a dish that has phosphate intake of less than 1,000 mg.		
3	A hypophosphate meal is defined as a dish that has high energy and is high in protein.		
4	The optimal amount of protein is 50g for women, 60 g for men.		
5	There is a lot of phosphorus in protein.		
6	40% of phosphate that is contained in a meal is absorbed from the intestine.		
7	A calcium-rich meal contains lots of phosphate.		
8	Dairy products contain a low level of phosphate.		
9	Rice contains more phosphate than bread.		
10	Take outs and ready made meals contain a high level of phosphate.		
11	Phosphate binders bind phosphate in your stomach and prevent its absorption into your body.		
12	Phosphate binders are effective even when you take them long after eating a meal.		
13	It is most effective to take medicines that decrease phosphate just before or after meals.		
14	If you forget to take the phosphate binders after meal, you should take twice as many of them after your next meal.		
15	One of the side effects of phosphate binders is constipation.		
16	One of the side effects of phosphate binders id diarrhea		
17	Medicine taken before meals should be done 10 min before.		
18	Medicine taken just after meals should be taken just after meals.		
19	Medicines taken just before and after meals such as phosphate binders can be done during meals.		
20	You should not take phosphate binders if you have eaten little.		
21	Hyperphosphatemia is defined as over 4 g/dl of serum phosphate level,		
22	Hyperphosphatemia is defined as over 5 g/dl of serum phosphate level,		
23	Hyperphosphatemia is defined as over 6 g/dl of serum phosphate level,		
24	Hyperphosphatemia has a bad effect on the heart.		
25	Hyperphosphatemia has a bad effect on muscle tissue.		
26	Hyperphosphatemia occurs due to deposits of phosphate and potassium		
27	Hyperphosphatemia occurs due to a lack of vitamin C.		
28	Supplementation with calcium is effective for the treatment of hyperphosphatemia.		
29	Phosphate is excreted.		
30	You can only remove phosphate by dialysis		

Academy of Nutrition and Dietetics in the USA proposed the Nutrition Care Process (NCP). This systematic approach provides high-quality nutrition care through the following four steps: (1) nutrition assessment and reassessment, (2) nutrition diagnosis, (3) nutrition intervention, and (4) nutrition monitoring and evaluation [40, 41]; Fig. 3.

A number of large studies have examined the association between educational attainment and outcomes in patients with kidney disease. In an analysis of 61,457 participants in the Kidney Early Evaluation Program, lower educational attainment was independently associated with reduced kidney function and increased mortality [42]. Several interrelated pathways have been proposed to explain the relationship between educational attainment and health including (a) health knowledge and behaviors, (b) employment and income [43], and (c) social and psychological factors. In particular, education contributes to health by improving health knowledge, affording adequate health literacy, and improving coping and problem-solving skills [44, 45]. These advantages allow patients to make better decisions about their health, engage in healthy behaviors, and self-manage their medical conditions [46].

Successful control of diet is often challenging, and the availability of a variety of educational resources is very beneficial when working with patients and their families [47]. In an ideal situation, patients are allowed to learn at their own speed. Many medical teams have developed an array of educational tools that include written, visual, or auditory programs to instruct patients on how to effectively modify their diets. Dietitians in our hospital also evaluate and educate MHD patients using original question sheets and tools (Additional file 1; Tables 2, 3, and 4; Figs. 4, 5, and 6). Many patients have noted that altering diet behavior is one of the hardest challenges in adjusting to dialysis. A recent survey of nutrition trends in CKD patients showed that the greatest perceived obstacles to positive dietary change included the fear of giving up favorite foods, confusion regarding dietary recommendations, and false beliefs regarding the length of time required to prepare healthy foods.

In addition to education, assessing patients' knowledge is an important factor in estimating patient compliance to the renal diet [46, 47]. Dietitians initiate the processes of assessment and education in order to (1) establish communication with patients and their families, (2) provide information to address any underlying nutritional issues, and (3) calm the fears that many patients have regarding the implementation of the many changes required in their lives [48]. In support of this approach, Reddy et al. [41] found that an education program significantly improved patients' general knowledge of phosphorus and phosphate binders and was associated with a significant reduction in serum phosphate in patients with hyperphosphatemia.

Knowledge of phosphate binders as common drugs prescribed to dialysis patients

Phosphate binders limit the absorption of dietary phosphorus into the body through the intestine, thus reducing the amount of phosphorus that enters the circulation. Usually, phosphate binders are taken 5–10 min before or immediately after meals and snacks. Dietitians should know that the combination of phosphate binders and adequate nutrition can help to avoid malnutrition. The two common types of phosphorus binders are calcium-based phosphate binders and calcium-free phosphate binders. New phosphate binders have been released recently, and dietitians also need to keep up with such developments [49].

Key points for patient education

In the first counseling session with a patient, dietitians should assess the patient's level of understanding regarding phosphorus and hyperphosphatemia. The dietitian should then instruct the patient to:

(a) Take vegetable-based protein rather than animal-based
(b) Check the ingredient list (do not forget the phosphorus in popular beverages)
(c) Reduce processed food consumption
(d) Prepare and cook foods to reduce phosphorus content
(e) Use food supplements to avoid PEW.

To convince patients to effectively control dietary phosphorus and protein intake, dietitians need to provide patients with educational resources, such as booklets or leaflets; demonstrate how to recognize and avoid inorganic phosphorus additives; show how to select protein sources and achieve protein adequacy; and explain to patients how to estimate the phosphorus content of chosen foods [50–53]. The dietitian should also advise that reading the additives listed in food labels on packages can help patients restrict consumption of phosphorus in processed and fast foods.

Monitoring of nutritional status

Regular evaluation of nutritional status includes the measurement of the percent usual body weight and percent standard body weight. Patients can also be evaluated using subjective global assessments, diet

Table 4 Phosphorus to protein ratio in dairy product

		P (mg/100g)	Protein (g/100g)	P to P ratio (mg/g)	Daily use (g)	P in daily use (mg)
A: Plain yogurt and milk						
Plain yogurt		100	3.6	27.8	80	80
Milk		93	3.3	28.2	210	195
B: Processed cheese and natural cheese						
Processed cheese		730	22.7	32.2	20	146
Natural Cheese	Cheddar	500	25.7	19.5	20	100
	Camembert	330	19.1	17.3	20	66
	Cottage	130	13.3	9.8	20	26

a **Phosphorus content in 1 bottle (420-500 ml)**

About 150 mg

About 100 mg

78 mg

<42 mg

35 mg

<5 mg

High **Low**

b **〈Japan McDonald's〉**

Egg McMuffin	Cheeseburger	Teriyaki McBurger	Hamburger
P : 267 mg	P : 190 mg	P : 153 mg	P : 114 mg
NaCl : 1.7 g	NaCl : 2.4 g	NaCl : 2.0 g	NaCl : 1.9 g

High **Low**

| McShake Vanilla Medium size | McChicken Nugget 5 pieces | French Fries Medium size | Hot Apple Pie |
| P : 304 mg NaCl : 0.6 g | P : 261 mg NaCl : 1.3 g | P : 174 mg NaCl : 0.6 g | P : 17 mg NaCl : 0.6 g |

c **〈Kentucky Fried Chicken Japan〉**

岩塩 チキン

レッドホット チキン

| Original Recipe Chicken | Savory Rock Salt Chicken | Red Hot Chicken |
| P : 200 mg NaCl : 1.7 g | P : 113 mg NaCl : 1.0 g | P : 108 mg NaCl : 1.4 g |

High **Low**

Fig. 4 Educational leaflets on dietary phosphorus made by the Kyoto working committee on food for dialysis patients. Leaflets address (**a**) carbonated beverages, (**b**) Japan McDonald's, and Kentucky Fried Chicken Japan (**c**). Food information is published with permission from these companies

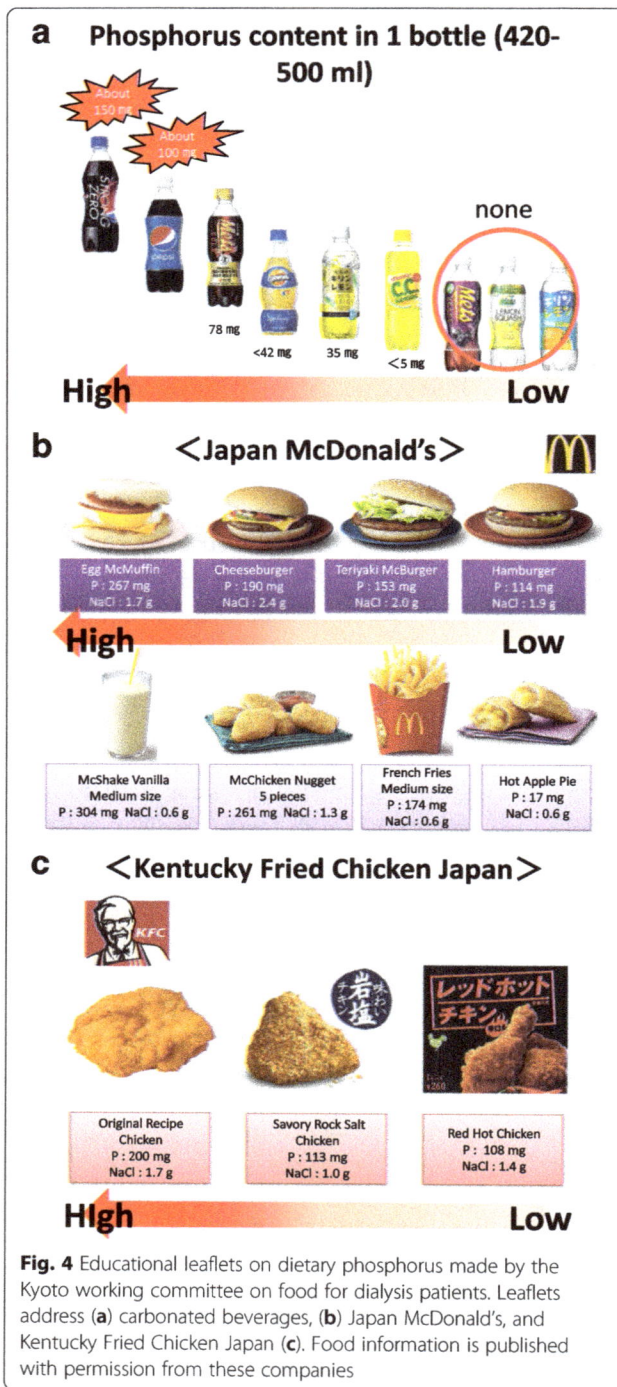

diaries, normalized protein catabolic rates, and renal laboratory evaluations. A renal laboratory evaluation should assay the following serum constituents: albumin, glucose, glycosylated hemoglobin and glycosylated albumin (for diabetic patients only), hematocrit, calcium, phosphate, calcium phosphate, potassium, and cholesterol. Results from these assays, when used with the national renal diet guidelines, can then assist renal dietitians in developing a nutrition plan that is appropriate for each patient [37].

Tools to measure body composition tools are extremely useful for the assessment of adult malnutrition at the bedside. Of the available tools, bioimpedance has been the most widely investigated in clinical research. This tool is used by clinicians for assessment purposes in Europe and elsewhere around the globe, in large part due to the affordability, portability, and ease of the use of bioimpedance devices [54]. A bioimpedance measurement takes less than 15 min and is completely noninvasive, making it advantageous for repeat measurements. We assess patient nutritional status using such impedance methods as those offered with the InBody bioimpedance device (InBody, Ltd., Tokyo, Japan).

Importance of avoiding PEW

Recent data indicate that imposed dietary phosphorus restriction may compromise the patient's ability to achieve adequate protein intake, thereby leading to PEW and possibly to increased mortality. Thus, nutritional management is a critical component in CKD treatment as there is a high prevalence of PEW. The concept of PEW was proposed in 2007 by the International Society of Renal Nutrition and Metabolism [55]. This state is characterized by the simultaneous loss of systemic body protein and energy stores in patients with CKD, leading to the loss of both muscle and fat mass and cachexia [56, 57]. PEW is caused by hypercatabolic status, uremic toxins, malnutrition, and inflammation and is both exceptionally common and closely associated with mortality and morbidity in CKD patients [58, 59]. In a recent study, patients with CKD who exhibited serum albumin concentrations below 3.5 mg/dl had a higher rate of mortality [11]. To avoid PEW, the nutritional modifications for CKD patients include adjustments in dietary protein, sodium, potassium, and phosphate intake based on the patient's nutritional status, which is regularly evaluated as described above.

The concept of PEW should be distinguished from malnutrition. CKD-related factors may contribute to the development of PEW; these factors occur in addition to or independent of inadequate nutrient intake due to anorexia and/or dietary restrictions.

Supplementation for MHD patients with malnutrition

The high prevalence of malnutrition in patients on dialysis, and the elevated protein requirements for patients on hemodialysis or peritoneal dialysis, have been documented [58, 59]. Poor appetite, inflammation, and protein loss during dialysis make it difficult for patients to achieve their nutritional targets, especially with regard to protein intake. Thus, we propose the use of protein

Let's reduce phosphorus intake!

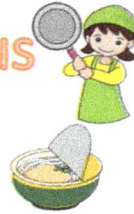

Point 1 : How to prepare instant noodles before eating

- A lot of phosphorus food additives containing phosphorus are included in instant noodles.
- When preparing instant noodles, throw away the hot water after boiling the noodles , and cook the soup with new hot water.
- Similarly for cup noodles, throw away the hot water used for boiling the noodles , and cook the soup with new water. Add the packet seasoning to the new hot water..
- Phosphorus additives melt in the hot water used for boiling noodles.
- You can reduce the amount of phosphorus additive by throwing away the hot water.
- Leave behind any excess soup!
- You can reduce your consumption of harmful excess salt, water and phosphorus additives which are harmful by doing this.

Point 2 : How to prepare processed food

★**Ham , Bacon**
Let's boil it.

★**Frankfurter**
Cut, and let's boil it.

★**Fish jelly product**
Slice it, and let's boil it.

※Phosphorus food additives will dissolve in hot water.

★**Canned food**
Throw away the juice.
Because a phosphorus additives are often added to the juice of in canned food, broth, let's get rid of the juice before cooking

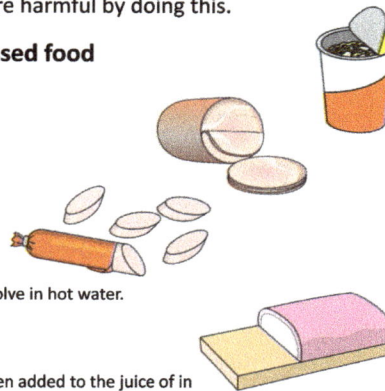

Fig. 5 Leaflet on preparation methods for reducing phosphorus in processed food

supplements such as Enjoyprotein® (Clinico Co., Ltd., Tokyo, Japan), which has less potassium, and mid-chain fatty acids (MCFAs), which are well-absorbed fatty acids.

1) Enjoyprotein®

This high-protein supplement has lower levels of both potassium and phosphorus, with a phosphate-to-protein ratio of 0.90 mg/g. The high amount of protein in this supplement helps CKD patients to take in adequate nutrition and to avoid PEW (Fig. 6).

2) MCFA

In contrast to longer fatty acids, MCFAs are readily absorbed from the gastrointestinal tract and directly enter the portal system. Furthermore, MCFA absorption does not require modification, unlike with the absorption of long-chain or very-long-chain fatty acids. In addition, the digestion of MCFA does not require bile salts. Thus, MCFA supplementation is attracting attention as a means for ensuring adequate nutrition in patients with malnutrition or malabsorption. For such patients in our hospital, we cook rice porridges with Enjoyprotein and MCT oil (The Nisshin Oillio Group, Ltd., Tokyo, Japan), as described below.

3) Chikara-gayu (rice porridge supplemented with Enjoyprotein® and MCT oil)

We cook chikara-gayu for malnutrition patients. This special porridge is prepared using the following ingredients (the taste is improved by adding salt):

1. Porridge 150 g
2. Nisshin MCT oil 9 g
3. Enjoyprotein® 5.5 g
4. Salt 0.42 g

Additional menu for malnutrition patients!

(1) How to get protein without increasing phosphorus intake!

Let's use Enjoyprotein®

①Rice Porridge (Okayu)
Mix a tablespoon of Enjoyprotein® into a bowl of rice porridge.

②Miso Soup
Dissolve a tablespoon of Enjoyprotein® into a cup of miso soup.

③Other uses
You can dissolve this supplement into a drink or use it in liquid for cooking.
For example, you can dissolve this into stock (dashi), which can be used to make a Japanese omelet, etc. The solution is tasteless and odorless, so is easy to use.

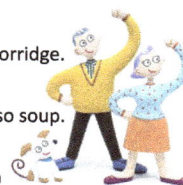

(2) How to increase energy intake!

How to use MCT oil & powder®
MCT oil & powder® are medium-chain fatty acids, which are efficiently digested and converted into energy.

①Rice
Mix two to three tablespoons of MCT powder or two teaspoons of MCT oil with 1 measure of rice (about 150 g), wash the rice beforehand. Add slightly more water.

②Rice Porridge (Okayu)
You can mix MCT oil & powder® in cooked rice porridge (okayu). A tablespoon of MCT powder or one to two teaspoons of MCT oil with a bowl of rice porridge (approx. 250 g).

③Other Dishes
You can use these for soup and salad dressing, but you can't use these for deep-fried food. Please be careful not to overheat the MCT oil because its boiling point is a lot lower than other cooking oils.

*Daily intake should be no more than 30 g for MCT oil, 40 g for MCT powder.

Fig. 6 Recipes on diet supplementation for avoiding PEW

Activities and approaches for dietitians

Team Kidney in Kyoto Katsura Hospital

Team Kidney was established in our hospital in 2015 as a team including nephrologists, pharmacists, nurses, clinical engineers, medical technologists, physiotherapists, dietitians, staffs of regional medical cooperative office, and medical secretaries. This multi-disciplinary team works cooperatively to prevent CKD progression by working with a regional medical network of general practitioners, planning educational events, and coordinating admissions to a nephrology ward. Figure 7 shows physiotherapists giving a lecture in a kidney disease seminar. As a part of the activities, nurses, dietitians, and sometimes medical doctors talk to hemodialysis patients about the importance of diet modification, particularly in terms of reducing phosphorus intake. To assess patient understanding, a questionnaire focused on phosphorus and hyperphosphatemia is administered to patients (Tables 2 and 3). Dietitians conduct counseling with the assistance of a handbook, and pharmacists educate the patients about effects of phosphorus-binding medications, vitamin D, cinacalcet, and other drugs.

Kyoto working committee on foods for dialysis patients

This society was established in 1973 in Kyoto for dietitians working at institutes with a dialysis unit and/or with MHD patients 5 years after renal replacement therapy was granted universal coverage under Japan's National Health Insurance. The society aims to conduct research by surveying CKD patients' nutrition and to identify meals suitable for MHD patients. Currently, 20 dietitians from 16 different institutes and dietitian training facilities belong to this society. One representative event is the annual cooking workshop for MHD patients (Fig. 8).

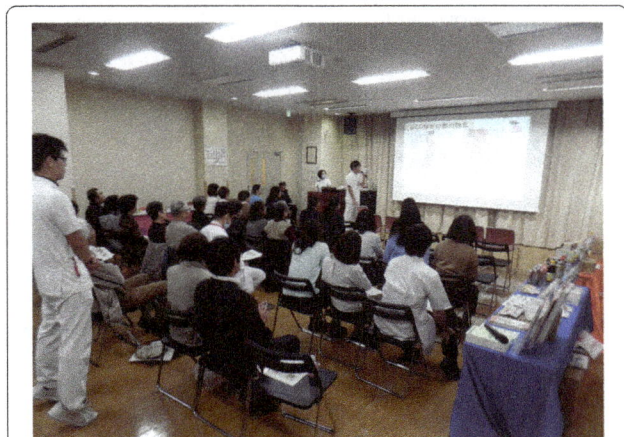

Fig. 7 Photo of a lecture by physiotherapists in Kyoto Katsura Hospital

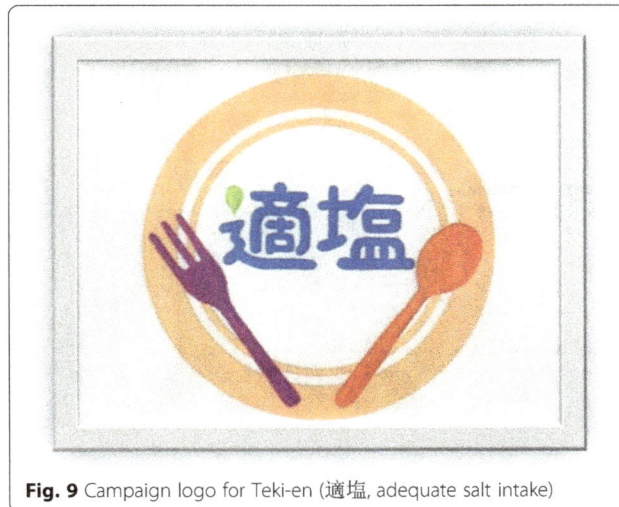

Fig. 9 Campaign logo for Teki-en (適塩, adequate salt intake)

Task force consortium for kidney disease in Kyoto

This society was established in 1979 to promote activities preventing CKD progression. Nephrologists, pharmacists, dietitians, and patients with CKD are the members of the executive committee, which organizes lectures open to the public and provides a site for individual dietary counseling by specialists such as dietitians. The committee also conducted a survey of institutes in Kyoto Prefecture on approaches for preventing renal replacement therapy in diabetes patients. In 2015, traditional Japanese cuisine (Washoku) was added to UNESCO Intangible Cultural Heritage List. Washoku is considered among the most highly rated foods in terms of providing a balanced level of nutrients with low fat. However, Kyo-ryori (local cuisine in Kyoto) tends to have a higher salt content, which is linked to accelerated progression of CKD. Therefore, the society recently developed a new logo indicating adequate salt intake, the "Teki-en" (適塩 in Japanese), which would be much more acceptable for patients rather than the logo for reduced salt intake, "Gen-enn" (減塩 in Japanese) (Fig. 9). The society is involved in campaigns to educate patients about managing salt reduction.

Conclusions

Diet therapy for MHD patients is as integral to maintaining patient health as taking drugs and receiving adequate dialysis. The dietitian should be one of the principal specialists for educating patients about diet and how best to prepare their food. Open communication and a good rapport between dietitian and patient are vital to improving the patient knowledge and diet compliance. Over time, the work of dietitians will positively change patients' lifestyles. We are confident that, through intensive nutritional intervention, we can prevent complications caused by hyperphosphatemia in ESKD.

Abbreviations
CKD: Chronic kidney disease; ESKD: End-stage kidney disease; MCFA: mid-chain fatty acid; MHD: Maintained hemodialysis; NCP: Nutrition Care Process; PDCAAS: Protein digestibility-corrected amino acid score; PEW: Protein energy wasting

Acknowledgements
We thank Prof. Kalantar-Zadeh for his kind advice and for providing his slides (which formed the basis of Fig. 1 and Table 1), Ms. Maureen and Dr. Steiber for their efforts as members of the American Academy of Nutrition and Dietetics to provide the NCP diagram (Fig. 3), all members of Team Kidney in Kyoto Katsura Hospital, and Dr. Marlini Muhamad (Physiology Department, NUI Galway, Ireland) for her advice on the English language used in this review.

Funding
None to declare

Authors' contributions
KY and HM wrote this article. Both authors read and approved the final manuscript.

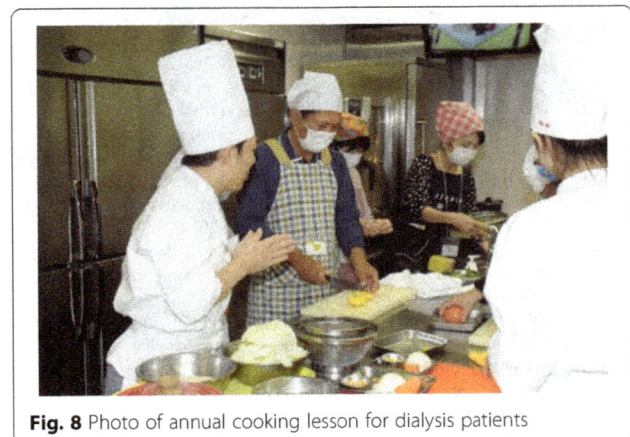

Fig. 8 Photo of annual cooking lesson for dialysis patients

Authors' information
Ms. Kawate is the head of the Div. of Nutrition, and Dr. Miyata is the director of the Dept. of Nephrology and Dialysis Unit in Kyoto Katsura Hospital.

Competing interests
The authors declare that they have no competing interests.

Author details
[1]Department of Nutrition, Kyoto Katsura Hospital, 17 Yamadahirao-cho Nishikyo-ku, Kyoto 615-8157, Japan. [2]Department of Nephrology, Kyoto Katsura Hospital, 17 Yamadahirao-cho Nishikyo-ku, Kyoto 615-8157, Japan.

References
1. Nakai S, Hanafusa N, Masakane I, Taniguchi M, Hamano T, Shoji T, et al. Overview of regular dialysis treatment in Japan (as of 31 December 2012). Ther Apheres Dial. 2014;18(6):535-602.
2. Overview of dietary reference intakes for Japanese (2015), http://www0.nih.go.jp/eiken/english/research/project_dris.html Accessed 1 Sep 2016.
3. Block GA, Hulbert-Shearon TE, Levin NW, Port FK. Association of serum phosphorus and calcium phosphate product with mortality risk in chronic hemodialysis patients: a national study. Am J Kidney Dis. 1998;31(4):607-17.
4. Tentri F, Blayney MJ, Albert JM, Gillespie BW, Kerr PG, Bommer J, et al. Mortality risk for dialysis patients with different levels of serum calcium, phosphorus, and PTH: the Dialysis Outcomes and Practice Patterns Study (DOPPS). Am J Kidney Dis. 2008;52(3):519-30.
5. Young EW, Akiba T, Albert JM, McCarthy JT, Kerr PG, Mendelssohn DC, et al. Magnitude and impact of abnormal mineral metabolism in hemodialysis patients in the Dialysis Outcomes and Practice Patterns Study (DOPPS). Am J Kidney Dis. 2004;44 Suppl 2:34-8.
6. Sullivan C, Sayre SS, Leon JB, Machekano R, Love TE, Poter D, et al. Effect of food additives on hyperphosphatemia among patients with end-stage renal disease: a randomized controlled trial. JAMA. 2009;301(6):629-35.
7. Bergwitz C, Juppner H. Regulation of phosphate homeostasis by PTH, vitamin D, and FGF23. Ann Rev Med. 2010;61:91-104.
8. Quarles LD. Endocrine functions of bone in mineral metabolism regulation. J Clin Invest. 2008;118(12):3820-28.
9. Isakova T, Xie H, Yang W, Xie D, Anderson AH, Scialla J, Chronic Renal Insufficiency Cohort (CRIC) Study Group, et al. Fibroblast growth factor 23 and risks of mortality and end-stage renal disease in patients with chronic kidney disease. JAMA. 2011;305(23):2432-9.
10. Palmer SC, Hyen A, Macaskill P, Pellegrini F, Craig JC, Elder GJ, et al. Serum levels of phosphorus, parathyroid hormone, and calcium and risks of death and cardiovascular disease in individuals with chronic kidney disease: a systematic review and meta-analysis. JAMA. 2011;305(11):1119-27.
11. Kalantar-Zadeh K, Gutenurnst L, Mehrotra R, Kovesdy CP, Bross R, Shinaberger CS, et al. Understanding sources of dietary phosphorus in the treatment of patients with chronic kidney disease. Clin J Am Soc Nephrol. 2010;5(3):519-30.
12. Combe C, McCullough KP, Asano Y, Ginsberg N, Maroni BJ, Pifer TB. Kidney Disease Outcomes Quality Initiative (K/DOQI) and the Dialysis Outcomes and Practice Patterns Study (DOPPS): nutrition guidelines, indicators, and practices. Am J Kidney Dis. 2004;44((5) Suppl 2):39-46.
13. Cannata-Andia JB, Fernandez-Martin JL, Locatelli F, London G, Gorriz JL, et al. Use of phosphate-binding agents is associated with a lower risk of mortality. Kidney Int. 2013;84(5):998-1008.
14. Caldeira D, Amaral T, David C, Sampaio C. Educational strategies to reduce serum phosphorus in hyperphosphatemic patients with chronic kidney disease: systemic review with meta-analysis. J Ren Nutr. 2011;21(4):285-94.
15. Ashurst Ide B, Dobbie H. A randomized controlled trial of an educational intervention to improve phosphate levels in hemodialysis patients. J Ren Nutr. 2003;13(4):267-74.
16. Kovesdy CP, Kalantar-Zadeh K. Bone and mineral disorders in pre-dialysis CKD. Int Urol Nephrol. 2008;40(2):427-40.
17. Sherman RA, Mehta O. Phosphorus and potassium content of enhanced meat and poultry products: implications for patients who receive dialysis. Clin J Am Soc Nephrol. 2009;4(8):1370-3.
18. Calvo MS, Urbarri J. Contribution to total phosphorus intake: all sources considered. Semin Dial. 2013;26(1):54-61.
19. Japanese Society of Nephrology. Dietary recommendations for chronic kidney disease, 2014. Nihon Jinzo Gakkai Shi. 2014;56(5):553-99. Japanese.
20. Capisti A, Kalantar-Zadeh K. Management of natural and added dietary phosphorus burden in kidney disease. Semin Nephrol. 2013;33(2):180-90.
21. Gonzalez-Parra E, Gracia-Iguacel C, Egido J, Ortiz A. Phosphorus and nutrient in chronic kidney disease. Int J Nephrol. 2012. doi:10.1155/2012/597605.
22. Kalantar-Zadeh K. Patient education for phosphorus management in chronic kidney disease. Patient Prefer Adherence. 2013;7:379-90.
23. Schaafsma G. The protein digestibility-corrected amino acid score. J Nutr. 2000;130(7):1865S-7S.
24. Noori N, Kalantar-Zadeh K, Kovesdy CP, Bross R, Benner D, Kopple JD. Association of dietary phosphorus intake and phosphorus to protein ratio with mortality in hemodialysis patients. Clin J Am Soc Nephrol. 2010;5(4):883-92.
25. Ando S, Sakuma M, Morimoto Y, Arai H. The effect of various boiling conditions on reduction of phosphorus and protein in meat. J Ren Nutr. 2015;6:504-9.
26. Moe SM, Zidehsarai MP, Chambers MA, Jackman LA, Radcliff JS, Trevino LL, et al. Vegetarian compared with meat dietary protein source and phosphorus homeostasis in chronic kidney disease. Clin J Am Soc Nephrol. 2011;6:257-64.
27. Kanno Y, Inoue T, Matsumoto G, Tanaka T, Mogi K, Suzuki H. The control of serum phosphate by pre-washed rice (Musenmai) for hemodialysis patients (in Japanese). J Jpn Soc Cli Nutr. 2004;25:219-21.
28. Watanabe S, Kannno Y, et al. The efficacy of pre-washed rice (Musenmai) on diet therapy for hemodialysis patients (in Japanese). J Jpn Soc Dial Ther. 2006;39(6):1187-90.
29. Uehara Y, Yanagisawa K, Takeuchi S, Suwa A, Uchiyama K, Iashida H, et al. The effectiveness and usefulness of washing rice five times to reduce serum phosphorus and potassium in hemodialysis patients (in Japanese). J Jpn Soc Dial Ther. 2015;48(7):423-9.
30. Takemasa M, Asahara A, Sugemasa M. Amount of phosphorus contained in some sausage samples from supermarkets. Kawasaki Medical Welfare Journal. 2015;25(1):227-33.
31. Noori N, Sims JJ, Kopple JD, Shah A, Colman S, Shinaberger CS, et al. Organic and inorganic dietary phosphorus and its management in chronic kidney disease. Ira J Kidney Dis. 2010;4(2):89-100.
32. Ohnishi R, et al. Management of phosphorus for CKD—the prevalence of phosphorus containing food additives. Jpn J Clin Nutr. 2014;124(3):317-24.
33. Urbarri J. Phosphorus additives in food and their effect in dialysis. Clin J Am Soc Nephrol. 2009;4(8):1290-2.
34. Ramierez JA, Emmett M, White MG, Faith N, Santa ACA, Morawski SG, et al. The absorption of dietary phosphorus and calcium in hemodialysis patients. Kidney Int. 1986;30:753-9.
35. Hoover H. Compliance in patients on hemodialysis: a review of literature. J Am Diet Assoc. 1989;89:957-9.
36. Japanese Society of Dialysis therapy. Dietary guideline for dialysis patients in Japan. J Jpn Soc Dial Ther. 2014;47(5):287-291. Japanese.
37. Japanese society of Nephrology. Special issue: evidence-based practice guideline for the treatment of CKD. Nihon Jinzo Gakkai Shi. 2013;55(5):585-860. Japanese.
38. Standard Tables of Food Composition in Japan, 2010. . 2010.
39. Beanlands H, Horsburgh ME, Fox S, Howe A, Heather LC, et al. Caregiving by family and friends of adults receiving dialysis. Neph Nurs J. 2005;32(6):621-31.
40. Kent PS, McCarthy MP, Burrowes JD, McCann L, Goeddeke-Merickel CM, et al. Academy of Nutrition and Diabetes and National Kidney Foundation: revised 2014 standards of practice and standards of professional performance for registered dietitian nutritionist (competent, proficient, and expert) in nephrology nutrition. J Acad Nutr Diet. 2014;114(9):1448-57.
41. Reddy V, Symes F, Sethi N, Scally AJ, Scott J, Mumtaz R, Stoves J. Dietitian-led education program to improve phosphate control in a single center hemodialysis population. J Ren Nutr. 2009;19(4):314-20.
42. Choi A, Weekley CC, Chen SC, Li S, Tamura MK, Norris KC, et al. Association of educational attainment with chronic disease and mortality: the Kidney Early Evaluation Program (KEEP). Am J Kidney Dis. 2011;58(2):228-34.
43. Gutierrez OM, Anderson C, Isakova T, Scialla J, Negrea L, Anderson AH, et al. Low socioeconomic status associates with higher serum phosphate irrespective of race. J Am Soc Nephrol. 2010;21(11):1953-60.

44. Locatelli F, Fouque D, Hemiburger O, Drueke TB, Cannata-Andia JB, Horl WH. Nutritional status in dialysis patients: a European consensus. Nephrol Dial Transplant. 2002;17:563–72.

45. Green JA, Cavanaugh KL. Understanding the influence educational attainment on kidney health and opportunities for improved care. Adv Chronic Kidney Dis. 2015;22(1):24–30.

46. Pollock J, Jaffery JB. Knowledge of phosphorus compared with other nutrients in maintenance dialysis patients. J Ren Nutr. 2007;17(5):323–8.

47. Yokum D, Glass G, Cheung DF, Cunningham J, Fan S, Madden AM. Evaluation of a phosphate management protocol to achieve optimum serum phosphate levels in hemodialysis patients. J Ren Nutr. 2008;18(6):521–9.

48. Packard DP, Milton JE, Shunler LA, Short RA, Tuttle RR. Implications of chronic kidney disease for dietary treatment in cardiovascular disease. J Ren Nutr. 2006; 16(3):259–68.

49. Gutekunst L. An update on phosphate binders: a dietitian's perspective. J Ren Nutr. 2016;26(4):209–18.

50. Clements L, Ashurst I. Dietary strategy to halt the progression of chronic kidney disease. J of Renal Care. 2006;32:192–7.

51. CI D, Holdsworth M, Atson V, Prsygodzka F. Knowledge of dietary restrictions and the medical consequence. J Am Diet Assoc. 2004;104:35–40.

52. Murphy-Gutekunst L. Hidden phosphorus in popular beverages. Nephrol Nurs J. 2005;32(4):443–5.

53. Sullivan CM, Leon JB, Sehgal AR. Phosphorus-containing food additives and the accuracy of nutrient databases: implications for renal patients. J Ren Nutr. 2007;17(5):350–4.

54. Russell MK. Functional assessment of nutrition status. Nutr Clin Pract. 2015; 30(2):211–8.

55. Fouque D, Kalantar-Zadeh K, Kopple J, Cano N, Chauveau P, Cuppari L, et al. A proposed nomenclature and diagnostic criteria for protein-energy wasting in acute and chronic kidney disease. Kidney Int. 2008;73(4):391–8.

56. Obi Y, Qader H, Kovesdy CP, Kalantar-Zadeh K. Latest consensus and update on protein-energy wasting in chronic kidney disease. Curr Opin Clin Nutr Metab Care. 2015;18(3):254–62.

57. Carrero JJ, Stenvinkel P, Cappari S, Ikizler TA, Kalantar-Zadeh K, Kaysen G, et al. Etiology of the protein-energy wasting syndrome in chronic kidney disease: a consensus statement from the international society of renal nutrition and metabolism (ISRNN). J Ren Nutr. 2013;23(2):77–90.

58. Kovesdy CP. Malnutrition in dialysis patients—the need for intervention despite uncertain benefits. Semin Dial. 2015;20(1):28–34.

59. Kovesdy CP, Shinaberger CS, Kalantar-Zadeh K. Epidemiology of dietary nutrient intake in ESRD. Semin Dial. 2010;23(4):353–8.

17

Efficacy and safety of plasma exchange for Kawasaki disease with coronary artery dilatation

Yusuke Kaida[1*], Takatoshi Kambe[1], Shintaro Kishimoto[2], Yusuke Koteda[2], Kenji Suda[2], Ryo Yamamoto[1], Tetsurou Imai[3], Takuma Hazama[1], Yoshimi Takamiya[1], Ryo Shibata[1], Hidemi Nishida[1], Seiya Okuda[1] and Kei Fukami[1]

Abstract

Background: The treatment of Kawasaki disease is controversial when intravenous immunoglobulin therapy fails, although it typically relies on combinations of prednisolone, infliximab, cyclosporine, and plasma exchange therapy. The goal of the treatment is no longer merely to reduce mortality but also to decrease the sequelae of coronary artery lesions, which are the most common and potentially life-threatening complications. Recently, plasma exchange therapy has been used to treat intravenous immunoglobulin-unresponsive Kawasaki disease with coronary artery lesions. When performed before coronary artery dilatation, the outcomes for plasma exchange are known to be excellent; however, when dilatation is already present, sequelae persist.

Methods: Between December 2006 and April 2015, we treated ten patients with Kawasaki disease complicated by coronary artery lesions that received plasma exchange because intravenous immunoglobulin therapy had proven to be ineffective. Here, we retrospectively review the efficacy and safety of plasma exchange therapy in such unresponsive cases against coronary artery lesions in patients with Kawasaki disease when plasma exchange performed after coronary artery dilatation.

Results: In nine of the ten patients (90.0%), the body temperature was confirmed to be < 37.5 °C at an average of 2.7 ± 1.4 days after starting plasma exchange. Serum C-reactive protein levels decreased significantly from 9.9 ± 4.9 mg/dL before exchange to 1.9 ± 2.9 mg/dL after exchange ($P < 0.05$). One year after plasma exchange treatment, the coronary artery lesions had regressed to within normal limits in six of the ten patients. Although lesions remained in three patients, all three of these patients were asymptomatic. In addition, there were no stenosis of the coronary artery in nine of the ten patients. One patient died due to a ruptured giant coronary aneurysm 1 day after starting plasma exchange.

Conclusions: In conclusion, plasma exchange may be effective in not only regressing coronary artery lesions but also preventing sequelae in patients with Kawasaki disease when plasma exchange is performed after coronary artery dilatation.

Keywords: Kawasaki disease, Plasma exchange, Coronary artery

Background

Kawasaki disease, first reported in 1967, is an acute systemic vasculitis of unknown etiology that predominantly occurs in infants and young children [1]. It is characterized by prolonged fever, rash, bilateral bulbar conjunctival injection, oral mucosal erythema, cervical lymphadenopathy, and hand and foot swelling. Clinically, the course of

Kawasaki disease is usually self-limiting, and most patients recover without any long-term sequelae. However, some patients develop complications, of which the most common and potentially life-threatening are cardiovascular manifestations. These cardiovascular manifestations include pericardial, myocardial, endocardial, and coronary artery lesions, such as dilation, aneurysm, and stenosis.

The current goal of Kawasaki disease treatment is no longer merely to reduce the death rate but also to decrease the coronary sequelae. To this end, early treatment with intravenous immunoglobulin (IVIG) is the

---

* Correspondence: kaida_yuusuke@kurume-u.ac.jp
[1]Division of Nephrology, Department of Medicine, Kurume University School of Medicine, 67 Asahi-machi, Kurume, Fukuoka 830-0011, Japan
Full list of author information is available at the end of the article

standard initial treatment. However, 15.8% of cases are unresponsive to IVIG, and 38.5% of them develop coronary artery abnormalities [2]. Patients with IVIG-unresponsive Kawasaki disease are currently treated with prednisolone, infliximab, and cyclosporine and plasma exchange therapy [3–6]. However, no optimal therapeutic regimen has yet been established.

Recent studies have reported the use of plasma exchange therapy in the treatment of IVIG-unresponsive Kawasaki disease [6–8]. When plasma exchange was initiated before the beginning of coronary artery dilatation, no sequelae developed in patients; however, when dilatation had already begun, sequelae developed in 30% of patients despite the plasma exchange [7]. Hokosaki et al. also reported that treatment outcomes tended to be better when plasma exchange was initiated before day 9 of the disease onset [7]. In this study, we retrospectively reviewed the efficacy and safety of plasma exchange against coronary artery lesions in patients with Kawasaki disease unresponsive to IVIG therapy when coronary artery dilatation had already started.

Methods

We retrospectively reviewed the clinical records of children with coronary artery lesions caused by Kawasaki disease that had been treated with plasma exchange after IVIG had been proven ineffective. Data from the Kurume University Hospital, for the period between December 2006 and April 2015, were used. IVIG responsiveness was defined as the resolution of fever (body temperature below 37.5 °C) within 24 h of initiating the IVIG treatment. Usually, plasma exchange is performed at least three times in patients with Kawasaki disease. However, if the high fever is not improved, additional plasma exchange might be performed. When the resolution of fever (body temperature below 37.5 °C) was observed, plasma exchange is discontinued. The study protocol was approved by the Institutional Ethics Committees of Kurume University School of Medicine (No16219).

Plasma exchange

Plasma exchange was generally conducted as a vein-to-vein procedure, although an artery-to-vein option was also used until 2006 [7]. For the procedure, a 6- or 7-Fr double-lumen catheter was inserted into the femoral vein. The replacement fluid contained 5% albumin or fresh frozen plasma, and the amount exchanged was approximately 1.0- to 1.5-fold the circulating blood plasma volume (mL), which was calculated as 1/13 body weight × [100 – hematocrit (%)]. An anticoagulant, heparin, was used at an appropriate dose to keep the activated clotting time in the range of 150 to 200 s. While this was being done, sedation was given as needed, and the patient was carefully secured to the bed to avoid movement.

Coronary artery evaluation

Echocardiography was used to evaluate both cardiac function and the coronary arteries. Dilatation of a coronary artery was diagnosed if the diameter of any artery was ≥ 3 mm in children younger than 5 years, ≥ 4 mm in children older than 5 years, or if the coronary artery size was 1.5 times that of neighboring coronary arteries. We diagnosed a coronary aneurysm if the artery diameter was ≥ 4 mm, and we diagnosed a giant coronary aneurysm if it was ≥ 8 mm [9].

Statistical analysis

Data are presented as mean ± standard deviations. Continuous variables were compared using a paired t test. All statistical analyses were performed using GraphPad Prism 5 software (GraphPad Software, Inc., La Jolla, CA, USA).

Results

Patient characteristics

We identified ten children with Kawasaki disease (eight boys and two girls) that met the inclusion criteria. The mean age at onset was 23.8 ± 20.8 months (range, 3–63 months), and the mean body weight was 10.8 ± 4.0 kg (range, 4.5–17.8 kg). The initial treatment was started after an average of 6.1 ± 5.3 days from disease onset. Typically, acetylsalicylic acid, prednisolone, or both were given as part of the initial treatment with IVIG (Table 1). Additional IVIG treatment was performed in five patients (Table 1). Case 10 was treated with infliximab (5 mg/kg) 1 day after plasma exchange due to elevated CRP levels.

Efficacy of plasma exchange

On average, plasma exchange was started 13.7 ± 5.7 days after onset and was given for 10.2 ± 4.7 h per treatment over 3.1 ± 0.9 days. The detail of the plasma exchange therapy is shown in Tables 2 and 3. In nine of the ten patients (90.0%), the body temperature was confirmed to be < 37.5 °C at an average of 2.7 ± 1.4 days after starting plasma exchange. Serum C-reactive protein levels decreased significantly from 9.9 ± 4.9 mg/dL before exchange to 1.9 ± 2.9 mg/dL after exchange ($P < 0.05$) (Fig. 1).

Table 4 shows the clinical courses of the coronary artery lesions identified in the patients from before plasma exchange. Coronary artery dilatations were seen in four cases, and aneurysms, in six. One year after plasma exchange treatment, the coronary artery lesions had regressed to within normal limits in six of the ten patients. However, lesions remained in three patients (1, 3, and 10). Right coronary artery lesions were present in patient 1 (4.2 mm) and patient 3 (4.6 mm) 7 years after plasma exchange, although these had regressed (Fig. 2). Patient 10 still had lesions of the right coronary

Table 1 Characteristics of patients

Patient	Gender	Age (months)	BW (kg)	Start of IVIG (day)	Treatment before PE	Dose of IVIG	Period of PSL (day)	Additional treatment of IVIG
1	M	7	7.5	6	ASA, PSL, IVIG × 3	1 g/kg × 2, 2 g/kg × 1	11–30	–
2	M	29	13.8	4	ASA, PSL, IVIG × 2	2 g/kg × 2	7.11	–
3	M	7	7.4	4	ASA, PSL, IVIG × 2	1 g/kg × 2	6–8	1 g/kg × 2 (days 9 and 10), 2 g/kg × 2 (day 11)
4	M	11	8.0	4	ASA, IVIG × 2	2 g/kg × 2	–	–
5	F	3	4.5	5	ASA, IVIG × 2	2 g/kg × 2	14–59	2 g/kg × 2 (days 14 and 18)
6	M	36	13.3	4	ASA, PSL, IVIG × 2	2 g/kg × 2	7,8	2 g/kg × 2 (day 13)
7	M	53	14.0	4	ASA, PSL, IVIG × 3	1 g/kg × 2, 2 g/kg × 1	6–8	–
8	M	17	10.2	4	PSL, IVIG × 2	2 g/kg × 2	6–27	2 g/kg × 2 (day 14)
9	F	12	11.9	21	ASA, PSL, IVIG × 1	1 g/kg × 1	4, 10, 11, 14	–
10	M	63	17.8	5	ASA, PSL, IVIG × 3	2 g/kg × 3	6, 8, 9	2 g/kg × 2 (days 10 and 20)

BW body weight, *ASA* acetylsalicylic acid, *PSL* prednisolone, *IVIG* intravenous immunoglobulin infusion, *PE* plasma exchange
Dose of IVIG: single dose × day

(6.7 mm) and left anterior descending (5.1 mm) arteries 1.5 years after plasma exchange. All three of these patients were asymptomatic. In addition, there were no stenosis of the coronary artery in nine of the ten patients. One patient (patient 9) died due to a ruptured giant coronary aneurysm 1 day after starting plasma exchange.

Adverse events

Sedation was given to all patients, but three required mechanical ventilation and one developed respiratory syncytial virus infection, which improved within a few days. No hemorrhage or infection was observed during plasma exchange. However, decreased blood pressure was often noted after initiating therapy, and two cases required vasopressor support. In both cases, the patients

were in a condition to allow the therapy to continue. Generally, plasma exchange could be safely implemented without causing any life-threatening or irreversible complications.

Discussion

The present study supports the possibility that outcomes are favorable in cases where plasma exchange is used to treat Kawasaki disease when coronary artery lesions have developed and the course is unresponsive to IVIG therapy. Moreover, we showed that plasma exchange could be safely performed in children with this disease.

Table 2 Technical characteristics of plasma exchange therapy 1

Patient	Vascular access	Start of PE (day)	Duration for PE (days)	Total operation time of PE (h)
1	A-V	27	3	19.5
2	7-Fr catheter (FV)	12	3	13.0
3	6-Fr catheter (FV)	9	4	15.0
4	8-Fr catheter (FV)	13	3	5.0
5	6-Fr catheter (FV)	11	3	8.0
6	6-Fr catheter (FV)	10	4	11.5
7	6-Fr catheter (FV)	12	3	8.0
8	6-Fr catheter (FV)	11	4	10.0
9	6-Fr catheter (FV)	21	1	4.5
10	8-Fr catheter (FV)	10	3	7.5

A-V artery-to-vein, *FV* femoral vein, *PE* plasma exchange

Table 3 Technical characteristics of plasma exchange therapy 2

Patient	Total volume of plasma removed (mL)	Plasma separator	Replacement fluid
1	1415	Plasma flow OP-05®	FFP
2	5394	Centrifugation	FFP
3	2692	Centrifugation	FFP
4	1540	Plasma flow OP-02®	5% albumin
5	1515	Plasma flow OP-02®	FFP, 5% albumin
6	3819	Plasma flow OP-02®	FFP, 5% albumin
7	2800	Plasma flow OP-02®	5% albumin
8	2780	Plasma flow OP-02®	FFP, 5% albumin
9	600	Plasma flow OP-02®	FFP
10	3000	Plasma flow OP-02®	5% albumin

FFP fresh frozen plasma

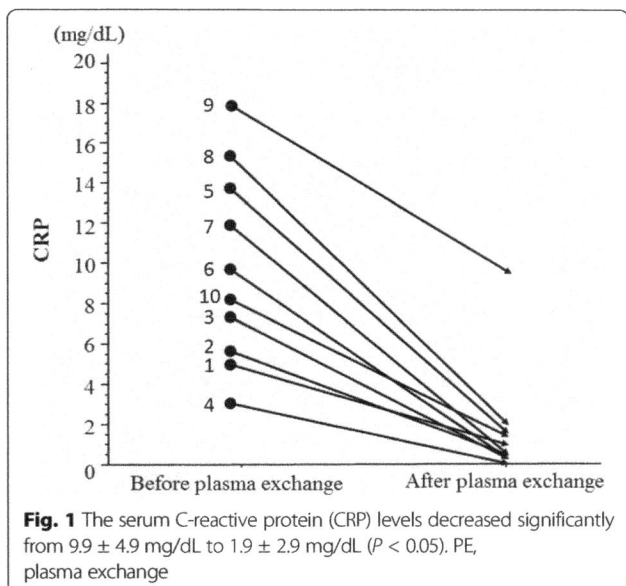

Fig. 1 The serum C-reactive protein (CRP) levels decreased significantly from 9.9 ± 4.9 mg/dL to 1.9 ± 2.9 mg/dL ($P < 0.05$). PE, plasma exchange

Recent reports have shown the effectiveness of plasma exchange in patients with IVIG-unresponsive Kawasaki disease [6, 8]. According to one report, plasma exchange therapy reduced the incidence of coronary artery lesions in Kawasaki disease to < 1% [8]. Hokosaki et al. described that there were no sequelae when plasma exchange was initiated before the beginning of coronary artery dilatation. However, when dilatation had already begun before the therapy, about 30% (6/20) patients showed persistent sequelae. Further, the size of aneurysms increased in all patients in whom sequelae remained and developed into

giant aneurysms in five of the six patients in the late period (≥1 year after onset) [7]. However, despite starting plasma exchange after the beginning of coronary artery expansion, we demonstrated that plasma exchange could improve the size of coronary artery lesions in almost all of the patients. For example, after plasma exchange, coronary artery lesions regressed to within normal limits in six of the ten patients and improved in another two patients. This is consistent with a previous case report that plasma exchange therapy significantly improved coronary artery lesions [10]. Furthermore, the aneurysms did not develop into giant aneurysms even in more than 1 year after onset in all of our patients. The period of until the start of the plasma exchange after onset was 13.7 ± 5.7 days in our study, whereas 8.1 ± 1.9 days reported by Hokosaki et al. [7]. Though plasma exchange was started late, coronary artery lesions regressed in almost all of our patients. In addition, there were no stenosis of the coronary artery. Therefore, plasma exchange may be effective not only in treating coronary artery lesions but also in preventing sequelae in patients with IVIG-unresponsive disease when plasma exchange performed after coronary artery dilatation.

In this study, one patient died due to a ruptured giant coronary aneurysm (patient 9), and another patient showed progression to a giant aneurysm (patient 1). In Japan, approximately 0.3–0.4% of patients are reported to develop giant coronary aneurysms [11, 12], and their formation is one of the most important factors affecting the prognosis of Kawasaki disease. Giant coronary aneurysms pose the greatest risk of thrombosis and stenosis (myocardial infarction). However, there is only a slight risk of rupture, and the incidence of rupture as a cause of death is very low compared with either myocardial infarction or myocarditis. There have been very few reports of ruptures of giant coronary aneurysms due to Kawasaki disease, although whenever reported, these were fatal [13]. Unfortunately, patient 9 died owing to a ruptured giant coronary aneurysm. Although plasma exchange basically should be indicated to IVIG-resistant patients, this patient had received IVIG and plasma exchange on the same day. Unstable circulation and anticoagulant associated with plasma exchange might influence the rupture of the aneurysm. In addition, it has been reported that the use of corticosteroids in the acute phase of Kawasaki disease for patients with evolving coronary artery aneurysms might be associated with worsening involvement and impaired vascular remodeling [14]. Therefore, plasma exchange and the use of corticosteroids may have serious concerns in some situation.

Recently, the age less than 1 year has been reported to be a significant risk factor for giant coronary aneurysms [15, 16], with increased likelihoods also associated with age more than 5 years, especially in males [16]. In the

Table 4 Patients with coronary artery lesions

Patient	Coronary artery size before PE (mm)	Coronary artery size after PE (mm)	Coronary artery size 1 year after treatment (mm)
1	RCA 6.9 LMT 5.0 LAD 4.0 LCx 3.6	RCA 13.1 LMT 6.9 LAD 7.0 LCx 7.0	RCA 4.9
2	RCA 3.3 LAD 4.1	Regression	Regression
3	RCA 3.6 LAD 3.4	RCA 5.0 LAD 5.6	RCA 5.9 LAD 5.1
4	RCA 4.1 LAD 4.9	RCA 3.4 LAD 4.4	Regression
5	RCA 3.1	Regression	Regression
6	LMT 4.3	LMT 4.7	Regression
7	RCA 3.1	RCA 3.0	Regression
8	RCA 3.0 LMT 3.2 LAD 3.0	RCA 4.4 LMT 3.5 LAD 5.0	Regression
9	RCA 15.1 LMT 3.5 LAD 18.2	Death due to ruptured coronary artery aneurysm	–
10	RCA 4.3 LMT 3.5 LAD 4.5	RCA 6.6 LAD 7.5	RCA 5.5 LAD 6.0

LCx left circumflex, *LAD* left descending artery, *LMT* left main trunk, *RCA* right coronary artery

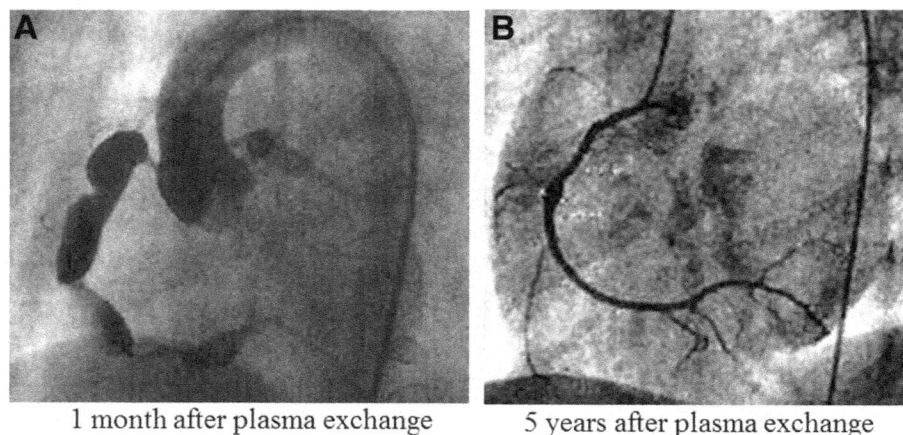

Fig. 2 Representative coronary angiography in patient 1. Coronary angiography in the right coronary artery 1 month (**a**) and 5 years (**b**) after plasma exchange in patient 1

present study, two cases of giant coronary aneurysms occurred in patients younger than 1 year. In addition, patient 3 was male and younger than 1 year, while patient 10 was older than 5 years and male. Therefore, both age and sex appear to be important for the management of Kawasaki disease and should be considered when stratifying the risk of developing coronary aneurysms.

When plasma exchange was started before coronary artery dilatation began, there were no sequelae [7]. Hokosaki et al. also found that the outcome of plasma exchange was better when plasma exchange started before day 9 after onset [7]. In the present study, two cases of giant coronary aneurysms were treated after more than 20 days had passed since the disease onset. These results are compatible with the view that plasma exchange should be started as early as possible, before coronary artery dilatation has started.

The pathogenesis of coronary artery aneurysm formation in Kawasaki disease remains unknown. It has been reported that elevations in proinflammatory cytokines, such as interleukin (IL)-6, tumor necrosis factor (TNF)-α, and IL-1β, are closely related to the pathogenesis of Kawasaki disease [17–19]. Fujimura et al. reported that IL-6, TNF-α (including TNF receptors 1 and 2), granulocyte colony-stimulating factor, and IL-17 were significantly decreased after plasma exchange treatment [20]. In particular, TNF-α has been shown to be necessary for the development of coronary artery lesions in Kawasaki disease [21]. Although we did not measure TNF-α in these patients, we did show that serum C-reactive protein levels and fever both improved rapidly after the initiation of plasma exchange treatment. Therefore, we speculate that the effect of plasma exchange might be related to the removal of these cytokines.

Adverse effects associated with plasma exchange, such as hypotension, bleeding, allergy, and infection, have been reported [22]. Although complications occurred in some patients, they were treatable and plasma exchange could be continued. Moreover, there were no deaths attributable to plasma exchange therapy. These findings indicate that plasma exchange is a safe treatment modality in children.

These results should, however, be considered in the context of the study's limitations. Notably, it had a small sample size and was not performed as a controlled clinical trial. We also did not compare plasma exchange with other therapies like infliximab, and the initial IVIG doses and timings may have differed from those used in other hospitals. A further clinical study that takes these issues into account might be needed.

Conclusions

In conclusion, plasma exchange may be effective in not only regressing coronary artery lesions but also preventing sequelae in patients with IVIG-unresponsive disease when plasma exchange is performed after coronary artery dilatation.

In addition, although plasma exchange generally appears to be safe, this study, in conjunction with other reports, indicates that outcomes are unfavorable if it is started when giant coronary aneurysms are present.

Acknowledgements
The authors would like to thank Enago (http://www.enago.jp) for the English language review.

Funding
None.

Authors' contributions
YKa, TK, and FK carried out the conception and design, data collection, data analysis, and manuscript writing. KS, YKo, KS, RY, TI, TH, YT, RS, HN, and SA participated in the design and coordination of the manuscript. All authors read and approved the final manuscript.

Competing interests

The authors declare that they have no competing interests.

Author details

[1]Division of Nephrology, Department of Medicine, Kurume University School of Medicine, 67 Asahi-machi, Kurume, Fukuoka 830-0011, Japan. [2]Department of Pediatrics and Child Health, Kurume University School of Medicine, Kurume, Japan. [3]Clinical Engineering Center, Kurume University Hospital, Kurume, Japan.

References

1. Kawasaki T. Acute febrile mucocutaneous syndrome with lymphoid involvement with specific desquamation of the fingers and toes in children. Arerugi. 1967;16:178–222.
2. Fukunishi M, Kikkawa M, Hamana K, Onodera T, Matsuzaki K, Matsumoto Y, et al. Prediction of non-responsiveness to intravenous high-dose gamma-globulin therapy in patients with Kawasaki disease at onset. J Pediatr. 2000;137:172–6.
3. Kobayashi T, Saji T, Otani T, Takeuchi K, Nakamura T, Arakawa H, et al. Efficacy of immunoglobulin plus prednisolone for prevention of coronary artery abnormalities in severe Kawasaki disease (RAISE study): a randomised, open-label, blinded-endpoints trial. Lancet. 2012;379:1613–20.
4. Burns JC, Mason WH, Hauger SB, Janai H, Bastian JF, Wohrley JD, et al. Infliximab treatment for refractory Kawasaki syndrome. J Pediatr. 2005;146:662–7.
5. Suzuki H, Terai M, Hamada H, Honda T, Suenaga T, Takeuchi T, et al. Cyclosporin A treatment for Kawasaki disease refractory to initial and additional intravenous immunoglobulin. Pediatr Infect Dis J. 2011;30:871–6.
6. Mori M, Imagawa T, Katakura S, Miyamae T, Okuyama K, Ito S, et al. Efficacy of plasma exchange therapy for Kawasaki disease intractable to intravenous gamma-globulin. Mod Rheumatol. 2004;14:43–7.
7. Hokosaki T, Mori M, Nishizawa T, Nakamura T, Imagawa T, Iwamoto M, et al. Long-term efficacy of plasma exchange treatment for refractory Kawasaki disease. Pediatr Int. 2012;54:99–103.
8. Imagawa T, Mori M, Miyamae T, Ito S, Nakamura T, Yasui K, et al. Plasma exchange for refractory Kawasaki disease. Eur J Pediatr. 2004;163:263–4.
9. Masuzawa Y, Mori M, Hara T, Inaba A, Oba MS, Yokota S. Elevated D-dimer level is a risk factor for coronary artery lesions accompanying intravenous immunoglobulin-unresponsive Kawasaki disease. Ther Apher Dial. 2015;19:171–7.
10. Mori M, Tomono N, Yokota S. Coronary arteritis of Kawasaki disease unresponsive to high-dose intravenous gammaglobulin successfully treated with plasmapheresis. Nihon Rinsho Meneki Gakkai Kaishi. 1995;18:282–8.
11. Nakamura Y, Yashiro M, Uehara R, Oki I, Kayaba K, Yanagawa H. Increasing incidence of Kawasaki disease in Japan: nationwide survey. Pediatr Int. 2008;50:287–90.
12. Nakamura Y, Yashiro M, Uehara R, Oki I, Watanabe M, Yanagawa H. Epidemiologic features of Kawasaki disease in Japan: results from the nationwide survey in 2005–2006. J Epidemiol. 2008;18:167–72.
13. Imai Y, Sunagawa K, Ayusawa M, Miyashita M, Abe O, Suzuki J, et al. A fatal case of ruptured giant coronary artery aneurysm. Eur J Pediatr. 2006;165:130–3.
14. Millar K, Manlhiot C, Yeung RS, Somji Z, McCrindle BW. Corticosteroid administration for patients with coronary artery aneurysms after Kawasaki disease may be associated with impaired regression. Int J Cardiol. 2012;154:9–13.
15. Sudo D, Monobe Y, Yashiro M, Sadakane A, Uehara R, Nakamura Y. Case-control study of giant coronary aneurysms due to Kawasaki disease: the 19th nationwide survey. Pediatr Int. 2010;52:790–4.
16. Nakamura Y, Yashiro M, Uehara R, Watanabe M, Tajimi M, Oki I, et al. Case-control study of giant coronary aneurysms due to Kawasaki disease. Pediatr Int. 2003;45:410–3.
17. Matsubara T, Furukawa S, Yabuta K. Serum levels of tumor necrosis factor, interleukin 2 receptor, and interferon-gamma in Kawasaki disease involved coronary-artery lesions. Clin Immunol Immunopathol. 1990;56:29–36.
18. Okada Y, Shinohara M, Kobayashi T, Inoue Y, Tomomasa T, Morikawa A, et al. Effect of corticosteroids in addition to intravenous gamma globulin therapy on serum cytokine levels in the acute phase of Kawasaki disease in children. J Pediatr. 2003;143:363–7.
19. Sohn MH, Noh SY, Chang W, Shin KM, Kim DS. Circulating interleukin 17 is increased in the acute stage of Kawasaki disease. Scand J Rheumatol. 2003;32:364–6.
20. Fujimaru T, Ito S, Masuda H, Oana S, Kamei K, Ishiguro A, et al. Decreased levels of inflammatory cytokines in immunoglobulin-resistant Kawasaki disease after plasma exchange. Cytokine. 2014;70:156–60.
21. Hui-Yuen JS, Duong TT, Yeung RS. TNF-alpha is necessary for induction of coronary artery inflammation and aneurysm formation in an animal model of Kawasaki disease. J Immunol. 2006;176:6294–301.
22. Shemin D, Briggs D, Greenan M. Complications of therapeutic plasma exchange: a prospective study of 1,727 procedures. J Clin Apher. 2007;22:270–6.

18

Dialysis-related factors affecting self-efficacy and quality of life in patients on haemodialysis: a cross-sectional study from Palestine

Ibrahim Mousa[1], Raed Ataba[1], Khaled Al-ali[1], Abdulsalam Alkaiyat[2] and Sa'ed H. Zyoud[3,4,5*]

Abstract

Background: Chronic kidney disease (CKD) is one of the main public health issues. It increases the morbidity and mortality of patients. Treatment includes multiple aspects such as dialysis and lifestyle modifications. The primary goal of this study was to determine factors associated with self-efficacy and health-related quality of life (HRQoL) among haemodialysis (HD) patients.

Methods: A cross-sectional descriptive correlation study was conducted on CKD patients undergoing HD at 12 different dialysis centres in Palestine. Self-efficacy was assessed by the Self-Efficacy for Managing Chronic Disease Six-Item Scale (SEMCD-6), and HRQoL was assessed using the Five-level EuroQol Five-Dimensions (EQ-5D-5L) tool. Multiple linear regression analysis was carried out to assess the association of factors with each of the SEMCD-6 and HRQoL scale scores.

Results: A total of 283 HD patients were included in the study. A correlation test revealed moderately positive association between the EQ-5D and SEMCD-6 scores ($r = 0.497$, p value < 0.001). In multiple linear regression analysis, age, living status, and number of co-morbid diseases were negatively associated with SEMCD-6 scores ($\beta = -2.66$, $p = 0.016$; $\beta = -5.71$, $p = 0.033$; $\beta = -1.84$, $p = 0.006$, respectively). Furthermore, there is a positive association between educational level and SEMCD-6 score with QoL score ($\beta = 0.05$, $p = 0.017$; $\beta = 0.01$, $p < 0.001$, respectively), while there is a negative association between the number of co-morbid diseases and QoL score ($\beta = -0.07$, $p = 0.001$).

Conclusions: This study assessed factors associated with impaired self-efficacy and HRQoL in HD patients. The results show that impaired self-efficacy was associated with the elderly, patients living with family, and patients with a high number of co-morbid diseases. Furthermore, this study found that the worst HRQoL was associated with patients with a low education level, lower levels of self-efficacy, and a high number of co-morbid diseases.

Keywords: Chronic kidney disease, Haemodialysis, Self-efficacy for managing chronic disease, Health-related quality of life

Background

Chronic kidney disease (CKD) is one of the major public health problems worldwide [1]. It is characterised by progressive loss in kidney function that gradually causes end-stage renal disease (ESRD) [2], which requires kidney transplantation or dialysis [3, 4]. ESRD is the last

---
* Correspondence: saedzyoud@yahoo.com; saedzyoud@najah.edu
[3]Poison Control and Drug Information Center (PCDIC), College of Medicine and Health Sciences, An-Najah National University, Nablus 44839, Palestine
[4]Department of Clinical and Community Pharmacy, College of Medicine and Health Sciences, An-Najah National University, Nablus 44839, Palestine
Full list of author information is available at the end of the article

stage of the National Kidney Foundation Kidney Disease Outcomes Quality [2]. In the last 10 years, the prevalence and frequency of ESRD has risen steadily by 4–8% per year throughout the world. Diabetes mellitus (DM) is the major predisposing factor for ESRD [5, 6], accounting for nearly 44% of new cases [6–8]. CKD has a major effect on the individual level by increasing the morbidity and mortality of patients and also increasing healthcare costs and the demand for healthcare services on a national level [1]. With this increasing rate of CKD, increased awareness and understanding of the overall

CKD burden is needed, which may lead to improvement in the knowledge, trust, and involvement in self-managing the disease [9]. Haemodialysis (HD) is the most common method of treatment, with approximately 90.6% of patients undergoing it. The difficulties faced by these patients are countless and influence their routine and the way they relate, as they often cause emotional difficulty and physical impairment [10]. Treatment of patients with ESRD has multiple aspects in addition to dialysis, as it requires total lifestyle changes that affect the social and psychological state of patients [4].

Self-management of adults with CKD has a positive relation with health outcomes. Perceived disease-related self-efficacy (DSE) is essential to self-managing chronic disease successfully [3]. Recent studies discuss how ESRD patients treated with HD carry out self-management activities in their daily life [11–16]. Patients should follow the treatment recommendations and learn to include them in their life circumstances in order to make CKD progress slowly and to have a stable life [3]. Generally, the concept of self-efficacy involves finding the limit at which the patients can achieve their desired outcomes. An association between self-efficacy and self-management in patients with CKD has been shown in previous researches [11, 17, 18]. HD patients with improved self-efficacy and self-care by empowerment programmes show an increased likelihood to get involved in self-management [19]. Higher perceived self-efficacy scores have shown a significant relation with quality of life (QoL) [6], a higher level of cooperation, self-care, communication, and medication-adherence behaviours [19]. Furthermore, high self-efficacy has an association with good changes in healthcare actions and health status. An improvement in deferent aspects of HD patients has been evidenced with increased self-efficacy, decreased hospitalisations, decreased amputations, control of interdialytic weight gain, and improved QoL in diabetic dialysis patients [11]. In order to attain a better QoL, patients with chronic renal disease should incorporate this goal in their daily life. The index of well-being or QoL is completely different from persons considered healthy, because CKD patients' health objectives concentrate on having a health level that secures an independent life [20].

Chronic kidney disease was ranked the six (3.6%) as the leading cause of the most burden disease, expressed as a percentage of disability-adjusted life years (DALYs) from reported chronic diseases in the West Bank/Palestine in 2010 [21]. According to the 2017 annual health report of the Palestinian Ministry of Health [22], there is an increasing number of patients with CKD who become dialysis dependent. The overall number of dialysis patients in the West Bank/Palestine has increased from 1014 patients in 2015 [23] to 1119 patients in 2016 which showed substantial trends in patients requiring haemodialysis [22]. A study by Younis et al. in 2015 [24] assessed the costs of HD in Palestine. The study found that the total cost per HD patient during visits to dialysis centres was an average of US$16085 per year which covered all medications, laboratory tests, and outpatient visits. The Palestinian government covered almost all of the costs of HD and transplantation [24].

Despite the assessment of self-management and self-efficacy in many studies [4, 9, 11–16, 19, 25–34], no studies have been performed to calculate the self-efficacy and QoL of HD patients in Palestine. Although several research has been carried out on HD patients and about CKD in Palestine [35–41], a literature review showed no previous studies on the association between the QoL and self-efficacy among HD patients in Palestine. This is important, because it is thought that religion and culture may play a significant role in health-related issues. Healthcare workers should cooperate with patients to build strategies and plans that will improve patients' health-related quality of life (HRQoL), like minimising depression as their disease progresses. Emphasis on the need to help healthcare workers to concentrate on improving knowledge, understanding, motivation, experience, self-trust, and the formation of self-efficacy and self-management for patients receiving HD by designing interventions and empowerment programmes for this purpose.

Methods

Purposes of the study

The primary goals of this study were (1) to describe the relation between HD patients' self-efficacy and their QoL, (2) to assess factors associated with self-efficacy among HD patients, and (3) to assess factors associated with QoL among HD patients. The results of this study will be used to provide recommendations that may aid healthcare workers to teach patients the self-management-related skills for their chronic disease to help them become more confident in many aspects, such as solving their problems, performing activities and skills on their own, and overcoming barriers that affect their ideal disease self-management in order to improve their QoL.

Study design

A cross-sectional study was conducted to achieve our objectives.

Setting

Patients included in the study were selected from every dialysis centre in the West Bank, Palestine. There are 12 dialysis centres in the West Bank: one is private (An-Najah University Hospital) and the others are governmental, including Al-Watani/Nablus, Tubas Turkish, Salfit (Yaser Arafat), Jenin (Khalil Souliman), Qalqiliya

(Darweesh Nazal), Hebron (Alia), Tulkarm (Thabet Thabet), Jericho, Beit Jala (Al Housain), Palestine Medical Complex/Ramallah, and Yatta (Abu Al Hassan Al Kassem) [23].

Study population
There were 1014 dialysis patients who came regularly to the dialysis centres in the West Bank, according to the 2015 annual health report of the Palestinian Ministry of Health which was published at the time of the study [23]. In West Bank/ Palestine, there are 12 kidney dialysis units (11 units in hospitals of the Ministry of Health and one unit in An-Najah National University hospital in Nablus) with a total of 183 machines [22]. According to the 2017 annual health report of the Palestinian Ministry of Health, a total of 147,494 HD sessions took place in 2016 [22].

Sampling procedure and sample size calculations
To achieve the goal of this study, we used a web-based calculator, which is called the Raosoft sample size calculator, to determine the sample size [42]. We decided that the sample size will be 279 patients to get a 95% confidence level and a 5% margin of error, depending on the assumption that half of the patients correctly answered every question. The HD patients from this cross-sectional study were chosen using a convenience sampling technique. HD patients were selected from all kidney dialysis units in West Bank/Palestine using the proportional quota sampling method to be representative of the general HD population (Table 1).

Inclusion and exclusion criteria
We included participants who met the following criteria: (1) patients older than 18 years of age, (2) confirmed diagnosis of ESRD, and (3) patients on regular HD therapy for at least 6 months. We excluded the patients who had major psychiatric disorders or were seriously ill at the time of the study. We also excluded patients if they were physically or mentally unable to communicate with the interviewer.

Data collection instrument
We used an instrument that contained four sections (see Additional file 1: English and Arabic version of the instrument):

The first section covered the social and demographic factors like age, sex, residency, occupational status, the dialysis centre visited, marital status, educational level, smoking status, and monthly income.

The second section discussed the clinical status of the patients, including questions such as how many hours per dialysis session, how many dialysis sessions per week, duration of disease in months, body mass index (BMI), how many medications they use regularly to calculate the total number of chronic medications, and how many chronic diseases they have to calculate the total number of co-morbid diseases. Therefore, the presence of one or more chronic diseases (co-morbidity) was calculated only for HD patients who had chronic diseases other than CKD. Furthermore, the total number of chronic medications used was defined as types of medication (i.e. prescriptions) used for certain chronic disease.

Table 1 Distribution of dialysis in hospitals, West Bank/Palestine, 2015 and 2016, and number of patients collected from each dialysis centre for the current study

Hospital's name	No. of patients in 2015[a]	No. of patients collected for the current study (%)	No. of patients in 2016[b]	No. of machines[b]
Jenin (Khalil Suliman)	113	30 (10.6)	120	16
Tubas Turkish	27	5 (1.8)	33	12
Tulkarm (Thabit Thabit)	78	22 (7.8)	71	13
Al Watani\ Nablus	0	0 (0.0)	0	1
Qalqiliya (Darwish Nazal)	47	13 (4.6)	51	12
Salfit (Yasser Arafat)	32	9 (3.2)	34	9
Ramallah's Sons Ward	137	45 (15.9)	157	21
Jericho	25	8 (2.8)	29	9
Beit Jala (Al Housein)	83	25 (8.8)	90	13
Hebron (Alia)	220	62 (21.9)	245	32
Yatta (Abu Alhasan Al Kassem)	42	10 (3.5)	52	10
An-Najah National University	210	54 (19.1)	237	35
Total	1014	283 (100)	1119	183

[a]The data adapted from the 2016 annual health report of the Palestinian Ministry of Health [23]
[b]The data adapted from the 2017 annual health report of the Palestinian Ministry of Health [22]

The third part used the Self-Efficacy for Managing Chronic Disease Six-Item Scale (SEMCD-6), which is applied commonly in many chronic illnesses and concentrates on the level of confidence that the patients have in each area depending on a six-item scale. These areas include symptom control, emotional functioning, role function, and communication with doctors [43]. Relying on a 10-point rating scale, each question has a score varying from 1 to 10 (1 = totally not confident; 10 = very confident).

The fourth part used the Five-level EuroQol Five-Dimensions (EQ-5D-5L) tool to assess the HRQoL. The Euro QoL Group developed this tool. It lets patients define their present health status during dialysis using a descriptive system of five items to measure the EQ-5D index score and the EQ visual analogue scale (EQ-VAS) [40]. We asked the patient to choose the most accurate sentence that describes his current health status, like the ability to walk: (1) I do not have any walking problems, (2) I have mild problems with walking, (3) I have moderate problems with walking, (4) I have severe problems with walking, and (5) I cannot walk. Permission to use the Arabic version of the EQ-5D [44] was offered by the Euro QOL Group, and it was scored according to Euro QOL guidelines [45]. The questionnaire was tested on a pilot sample of 15 HD patients to evaluate comprehension. The pilot sample was not included in the final sample of the study. Face and content validity of the final data collection form was evaluated by a panel of three researchers who are experts in the field of QoL for assessing the preparation, organisation, translation, and evaluation. Some items were modified as necessary. Cronbach's alpha of the SEMCD-6 was 0.753, indicating acceptable internal consistency reliability. Additionally, Cronbach's alpha of five dimensions of the EQ-5D index was 0.771, indicating acceptable internal consistency reliability.

Ethical approval

Ethical approval for the study was obtained from the local health authorities that had control and rule over the local study population and from An-Najah National University's Ethics Committee. We described the interview content to the respondents, and before the start of the interview, we obtained verbal consent from each participant.

Statistical analysis

Data analysis was performed using the Statistical Package for Social Sciences programme, version 15 (SPSS). Data for categorical variables were presented as frequencies (percentages), and data for continuous variables were presented as mean ± SD or as medians (lower-upper quartiles). We utilised the Kolmogorov–Smirnov test to assess variables for normality use. The Kruskal–Wallis test and Mann–Whitney test were used to test for differences in the medians between groups. Correlation between SEMCD-6 and HRQoL scale scores was investigated using Spearman's correlation coefficient. Linear regression analysis was carried out to assess the association of factors with each of the SEMCD-6 and HRQoL scale scores. The significance level was set at a p value < 0.05. Internal consistency reliability for all scales was calculated using Cronbach's alpha.

Results

Participants' characteristics

A total of 301 individuals were interviewed within 7 months from November 2016 to June 2017. Eighteen patients refused to participate, giving a response rate of 94%. After excluding non-responses, the final sample was 283. The majority of patients were aged between 30 and 60 years (61.1%), and the patients' mean age was 50. 3 ± 16 years. Most participants were male (61.8%), married (74.2%), unemployed (79.9%), and living with their families (94.3%). Nearly half (44.5%) of the patients were categorised with a higher educational level (i.e. university level and above) and with less than 2000 New Israeli Shekel (NIS) monthly income (50.9%) (Table 2).

In terms of their medical aspect, the length of dialysis ranged from 6 months to 252 months, with the majority at less than 48 months (72.4%) and three dialysis sessions weekly (88%). Regarding the dialysis sessions' duration, about half of the patients took more than 3 hours (51.6%). Eighty-seven percent of patients did not have a kidney transplant history. Most had at least one chronic co-morbid disease (83.3%) and were on regular medications (78.4%) (Table 2).

Self-efficacy scale

The mean and median of the SEMCD-6 were 38.70 ± 11. 1 and 39 (interquartile range: 31–47), respectively. Table 3 presents the factors associated with the SEMCD score. We found a significant association between age and SEMCD score (p value< 0.05), where younger ages had better scores. There was also a significantly better SEMCD score with graduated patients than more uneducated ones, and the same for those who live alone, patients with high income, and employed patients. Other sociodemographic factors, such as BMI, residency, marital status, and smokers, were not significantly associated with SEMCD score (p value > 0.05).

Patients without any co-morbid conditions or low rates of co-morbid conditions in patients with HD and a low number of chronic medications were significantly associated with a high SEMCD score (p value < 0.05). Other clinical factors such as dialysis vintage, dialysis per week, dialysis duration, and history of kidney

Table 2 Sociodemographic and clinical characteristics of participants

Variable	Frequency (%) N (283)
Age category (years)	
< 30	36(12.7)
30–60	173(61.1)
> 60	74(26.1)
Gender	
Male	175(61.8)
Female	108(38.2)
BMI[a]	
Underweight	16(5.7)
Normal	107(37.8)
Overweight	92(32.5)
Obese	68(24)
Education	
No formal education	20(7.1)
Elementary school (primary)	63(22.3)
High school (secondary school)	74(26.1)
Graduated (university and above)	126(44.5)
Household income (month)[a]	
High (more than 5000 NIS)	16(5.7)
Moderate (2000–5000 NIS)	123(43.5)
Low (less than 2000 NIS)	144(50.9)
Residency	
City and refugee camps	115(40.6)
Village	168(59.4)
Living status	
Alone	16(5.7)
With family	267(94.3)
Marital status	
Single, divorced, widowed	73(25.8)
Married	210(74.2)
Occupation	
Employed	57(20.1)
Unemployed	226(79.9)
Dialysis vintage (months)	
< 48	205(72.4)
≥ 48	78(27.6)
Dialysis per week	
≤ 2	29(10.2)
3	249(88.0)
≥ 4	5(1.8)
Dialysis session duration (hours)	
≤ 3	137(48.4)
> 3	146(51.6)

Table 2 Sociodemographic and clinical characteristics of participants (Continued)

Variable	Frequency (%) N (283)
Transplantation history	
Yes	35(12.4)
No	248(87.6)
Total chronic co-morbid diseases	
None	47(16.6)
1	74(26.1)
2	68(24.0)
≥ 3	94(33.2)
Chronic medications	
< 4	61(21.6)
≥ 4	222(75.4)

Abbreviations: BMI body mass index, NIS New Israeli Shekel
[a]1 Israeli New Shekel equals 0.29 US Dollar

transplant were not significantly associated with SEMCD score (p value > 0.05).

EQ-5D index values and EQ-VAS score

The mean and median of the EQ-5D index value were 0.46 ± 0.35 and 0.53 (interquartile range, 0.22–0.74), respectively. The mean and median of the EQ-VAS were 65.5 ± 21.9 and 70 (interquartile range, 50–80), respectively. Table 4 presents the factors associated with EQ-5D score. We found that factors such as age, education level, income, living status, occupation, dialysis session duration, transplantation history, total number of co-morbid diseases, and number of medications were significantly associated with EQ-5D score (p value < 0.05). Correlation tests revealed moderately positive association between the EQ-5D score and the EQ-VAS ($r = 0.486$, p value < 0.001) and SEMCD-6 ($r = 0.497$, p value < 0.001).

Multiple linear regression analysis

The multiple linear regression model of the SEMCD-6 scale is shown in Table 5. Age, education level, income, living status, occupation, total number of co-morbid diseases, and number of medications were included as independent variables. Table 5 shows that age, living status, and number of co-morbid diseases were negatively associated with SEMCD-6 score ($\beta = -2.66$, $p = 0.016$; $\beta = -5.71$, $p = 0.033$; $\beta = -1.84$, $p = 0.006$, respectively). More specifically, being younger, living alone, and having a low number of co-morbid diseases were associated with a higher SEMCD-6 score.

The multiple linear regression model of the HRQoL scale is shown in Table 6. Age, education level, income, living status, occupation, dialysis session duration, transplantation history, total number of co-morbid diseases,

Table 3 Association of sociodemographic and clinical characteristics with self-efficacy score in haemodialysis patients with chronic kidney disease

Variable	Frequency (%) N (283)	Median (Q1–Q3)	P value[a]
Age category (years)			
< 30	36(12.7)	46(36–52.75)	< 0.001[b]
30–60	173(61.1)	40(33–47.5)	
> 60	74(26.1)	33(26–41.25)	
Gender			
Male	175(61.8)	38(32–47)	0.958[c]
Female	108(38.2)	40(31–48.75)	
BMI[a]			
Underweight	16(5.7)	37(31–48.5)	0.206[b]
Normal	107(37.8)	41(33–50)	
Overweight	92(32.5)	39(29–46)	
Obese	68(24)	37(31–45)	
Education			
No formal education	20(7.1)	34.5(28–48)	0.014[b]
Elementary school (primary)	63(22.3)	35(27–43)	
High school (secondary school)	74(26.1)	39.5(31–49)	
Graduated (university and above)	126(44.5)	41(34–48.25)	
Household income (month)[d]			
High (more than 5000 NIS)	16(5.7)	43(34–50.5)	0.005[b]
Moderate (2000–5000 NIS)	123(43.5)	42(34–49)	
Low (less than 2000 NIS)	144(50.9)	37(29.25–45)	
Residency			
City and refugee camps	115(40.6)	39(31–47)	0.995[c]
Village	168(59.4)	39(31–47.75)	
Living status			
Alone	16(5.7)	45(38–54.25)	0.031[c]
With family	267(94.3)	39(31–47)	
Marital status			
Single, divorced, widowed	73(25.8)	40(31.5–49)	0.438[c]
Married	210(74.2)	38.5(31–47)	
Occupation			
Employed	57(20.1)	45(37–50)	< 0.001[c]
Unemployed	226(79.9)	38(30–46)	
Dialysis vintage (months)			
< 48	205(72.4)	39(31–47)	0.905 [c]
≥ 48	78(27.6)	38.5(32.75–47)	
Dialysis per week			
≤ 2	29(10.2)	40(27.5–48.5)	0.908 [b]
3	249(88.0)	39(31–47)	
≥ 4	5(1.8)	37(19–48)	
Dialysis session duration (hours)			
≤ 3	137(48.4)	38(32–46)	0.482[c]
> 3	146(51.6)	40(30–48.25)	

Table 3 Association of sociodemographic and clinical characteristics with self-efficacy score in haemodialysis patients with chronic kidney disease (Continued)

Variable	Frequency (%) N (283)	Median (Q1–Q3)	P value[a]
Transplantation history			
Yes	35(12.4)	39(34–52)	0.108[c]
No	248(87.6)	39(31–47)	
Total chronic co-morbid diseases			
None	47(16.6)	44(37–51)	*<0.001*[b]
1	74(26.1)	42(33.75–50)	
2	68(24.0)	39.5(31–48.75)	
≥ 3	94(33.2)	35(28–41)	
Chronic medications			
< 4	61(21.6)	42(34–51)	*0.004*[c]
≥ 4	222(75.4)	38(30–46)	

Abbreviations: BMI body mass index, *NIS* New Israeli Shekel
[a]The p values are italicized where they are less than the significance level cut-off of 0.05
[b]Statistical significance of differences calculated using the Kruskal–Wallis test
[c]Statistical significance of differences calculated using the Mann–Whitney U test
[d]1 Israeli New Shekel equals 0.29 US Dollar

number of medications, and SEMCD-6 score were included as independent variables once interactions such as EQ-VAS were excluded. As shown in Table 6, there is a positive association between the educational level and the SEMCD-6 score with the QoL score ($\beta = 0.05$, $p = 0.017$; $\beta = 0.01$, $p < 0.001$, respectively), while there is a negative association between the number of co-morbid diseases and the QoL score ($\beta = -0.07$, $p = 0.001$). More specifically, patients with a high education level, greater levels of self-efficacy, and a low number of co-morbid diseases were associated with a higher QoL score.

Discussion

In the current study, we examined HD patients on different levels demographically and clinically using SEMCD-6 scores, EQ5D scores, and EQ-VAS scores. We found a significant relation between SEMCD-6 score and age, education status, monthly household income, living status, occupation, total chronic co-morbid diseases, and regular medications. There was a significant relation between age, monthly household income, occupation, total chronic co-morbid diseases, and regular medications and EQ-VAS score. Moreover, a significant relation was found between age, education status, monthly household income, living status, occupation, current smoking status, dialysis session duration, transplantation history, total chronic co-morbid diseases, and chronic medications and EQ-5D score.

In the current study, the mean of SEMCD-6 was 38.70, SD = 11.06. Surprisingly, the mean score was found to be a little bit lower in comparison to that in a previous American study's mean and SD = 48.66 (10.79) [11]. The results of our study showed that a younger age is

significantly associated with better self-efficacy. This finding supports previous research in this area that links age and self-efficacy [11]. It is important to note that the mean age of participants for the American study's was 50.9 years [11] which is considered close to the mean age in our sample.

Employed patients with a higher monthly income are strongly associated with a better self-efficacy score. This result is in accordance with a previous Turkish study [26] and Callaghan's study [46]. In the current study, we found that patients with more education have a better SEMCD-6 score. This result is in agreement with results obtained by Curtin et al. [11]. It is also consistent with Kav et al.'s research, which studied the self-efficacy of diabetic patients [47].

We obtained from our results a significant relation between living status and SEMCD-6 score. People who live alone have better self-efficacy than those who live with their families. This result seems to be consistent with another Turkish study, which found the same result in diabetic patients [47]. It is interesting to note that in this study, self-efficacy was inversely associated with the number of co-morbid diseases and medications. Patients who have no or fewer medications or co-morbid diseases have better self-efficacy. However, this result has not previously been described. This is an important issue for future research.

In our study, the EQ-5D score showed a mean of 0.46 (SD = 0.35), which is lower than other studies' means, such as a Swiss study that had a mean of 0.62 (SD = 0.30) [48], an English and Welsh study with a mean of 0.60 (SD = 0.28) [49], and a Japanese study with a mean of 0.75 (SD = 0.17) [50].

Table 4 Association of sociodemographic and clinical characteristics with health-related quality of life in haemodialysis patients with chronic kidney disease

Variable	Frequency (%) N (283)	Median (Q1–Q2)	P value[a]
Age category (years)			
< 30	36(12.7)	0.74(0.43–0.84)	< 0.001[b]
30–60	173(61.1)	0.55(0.25–0.74)	
> 60	74(26.1)	0.31(0.06–0.59)	
Gender			
Male	175(61.8)	0.52(0.19–0.73)	0.965[c]
Female	108(38.2)	0.55(0.25–0.74)	
BMI[a]			
Underweight	16(5.7)	0.33(−0.03–0.76)	0.070[b]
Normal	107(37.8)	0.59(0.26–0.78)	
Overweight	92(32.5)	0.54(0.29–0.73)	
Obese	68(24)	0.41(0.12–0.70)	
Education			
No formal education	20(7.1)	0.28(− 0.05–0.63)	< 0.001[b]
Elementary school (primary)	63(22.3)	0.36(0.08–0.62)	
High school (secondary school)	74(26.1)	0.48(0.16–0.74)	
Graduated (university and above)	126(44.5)	0.67(0.39–0.80)	
Household income (month)[d]			
High (more than 5000 NIS)	16(5.7)	0.67(0.56–0.87)	0.001[b]
Moderate (2000–5000 NIS)	123(43.5)	0.66(0.29–0.77)	
Low (less than 2000 NIS)	144(50.9)	0.44(0.13–0.68)	
Residency			
City and refugee camps	115(40.6)	0.55(0.21–0.77)	0.566[c]
Village	168(59.4)	0.52(0.22–0.71)	
Living status			
Alone	16(5.7)	0.73(0.53–0.87)	0.007[c]
With family	267(94.3)	0.50(0.19–0.73)	
Marital status			
Single, divorced, widowed	73(25.8)	0.60(0.25–0.74)	0.453[c]
Married	210(74.2)	0.50(0.19–0.74)	
Occupation			
Employed	57(20.1)	0.71(0.50–0.80)	< 0.001[c]
Unemployed	226(79.9)	0.45(0.17–0.71)	
Dialysis vintage (months)			
< 48	205(72.4)	0.53(0.20–0.74)	0.741[c]
≥ 48	78(27.6)	0.48(0.28–0.73)	
Dialysis per week			
≤ 2	29(10.2)	0.40(0.06–0.74)	0.391[b]
3	249(88.0)	0.54(0.24–0.74)	
≥ 4	5(1.8)	0.43(0.01–0.73)	
Dialysis session duration (hours)			
≤ 3	137(48.4)	0.45(0.15–0.69)	0.012[c]
> 3	146(51.6)	0.61(0.27–0.77)	

Table 4 Association of sociodemographic and clinical characteristics with health-related quality of life in haemodialysis patients with chronic kidney disease *(Continued)*

Variable	Frequency (%) N (283)	Median (Q1–Q2)	P value[a]
Transplantation history			
Yes	35(12.4)	0.71(0.48–0.80)	*0.001*[c]
No	248(87.6)	0.48(0.19–0.71)	
Total chronic co-morbid diseases			
None	47(16.6)	0.71(0.53–0.84)	*< 0.001*[b]
1	74(26.1)	0.69(0.34–0.84)	
2	68(24.0)	0.45(0.21–0.70)	
≥ 3	94(33.2)	0.29(0.06–0.55)	
Chronic medications			
< 4	61(21.6)	0.70(0.29–0.78)	*0.007*[c]
≥ 4	222(75.4)	0.48(0.19–0.71)	

Abbreviations: BMI body mass index, *NIS* New Israeli Shekel
[a]The *p* values are italicized where they are less than the significance level cut-off of 0.05
[b]Statistical significance of differences calculated using the Kruskal–Wallis test
[c]Statistical significance of differences calculated using the Mann–Whitney *U* test
[d]1 Israeli New Shekel equals 0.29 US Dollar

In the present study, we found a significant association between higher QoL and younger age. This finding is in agreement with that obtained by an Iranian study [51]. This contrasts with the study of O'Reilly et al., which explained that HRQoL gets better when the patient is older in age [52]. A higher education level was associated with better QoL. This result is consistent with data obtained in a previous Iranian study [51]. A study in the United Arab Emirates, which used another score for QoL measurement, matches our result [53]. Our study revealed that the total number of co-morbid diseases was inversely associated with QoL. This finding is in agreement with two Iranian studies that showed a strong relation between the number of co-morbid diseases and poor QoL [54, 55].

One interesting finding associated with the dialysis session duration is that QoL is better with longer session duration. Dialysis adequacy may be the answer because shorter dialysis session may result in inadequate dialysis [56]. This suggestion reflects those of Adas et al. [35]

who also found that most patients in Palestine were inadequately dialyzed and a high percentage of the HD patients did not achieve the targets. This result seems to be consistent with other research, which found that initiating HD at longer session duration is associated with less mortality [57]. This result is also in agreement with results obtained by a Belgian study that found a longer duration improves the well-being of patients due to more removal of solutes from patients in the interdialytic period [58]. In our data, high income was associated with better QoL, which supports a previous Iranian study by Pakpour et al. [54]. Another study was conducted by Marinovich et al. [59], which further supports the association between high income and better QoL.

Another important finding was that patients who have undergone kidney transplantation have higher QoL. This result is in accordance with a recent study by Fiebiger et al. [60]. This corroborate the ideas of Laupacis et al. [61], who suggested that renal transplantation improves the HRQoL of patients on dialysis.

Table 5 Patients characteristics associated with self-efficacy in multiple linear regression

Variables[a]	Unstandardised coefficients (β)	S.E	Standardised coefficients (β)	P value[b]	95% confidence interval for β
Age	− 2.66	1.10	− 0.15	*0.016*	− 4.83 to − 0.50
Education level	0.49	0.69	0.04	0.482	− 0.87 to 1.84
Income	1.91	1.14	0.10	0.095	− 0.34 to 4.15
Living status	− 5.71	2.66	− 0.12	*0.033*	− 10.95 to − 0.48
Occupation	3.04	1.67	0.11	0.070	− 0.25 to 6.33
Number of co-morbid diseases	− 1.84	0.66	− 0.18	*0.006*	− 3.15 to − 0.54
Number of chronic medications	− 1.75	1.65	− 0.07	0.290	− 5.01 to 1.50

[a]Univariate factors with *p* values < 0.05 were entered into the multiple linear regression
[b]The *p* values are italicized where they are less than the significance level cut-off of 0.05

Table 6 Patients characteristics associated with quality of life in multiple linear regression

Variables [a]	Unstandardised coefficients (β)	S.E	Standardised coefficients (β)	P value [b]	95% confidence interval for β
Age	− 0.03	0.03	− 0.05	0.402	− 0.09 to 0.04
Education level	0.05	0.02	0.13	*0.017*	0.01 to 0.09
Income	0.04	0.03	0.06	0.257	− 0.03 to 0.10
Living status	− 0.15	0.08	− 0.09	0.062	− 0.30 to 0.01
Occupation	0.04	0.05	0.04	0.449	− 0.06 to 0.13
Dialysis session duration (hours)	0.03	0.04	0.05	0.356	− 0.04 to 0.11
Transplantation history	− 0.04	0.06	− 0.04	0.495	− 0.15 to 0.07
Number of co-morbid diseases	− 0.07	0.02	− 0.21	*0.001*	− 0.11 to − 0.03
Number of chronic medications	0.03	0.05	0.04	0.512	− 0.06 to 0.13
Self-Efficacy for Managing Chronic Disease score	0.01	0.00	0.37	*< 0.001*	0.01 to 0.02

[a]Univariate factors with p values < 0.05 were entered into the multiple linear regression
[b]The p values are bold where they are less than the significance level cut-off of 0.05

The most important finding in our study was the significant relation between self-efficacy and QoL. Patients with a higher self-efficacy score had better QoL. This result is in accordance with a previous Taiwanese study by Tsay and Healstead [4]. It is also in agreement with Lev and Owen's research [62], which showed that QoL is positively related to self-efficacy.

Strength and limitations
The key strengths of this study are the collection of data from all dialysis centres in the West Bank, which means a relatively large sample, as well as the performance of direct interviews with the patients to collect more realistic and valid information. However, no studies have been performed to calculate the self-efficacy and QoL of HD patients in Palestine. This is the first study to evaluate the association between SEMCD-6 and QoL among HD patients in Palestine.

The study is limited by a number of restrictions that should be discussed. The first limitation is that the generalisability of the study's results to other CKD patients is reduced, because we used a convenience sampling method. The second limitation is that the cross-sectional design precludes any statements about causal associations between study variables. The third limitation is that related to selection bias that may have been introduced into the sample due to the non-response rate among eligible participants, inclusion or exclusion patients according to eligible criteria, or due to the non-random selection of initial participants. Additionally, our result may be confounded by survivor bias, e.g. those patients who live alone with a poor SEMCD score may die very quickly without help from their family and some degree of survivor bias cannot be excluded.

Conclusions
This study assessed factors associated with impaired self-efficacy and HRQoL in HD patients. The results of this investigation show that impaired self-efficacy was associated with the elderly, patients living with family, and patients with a high number of co-morbid diseases. Furthermore, this study found that the worst HRQoL was associated with patients with low education level, lower levels of self-efficacy, and a high number of co-morbid diseases. The results of this investigation show that assessment of the self-efficacy of patients receiving HD is crucial in clinical practice. Doctors may require self-efficacy trainings to strengthen HD patients' trust in carrying out self-care behaviours, which can lead to improvement in their QoL. Future studies that examine the effect of dialysis adequacy by calculating the Kt/V or urea reduction ratio on QoL in HD patients are needed.

Abbreviations
BMI: Body mass index; DM: Diabetes mellitus; EQ-5D-5L: Five-Level EuroQol Five-Dimensions; EQ-VAS: EuroQol visual analogue scale; ESRD: End-stage renal disease; HRQoL: Health-related quality of life; NIS: New Israeli Shekel; SD: Standard deviation; SEMCD-6: Self-Efficacy for Managing Chronic Disease Six-Item Scale; US$: The United States dollar

Acknowledgements
The authors would like to thank An-Najah National University for providing the opportunity to conduct this study.

Authors' contributions

IM, RA, and KA collected data, performed the analyses, searched the literature, and drafted the manuscript. AA participated in the field study and in the development of the final version of the manuscript. SZ conceptualised and designed the study; coordinated, supervised, and analysed the data; critically reviewed the manuscript and the interpretation of the results; and assisted in the final write-up of the manuscript and the revised manuscript. All authors read and approved the final manuscript.

Competing interests

The authors declare that they have no competing interests.

Author details

[1]Department of Medicine, College of Medicine and Health Sciences, An-Najah National University, Nablus 44839, Palestine. [2]Public Health Department, College of Medicine and Health Sciences, An-Najah National University Hospital, An-Najah National University, Nablus 44839, Palestine. [3]Poison Control and Drug Information Center (PCDIC), College of Medicine and Health Sciences, An-Najah National University, Nablus 44839, Palestine. [4]Department of Clinical and Community Pharmacy, College of Medicine and Health Sciences, An-Najah National University, Nablus 44839, Palestine. [5]Division of Clinical and Community Pharmacy, Department of Pharmacy, College of Medicine and Health Sciences, An-Najah National University, Nablus 44839, Palestine.

References

1. Bruck K, Jager KJ, Dounousi E, Kainz A, Nitsch D, Arnlov J, Rothenbacher D, Browne G, Capuano V, Ferraro PM, et al. Methodology used in studies reporting chronic kidney disease prevalence: a systematic literature review. Nephrol Dial Transplant. 2015;30(Suppl 4):iv6–16.
2. Khader MI, Snouber S, Alkhatib A, Nazzal Z, Dudin A. Prevalence of patients with end-stage renal disease on dialysis in the West Bank, Palestine. Saudi J Kidney Dis Transpl. 2013;24:832–7.
3. Lin CC, Wu CC, Anderson RM, Chang CS, Chang SC, Hwang SJ, Chen HC. The chronic kidney disease self-efficacy (CKD-SE) instrument: development and psychometric evaluation. Nephrol Dial Transplant. 2012;27:3828–34.
4. Tsay SL, Healstead M. Self-care self-efficacy, depression, and quality of life among patients receiving hemodialysis in Taiwan. Int J Nurs Stud. 2002;39:245–51.
5. Coentrao L, Van Biesen W, Nistor I, Tordoir J, Gallieni M, Marti Monros A, Bolignano D. Preferred haemodialysis vascular access for diabetic chronic kidney disease patients: a systematic literature review. J Vasc Access. 2015; 16:259–64.
6. Caramori ML, Mauer M. Diabetes and nephropathy. Curr Opin Nephrol Hypertens. 2003;12:273–82.
7. Lim A. Diabetic nephropathy—complications and treatment. Int J Nephrol Renovasc Dis. 2014;7:361–81.
8. Dabla PK. Renal function in diabetic nephropathy. World J Diabetes. 2010;1:48–56.
9. Johnson ML, Zimmerman L, Welch JL, Hertzog M, Pozehl B, Plumb T. Patient activation with knowledge, self-management and confidence in chronic kidney disease. J Ren Care. 2016;42:15–22.
10. Oller GA, Ribeiro Rde C, Travagim DS, Batista MA, Marques S, Kusumota L. Functional independence in patients with chronic kidney disease being treated with haemodialysis. Rev Lat Am Enfermagem. 2012;20:1033–40.
11. Curtin RB, Walters BA, Schatell D, Pennell P, Wise M, Klicko K. Self-efficacy and self-management behaviors in patients with chronic kidney disease. Adv Chronic Kidney Dis. 2008;15:191–205.
12. Zrinyi M, Juhasz M, Balla J, Katona E, Ben T, Kakuk G, Pall D. Dietary self-efficacy: determinant of compliance behaviours and biochemical outcomes in haemodialysis patients. Nephrol Dial Transplant. 2003;18:1869–73.
13. Tsay SL. Self-efficacy training for patients with end-stage renal disease. J Adv Nurs. 2003;43:370–5.
14. Lindberg M, Fernandes MA. Self-efficacy in relation to limited fluid intake amongst Portuguese haemodialysis patients. J Ren Care. 2010;36:133–8.
15. Winters AM, Lindberg M, Sol BG. Validation of a Dutch self-efficacy scale for

16. Oka M, Chaboyer W. Influence of self-efficacy and other factors on dietary behaviours in Japanese haemodialysis patients. Int J Nurs Pract. 2001;7:431–9.
17. Balaga PAG. Self-efficacy and self-care management outcome of chronic renal failure patients. Asian J Health. 2012;2:111–29.
18. Lin CC, Tsai FM, Lin HS, Hwang SJ, Chen HC. Effects of a self-management program on patients with early-stage chronic kidney disease: a pilot study. Appl Nurs Res. 2013;26:151–6.
19. Moattari M, Ebrahimi M, Sharifi N, Rouzbeh J. The effect of empowerment on the self-efficacy, quality of life and clinical and laboratory indicators of patients treated with hemodialysis: a randomized controlled trial. Health Qual Life Outcomes. 2012;10:115.
20. Barata NE. Dyadic relationship and quality of life patients with chronic kidney disease. J Bras Nefrol. 2015;37:315–22.
21. Mosleh M, Dalal K, Aljeesh Y. Burden of chronic diseases in the Palestinian health-care sector using disability-adjusted life-years. Lancet. 2018;391:S21.
22. Ministry of Health, Palestinian Health Information Center. Health Annual Report, Palestine 2016. 2017 [cited 2018 January 20]; Available from: http://www.moh.ps/Content/Books/ZxRcynmiUofNqt66u4CrHRgm JR6Uv7z77srjjIEAho6xnz5V3rgLTu_RhO7xf2j2VusNiIvWkjwp84yXHLdGleB 97gKrHHI5iZ9oPJ25owGEN.pdf.
23. Ministry of Health, Palestinian Health Information Center. Health Status, Palestine, 2015. 2016 [cited 2017 February 17]; Available from: http://www.moh.ps/Content/Books/ NWNJXX7RJ92Bn4f5EGYiH43a2tjAAzKBnseGnEUCaqWqYZndsbCcPy_ JQWguvkHTR4Xk4zUpdT45ooWxH11BhIbVAxwpGWy2wiwHdGcM5K7aZ.pdf.
24. Younis M, Jabr S, Al-Khatib A, Forgione D, Hartmann M, Kisa A. A cost analysis of kidney replacement therapy options in Palestine. Inquiry. 2015;52 https://doi.org/10.1177/0046958015573494.
25. Hutchison AJ, Courthold JJ. Enabling self-management: selecting patients for home dialysis? NDT Plus. 2011;4:iii7–iii10.
26. Bag E, Mollaoglu M. The evaluation of self-care and self-efficacy in patients undergoing hemodialysis. J Eval Clin Pract. 2010;16:605–10.
27. Clark-Cutaia MN, Ren D, Hoffman LA, Burke LE, Sevick MA. Adherence to hemodialysis dietary sodium recommendations: influence of patient characteristics, self-efficacy, and perceived barriers. J Ren Nutr. 2014;24:92–9.
28. Clark-Cutaia MN, Ren D, Hoffman LA, Snetselaar L, Sevick MA. Psychometric validation of the self-efficacy for restricting dietary salt in hemodialysis scale. Top Clin Nutr. 2013;28:384–91.
29. Kim JY, Kim B, Park KS, Choi JY, Seo JJ, Park SH, Kim CD, Kim YL. Health-related quality of life with KDQOL-36 and its association with self-efficacy and treatment satisfaction in Korean dialysis patients. Qual Life Res. 2013;22:753–8.
30. Krespi Boothby MR, Salmon P. Self-efficacy and hemodialysis treatment: a qualitative and quantitative approach. Turk Psikiyatri Derg. 2013;24:84–93.
31. Takaki J, Nishi T, Shimoyama H, Inada T, Matsuyama N, Kumano H, Kuboki T. Interactions among a stressor, self-efficacy, coping with stress, depression, and anxiety in maintenance hemodialysis patients. Behav Med. 2003;29:107–12.
32. Tanner JL, Craig CB, Bartolucci AA, Allon M, Fox LM, Geiger BF, Wilson NP. The effect of a self-monitoring tool on self-efficacy, health beliefs, and adherence in patients receiving hemodialysis. J Ren Nutr. 1998;8:203–11.
33. Wright LS, Wilson L. Quality of life and self-efficacy in three dialysis modalities: incenter hemodialysis, home hemodialysis, and home peritoneal dialysis. Nephrol Nurs J. 2015;42:463–76. quiz 77
34. Slesnick N, Pienkos S, Sun S, Doss-McQuitty S, Schiller B. The chronic disease self-management program—a pilot study in patients undergoing hemodialysis. Nephrol News Issues. 2015;29:22–3. 7-8, 30-2
35. Adas H, Al-Ramahi R, Jaradat N, Badran R. Assessment of adequacy of hemodialysis dose at a Palestinian hospital. Saudi J Kidney Dis Transpl. 2014; 25:438–42.
36. Al Zabadi H, Rahal H, Fuqaha R. Hepatitis B and C prevalence among hemodialysis patients in the West Bank hospitals, Palestine. BMC Infect Dis. 2016;16:41.
37. Al-Ramahi R, Raddad AR, Rashed AO, Bsharat A, Abu-Ghazaleh D, Yasin E, Shehab O. Evaluation of potential drug–drug interactions among Palestinian hemodialysis patients. BMC Nephrol. 2016;17:96.
38. Naalweh KS, Barakat MA, Sweileh MW, Al-Jabi SW, Sweileh WM, Zyoud SH. Treatment adherence and perception in patients on maintenance hemodialysis: a cross-sectional study from Palestine. BMC Nephrol. 2017;18:178.
39. Zyoud SH, Al-Jabi SW, Sweileh WM, Tabeeb GH, Ayaseh NA, Sawafta MN, Khdeir RL, Mezyed DO, Daraghmeh DN, Awang R. Use of

complementary and alternative medicines in haemodialysis patients: a cross-sectional study from Palestine. BMC Complement Altern Med. 2016;16:204.

40. Zyoud SH, Daraghmeh DN, Mezyed DO, Khdeir RL, Sawafta MN, Ayaseh NA, Tabeeb GH, Sweileh WM, Awang R, Al-Jabi SW. Factors affecting quality of life in patients on haemodialysis: a cross-sectional study from Palestine. BMC Nephrol. 2016;17:44.

41. Khatib ST, Hemadneh MK, Hasan SA, Khazneh E, Zyoud SH. Quality of life in hemodialysis diabetic patients: a multicenter cross-sectional study from Palestine. BMC Nephrol. 2018;19:49.

42. Raosoft. Sample Size Calculator. [cited 2016 September 23]; Available from: http://www.raosoft.com/samplesize.html.

43. Lorig KR, Sobel DS, Ritter PL, Laurent D, Hobbs M. Effect of a self-management program on patients with chronic disease. Eff Clin Pract. 2001; 4:256–62.

44. Horowitz E, Abadi-Korek I, Shani M, Shemer J. EQ-5D as a generic measure of health-related quality of life in Israel: reliability, validity and responsiveness. Isr Med Assoc J. 2010;12:715–20.

45. Euro QOL Group EQ-5D-5L User Guide Basic information on how to use the EQ-5D-5L instrument. 2013 [cited 2015 April 1]; Available from: http://www.euroqol.org/fileadmin/user_upload/Documenten/PDF/Folders_Flyers/UserGuide_EQ-5D-5L_v2.0_October_2013.pdf.

46. Callaghan DM. Health-promoting self-care behaviors, self-care self-efficacy, and self-care agency. Nurs Sci Q. 2003;16:247–54.

47. Kav S, Yilmaz AA, Bulut Y, Dogan N. Self-efficacy, depression and self-care activities of people with type 2 diabetes in Turkey. Collegian. 2017;24:27–35.

48. Wasserfallen JB, Halabi G, Saudan P, Perneger T, Feldman HI, Martin PY, Wauters JP. Quality of life on chronic dialysis: comparison between haemodialysis and peritoneal dialysis. Nephrol Dial Transplant. 2004;19:1594–9.

49. Roderick P, Nicholson T, Armitage A, Mehta R, Mullee M, Gerard K, Drey N, Feest T, Greenwood R, Lamping D, et al. An evaluation of the costs, effectiveness and quality of renal replacement therapy provision in renal satellite units in England and Wales. Health Technol Assess. 2005; 9:1–178.

50. Katayama A, Miyatake N, Nishi H, Uzike K, Sakano N, Hashimoto H, Koumoto K. Evaluation of physical activity and its relationship to health-related quality of life in patients on chronic hemodialysis. Environ Health Prev Med. 2014;19:220–5.

51. Javanbakht M, Abolhasani F, Mashayekhi A, Baradaran HR, Jahangiri noudeh Y. Health related quality of life in patients with type 2 diabetes mellitus in Iran: a national survey. PLoS One. 2012;7:e44526.

52. O'Reilly DJ, Xie F, Pullenayegum E, Gerstein HC, Greb J, Blackhouse GK, Tarride JE, Bowen J, Goeree RA. Estimation of the impact of diabetes-related complications on health utilities for patients with type 2 diabetes in Ontario, Canada. Qual Life Res. 2011;20:939–43.

53. Ayoub AM, Hijjazi KH. Quality of life in dialysis patients from the United Arab Emirates. J Fam Commun Med. 2013;20:106–12.

54. Pakpour AH, Saffari M, Yekaninejad MS, Panahi D, Harrison AP, Molsted S. Health-related quality of life in a sample of Iranian patients on hemodialysis. Iran J Kidney Dis. 2010;4:50–9.

55. Saffari M, Pakpour AH, Naderi MK, Koenig HG, Baldacchino DR, Piper CN. Spiritual coping, religiosity and quality of life: a study on Muslim patients undergoing haemodialysis. Nephrology (Carlton). 2013;18:269–75.

56. Manns BJ, Johnson JA, Taub K, Mortis G, Ghali WA, Donaldson C. Dialysis adequacy and health related quality of life in hemodialysis patients. ASAIO J. 2002;48:565–9.

57. Swaminathan S, Mor V, Mehrotra R, Trivedi AN. Initial session duration and mortality among incident hemodialysis patients. Am J Kidney Dis. 2017;70:69–75.

58. Eloot S, Van Biesen W, Dhondt A, Van de Wynkele H, Glorieux G, Verdonck P, Vanholder R. Impact of hemodialysis duration on the removal of uremic retention solutes. Kidney Int. 2008;73:765–70.

59. Marinovich S, Lavorato C, Rosa-Diez G, Bisignano L, Fernandez V, Hansen-Krogh D. The lack of income is associated with reduced survival in chronic haemodialysis. Nefrologia. 2012;32:79–88.

60. Fiebiger W, Mitterbauer C, Oberbauer R. Health-related quality of life outcomes after kidney transplantation. Health Qual Life Outcomes. 2004;2:2.

61. Laupacis A, Keown P, Pus N, Krueger H, Ferguson B, Wong C, Muirhead N. A study of the quality of life and cost-utility of renal transplantation. Kidney Int. 1996;50:235–42.

62. Lev EL, Owen SV. A measure of self-care self-efficacy. Res Nurs Health. 1996; 19:421–9.

19

Effects of supervised exercise on depressive symptoms in hemodialysis patients: a systematic review and meta-analysis of randomized controlled trials

Takahiro Shimoda[1], Ryota Matsuzawa[2], Keika Hoshi[3], Kei Yoneki[1], Manae Harada[1], Takaaki Watanabe[1] and Atsuhiko Matsunaga[1*]

Abstract

Background: The reported prevalence rate of depressive symptoms in hemodialysis patients is 40%. Although appropriate management of these symptoms is important, they remain under-recognized and under-treated in hemodialysis patients. Here, we systematically reviewed relevant randomized controlled trials (RCTs) investigating the effects of supervised exercise training on depressive symptoms in hemodialysis patients.

Methods: MEDLINE, Embase, the Cochrane Central Register of Controlled Trials, the Cochrane Database of Systematic Reviews, CINAHL, Web of Science, PsycINFO, and PEDro databases were searched from the start until June 2016 for RCTs published in English evaluating the effects of supervised exercise training in hemodialysis patients. The main outcome measures were depressive symptoms.

Results: From a total of 10,923 screened references, five trials were included in the analysis. Exercise training was shown to significantly improve depressive symptoms in comparison with controls (standardized mean difference, SMD = $-$ 1.19; $P < 0.001$) under a random effects model. Subgroup analyses indicated that aerobic exercise and interventions lasting $\geq$ 6 months significantly reduced depressive symptoms in hemodialysis patients ($P = 0.016$, $P < 0.001$, respectively).

Conclusions: The meta-analysis found that supervised exercise training tends to alleviate depressive symptoms in hemodialysis patients. As our database search identified only a small number of studies on the association between exercise and depressive symptoms, we would surmise that additional high-quality studies are required to explore further this association.

Keywords: Chronic kidney disease, Hemodialysis, Depressive symptoms, Exercise, Meta-analysis

Background

With the increasing prevalence of lifestyle-related diseases, such as diabetes, hypertension, and arteriosclerosis, there are more than 2 million patients undergoing hemodialysis worldwide [1]. Depressive symptoms are common among hemodialysis patients, with a prevalence rate of 40% according to the Dialysis Outcomes and Practice Patterns Study (DOPPS) [2]. Depression is one of the most serious comorbidities among hemodialysis patients [2–4] and is associated with elevated mortality risk [2, 5, 6] and reduced quality of life (QOL) [7, 8]. Although the appropriate management of depressive symptoms as a patient-reported outcome (PRO) is known to be clinically important, these symptoms remain under-recognized and under-treated in dialysis patients [9–11]. Exercise training is an effective non-pharmacological means of reducing depressive symptoms among people dwelling in the community [12, 13], cancer survivors [14, 15], multiple

* Correspondence: atsuhikonet@gmail.com
[1]Department of Rehabilitation Sciences, Graduate School of Medical Sciences, Kitasato University, 1-15-1 Kitasato, Sagamihara, Kanagawa 252-0373, Japan
Full list of author information is available at the end of the article

sclerosis patients [16], stroke patients [17], and patients with chronic illness [18].

Although supervised exercise training has been suggested to improve exercise capacity, muscular strength, and QOL in hemodialysis patients [19–22], it remains unclear whether such exercise regimes can ameliorate depressive symptoms in these patients. Systematic reviews with meta-analyses are generally considered good means of determining the efficacy and effectiveness of treatments on selected outcomes.

This study was performed to systematically review relevant randomized controlled trials (RCTs) investigating the effects of supervised exercise training on depressive symptoms in hemodialysis patients. In addition, we performed subgroup analyses to examine the differences in efficacy related to the training program.

Methods

This review is reported in accordance with Preferred Reporting Items for Systematic Reviews and Meta-Analyses (PRISMA) guidelines (Additional file 1) and is one of a series of systematic reviews regarding the effects of exercise on depressive symptoms in hemodialysis patients. The protocol used for the systematic review and meta-analysis was registered with the International Prospective Register of Systematic Reviews (PROSPERO) (registration number: PROSPERO 2015: CRD4201502 0701), and our protocol has already been published (http://bmjopen.bmj.com/content/6/5/e010990.long) [23]. No ethical approval was required because this study did not include confidential personal data and did not involve patient intervention.

Study selection and data management

An electronic database search was performed in MEDLINE, Embase, the Cochrane Central Register of Controlled Trials, the Cochrane Database of Systematic Reviews, CINAHL, Web of Science, PsycINFO, and PEDro using the following terms: "dialysis," "renal replacement therapy," "exercise," "physical fitness," "cycling," "walking," and "physical therapy." The full strategy is described in Additional file 2. To identify any articles missed by the initial search, the reference lists of previously reported systematic reviews were also evaluated in addition to our electronic database search. EndNote X7 for Windows (Thompson Reuters, Philadelphia, PA) was used to manage literature records and data. Reviewers screened all titles, abstracts, and the full texts of the selected publications. In cases where required data were not available, the study authors were contacted by email.

Inclusion and exclusion criteria

Only RCTs published in English that evaluated the effects of supervised exercise training on at least depressive symptoms were included. Supervised exercise included resistance training, aerobic exercise, or combined exercise. Only RCTs treating patients at least 18 years of age and on hemodialysis were included in this meta-analysis. Patients affected by acute kidney failure were also excluded. The main outcome of the study was depressive symptoms.

Risk of bias

The methodological quality of trials included in the review was assessed independently using the Cochrane Collaboration tool [24] by three reviewers to determine the risk of bias. Studies were graded as having a "low risk," "high risk," or "unclear risk" of bias across the seven specified domains: random sequence generation, allocation concealment, participant and personnel blinding, outcome assessment blinding, incomplete outcome data, selective reporting, and other sources of bias. Furthermore, the risk of bias of references was assessed using the Tool for the assEssment of Study qualiTy and reporting in EXercise (TESTEX) [25], which consists of 15 different items and shows reliable performance for comprehensive review of exercise 1 training trials.

Data analysis and statistical methods

The effect sizes obtained from the RCTs are reported as mean change scores (Cohen's d). Although some of the included studies reported change scores and the standard deviations (SDs), we calculated change scores for those that did not by subtracting the mean baseline score from the mean follow-up score and calculated the change score SD. A random effects model was used to compute the overall or mean effect size (ES), as this model assumes that the samples are from populations with different ESs and that the true effect differs between studies. We used fixed effect models in cases in which the degree of statistical heterogeneity was low, while random effect models were used in all other cases. The 95% confidence interval (CI) around the mean ES was further calculated. To test for homogeneity of variance among ESs, we calculated the overall I^2 values, which represent the magnitude of heterogeneity where a larger number indicates greater heterogeneity; I^2 values of 25, 50, and 75% are related to low, moderate, and high degrees of heterogeneity, respectively.

Subgroup analyses were performed based on the categorical variables of exercise mode (i.e., Aerobic vs. Other), exercise duration (≥6 months vs. < 6 months), and type of exercise intervention (intradialytic exercise vs. non-intradialytic exercise). These were identified based on clinical relevance and experience with the characteristics of exercise training interventions. The analyses were performed using R version 3.3.0 (R Foundation for Statistical

Computing, Vienna, Austria). In all analyses, $P < 0.05$ was taken to indicate statistical significance [26].

Results

A total of 10,923 references were initially screened, of which 7640 had no duplicates and 7307 were rejected at the title and abstract stage. We then identified 333 studies for potential inclusion and full-text review, and five trials were finally entered into the analysis [27–31] (Fig. 1).

Participants and interventions

The trials included in the analysis are summarized in Table 1. The studies assessed depressive symptoms using the Center for Epidemiologic Studies Depression Questionnaire [27], Self-rating Depression Scale [28, 29], or the Beck Depression Inventory [30, 31]. Three of the studies used an intradialytic exercise program with interventions ranging in duration from 10 weeks to 6 months. Four studies used aerobic training, and one study used a combined exercise program that included calisthenics, steps, flexibility, and low weight resistance training. The interventions were performed two to four times per week in five studies.

Depressive symptoms

Comparison of exercise intervention groups and control groups indicated a small but significant overall standardized mean difference (SMD) = − 0.67 (CI, − 0.97 to − 0.36; $P < 0.001$) under a fixed effects model (Fig. 2). The mean ES was slightly smaller, but still statistically significant, under a random effects model (SMD = − 1.19; CI, − 2.17 to − 0.22; $P < 0.017$).

Subgroup analyses indicated significant reductions in depressive symptoms among hemodialysis patients associated with aerobic exercise and interventions lasting ≥ 6 months ($P = 0.016$, $P < 0.001$, respectively). However, no significant difference was seen in the remedial effects on depressive symptom between intradialytic and pre- or post-dialysis exercise programs (Figs. 3, 4, 5).

Assessment of bias risks

In the studies included in the analysis, the risks of bias were frequently high or unclear (Table 2). The methods used for random sequence generation, patient allocation, and assessor blinding to patient allocation were unclear in all studies. All trials clearly documented no blinding of participants and personnel. The outcome data were incomplete in one study and were reported only selectively in another study. The total TESTEX score, study quality score, and study reporting score of 5 studies were 7.40 ± 0.89, 1.80 ± 0.48, and 5.60 ± 1.14, respectively.

Discussion

The present meta-analysis was performed to determine the efficacy of supervised exercise training for reducing depressive symptoms in hemodialysis patients. The overall analysis tends to that exercise contributed to a reduction in depressive symptoms, and subgroup analyses showed that aerobic exercise and interventions lasting ≥

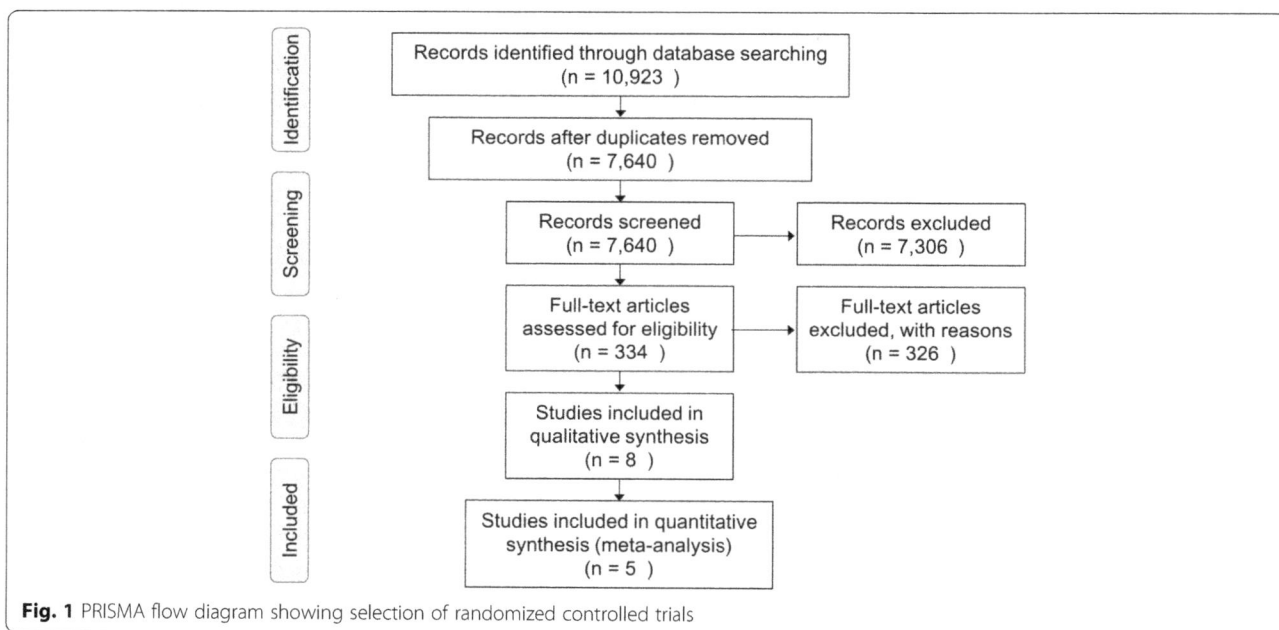

Fig. 1 PRISMA flow diagram showing selection of randomized controlled trials

Table 1 Characteristics of included studies

Studies	Year	Location	Mean age (SD)	Mean duration of dialysis therapy (SD), years	No. in groups (control, training)	Duration of intervention (weeks or months)	Type of intervention in control group	Type of intervention in exercise group	Training program	Intensity of program	Measure
Carmack et al. [26]	1995	USA	All 44.1	No data	Ex 23 Con 25	10 weeks	Usual care	Intradialytic	Aerobic exercise for 20–30 min using cycle ergometer 3 times per week	No data	CES-D
Giannaki et al. [27]	2013	Greece	Ex 56.4 (12.5) Con 55.7 (10.4) Total: no data	Ex 3.9 (1.3) Con 4.0 (1.7) Total: no data	Ex 15 Con 7	6 months	Placebo	Intradialytic	Progressive aerobic exercise training using a recumbent cycle ergometer 3 times a week	60–65% of the patient's maximal exercise capacity (in Watts)	SDS
van Vilsteren et al. [28]	2005	The Netherlands	Ex 52 (15) Con 58 (16)	Ex 3.22 (4.08) years Con 3.90 (4.41) years	Ex 53 Con 43	12 weeks	Usual care	Pre-dialysis strength training Intradialytic Exercise counseling	A 5–10-min warm up and cool down A 20-min exercise program including calisthenics, steps, flexibility, and low weight resistance training Cycling 20–30 min 2–3 times per week Techniques based on the transtheoretical model, motivational interviews, and health counseling	Borg scale 12-16 (< 60% maximal capacity)	SDS
Kouidi et al. [29]	1997	Greece	Ex 49.6 (12.1) Con 52.8 (10.2)	Ex 5.9 (4.9) Con 6.2 (5.4)	Ex 20 Con 11	6 months	Usual care	Non-dialysis days	Supervised exercise (stationary cycling, walking or jogging, calisthenics, aerobics, swimming, and/or game sports) 90 min 3–4 times weekly	50–60% of their VO$_2$max or 60–70% of their HRmax	BDI
Ouzouni et al. [30]	2009	Greece	Ex 47.4 (15.7) Con 50.5 (11.7)	Ex 7.7 (7.0) Con 8.6 (6.0)	Ex 19 Con 14	10 months	Usual care	Intradialytic	60–90 min 3 times weekly (cycling: 30 min; strength training: 30 min; flexibility exercise: 30 min)	Borg scale 13-14 ("somewhat hard")	BDI

SD standard deviation, *Ex* exercise, *Con* control, *CES-D* Center for Epidemiologic Studies Depression Scale, *SDS* Self-rating Depression Scale, *BDI* Beck Depression Inventory

Study	Experimental Total	Mean	SD	Control Total	Mean	SD	SMD	95%-CI	W(fixed)	W(random)
Carmack CL, 1995	10	-5.10	14.3693	11	-3.00	8.5871	-0.17	[-1.03; 0.69]	12.4%	19.9%
Giannaki CD, 2013	15	-8.28	7.9100	7	5.85	6.4100	-1.81	[-2.89; -0.74]	7.9%	18.3%
van Vilsteren Mcba, 2005	53	1.00	11.3897	43	2.40	12.9555	-0.11	[-0.52; 0.29]	56.2%	22.7%
Kouidi E, 1997	20	-7.30	2.1500	11	2.55	4.9400	-2.84	[-3.89; -1.78]	8.2%	18.5%
Ouzouni 2009	19	-7.60	6.0802	14	0.20	5.1856	-1.33	[-2.10; -0.56]	15.4%	20.6%
Fixed effect model	117			86			-0.67	[-0.97; -0.36]	100%	--
Random effects model							-1.19	[-2.17; -0.22]	--	100%

Heterogeneity: I-squared=87.5%, tau-squared=1.049, p<0.0001

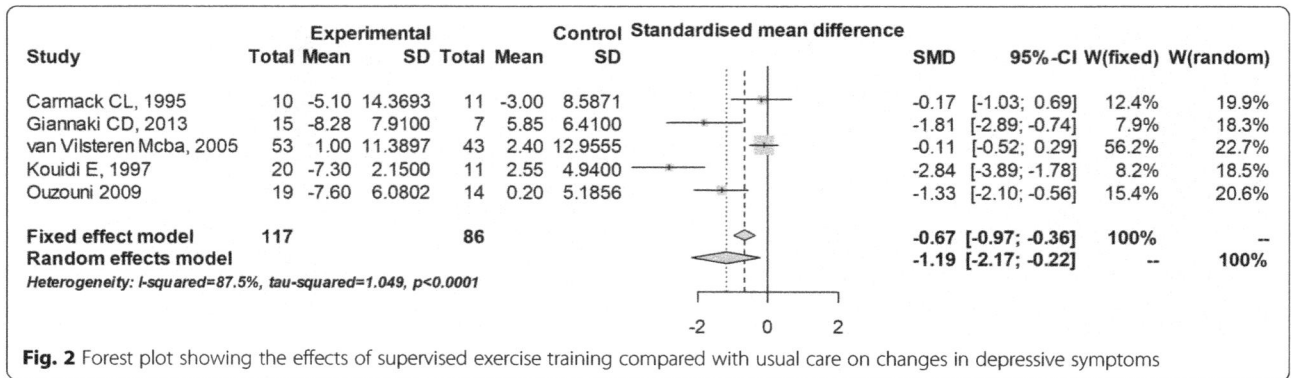

Fig. 2 Forest plot showing the effects of supervised exercise training compared with usual care on changes in depressive symptoms

6 months had greater probabilities of reducing the depressive symptoms in these patients. However, the results of the present study and other high-quality studies are required in order to clarify how exercise affects depressive symptoms in hemodialysis patients. To our knowledge, this is the first systematic review and meta-analysis regarding the efficacy of supervised exercise training for depression in hemodialysis patients taking the forms of exercise used and intervention durations into consideration.

The results presented here were consistent with previous meta-analyses regarding the effects of exercise on depression and depressive symptoms in other populations [32, 33]. A previous meta-analysis of 90 RCTs indicated that exercise reduces depressive symptoms among patients with various chronic illnesses, including chronic obstructive pulmonary disease, cardiovascular, fibromyalgia, multiple sclerosis, cancer, and chronic pain disorder [18]. However, it was unclear whether supervised exercise training could reduce depressive symptoms in hemodialysis patients due to major differences from those in populations including cancer survivors, stroke survivors, those with multiple sclerosis, those with other chronic illnesses, and the population in general. There are obvious differences with respect to age, prevalence of comorbidities, the presence of dialysis-related symptoms, and the overlap between symptoms of advanced kidney disease and those of depression. Therefore, the present study was performed using data from trials conducted only in hemodialysis patients, and our results indicated that, consistent with those in other populations, supervised exercise has a positive effect on depressive symptoms in these patients.

Observations regarding the release of monoamine neurotransmitters (i.e., serotonin, dopamine, and norepinephrine) and endorphins during aerobic exercise provided preliminary mechanistic support for the use of aerobic exercise to reduce and manage depressive symptoms [34, 35], and thus avoiding the common side effects associated with antidepressant medications [36]. Physical activity is associated with improved neurological function, with increased levels of neurotropic factors in the brain and improvements in mood [37]. However,

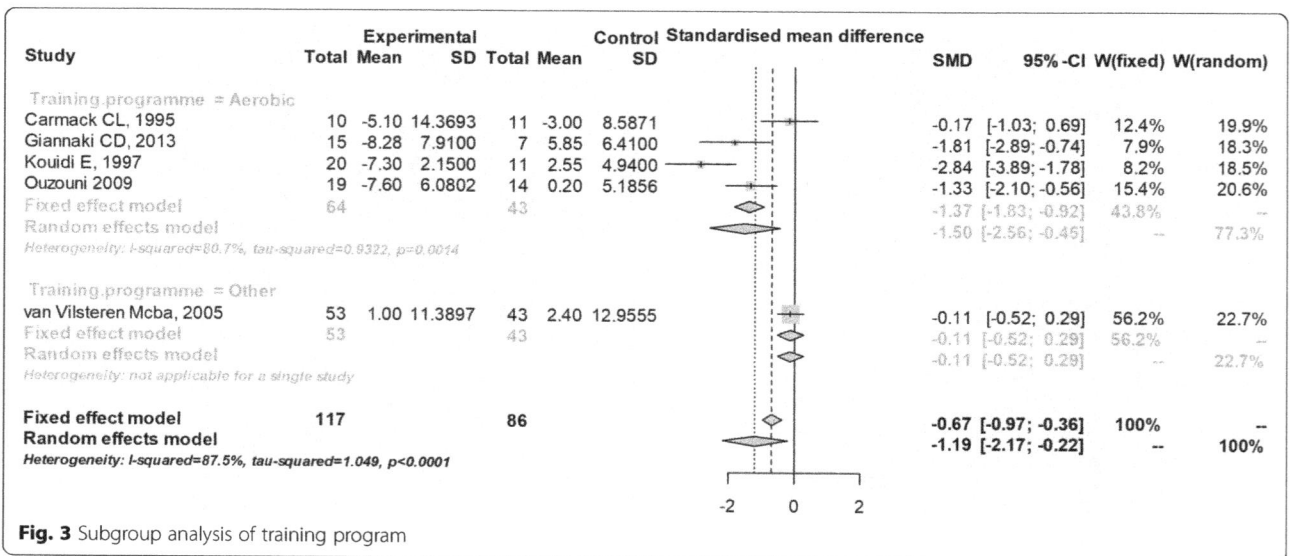

Study	Experimental Total	Mean	SD	Control Total	Mean	SD	SMD	95%-CI	W(fixed)	W(random)
Training.programme = Aerobic										
Carmack CL, 1995	10	-5.10	14.3693	11	-3.00	8.5871	-0.17	[-1.03; 0.69]	12.4%	19.9%
Giannaki CD, 2013	15	-8.28	7.9100	7	5.85	6.4100	-1.81	[-2.89; -0.74]	7.9%	18.3%
Kouidi E, 1997	20	-7.30	2.1500	11	2.55	4.9400	-2.84	[-3.89; -1.78]	8.2%	18.5%
Ouzouni 2009	19	-7.60	6.0802	14	0.20	5.1856	-1.33	[-2.10; -0.56]	15.4%	20.6%
Fixed effect model	64			43			-1.37	[-1.83; -0.92]	43.8%	--
Random effects model							-1.50	[-2.56; -0.45]	--	77.3%

Heterogeneity: I-squared=80.7%, tau-squared=0.9322, p=0.0014

Training.programme = Other										
van Vilsteren Mcba, 2005	53	1.00	11.3897	43	2.40	12.9555	-0.11	[-0.52; 0.29]	56.2%	22.7%
Fixed effect model	53			43			-0.11	[-0.52; 0.29]	56.2%	--
Random effects model							-0.11	[-0.52; 0.29]	--	22.7%

Heterogeneity: not applicable for a single study

Fixed effect model	117			86			-0.67	[-0.97; -0.36]	100%	--
Random effects model							-1.19	[-2.17; -0.22]	--	100%

Heterogeneity: I-squared=87.5%, tau-squared=1.049, p<0.0001

Fig. 3 Subgroup analysis of training program

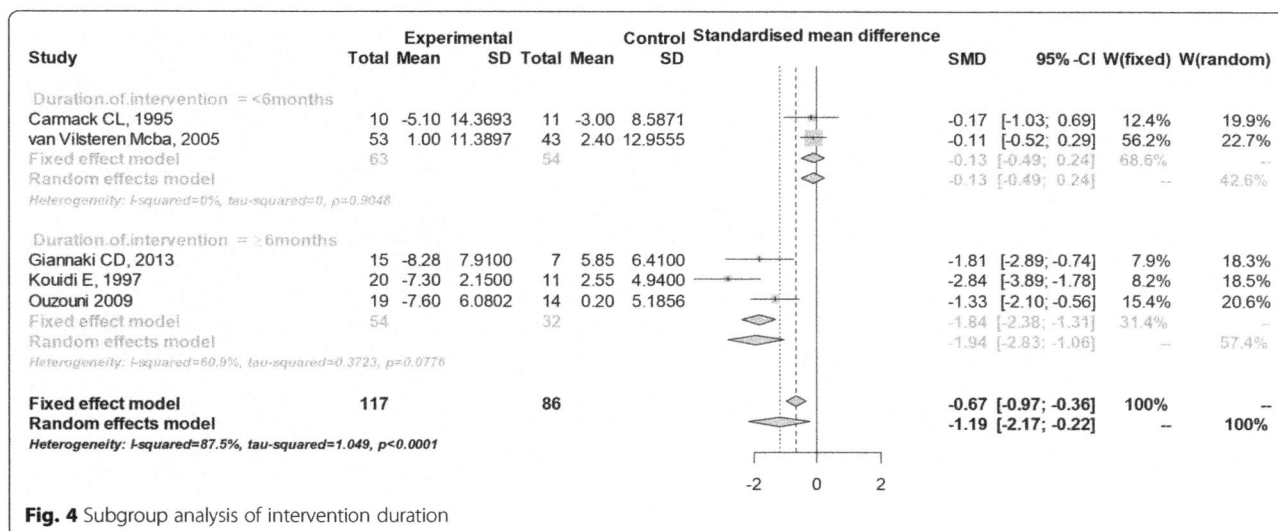

Fig. 4 Subgroup analysis of intervention duration

these hypotheses cannot fully explain the complex physiological and psychosocial etiologies of depressive symptoms, because the studies included in our meta-analysis rarely reported physiological measures. Further studies are therefore needed to examine the mechanisms underlying the exercise-induced reduction of depressive symptoms.

Based on the results of this study, we may be possible to recommend a structured, supervised aerobic exercise program for at least 6 months to manage or reduce depressive symptoms in hemodialysis patients. Exercise programs of 10–16 weeks produced greater effects in the general population than those lasting < 9 weeks [38]. In addition, Craft and Landers reported that interventions of longer duration resulted in greater decreases in depressive scores [39]. Therefore, further studies are required to examine not only the various effects of exercise on outcomes, but also how best to improve adherence to participation in exercise programs and which types of intervention have the greatest efficacy in hemodialysis patients with depressive symptoms.

Many Cochrane reviews have included cases that analyzed low-quality studies. The analysis of the present study ultimately included five studies with high inconsistency, imprecision, and high risk for bias. Implication for practice, we rated the quality of the body of evidence concerning the effects of exercise on depressive symptoms as low. However, this study helped to confirm that further investigation is necessary, as it clarified that the evidence is poor. It will be important for future studies to calculate sample size according to optimal information size and to report the risk of bias with regard to random sequence generation, allocation concealment, incomplete outcome data, selective reporting, and other sources of bias. Finally, we would suggest that many additional studies are required to examine different variables such as exercise mode, exercise duration, and type of exercise intervention.

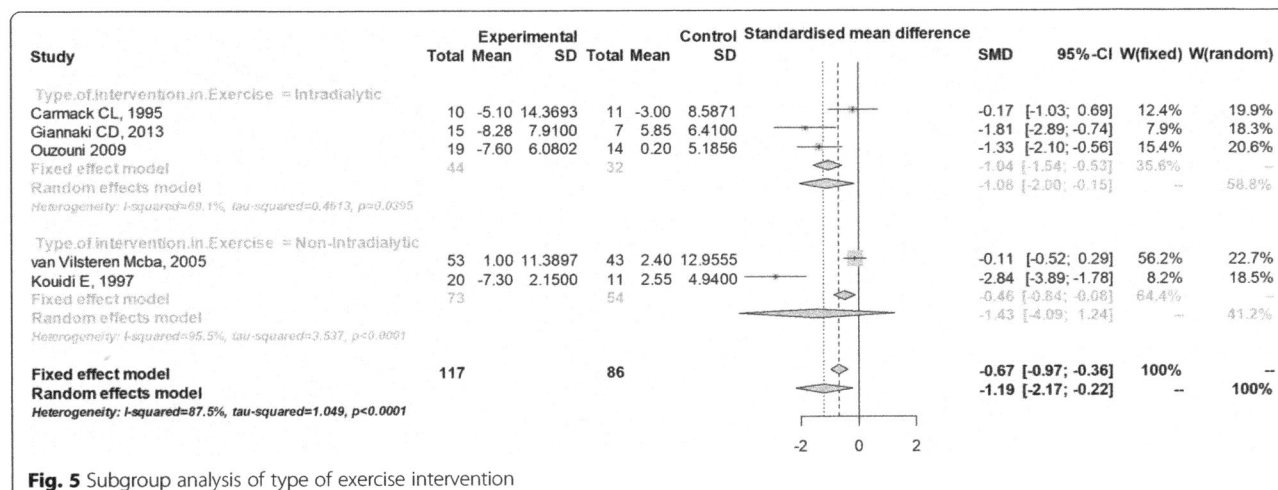

Fig. 5 Subgroup analysis of type of exercise intervention

Table 2 Summary of risk of bias assessment

Studies	Cochrane Collaboration tool							TESTEX		
	Random sequence generation	Allocation concealment	Blinding of participants and personnel	Blinding of outcome assessment	Incomplete outcome data	Selective reporting	Other sources of bias	Total score (15 points)	Study quality score (5 points)	Study reporting score (10 points)
Carmack et al. [26]	Unclear	Unclear	Unclear	Unclear	Unclear	Unclear	Unclear	6	2	4
Giannaki et al. [27]	Unclear	Unclear	High bias	Unclear	Low bias	Low bias	Unclear	7	2	5
van Vilsteren et al. [28]	Unclear	Unclear	Unclear	Unclear	High bias	Unclear	Low bias	8	1	7
Kouidi et al. [29]	Unclear	Unclear	Unclear	Unclear	Unclear	Unclear	Unclear	8	2	6
Ouzouni et al. [30]	Unclear	Unclear	Unclear	Unclear	Unclear	Unclear	Unclear	8	2	6

This study had a number of limitations due to the original studies and the paucity of data. First, the number of eligible studies investigating the associations between exercise and depressive symptoms was small. And we could not assess publish bias. Second, the studies included in the analyses used a number of different methods to evaluate depressive symptoms. Third, the included studies had high degrees of heterogeneity with regard to the exercise interventions (i.e., differences in modality, duration, volume, and intensity). Therefore, additional RCTs are required to establish adequate evidence. Fourth, the studies eligible for the meta-analysis examined the effects only of exercise therapy. Further randomized control trials and meta-analyses are required to evaluate the effects of exercise in hemodialysis patients with high depressive scores in comparison to other treatment modalities, including cognitive-behavioral therapy and antidepressant medication. Bridle et al. suggested that new RCTs should stratify randomization by severity of depression, receipt of antidepressant medications, and/or level of regular exercise [40]. In fact, appropriate antidepressant treatment may be necessary in chronic hemodialysis patients [41, 42].

Conclusions

The meta-analysis found that supervised exercise training tends to alleviate depressive symptoms in hemodialysis patients. As our database search identified only a small number of studies on the association between exercise and depressive symptoms, we would surmise that additional high-quality studies are required to explore further this association.

Abbreviations
CI: Confidence interval; DOPPS: Dialysis Outcomes and Practice Patterns Study; ES: Effect size; PRISMA: Preferred Reporting Items for Systematic Reviews and Meta-Analyses; PROSPERO: International Prospective Register of Systematic Reviews; PRO: Patient-reported outcome; QOL: Quality of life; RCTs: Randomized controlled trials; SDs: Standard deviations; SMD: Standardized mean difference; TESTEX: Tool for the assEssment of Study qualiTy and reporting in EXercise

Acknowledgements
We thank all of the investigators and contributors to our study.

Funding
Funding for this study was provided by Kitasato University Research Grant.

Authors' contributions
TS, RM, KH, and AM contributed to the research idea and study design; TS, RM, KY, MH, and TW contributed to the data acquisition; RM, MH, and TW contributed to the quality assessment of a risk of bias; TS, RM, KH, and AM contributed to the data analysis/interpretation; TS, RM, and KH contributed to the statistical analysis; AM contributed to the supervision or mentorship. Each author contributed important intellectual content during manuscript drafting or revision. All authors read an approved the final manuscript.

Competing interests
The authors declare that they have no competing interests.

Author details
[1]Department of Rehabilitation Sciences, Graduate School of Medical Sciences, Kitasato University, 1-15-1 Kitasato, Sagamihara, Kanagawa 252-0373, Japan. [2]Department of Rehabilitation, Kitasato University Hospital,

Sagamihara, Japan. [3]Department of Hygiene, Kitasato University School of Medicine, Sagamihara, Japan.

References

1. Liyanage T, Ninomiya T, Jha V, et al. Worldwide access to treatment for end-stage kidney disease: a systematic review. Lancet (London, England). 2015;385:1975–82.
2. Lopes AA, Albert JM, Young EW, et al. Screening for depression in hemodialysis patients: associations with diagnosis, treatment, and outcomes in the DOPPS. Kidney Int. 2004;66:2047–53.
3. Kimmel PL. Depression in patients with chronic renal disease: what we know and what we need to know. J Psychosom Res. 2002;53:951–6.
4. Kimmel PL, Peterson RA. Depression in end-stage renal disease patients treated with hemodialysis: tools, correlates, outcomes, and needs. Semin Dial. 2005;18:91–7.
5. Farrokhi F, Abedi N, Beyene J, et al. Association between depression and mortality in patients receiving long-term dialysis: a systematic review and meta-analysis. Am J Kidney Dis. 2014;63:623–35.
6. Fan L, Sarnak MJ, Tighiouart H, et al. Depression and all-cause mortality in hemodialysis patients. Am J Nephrol. 2014;40:12–8.
7. Lopes GB, Matos CM, Leite EB, et al. Depression as a potential explanation for gender differences in health-related quality of life among patients on maintenance hemodialysis. Nephron Clin Pract. 2010;115:c35–40.
8. Weisbord SD, Fried LF, Arnold RM, et al. Prevalence, severity, and importance of physical and emotional symptoms in chronic hemodialysis patients. J Am Soc Nephrol. 2005;16:2487–94.
9. Ma TK, Li PK. Depression in dialysis patients. Nephrology (Carlton, Vic). 2016;21:639–46.
10. Hedayati SS, Yalamanchili V, Finkelstein FO. A practical approach to the treatment of depression in patients with chronic kidney disease and end-stage renal disease. Kidney Int. 2012;81:247–55.
11. Ohtake Y. Psychonephrology in Japan. Ren Replace Ther. 2017;3:25.
12. Catalan-Matamoros D, Gomez-Conesa A, Stubbs B, et al. Exercise improves depressive symptoms in older adults: an umbrella review of systematic reviews and meta-analyses. Psychiatry Res. 2016;244:202–9.
13. Radovic S, Gordon MS, Melvin GA. Should we recommend exercise to adolescents with depressive symptoms? A meta-analysis. J Paediatr Child Health. 2017;53:214–20.
14. Craft LL, Vaniterson EH, Helenowski IB, et al. Exercise effects on depressive symptoms in cancer survivors: a systematic review and meta-analysis. Cancer Epidemiol Biomarkers Prev. 2012;21:3–19.
15. Brown JC, Huedo-Medina TB, Pescatello LS, et al. The efficacy of exercise in reducing depressive symptoms among cancer survivors: a meta-analysis. PLoS One. 2012;7:e30955.
16. Ensari I, Motl RW, Pilutti LA. Exercise training improves depressive symptoms in people with multiple sclerosis: results of a meta-analysis. J Psychosom Res. 2014;76:465–71.
17. Eng JJ, Reime B. Exercise for depressive symptoms in stroke patients: a systematic review and meta-analysis. Clin Rehabil. 2014;28:731–9.
18. Herring MP, Puetz TW, O'Connor PJ, et al. Effect of exercise training on depressive symptoms among patients with a chronic illness: a systematic review and meta-analysis of randomized controlled trials. Arch Intern Med. 2012;172:101–11.
19. Groussard C, Rouchon-Isnard M, Coutard C, et al. Beneficial effects of an intradialytic cycling training program in patients with end-stage kidney disease. Appl Physiol Nutr Metab. 2015;40:550–56.
20. Wu Y, He Q, Yin X, et al. Effect of individualized exercise during maintenance haemodialysis on exercise capacity and health-related quality of life in patients with uraemia. J Int Med Res. 2014;42:718–27.
21. DePaul V, Moreland J, Eager T, et al. The effectiveness of aerobic and muscle strength training in patients receiving hemodialysis and EPO: a randomized controlled trial. Am J Kidney Dis. 2002;40:1219–29.
22. Chen JL, Godfrey S, Ng TT, et al. Effect of intra-dialytic, low-intensity strength training on functional capacity in adult haemodialysis patients: a randomized pilot trial. Nephrol Dial Transplant. 2010;25:1936–43.
23. Matsuzawa R, Hoshi K, Yoneki K, et al. Evaluating the effectiveness of exercise training on elderly patients who require haemodialysis: study
24. Savovic J, Weeks L, Sterne JA, et al. Evaluation of the Cochrane Collaboration's tool for assessing the risk of bias in randomized trials: focus groups, online survey, proposed recommendations and their implementation. Syst Rev. 2014;3:37.
25. Smart NA, Waldron M, Ismail H, et al. Validation of a new tool for the assessment of study quality and reporting in exercise training studies: TESTEX. Int J Evid Based Healthc. 2015;13:9–18.
26. Kanda Y. Investigation of the freely available easy-to-use software 'EZR' for medical statistics. Bone Marrow Transplant. 2013;48:452–8.
27. Carmack CL, Amaral-Melendez M, Boudreaux E, et al. Exercise as a component in the physical and psychological rehabilitation of hemodialysis patients. Int J Rehabilitation Health. 1995;1:13–23.
28. Giannaki CD, Sakkas GK, Karatzaferi C, et al. Effect of exercise training and dopamine agonists in patients with uremic restless legs syndrome: a six-month randomized, partially double-blind, placebo-controlled comparative study. BMC Nephrol. 2013;14 Epub
29. van Vilsteren M, de Greef MHG, Huisman RM. The effects of a low-to-moderate intensity pre-conditioning exercise programme linked with exercise counselling for sedentary haemodialysis patients in The Netherlands: results of a randomized clinical trial. Nephrology Dialysis Transplantation. 2005;20:141–6.
30. Kouidi E, Iacovides A, Iordanidis P, et al. Exercise renal rehabilitation program: psychosocial effects. Nephron. 1997;77:152–8.
31. Ouzouni S, Kouidi E, Sioulis A, et al. Effects of intradialytic exercise training on health-related quality of life indices in haemodialysis patients. Clin Rehabil. 2009;23:53–63.
32. Conn VS. Depressive symptom outcomes of physical activity interventions: meta-analysis findings. Ann Behav Med. 2010;39:128–38.
33. Dalgas U, Stenager E, Sloth M, et al. The effect of exercise on depressive symptoms in multiple sclerosis based on a meta-analysis and critical review of the literature. Eur J Neurol. 2015;22:443–e434.
34. Brosse AL, Sheets ES, Lett HS, et al. Exercise and the treatment of clinical depression in adults: recent findings and future directions. Sports Med. 2002;32:741–60.
35. Thoren P, Floras JS, Hoffmann P, et al. Endorphins and exercise: physiological mechanisms and clinical implications. Med Sci Sports Exerc. 1990;22:417–28.
36. Papakostas GI. Tolerability of modern antidepressants. J Clin Psychiatry. 2008;69(Suppl E1):8–13.
37. Greenwood BN, Fleshner M. Exercise, stress resistance, and central serotonergic systems. Exerc Sport Sci Rev. 2011;39:140–9.
38. Rethorst CD, Wipfli BM, Landers DM. The antidepressive effects of exercise: a meta-analysis of randomized trials. Sports Med. 2009;39:491–511.
39. Craft L, Landers D. The effect of exercise on clinical depression and depression resulting from mental illness: a meta-analysis. J Sport Exerc Psychol. 1998;20:339–57.
40. Bridle C, Spanjers K, Patel S, et al. Effect of exercise on depression severity in older people: systematic review and meta-analysis of randomised controlled trials. Br J Psychiatry. 2012;201:180–5.
41. Finkelstein FO, Finkelstein SH. Depression in chronic dialysis patients: assessment and treatment. Nephrol Dial Transplant. 2000;15:1911–3.
42. Koo JR, Yoon JY, Joo MH, et al. Treatment of depression and effect of antidepression treatment on nutritional status in chronic hemodialysis patients. Am J Med Sci. 2005;329:1–5.

protocol for a systematic review and meta-analysis. BMJ Open. 2016;6: e010990.

20

Comparison of two polysulfone membranes for continuous renal replacement therapy for sepsis: a prospective cross-over study

Hideto Yasuda[1,2,3]* , Kosuke Sekine[4], Takayuki Abe[3,5], Shinichiro Suzaki[2], Atsushi Katsumi[2], Naoshige Harada[2], Hidenori Higashi[2], Yuki Kishihara[2], Hidetaka Suzuki[2] and Toru Takebayashi[3]

Abstract

Background: In Japan, the most commonly used hemofilters for patients with acute kidney injury (AKI) treated with continuous renal replacement therapy (CRRT) are made of polysulfone membranes. The aim of this study was to compare the efficacy of two commercially available polysulfone membranes for the removal of solutes.

Methods: This single-institution, prospective cross-over study was conducted between December 2010 and January 2012. Two polysulfone membranes, Hemofeel SHG (Toray) and Excelflo AEF (Asahi Kasei Medical), were compared in eight intensive care unit patients (median age, 80 years; seven men) who had severe sepsis that required CRRT and who required vasopressor treatment to maintain their mean blood pressure above 65 mmHg. The primary outcome measure was the efficacy of solute removal, evaluated for high-mobility group protein 1 (HMGB-1) and myoglobin.

Results: The main cause of sepsis was abdominal infection (50%); the mortality was 62.5%. Blood clearance of myoglobin in 1 h was significantly greater with SHG ($p = 0.02$), particularly at 24 h ($p = 0.17$). Blood creatinine clearance did not differ significantly between the two membranes after 1 h, but SHG demonstrated slightly greater appearance at 24 h. There were no significant differences between the two membranes in the clearance of other solutes including HMGB-1.

Conclusions: This preliminary study compared the use of two polysulfone membranes in patients with sepsis requiring CRRT and showed that the polysulfone membrane SHG was capable of removing myoglobin with greater efficacy.

Keywords: Acute kidney injury, Membranes, Myoglobin, Renal replacement therapy, Sepsis, Shock

Background

In Japan, the most commonly used hemofilters for patients with acute kidney injury (AKI) who are undergoing treatment for continuous renal replacement therapy (CRRT) are made of polysulfone membranes [1]. Sepsis is a life-threatening condition with a prevalence of 288 hospital-treated sepsis cases per 100,00 person years; in-hospital mortality has been reported as 17% for sepsis and 26% for severe sepsis [2]. The progression of AKI stage and newly developed AKI after hospital admission in patients with severe sepsis and septic shock increased 28-day mortality [3]. CRRT is used not only for hemodynamically

unstable patients with AKI and chronic kidney disease (CKD), such as for correcting electrolyte and acid–base balance abnormalities or removing solutes and extra fluid, but also for patients suffering from severe sepsis and septic shock, to remove various inflammatory cytokines [4, 5]. However, CRRT is often performed under more limited treatment conditions than those for intermittent renal replacement therapy (IRRT) in critically ill patients [4, 6–8]. Unlike IRRT, there are restrictions on blood and dialysate flow rates in CRRT, and its efficiency is often influenced by the dialysis membrane used.

The solute removal efficacy during renal replacement therapy depends not only on blood flow rate, dialysate flow rate, and solute concentration, but also on the dialysis membrane used [9]. Several types of CRRT dialysis membranes have been developed over the history of hemodialysis therapy, and these differ in their ability to

* Correspondence: yasudahideto@me.com
[1]Department of Intensive Care Unit, Kameda Medical Center, 929 Higashi-chou, Kamogawa-shi, Chiba 296-8602, Japan
[2]Intensive Care Unit, Department of Emergency and Critical Care Medicine, Japanese Red Cross Musashino Hospital, Tokyo, Japan
Full list of author information is available at the end of the article

remove solutes [10–16]. This depends on the membrane's composition and morphology, such as its inner diameter, the pore size (either radius or diameter), thickness of the skin layer, and the surface porosity of membrane. These differences may affect the blood concentrations of several drugs, including antibiotics, and so clinical outcome can be influenced by both the type of dialysis and the dialysis membrane used [17, 18]. There is one study on the removal of solutes by membranes such as high flux membranes [19], but, as yet, differences in dialysis efficacy between different polysulfone membranes have not been reported. The aim of this study was to compare the efficacy of solute removal of two commercially available polysulfone membranes mostly used in Japan.

Methods

Study design and setting

This prospective cross-over study was conducted in an eight-bed intensive care unit (ICU) at a single center of the Advanced Emergency Medical Center in Japan (Japanese Red Cross Musashino Hospital, Tokyo, Japan) between December 2010 and January 2012. This study protocol was approved by the local ethics committee, and the study was conducted in accordance with the principles of the Helsinki Declaration. Informed consent was obtained from all the participants or their surrogate decisionmakers. This study is described according to the Strengthening the Reporting of Observational Studies (STROBE) guidelines.

Subjects

Patients were eligible for inclusion in this study if they were in severe sepsis or septic shock, in need of CRRT, admitted to ICU, and needing a vasopressor to maintain their mean blood pressure at over 65 mmHg (within a suitable range). The definitions of sepsis, severe sepsis, and septic shock followed those of the American College of Chest Physicians and the Society of Critical Care Medicine [20]. The criteria for the initiation of CRRT were the following: (1) uncontrolled acidosis, (2) uremia, (3) uncontrolled hyperkalemia, and (4) volume overload. Patients were excluded from this study if they were younger than 15 years, pregnant, their physician decided they should be excluded, or they did not agree to participate.

During the study period, eight patients who met these criteria were included in the study. Seven were men and the median age was 80 years (interquartile range (IQR) 76–81 years).

Operational conditions for CRRT

Two polysulfone membranes, Hemofeel SHG 1.3 m^2 (SHG; Toray, Tokyo, Japan) and Excelflo AEF 1.3 m^2 (AEF; Asahi Kasei Medical, Tokyo, Japan) were used for

CRRT in this study (Table 1). To create the vascular access, ICU physicians inserted a 12-Fr flexible triple-lumen catheter (GamCath Catheter, Baxter, Japan) into the internal jugular or the femoral vein, if the patient did not have shunt for hemodialysis. The operation of the hemodiafiltration system was monitored with a personal bedside console (ACH-10 Asahi Kasei Medical, Tokyo, Japan). The CRRT mode used was continuous venovenous hemodiafiltration as follows: blood flow, 100 mL/min; dialysate, substitution solution and filtrate flow rates, all 400 mL/h. We used nafamostat mesilate for anticoagulation, with a protocol that maintained the activated partial thromboplastin time (APTT) at 60–80 s. The decision about whether to remove water by CRRT was left to the discretion of the individual physicians.

Study protocol and data collection

The study protocol is shown in Fig. 1. In this cross-over protocol, the patients underwent CRRT with either the SHG or the AEF hemofilter for 24 h, and this was then replaced with the other type for a further 24 h. Blood and effluent samples were drawn from the inlet and outlet of the hemofilter at the start of CRRT and after 1, 24, 25, and 48 h. The following data were recorded for each time point: vital signs (Glasgow Coma Scale score, mean arterial pressure, heart rate, respiratory rate, body temperature, and urine volume), the vasopressor dose (dopamine, dobutamine, noradrenaline, adrenaline, and vasopressin), blood sample results (white and red blood cell counts, hematocrit, platelet count, sodium, potassium, bilirubin, urea, creatinine, creatine kinase, myoglobin, and HMGB-1), and arterial blood gas analysis results (fraction of inspiratory oxygen, pH, PaO$_2$, HCO$_3$, and lactate). The following data were obtained for each subject: age, sex, comorbidity, date of hospital admission, date of ICU admission, acute physiology, and chronic health evaluation (APACHE) II score, sequential organ failure assessment (SOFA) score on the day of ICU admission, and primary diagnosis at the time they were included in this study. In addition, the date of ICU discharge and the patient's outcome (discharge alive or death in hospital) were recorded.

Table 1 Comparison of SHG and AEF

	SHG	AEF
Membrane manufacturer	Toray Medical Co. Ltd., Tokyo, Japan	Asahi Kasei Medical, Tokyo, Japan
Hemofilter	Polysulfone membrane	Polysulfone membrane
Membrane surface area, m^2	1.3	1.3
Inside diameter, μm	200	225
Thickness of membrane, μm	40	45

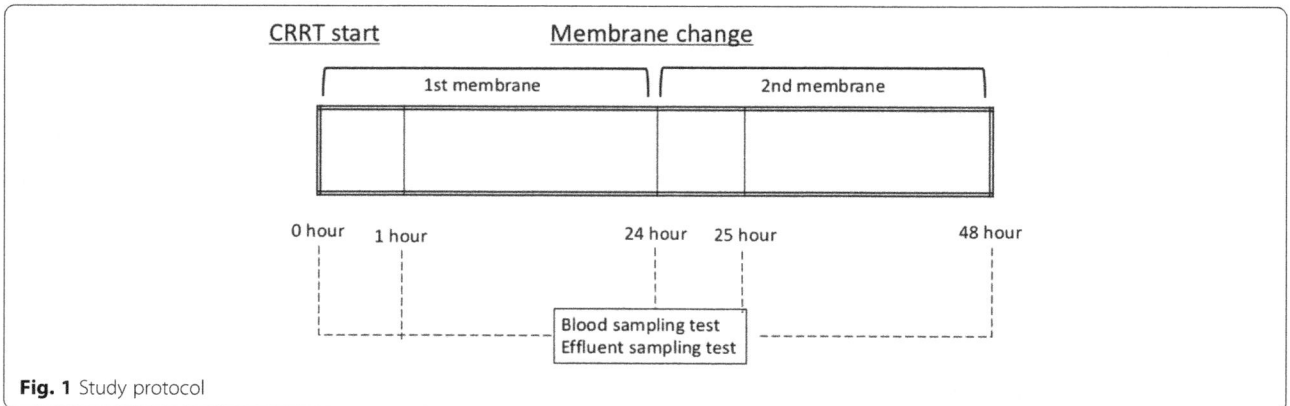

Fig. 1 Study protocol

Calculations

Blood clearance (Kb) and effluent clearance (KE) were calculated for each solute using the following formulas:

$$Kb = \{(QBin \times CBin)-(QBin-QF) \times CBout\}/CBin$$

$$KE = (CE/CBin) \times (QDin + QF)$$

where QBin, QDin, and QF are the inlet blood flow rate, inlet dialysate flow rate, and filtration rate of the hemofilter, respectively, CBin and CBout are the plasma concentrations of the solute in inlet and outlet blood of the hemofilter, and CE is the concentration of the effluent dialysate of the hemofilter.

Outcome measures

The primary outcome measure was the removal efficacy for the medium-sized solute molecules myoglobin and HMGB-1 between two membrane types. The secondary outcome was its efficacy for removing small and other medium-sized solute molecules.

Statistical analysis

The data are presented as mean and standard deviation (SD) or median with interquartile range (IQR) for continuous variables and as number and percentages for categorical variables. Paired *t* tests and the mixed-effect model were used for comparisons between the membranes for the clearance of solutes and to investigate the possible carry-over effect of the hemofilter, using Holm's procedure. Mean differences with 95% confidence intervals were also calculated. No missing data were imputed; if any cases were lost to follow-up, they were to be excluded. The significance level for all tests was two-sided 5%. All statistical analyses except for the mixed-effect model were performed using JMP software, version 11 (SAS Inc., Cary, NC); the mixed-effect model was performed using SAS (SAS Inc., Cary, NC).

Results

The demographic characteristics of the eight patients are shown in Tables 2 and 3. In four patients (50%), the cause of sepsis was abdominal infection; five of the patients (63%) died. There was no case of loss to follow-up.

Figures 2 and 3 show the results for each of the two membranes for blood clearance and effluent clearance of each solute at 1 and 24 h after the start of CRRT using the SHG and AEF membranes. There were no significant differences in the blood clearance of blood urea, creatine kinase, and HMGB-1 in 1 or 24 h. However, the blood clearance of myoglobin in 1 h was significantly higher when using the SHG membrane (mean difference, 8.0 ml/min; 95% CI 1.8 to 14.1 ml/min; $p = 0.02$). Over 24 h, blood clearance with the SHG membrane tended to be higher, but the difference did not achieve statistical significance (mean difference, 7.4 ml/min; 95% CI – 4.1 to 18.7 ml/min; $p = 0.17$). The blood clearance of creatinine showed the opposite tendency, with no significant difference in 1 h (mean difference, – 2.0 ml/min; 95% CI – 6.2 to 2.2 ml/min; $p = 0.29$) but slightly higher clearance with SHG in 24 h (mean difference 3.6 ml/min; 95% CI 0.6 to 6.6 ml/min; $p = 0.02$). Effluent clearance showed similar results to blood clearance: the effluent clearance of myoglobin in 1 h was significantly higher with SHG than that with AEF (mean difference, 1.0 ml/min; 95% CI 0.60 to 1.41 ml/min; $p < 0.01$).

No significant difference was found between the SHG and AEF membranes in the change of clearance between 1 and 24 h after the start of CRRT, except for the blood clearance of creatinine (mean difference, 5.6 ml/min; 95% CI 1.7 to 9.5 ml/min, $p = 0.01$) (Table 4). However, although there was a significant difference in the change of blood clearance for creatinine from 1 to 24 h after the start of CRRT between the two types of membrane, the difference was negligible.

There was no carry-over effect due to the difference in membrane in any solute, except for the effluent clearance of creatinine in 24 h (Table 5).

Table 2 Patient characteristics

	Total (n = 8)	SHG → AEF (n = 4)	AEF → SHG (n = 4)
Age, median (IQR), years	80 (76–81)	80 (78–83)	78 (74–81)
Gender, male (number, %)	7 (87.5%)	3 (75%)	4 (100%)
Height, median (IQR), cm	167 (153–170)	167 (149–172)	166 (153–170)
Weight, median (IQR), kg	56 (46–71)	51 (44–58)	65 (48–82)
Body mass index, median (IQR), kg/m²	20.5 (15.1–25.6)	17.1 (14.4–20.9)	25.2 (19.1–28.5)
Source of sepsis, n, (%)			
Intrathoracic	2 (25%)	1 (25%)	1 (25%)
Intraabdominal	4 (50%)	3 (75%)	1 (25%)
Urogenital	1 (25%)	0 (0%)	1 (25%)
Skin/soft tissue/bone/joint	1 (25%)	0 (0%)	1 (25%)
APACHE II score, median (IQR)	21 (16–26)	23 (14–28)	19 (16–25)
SOFA score, median (IQR)	11 (9–13)	12 (10–14)	10 (8–13)
ICU stay, median (IQR), day	4.5 (4.0–27.8)	7 (4.3–30.8)	4.0 (4.0–26.5)
Hospital mortality, n, (%)	5 (62.5%)	3 (75%)	2 (50%)
Acute kidney injury, n, (%)	3 (37.5%)	1 (25%)	2 (50%)
Lactate, median (IQR), mg/dL	34.7 (19.0–65.7)	45.7 (27.3–65.7)	22.0 (15.0–181.1)
Procalcitonin, median (IQR), ng/mL	5.2 (3.8–17.2)	12.8 (4.8–46.7)	4.2 (1.5–8.3)
Glasgow Coma Scale, median (IQR)	13 (6–15)	10 (4–15)	14 (8–15)
Noradrenaline, median (IQR), μg/kg/min	0.3 (0.2–0.35)	0.28 (0.20–0.47)	0.30 (0.11–0.4)

Data are presented as median (IQR) or n (%)
APACHE acute physiology and chronic health evaluation, *SOFA* sequential organ failure assessment, *ICU* intensive care unit, *IQR* interquartile range

Discussion

The results of this study showed that the use of the SHG membrane resulted in higher blood clearance of myoglobin and creatinine than using the AEF membrane. There was no difference between the two types of membrane in the clearance of other solutes, and no carry-over effect was observed for any solute.

Few such studies involving CRRT have been reported. One study in critically ill patients with acute renal failure treated with CRRT investigated solute clearance and compared different kinds of membranes [11]. It reported that some dialysis membranes produced high creatinine and bicarbonate clearance, but it did not statistically verify the differences in clearance. In general, though,

Table 3 Baseline serum parameters in each homofilter

Serum parameters	Total (n = 8)	SHG → AEF (n = 4)	AEF → SHG (n = 4)
PaO₂/FiO₂ ratio, Torr	260 (180–375)	260 (191–273)	309 (171–456)
pH	7.38 (7.26–7.44)	7.40 (7.31–7.50)	7.32 (7.22–7.43)
Bicarbonate	18.9 (16.7–23.7)	18.7 (16.7–21.3)	21.0 (12.1–35.9)
Bilirubin, mmol/L	0.8 (0.2–1.6)	1.1 (0.3–1.6)	0.5 (0.2–2.7)
Creatinine, mg/dL (μmol/L)	2.3 (1.3–3.3)	1.8 (0.9–2.5)	2.9 (1.5–4.8)
Urea, mg/dL	66 (33–76)	51 (23–79)	70 (41–76)
Sodium, mEq/L	142 (136–147)	142 (137–142)	143 (136–150)
Potassium, mEq/L	4.0 (3.1–4.6)	3.5 (3.1–4.4)	4.3 (3.3–5.6)
Creatine kinase, IU/L	618 (117–1319)	871 (203–3717)	512 (100–974)
Myoglobin, ng/ml	3059 (478–6528)	3609 (1242–11,901)	1745 (389–6253)
HMGB-1, ng/ml	6.9 (5.6–13.0)	9.2 (6.4–13.0)	5.7 (4.8–85.4)
Hematocrit, %	30.8 (25.1–36.4)	34.0 (26.5–37.6)	28.0 (25.1–33.3)
Plate count, 10³/μL	9.8 (7.6–16.3)	9.2 (6.9–14.5)	13.2 (7.8–21.0)

Data are presented as median (IQR) or n (%)
HMGB-1 high mobility group box-1, *IQR* interquartile rang

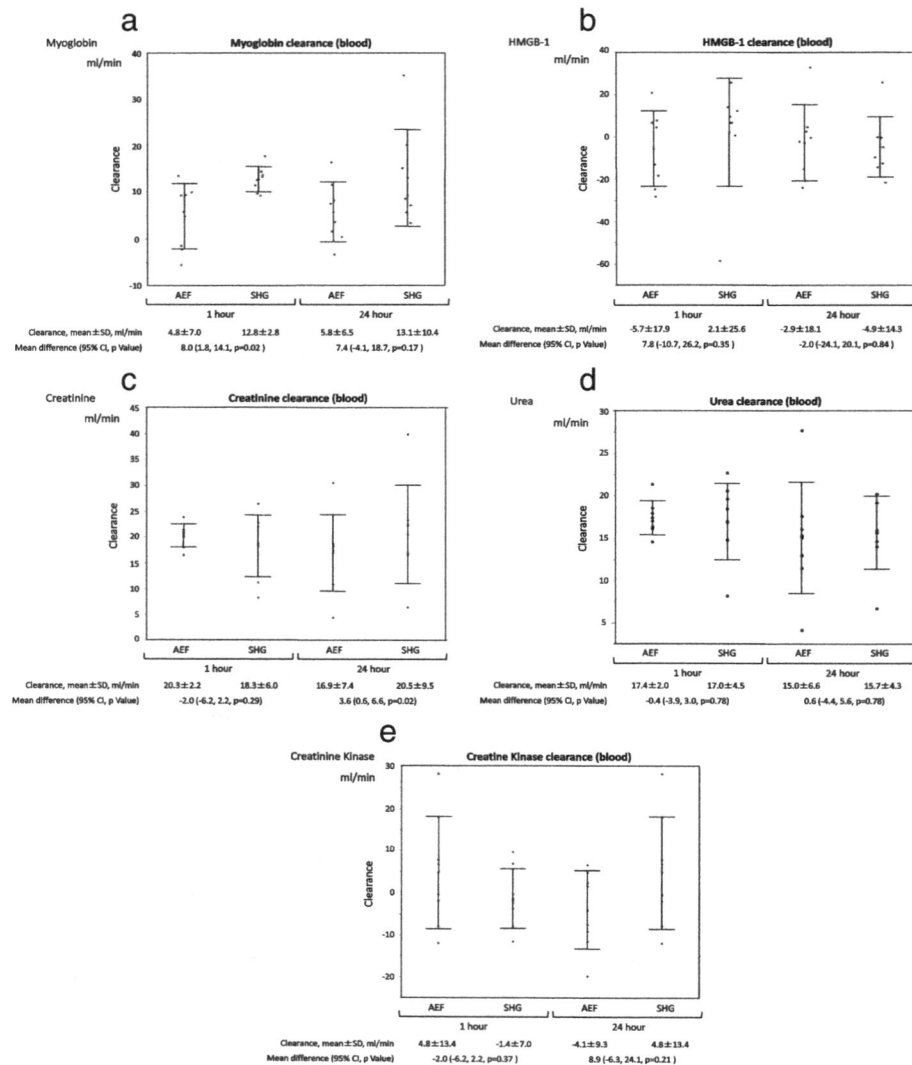

Fig. 2 Comparison between the two membranes (SHG and AEF) of the blood clearance of various solutes. **a** Myoglobin, **b** HMGB-1, **c** creatinine, **d** urea, and **e** creatine kinase

most studies of dialysis membranes so far have reported results obtained during IRRT with maintenance dialysis patients. The results of such studies cannot be applied to the membranes used during CRRT for patients in the acute phase. Unlike CRRT, the solute removal during IRRT depends not only on the dialysis membrane but also on the blood and dialysate flow rates. However, in Japan, the dialysate flow rate during CRRT is less than 5% of that during IRRT [21], and so the dialysis membrane makes a greater difference to dialysis efficiency with CRRT. Thus, the results of comparisons of dialysis membranes made during IRRT cannot be directly applied to membranes used in CRRT.

However, there have not previously been any studies that compared the solute removal efficacy of dialysis

membranes, particularly polysulfone membranes, during CRRT. The present study, for the first time, compared the use of two dialysis membranes with patients and showed that SHG had a significantly higher ability than AEF to remove myoglobin and creatinine. However, because there has been no other study that compared polysulfone membranes in patients, these differences cannot yet be concluded. Nor is it possible to clarify the mechanism underlying the differences between the two membranes from the results of this study. All commercial polysulfone membranes include different amounts of and different kinds of polyvinylpyrrolidon as a hydrophilic agent. One possible explanation is structural differences between the two types of membrane, such as inside diameters of the hollow fiber, effective length of

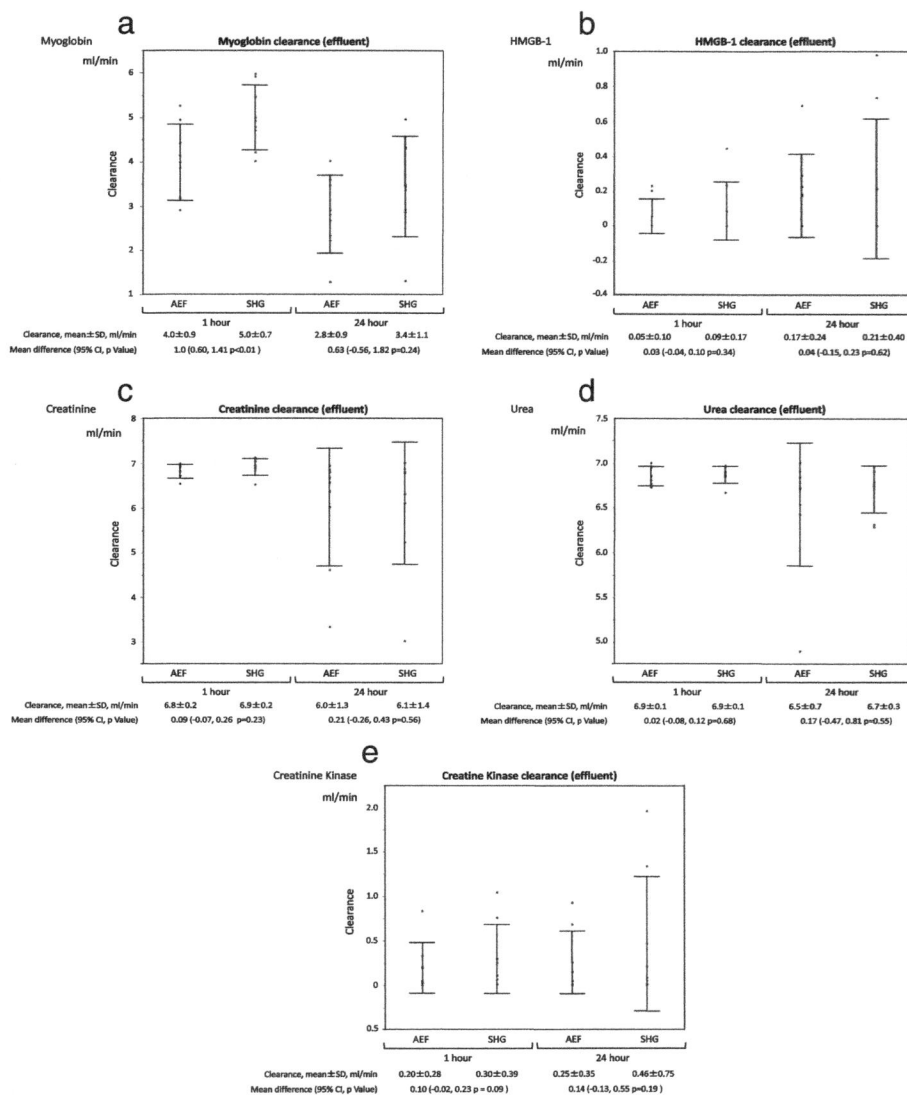

a Myoglobin, ml/min — Myoglobin clearance (effluent)

	1 hour		24 hour	
	AEF	SHG	AEF	SHG
Clearance, mean±SD, ml/min	4.0±0.9	5.0±0.7	2.8±0.9	3.4±1.1
Mean difference (95% CI, p Value)	1.0 (0.60, 1.41 p<0.01)		0.63 (-0.56, 1.82 p=0.24)	

b HMGB-1, ml/min — HMGB-1 clearance (effluent)

	1 hour		24 hour	
	AEF	SHG	AEF	SHG
Clearance, mean±SD, ml/min	0.05±0.10	0.09±0.17	0.17±0.24	0.21±0.40
Mean difference (95% CI, p Value)	0.03 (-0.04, 0.10 p=0.34)		0.04 (-0.15, 0.23 p=0.62)	

c Creatinine, ml/min — Creatinine clearance (effluent)

	1 hour		24 hour	
	AEF	SHG	AEF	SHG
Clearance, mean±SD, ml/min	6.8±0.2	6.9±0.2	6.0±1.3	6.1±1.4
Mean difference (95% CI, p Value)	0.09 (-0.07, 0.26 p=0.23)		0.21 (-0.26, 0.43 p=0.56)	

d Urea, ml/min — Urea clearance (effluent)

	1 hour		24 hour	
	AEF	SHG	AEF	SHG
Clearance, mean±SD, ml/min	6.9±0.1	6.9±0.1	6.5±0.7	6.7±0.3
Mean difference (95% CI, p Value)	0.02 (-0.08, 0.12 p=0.68)		0.17 (-0.47, 0.81 p=0.55)	

e Creatinine Kinase, ml/min — Creatine Kinase clearance (effluent)

	1 hour		24 hour	
	AEF	SHG	AEF	SHG
Clearance, mean±SD, ml/min	0.20±0.28	0.30±0.39	0.25±0.35	0.46±0.75
Mean difference (95% CI, p Value)	0.10 (-0.02, 0.23 p = 0.09)		0.14 (-0.13, 0.55 p=0.19)	

Fig. 3 Comparison between the two membranes (SHG and AEF) of the effluent clearances of various solutes. **a** Myoglobin, **b** HMGB-1, **c** creatinine, **d** urea, and **e** creatine kinase

the module, thickness of the skin layer, the pore size (either radius or diameter), and the surface porosity of the membrane, as well as the difference in chemical composition between them [22, 23]. The physicochemical heterogeneity provided by the hydrophilic–hydrophobic microdomains present at the surface of the SHG membrane impedes the formation of stable hydrophobic interactions between the various solutes and the membrane surface. Medium-sized molecules may be more susceptible than small molecules to this physicochemical heterogeneity, which may explain why there were no differences between the two membranes in this study in the clearance of small-molecule solutes. However, this is no more than a hypothesis, and a future study is needed to confirm it.

According to the results of the present study, SHG may provide better dialysis efficiency for the removal of medium-sized molecules, which may result in a decrease in the number of dialyzers needed and the dialysis time; this in turn may lead to a reduction in dialysis costs. This may be advantageous not only for health care workers but also for patients and stakeholders.

This study had several limitations. First, it included only eight patients and 16 dialysis membranes and was conducted in single center; the sample size was therefore not optimal for comparing solute clearance between two membranes. It is possible that a large difference in solute removal could not be recognized between the two dialysis membranes. Second, in this study, statistically significant differences in myoglobin clearance were observed

Table 4 Change of clearance in 24 h

	SHG	AEF	Mean difference	95% CI	p value
Blood clearance					
Myoglobin, median (IQR), ml/min	0.3 (− 9.0, 9.6)	1.0 (− 5.1, 7.0)	− 0.63	− 12.8, 11.6	0.91
HMGB-1, median (IQR), ml/min	− 7.0 (−27.0, 13.1)	2.8 (− 18.3, 23,9)	− 9.7	− 38.7, 19.3	0.45
Creatinine, median (IQR), ml/min	2.2 (− 4.6, 9.0)	− 3.4 (− 9.8, 3.1)	5.6	1.7, 9.5	0.012
Urea, median (IQR), ml/min	− 1.3 (− 2.5, − 0.2)	− 2.4 (− 7.9, 3.2)	1.1	− 4.5, 6.6	0.67
Creatine kinase, median (IQR), ml/min	6.2 (− 7.7, 20.1)	− 8.9 (− 24.1, 6.3)	15.1	− 13.4, 43.6	0.25
Effluent clearance					
Myoglobin, median (IQR), ml/min	− 1.55 (− 2.59, − 0.52)	− 1.18 (− 1.63, − 0.73)	− 0.38	− 1.65, 0.90	0.51
HMGB-1, median (IQR), ml/min	0.13 (− 0.07, 0.33)	0.12 (− 0.03, 0,27)	0.01	− 1.57, 0.18	0.90
Creatinine, median (IQR), ml/min	− 0.81 (− 1.96, 0.35)	− 0.80 (− 1.06, 0.35)	− 0.01	− 0.29, 0.28	0.97
Urea, median (IQR), ml/min	− 0.16 (− 0.42, 0.10)	− 0.31 (− 0.86, 0.24)	0.15	− 0.44, 0.74	0.56
Creatine kinase, median (IQR), ml/min	0.17 (− 0.14, 0.48)	− 0.06 (− 0.05, 0.17)	0.11	− 0.15, 0.36	0.36

HMGB-1 high mobility group box-1, *IQR* interquartile range, *CI* confidence interval

between the two membranes, but it is unclear whether this difference was clinically important. It may be possible to evaluate the effectiveness of the membrane by verifying how much the solute concentration has decreased after a certain time has elapsed. However, rather than basing the evaluation on the change in solute

Table 5 Carry-over effect

		p value
Blood clearance		
Clearance 1 h	Myoglobin	0.56
	HMGB-1	0.30
	Creatinine	0.60
	Urea	0.99
	Creatine kinase	0.54
Clearance 24 h	Myoglobin	0.56
	HMGB-1	0.81
	Creatinine	0.61
	Urea	0.69
	Creatine kinase	0.71
Effluent clearance		
Clearance 1 h	Myoglobin	0.67
	HMGB-1	0.72
	Creatinine	0.84
	Urea	0.07
	Creatine kinase	0.23
Clearance 24 h	Myoglobin	0.77
	HMGB-1	0.99
	Creatinine	0.01
	Urea	0.26
	Creatine kinase	0.23

HMGB-1 high mobility group box-1

concentration before and after using the membrane, one problem with this method is that the solute concentration may be influenced by the patient's residual renal function and underlying disease. It would therefore not be possible to estimate the performance of the dialysis membrane unconditionally. Finally, the types of solute examined in this study may not have been sufficient to verify the difference in clearance between the two membranes. For example, we did not consider solutes such as β2 microglobulin or inflammatory cytokines, which have been well validated in recent years [24–26]. However, we examined the difference in the clearance of HMGB-1, which has been the focus of attention in recent years, and reported a difference between the two polysulfone membranes in its clearance. There has been no previous report on the clearance of HMGB-1 in polysulfone membranes, and so the usefulness of HMGB-1 is not known. Because the clearance of this solute is also influenced by the protein binding rate, its clearance is not necessarily constant. Thus, there is a possibility that the differences between the membranes may be underestimated.

Conclusions
In conclusion, this preliminary study comparing the use of two polysulfone membranes in patients with sepsis requiring CRRT and showed that the SHG membrane was capable of removing myoglobin with greater efficacy then the AEF membrane. However, it remains unclear whether the differences were clinically meaningful, and further study is needed.

Abbreviations
AKI: Acute kidney injury; APACHE: Acute physiology, and chronic health evaluation; APTT: Activated partial thromboplastin time; CI: Confidence interval; CKD: Chronic kidney disease; CRRT: Continuous renal replacement therapy; HMGB-1: High-mobility group protein 1; ICU: Intensive care unit; IQR: Interquartile range; IRRT: Intermittent renal replacement therapy;

SD: Standard deviation; SOFA: Sequential organ failure assessment; STROBE: Strengthening the Reporting of Observational Studies

Acknowledgements
The authors would like to thank all study participants.
The authors would like to thank Enago (www.enago.jp) for the English language review.

Funding
This study was supported by Toray Medical.

Authors' contributions
HY is the guarantor of the content of the manuscript, including the data and analysis. He had full access to all of the data in the study and takes responsibility for the integrity of the data and the accuracy of the data analysis, including especially the adverse effects. SS contributed substantially to the study concept and design, data analysis and interpretation, and critical revision of the manuscript for important intellectual content. TA contributed to the accuracy of the data analysis. KS, AK, NH, HH, YK, and HS contributed to the study design, the acquisition and the interpretation of data, and drafting of the manuscript. TT contributed to the study design and drafting of the manuscript. All authors read and approved the final manuscript.

Competing interests
The authors declare that they have no competing interests.

Author details
[1]Department of Intensive Care Unit, Kameda Medical Center, 929 Higashi-chou, Kamogawa-shi, Chiba 296-8602, Japan. [2]Intensive Care Unit, Department of Emergency and Critical Care Medicine, Japanese Red Cross Musashino Hospital, Tokyo, Japan. [3]Department of Preventive Medicine and Public Health, Keio University School of Medicine, Tokyo, Japan. [4]Department of Medical Engineer, Kameda Medical Center, Chiba, Japan. [5]Biostatistics Unit at Clinical and Translational Research Center, Keio University Hospital, Tokyo, Japan.

References
1. Japanese Society of Education for Physicians and Trainees in Intensive Care (JSEPTIC): Available at<http://www.jseptic.com/rinsho/pdf/questionnaire_120325.pdf>. Accessed 25 Nov 2017.
2. Fleischmann C, Scherag A, Adhikari NK, et al. Assessment of global incidence and mortality of hospital-treated sepsis. Current estimates and limitations. Am J Respir Crit Care Med. 2016;193:259–72.
3. Kim WY, Huh JW, Lim CM, Koh Y, Hong SB. Analysis of progression in risk, injury, failure, loss, and end-stage renal disease classification on outcome in patients with severe sepsis and septic shock. J Crit Care. 2012;27:104. e101-107
4. Ronco C. Continuous renal replacement therapies for the treatment of acute renal failure in intensive care patients. Clin Nephrol. 1993;40:187–98.
5. Hoffmann JN, Hartl WH, Deppisch R, Faist E, Jochum M, Inthorn D. Hemofiltration in human sepsis: evidence for elimination of immunomodulatory substances. Kidney Int. 1995;48:1563–70.
6. Forni LG, Hilton PJ. Continuous hemofiltration in the treatment of acute renal failure. N Engl J Med. 1997;336:1303–9.
7. Vinsonneau C, Camus C, Combes A, et al. Continuous venovenous haemodiafiltration versus intermittent haemodialysis for acute renal failure in patients with multiple-organ dysfunction syndrome: a multicentre randomised trial. Lancet. 2006;368:379–85.
8. Schefold JC, von Haehling S, Pschowski R, et al. The effect of continuous versus intermittent renal replacement therapy on the outcome of critically ill patients with acute renal failure (CONVINT): a prospective randomized controlled trial. Crit Care. 2014;18:R11.
9. Keshaviah P. Technology and clinical application of hemodialysis. In: Striker GE, Klahr S, Decker BC, editors. The principles and practice of nephrology. Philadelphia: 2nd edition Mosby. 1991. p. 740. ISBN-10:1556641494. ISBN-13: 978-1556641497
10. Palmer SC, Rabindranath KS, Craig JC, Roderick PJ, Locatelli F, Strippoli GF. High-flux versus low-flux membranes for end-stage kidney disease. Cochrane Database Syst Rev. 2012:CD005016. https://doi.org/10.1002/14651858.CD005016.pub2.
11. Ifediora OC, Teehan BP, Sigler MH. Solute clearance in continuous venovenous hemodialysis. A comparison of cuprophane, polyacrylonitrile, and polysulfone membranes. ASAIO J. 1992;38:M697–701.
12. Ingram AJ, Parbtani A, Churchill DN. Effects of two low-flux cellulose acetate dialysers on plasma lipids and lipoproteins—a cross-over trial. Nephrol Dial Transplant. 1998;13:1452–7.
13. Krieter DH, Lemke HD. Polyethersulfone as a high-performance membrane. Contrib Nephrol. 2011;173:130–6.
14. Mudge DW, Rogers R, Hollett P, et al. Randomized trial of FX high flux vs standard high flux dialysis for homocysteine clearance. Nephrol Dial Transplant. 2005;20:2178–85.
15. Ouseph R, Hutchison CA, Ward RA. Differences in solute removal by two high-flux membranes of nominally similar synthetic polymers. Nephrol Dial Transplant. 2008;23:1704–12.
16. Lee D, Haase M, Haase-Fielitz A, Paizis K, Goehl H, Bellomo R. A pilot, randomized, double-blind, cross-over study of high cut-off versus high-flux dialysis membranes. Blood Purif. 2009;28:365–72.
17. Jamal JA, Mueller BA, Choi GY, Lipman J, Roberts JA. How can we ensure effective antibiotic dosing in critically ill patients receiving different types of renal replacement therapy? Diagn Microbiol Infect Dis. 2015;82:92–103.
18. Philip KNL, Tian Q, Ip M, Gomersall CD. In vitro adsorption of gentamicin and netilmicin by polyacrylonitrile and polyamide hemofiltration filters. Antimicrob Agents Chemother. 2010;54:963–5.
19. Villa G, Zaragoza JJ, Sharma A, Neri M, De Gaudio AR, Ronco C. Cytokine removal with high cut-off membrane: review of literature. Blood Purif. 2014; 38:167–73.
20. American College of Chest Physicians/Society of Critical Care Medicine Consensus Conference: definitions for sepsis and organ failure and guidelines for the use of innovative therapies in sepsis. Crit Care Med. 1992; 20:864–74.
21. Uchino S, Toki N, Takeda K, et al. Validity of low-intensity continuous renal replacement therapy. Crit Care Med. 2013;41:2584–91.
22. Excelflo AEFAEF: Available at<http://www.asahi-kasei.co.jp/medical/pdf/apheresis/excelflo-aef_document.pdf>. Accessed 22 Apr 2017.
23. Hemofeel SHG: Available athttp://www.info.pmda.go.jp/downfiles/md/PDF/480220/480220_22100BZX01046000_A_01_03.pdf. Accessed 19 Jan 2018.
24. Ahrenholz PG, Winkler RE, Michelsen A, Lang DA, Bowry SK. Dialysis membrane-dependent removal of middle molecules during hemodiafiltration: the beta2-microglobulin/albumin relationship. Clin Nephrol. 2004;62:21–8.
25. Lian JD, Cheng CH, Chang YL, Hsiong CH, Lee CJ. Clinical experience and model analysis on beta-2-microglobulin kinetics in high-flux hemodialysis. Artif Organs. 1993;17:758–63.
26. Pellicano R, Polkinghorne KR, Kerr PG. Reduction in beta2-microglobulin with super-flux versus high-flux dialysis membranes: results of a 6-week, randomized, double-blind, crossover trial. Am J Kidney Dis. 2008;52:93–1.

21

Development of prognostic model for fistula maturation in patients with advanced renal failure

Muhammad A. Siddiqui[1,2*], Suhel Ashraff[3], Derek Santos[4], Robert Rush[4], Thomas E. Carline[4] and Zahid Raza[5]

Abstract

Background: This study aimed to explore the role of patient's characteristic and haematological factors as predictive on the maturation of arteriovenous fistulae in patients who underwent vascular access surgery at the Royal Infirmary of Edinburgh.

Methods: Retrospective data from 300 patients who had undergone fistula creation between February 2007 and October 2010 was examined. A predictive logistic regression model was developed using the backward stepwise procedure. Model performance, discrimination and calibration, was assessed using the receiver operating characteristics (ROC) curve and Hosmer and Lemeshow goodness of fit test.

Results: Three variables were identified which independently influenced fistula maturation. Males were twice as likely to undergo fistula maturation, compared to that of females (odds ratio (OR) 0.514; 95% confidence interval (CI) 0.308–0.857), patients with no evidence of peripheral vascular disease (PVD) were three times more likely to mature their fistula (OR 3.140; 95% CI 1.596–6.177) and a pre-operative vein diameter > 2.5 mm resulted in a fivefold increase in fistula maturation compared to a vein size less than 2.5 mm (OR 4.532; 95% CI 2.063–9.958). The model for fistula maturation had fair discrimination as indicated by the area under the ROC curve (0.68; 95% CI 0.615–0.738) but good calibration indicated by Hosmer and Lemeshow test ($p = 0.79$).

Conclusion: Gender, PVD and vein size are independent predictors of arteriovenous fistula maturation. The clinical utility of these risk equation in the maturation of arteriovenous fistulae requires further validation in the newly treated patients.

Keywords: Vascular access, Arteriovenous fistula, Maturation, Haemodialysis, Success of AVF

Background

Chronic kidney disease (CKD) is a critical condition with considerable public health implications. It affects a significant proportion of the general population and, when progressive, has an increasing influence on morbidity and mortality. In the USA, it is reported that 10% (more than 20 million adults) are affected with CKD [1]. In the UK, the prevalence of stage 3–5 CKD is 1.7 million adults [2] with an annual incidence of stage 5 CKD of 100 per million of the population [3]. Once a patient reaches end-stage kidney disease, their quality of life

becomes poor and the life expectancy is considerably shortened [4]. According to the United States Renal Data System [5], more than 87,000 people die from causes related to kidney failure each year.

Through the provision of renal replacement therapy, survival and quality of life of the patients can be markedly improved [6]. The efficiency of haemodialysis treatment relies on a functional status of vascular access, and complications here represent the main factor that determines a rise in the morbidity among haemodialysis patients and consequently, a rise in the healthcare expenses [7]. In the UK, renal replacement therapy utilizes up to 2% of its financial resources [8]. To ensure that the dialysis therapy can be efficiently undertaken, all patients have to have a fully developed fistula appropriate

* Correspondence: drasadi@hotmail.com
[1]Department of Research and Performance Support, Saskatchewan Health Authority, Regina, Saskatchewan, Canada
[2]School of Health Sciences, Queen Margaret University, Edinburgh, UK
Full list of author information is available at the end of the article

for cannulation. The percentage of arteriovenous fistulae (AVF) that fail to mature for haemodialysis is 28–53% [9]. The dialysis therapy is often postponed for up to 6 months or more to allow extra time for the fistula to develop; if this does not happen, the AVF is declared as 'failed to mature'. The development process of AVF is complicated, and it is difficult to settle on the precise length of time it requires to mature [10]. Several researchers [11–16] have recommended a number of pre-surgical principles relying on invasive and non-invasive procedures; however, factors, such as cost, time and complexity, hinder the widespread application of these principles.

It may be possible to improve the end results of vascular access by gaining a more comprehensive picture about the various factors involved in the maturation of fistulae. This could then in turn provide important information during the pre-surgical evaluation that surgeons can base their decisions on. Independent predictive factors may be beneficial in anticipating successful fistula maturation without the use of invasive tests, and this could be cost-effective. The objective of the study was to assess factors which are important in the successful maturation of AVF. These were used to formulate a simple and economical prognostic model on the maturation of AVF.

Methods

Research design
This is a single-centre exploratory study that involved the collection of retrospective data from the Royal Infirmary of Edinburgh and identification of those independent predictors for a predictive model of fistula maturation. A favourable ethical opinion was obtained from the NHS Lothian ethics committee and Queen Margaret University ethics committee for the study.

Using the retrospective clinical database of patients with ESRD, we identified 300 patients between February 2007 and October 2010 who had undergone vascular access surgery for first-time AVF creation. Patients who underwent a repeat AVF creation (second and further fistula creations) were not included in this study. Purposive sampling technique was used for patient's recruitment. Study was performed systematically in different steps from identification, screening, recruitment, data collection of potential participants and finally data analysis by using appropriate statistical test (Fig. 1).

A retrospective case note review was performed on all patients identified from the hospital vascular access database as having undergone construction of AVF. The medical case files of the patients who had undergone fistula surgery between 2007 and 2010 were retrieved from the medical records (Proton® software and Apex® software) at the Royal Infirmary Edinburgh. At the beginning, all potential participants' records were screened comprehensively. From the data, reports of patients were developed from the pre-operative assessment papers and the clinical results of their operation obtained from the clinical records and follow-up case notes.

The details of patient's factor and blood markers were explored by complete review of the patient's inpatient and outpatient medical record (containing all information pertaining to medical and surgical consultations and all previous hospital admissions and management) via an electronic database. All the data was entered into an Excel spreadsheet (Microsoft, USA).

The patient record including age, gender and risk factors; peripheral vascular disease (PVD); diabetes mellitus (DM); hypertension (HTN); smoking (ever versus never); and dialysis (ever versus never). Patients were defined as obese when their body mass index was > 30, consistent with the World Health Organization classification [17]. Fistula characteristics that were ascertained included fistula type and its location (right or left). Clinically important biomedical factors including estimated glomerular filtration rate (eGFR); creatinine; blood urea; serum potassium (K); sodium (Na); calcium (Ca); bicarbonate (HCO_3); prothrombin time (PT); international normalization ratio (INR); high-density lipoprotein (HDL); triglyceride (TG); total cholesterol (TC); and vein diameter were also included in the analysis. Duplex investigation of the veins was performed to measure the diameter of arm veins according to a standard protocol by vascular scientists in the vascular clinic of Royal Infirmary Edinburgh. All procedures such as general physical examination consisted of inspection and palpation of the vessels of the upper arm and forearm and measurement of brachial artery blood pressure. Subsequently, height and weight details were recorded in order to calculate the BMI values and blood samples were obtained by the regular NHS staff. PVD was identified through a physical examination and by comparing the blood pressure in the arm and ankle. Ankle-brachial pressure index (ABPI) ≤ 0.90 reliably identifies 95% of symptomatic arteriogram-positive PVD individuals and almost 100% of healthy controls [18].

Outcome definition
Maturation was defined as the ability to provide ongoing functional haemodialysis at the sixth week [19, 20] from the access procedure. An experienced dialysis specialist nurse determined when the fistula was ready for an attempt at cannulation and then attempted initial cannulation of the fistula; if unsuccessful, the fistula then was evaluated by the vascular surgeon at the Royal Infirmary of Edinburgh.

Statistical analysis
Statistical analysis was performed using SPSS (IBM SPSS Statistics 20.0). Data was expressed as mean, standard

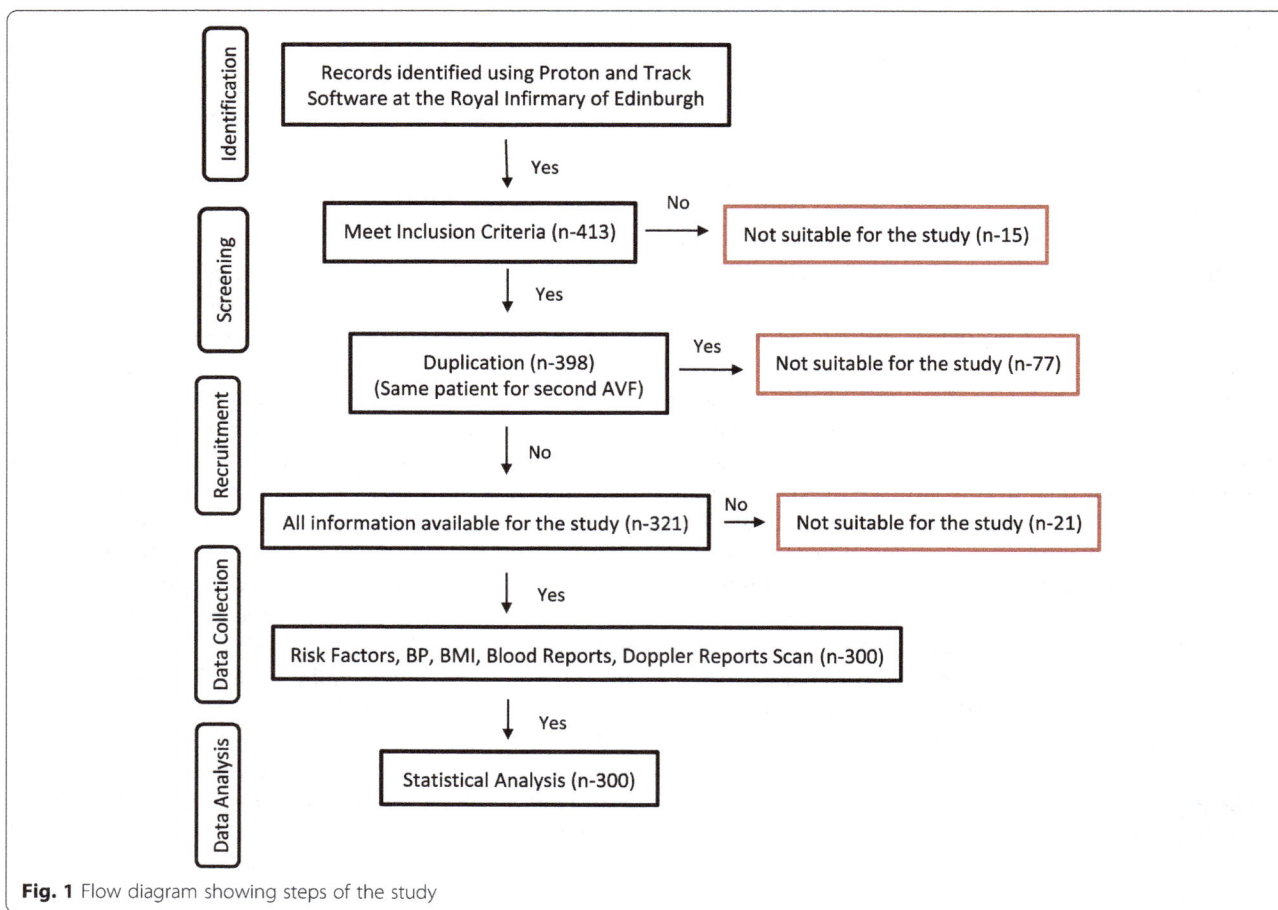

Fig. 1 Flow diagram showing steps of the study

deviation (SD) and 95% confidence interval (CI) or as proportions. The association between the independent factors and outcome, i.e. mature fistula, was assessed initially employing univariable logistic regression, and following this, a multivariable model was produced utilizing backward stepwise logistic regression with those variables found to be significant in the univariable regression at $p < 0.25$. The odds ratios and associated 95% confidence intervals for variables in the final model were reported. The significance level for the multivariable model was set at $p < 0.05$. Multicollinearity in the model was investigated to assess the relationship between the independent factors. We evaluated the calibration and discrimination performance of the model. For the calibration, the Hosmer-Lemeshow test was employed to investigate how well the predicted probabilities agreed with the observed probabilities. Discrimination, which refers to the ability of a model to distinguish between the maturation and immaturation of the AVF, was quantified using the ROC curve. The ROC curve plots the sensitivity (true positive rate) against 1—specificity (false positive rate) for consecutive cut-offs for the probability of an outcome [21].

Results

Retrospective data was obtained for 300 patients who underwent vascular access surgery. Ages ranged from 19 to 87 years, with a mean age of 60.5 (16) years. Successful maturation of the AVF was achieved in 168 (56%) patients as assessed by dialysis specialist nurses.

Univariable associations

AVF characteristics and univariable analysis of clinical variables for the prediction of maturation of fistula are shown in Table 1. Univariable analysis found nine variables to be associated with maturation of AVF: gender, side of arm, type of fistulae, PVD, diabetes, SBP, INR, TG and vein size. In addition to the above variables, a further two statistically non-significant variables, i.e. dialysis [22, 23] (ever versus never) and eGFR [24], were added to the model due to their possible clinical association with the maturation of AVF as suggested by the vascular surgeons.

Multivariable associations

Three variables were identified which were independently associated with fistula maturation using

Table 1 Univariable analysis of independent factors to maturation of AVF

Clinical characteristics	Mature AVF %	Total %	Crude OR (95% CI)	p value
Age				0.45
> 50 years	57.2	76.3		
≤ 50 years	52.1	23.7	0.814 (0.477–1.389)	
Gender				0.049*
Male	60	66.7		
Female	48	33.3	0.615 (0.379–0.998)	
Arm				0.129*
Left	53.4	73.7		
Right	63.3	26.3	1.505 (0.887–2.553)	
Fistula				0.115*
BC	60.1	62.7		
RC	51.9	27	0.715 (0.423–1.208)	
BB	41.9	10.3	0.479 (0.222–1.036)	
Surgeons				0.788
Surgeon A	56.4	68.0		
Surgeon B	56	25.0	0.985 (0.578–1.679)	
Surgeon C	71.4	2.3	1.935 (0.367–10.206)	
Surgeon D	40	1.7	0.516 (0.084–3.154)	
Surgeon E	44.4	3	0.619 (0.162–2.373)	
PVD				0.001*
Yes	33.3	16		
No	60.3	84	3.04 (1.585–5.829)	
DM				0.102*
Yes	50	38		
No	59.7	62	1.48 (0.925–2.367)	
Smoker				0.49
Yes	61	13.7		
No	55.2	86.3	0.789 (0.402–1.547)	
HTN				0.406
Yes	57.3	78		
No	51.5	22	0.793 (0.458–1.371)	
Dialysis				0.513
Yes	53.6	37.3		
No	57.4	62.7	1.17 (0.731–1.873)	
K^+ (mmol/L)				0.948
Normal	56.2	54.3		
Abnormal	55.8	45.7	1.015 (0.642–1.605)	
Na^+ (mmol/L)				0.439
Normal	55.1	85.3		
Abnormal	61.4	14.7	1.295 (0.673–2.494)	
Ca^{++} (mmol/L)				0.525
≤ 2.5	56.7	87		
> 2.5	51.3	13	0.804 (0.41–1.577)	
HCO3 (mmol/L)				0.743

Table 1 Univariable analysis of independent factors to maturation of AVF *(Continued)*

Clinical characteristics	Mature AVF %	Total %	Crude OR (95% CI)	p value
≤ 23	57	45		
> 23	55.2	55	0.926 (0.586–1.465)	
Creatinine (mmol/L)				0.676
> 400	57.5	44.7		
> 120 ≤ 400	55.2	54.3	0.913 (0.576–1.447)	
≤ 120	33.3	1	0.37 (0.033–4.182)	
Urea (mmol/L)				0.949
> 15	55.3	65.7		
> 6.6–≤ 15	57.1	18.7	1.076 (0.591–1.960)	
≤ 6.6	57.4	15.7	1.09 (0.73–2.073)	
eGFR (ml/min/1.73m^2)				0.459
≤ 15	57.4	64.6		
> 15	52.9	35.4	0.834 (0.516–1.349)	
SBP (mm of Hg)				0.101*
≤ 130	51.6	53		
> 130	48.4	47	1.468 (0.927–2.325)	
DBP (mm of Hg)				0.786
≤ 85	56.3	90.7		
> 85	53.6	9.3	0.897 (0.411–1.958)	
BMI (kg/m^2)				0.563
≤ 30	55	73.3		
> 30	58.8	26.7	1.165 (0.694–1.957)	
PT (s)				0.413
≤ 13.4	56.9	86.6		
> 13.5	50	13.4	0.757 (0.389–1.474)	
INR (ratio)				0.140*
≤ 1.2	57.6	88		
> 1.2	44.4	12	0.589 (0.292–1.189)	
TC (mmol/L)				0.24*
≤ 5	57.9	76		
> 5	50	24	1.294 (0.804–2.084)	
TG (mmol/L)				0.289
≤ 2.1	53.7	63.3		
> 2.1	60	36.7	0.773 (0.48–1.244)	
HDL (mmol/L)				0.874
≤ 1.1	55.6	51		
> 1.1	56.5	49	1.037 (0.658–1.637)	
Vein size (mm)				< 0.001*
≤ 2.5	26.3	12.6		
> 2.5	60.3	87.4	4.254 (1.983–9.126)	

Independent patient factors and blood markers that underwent in univariate analysis and their association with the maturation of AVF. Data values are expressed as value (%), odds ratio (OR), confidence interval (CI) and level of significance (p)

BC brachiocephalic, *RC* radiocephalic, *BB* bicarbonate, *PVD* peripheral vascular disease, *DM* diabetes mellitus, *HTN* hypertension, *K* potassium, *Na* sodium, *Ca* calcium, *HCO3* bicarbonate, *e-GFR* estimated glomerular filtration rate, *SBP* systolic blood pressure, *DBP* diastolic blood pressure, *BMI* body mass index, *PT* prothrombin time, *INR* international normalization ratio, *TC* total cholesterol, *TG* triglyceride, *HDL* high density lipoprotein
*Significant variables having p value < 0.25

multivariable logistic regression analysis (Table 2). Males were twice as likely to undergo fistula maturation, compared to females (OR 0.514; 95% CI 0.308–0.857; $p = 0.011$) with patients who had no evidence of PVD being three times more likely to mature their fistula (OR 3.140; 95% CI 1.596–6.177; $p < 0.001$) and those with a pre-operative vein diameter greater than 2.5 mm [25, 26] resulting in a fivefold increase in fistula maturation compared to a vein size less than 2.5 mm (OR 4.532; 95% CI 2.063–9.958; $p < 0.001$). No multicollinearity was observed between the independent factors.

The overall risk score for each patient was estimated by summing the scores of each significant independent variable. Using the prediction model, the following prognostic equation was developed:

$$\text{Risk score}\,(-\log \text{odds}) = \beta_0 + \beta_1 X_1 + \beta_2 X_2 + \ldots\ldots + \beta_n X_n$$

where β_0 is the intercept, β_1 till β_n are the regression coefficients and X_1 to X_n are independent variables.

$$\text{Risk score}\,(-\log \text{odds of failure of AVF maturation}) = 00.182 + (-0.666 \times \text{gender}) + (1.144 \times \text{PVD}) + (1.511 \times \text{vein size})$$

where all variables are coded 0 for no or 1 for yes. The value – 0.182 is called the intercept, and the other numbers are the estimated regression coefficients for the predictors, which indicate their mutually adjusted relative contribution to the outcome risk.

The performance of the final prognostic model assessed in terms of calibration using Hosmer-Lemeshow test was not significant ($p = 0.79$). This suggests that there was no statistically significant difference between predicted and observed outcomes. The area under the ROC curve for prediction of maturation of fistula was 0.68 (95% bias-corrected CI 0.615, 0.738), which indicates fair [27] discrimination (Fig. 2).

Discussion

The results of this study identify three clinical factors, each of which was independently associated with maturation of AVF: male gender, PVD and vein diameter. AVF

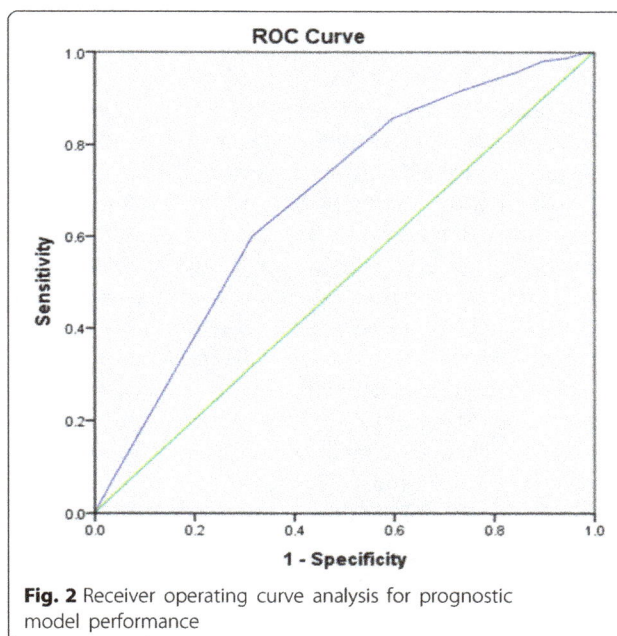

Fig. 2 Receiver operating curve analysis for prognostic model performance

successfully matured in 168 patients, accounting for 56% of the total number of patients. Similar results have been obtained by Feldman et al. [28], with 55.5% out of a total of 348 patients exhibiting successful AVF maturation.

The study result showed a gender difference, mature rates of 60% for men and of 48% for women. Miller et al. [29] found Ithat the AVF maturation is more successful in men than in women. Similar results were obtained by Gibbons [30] and Iyem [31]. In our study, males were twice as likely to undergo fistula maturation, compared to that of females; the most rational explanation for this difference is the smaller size of vessels in women. Some studies also found female gender to be associated with immature fistula [12, 13, 15, 32]. However, there are also studies that did not show a gender difference. Jennings et al. [26] involved the creation of AVFs on 114 participants and did not observe any gender difference in the maturation of AVF [33, 34].

Out of 300 patients, 38% were diabetic and 16% had clinical evidence of PVD. In a number of studies, it has been reported that more than 50% of North American dialysis patients had diabetes, and approximately one

Table 2 Multivariable predictors of AVF maturation

Predictors of AVF maturation	Test statistics and associated degree of freedom	Adjusted OR (95% CI)	p value
Gender (male)	$\chi^2(1) = 3.896, p = 0.048$	0.514 (0.308–0.857)	0.011
PVD (no)	$\chi^2(1) = 11.91, p = 0.001$	3.140 (1.596–6.177)	< 0.001
V. size (> 2.5)	$\chi^2(1) = 15.56, p < 0.001$	4.532 (2.063–9.958)	< 0.001
Model summary −2 log-likelihood	Cox and Snell R^2	Nagelkerke R^2	
378.714	0.104	0.139	

third had PVD [35–37]. In our study, fistula maturation was 59.7% in a group with no history of PVD and 33.3 in patients with PVD. This emerged as one of the predictive factors in the maturation of fistulae in the multivariable analysis. Patients with no evidence of PVD were three times more likely to mature their fistula. Our data is consistent with other studies in which PVD was associated with AVF failure [38, 39]. Chan et al. conducted a retrospective cohort analysis using 1486 patients' data [40]. It was revealed that patients who suffer from PVD are more likely to experience non-maturation of AVF (OR 2.78, 95% CI 1.01–7.63, $p = 0.047$). Fistula failure is consistent with the underlying need for adequate arterial vessels, which deteriorate with the normal aging process and are damaged by concurrent disease; this finding is supported by other studies [11, 41].

Our data are consistent with other studies in which vein size was associated with successful maturation of fistulae. Mendes et al. reported that if the diameter of the cephalic veins exceeds 2 mm, there is a 76% success rate of functional dialysis access, whereas if the diameter is less than 2 mm, there is only a 16% success rate [14]. In this study, a pre-operative vein diameter greater than 2.5 mm resulted in a fivefold increase in fistula maturation compared to a vein size less than 2.5 mm. Our data is consistent with other studies in which vein size is associated with successful fistula maturation [41, 42]. The cut-off value identified by Brimble et al. was 2.6 mm; however, only women exhibited a substantial discrepancy between AVF success and failure with regard to vein diameter [43]. In contrast, Wong et al. did not observe any discrepancies between AVF success and failure in the mean vein diameter at the wrist but indicated AVF failure in all cases where the vein diameter was below 1.6 mm [44].

This study hypothesized that blood and patient factors could be used to stratify risk of self-report of maturation of AVF. In brief, using the development dataset of 300 subjects, we identified three variables associated with maturation of fistula: gender, PVD and vein size. The performance of the developed model in this study was assessed by discrimination and calibration of the model. The area under the ROC curve for a prognostic model is classically between 0.6 and 0.85 [45]. In our study, ROC curve was primarily designed for prognostic models, rather for diagnostic models. ROC curve was 0.68 in the development model and 0.59 in the validation stage, meaning that the model had limited capacity to correctly distinguish between mature and immature fistulae.

The present study has a number of limitations. The connection between artery diameter and blood inflow rate was emphasized by a number of studies [42, 46, 47]. However, we did not included artery diameter and arterial blood flow in our study due to the unavailability of

retrospective data. Another limitation were the duplex measurements of the vein diameter and measurements of vessel diameter carried out by vascular scientists who had a great deal of experience and were familiar with the procedure. The objective of the scientist was to carry out the measurements in spite of the differences between pre-surgery examination and the actual intervention. However, there were few staff changes during the 5 years when the fistulae were constructed. As argued by Pisoni et al. [48], it is important to take into consideration non-measurable elements, such as measurement techniques and principles of care, apart from ample case-mix adaptations highlighted by other studies.

Conclusion

A preoperative, clinical prediction model to determine fistulae that are likely to mature was created. It was found to be simple and easily reproducible and applied to predictive risk categories. Gender, PVD and vein size are useful predictors of arteriovenous fistula maturation. The clinical utility of these risk categories in the maturation of arteriovenous fistula requires further validation in the newly treated patients.

Abbreviations
ABPI: Ankle-brachial pressure index; AVF: Arteriovenous fistula; BMI: Body mass index; Ca: Calcium; CI: Confidence interval; CKD: Chronic kidney disease; DM: Diabetes mellitus; eGFR: Estimated glomerular filtration rate; ESRD: End-stage renal disease; HCO_3: Bicarbonate; HDL: High-density lipoprotein; HTN: Hypertension; INR: International normalized ratio; K: Potassium; Na: Sodium; NHS: National Health System; NICE: National Institute for Health and Care Excellence; OR: Odds ratio; PT: Prothrombin time; PVD: Peripheral vascular disease; ROC: Receiver operating curve; SD: Standard deviation; SPSS: Statistical Package for the Social Science; TC: Total cholesterol; TG: Triglyceride; USRDS: United States Renal Data System

Acknowledgements
We appreciate Rona Lochiel, a vascular access nurse specialist, Royal Infirmary, Edinburgh, for her assistance in the recruitment and follow-up of the patients. We also like to thank statistician Catriona Graham (Wellcome Trust Clinical Research Facility, University of Edinburgh) for her advice in the data analysis.

Funding
No funding was obtained.

Authors' contributions
MAS conceived the study and collected the data. MAS and RR analysed the data. MAS and SA drafted the manuscript while DS, TC and ZR revised and reviewed the whole manuscript. All authors read and approved the final manuscript.

Competing interests

The authors declare that they have no competing interests.

Author details

[1]Department of Research and Performance Support, Saskatchewan Health Authority, Regina, Saskatchewan, Canada. [2]School of Health Sciences, Queen Margaret University, Edinburgh, UK. [3]Department of Diabetes and Endocrinology, Royal Victoria Infirmary, Newcastle, UK. [4]School of Health Sciences, Queen Margaret University, Edinburgh, UK. [5]Department of Vascular Surgery, Royal Infirmary, Edinburgh, UK.

References

1. Centres for Disease Control and Prevention (CDC). National chronic kidney disease fact sheet: general information and national estimates on chronic kidney disease in the United States. Atlanta, GA: US Department of Health and Human Services, Centres for Disease Control and Prevention; 2014.

2. NHS Kidney Care. Kidney Disease: Key Facts and Figures. [Online]. East Midlands Public Health Observatory (EMPHO), East Midlands. 2011. Available from: http://patientsafety.health.org.uk/sites/default/files/resources/diabeteswithkidneydiseasekeyfacts.pdf. Accessed May 2014.

3. Hamer RA, El Nahas AM. The burden of chronic kidney disease: Is rising rapidly worldwide. BMJ :British Medical Journal. 2006;332(7541):563–564.

4. Noble H, Lewis R. Acceptance and rejection of dialysis—the need for patient evaluation. Journal of renal care 2008;34(1):45. Epub 2008/03/14. https://doi.org/10.1111/j.1755-6686.2008.00011.x. PubMed PMID: 18336524.

5. (System) UURD. Annual data report: atlas of chronic kidney disease and end-stage renal disease in the United States, National Institutes of Health, National Institute of Diabetes and Digestive and Kidney Diseases, Bethesda, MD. 2011.

6. Mazzuchi N, Carbonell E, Fernandez-Cean J. Importance of blood pressure control in hemodialysis patient survival. Kidney Int 2000;58(5):2147–2154. Epub 2000/10/24. https://doi.org/10.1111/j.1523-1755.2000.00388.x. PubMed PMID: 11044236.

7. NICE, National Institute for Health and Clinical Excellence. Chronic kidney disease in adults: assessment and management. NICE clinical guideline 73. London: National Institute for Health and Clinical Excellence; 2014.

8. NICE, National Institute for Health and Clinical Excellence. Chronic kidney disease: early identification and management of chronic kidney disease in adults in primary and secondary care. NICE clinical guideline 73. London: National Institute for Health and Clinical Excellence; 2008.

9. Asif A, Cherla G, Merrill D, Cipleu CD, Briones P, Pennell P. Conversion of tunneled hemodialysis catheter-consigned patients to arteriovenous fistula. Kidney Int 2005;67(6):2399–2406. Epub 2005/05/11. https://doi.org/10.1111/j.1523-1755.2005.00347.x. PubMed PMID: 15882285.

10. Corpataux JM, Haesler E, Silacci P, Ris HB, Hayoz D. Low-pressure environment and remodelling of the forearm vein in Brescia–Cimino haemodialysis access. Nephrol Dial Transplant. 2002;17(6):1057–62. Epub 2002/05/29. PubMed PMID: 12032197.

11. Feldman HI, Joffe M, Rosas SE, Burns JE, Knauss J, Brayman K. Predictors of successful arteriovenous fistula maturation. Am J Kidney Dis. 2003;42(5):1000–12. Epub 2003/10/29. PubMed PMID: 14582044.

12. Huber TS, Ozaki CK, Flynn TC, Lee WA, Berceli SA, Hirneise CM, et al. Prospective validation of an algorithm to maximize native arteriovenous fistulae for chronic hemodialysis access. J Vasc Surg. 2002;36(3):452–9. Epub 2002/09/10. PubMed PMID: 12218966.

13. Lok CE, Allon M, Moist L, Oliver MJ, Shah H, Zimmerman D. Risk equation determining unsuccessful cannulation events and failure to maturation in arteriovenous fistulas (REDUCE FTM I). J Am Soc Nephrol 2006;17(11):3204–3212. Epub 2006/09/22. https://doi.org/10.1681/asn.2006030190. PubMed PMID: 16988062.

14. Mendes RR, Farber MA, Marston WA, Dinwiddie LC, Keagy BA, Burnham SJ. Prediction of wrist arteriovenous fistula maturation with preoperative vein mapping with ultrasonography. J Vasc Surg. 2002;36(3):460–3. Epub 2002/09/10. PubMed PMID: 12218967.

15. Robbin ML, Chamberlain NE, Lockhart ME, Gallichio MH, Young CJ, Deierhoi MH, et al. Hemodialysis arteriovenous fistula maturity: US evaluation. Radiology 2002;225(1):59–64. Epub 2002/10/02. https://doi.org/10.1148/radiol.2251011367. PubMed PMID: 12354984.

16. Rooijens PP, Burgmans JP, Yo TI, Hop WC, de Smet AA, van den Dorpel MA, et al. Autogenous radial-cephalic or prosthetic brachial-antecubital forearm loop AVF in patients with compromised vessels? A randomized, multicenter study of the patency of primary hemodialysis access. J Vasc Surg. 2005;42(3):481–486; discussions 7. Epub 2005/09/21. https://doi.org/10.1016/j.jvs.2005.05.025. PubMed PMID: 16171591.

17. World Health Organisation. Global database on basal metabolic index. 2004. [online]. Available from: http://apps.who.int/bmi/index.jsp?introPage=intro_3.html. Accessed 12 Sept 2016.

18. Norgren L, Hiatt WR, Dormandy JA, Nehler MR, Harris KA, Fowkes FG. Inter-society consensus for the management of peripheral arterial disease (TASC II). J Vasc Surg. 2007;45 Suppl S:S5–67. Epub 2007/01/16. https://doi.org/10.1016/j.jvs.2006.12.037. PubMed PMID: 17223489.

19. Clinical practice guidelines for hemodialysis adequacy, update 2006. Am J Kidney Dis. 2006;48 Suppl 1:S2–90. Epub 2006/07/04. https://doi.org/10.1053/j.ajkd.2006.03.051. PubMed PMID: 16813990.

20. Patel ST, Hughes J, Mills JL Sr. Failure of arteriovenous fistula maturation: an unintended consequence of exceeding dialysis outcome quality initiative guidelines for hemodialysis access. J Vasc Surg. 2003;38(3):439–45. discussion 45. Epub 2003/08/30. PubMed PMID: 12947249.

21. Steyerberg EW, Vickers AJ, Cook NR, Gerds T, Gonen M, Obuchowski N, et al. Assessing the performance of prediction models: a framework for traditional and novel measures. Epidemiology. 2010;21(1):128–138. Epub 2009/12/17. https://doi.org/10.1097/EDE.0b013e3181c30fb2. PubMed PMID: 20010215; PubMed Central PMCID: PMCPMC3575184.

22. Weale AR, Bevis P, Neary WD, Boyes S, Morgan JD, Lear PA, et al. Radiocephalic and brachiocephalic arteriovenous fistula outcomes in the elderly. J Vasc Surg 2008;47(1):144–150. Epub 2008/01/08. https://doi.org/10.1016/j.jvs.2007.09.046. PubMed PMID: 18178467.

23. Zeebregts C, van den Dungen J, Bolt A, Franssen C, Verhoeven E, van Schilfgaarde R. Factors predictive of failure of Brescia-Cimino arteriovenous fistulas. Eur J Surg 2002;168(1):29–36. Epub 2002/05/23. https://doi.org/10.1080/110241502317307544. PubMed PMID: 12022368.

24. Jindal K, Chan CT, Deziel C, Hirsch D, Soroka SD, Tonelli M, et al. Hemodialysis clinical practice guidelines for the Canadian Society of Nephrology. J Am Soc Nephrol 2006;17(3 Suppl 1):S1–27. Epub 2006/02/25. https://doi.org/10.1681/asn.2005121372. PubMed PMID: 16497879.

25. Jennings WC. Creating arteriovenous fistulas in 132 consecutive patients: exploiting the proximal radial artery arteriovenous fistula: reliable, safe, and simple forearm and upper arm hemodialysis access. Arch Surg. 2006;141(1):27–32; discussion Epub 2006/01/18. https://doi.org/10.1001/archsurg.141.1.27. PubMed PMID: 16415408.

26. Jennings WC, Kindred MG, Broughan TA. Creating radiocephalic arteriovenous fistulas: technical and functional success. J Am Coll Surg 2009;208(3):419–425. Epub 2009/03/26. doi: https://doi.org/10.1016/j.jamcollsurg.2008.11.015. PubMed PMID: 19318004.

27. Brubaker PH. Do not be statistically cenophobic: time to roc and roll! J Cardiopulm Rehabil Prev 2008;28(6):420–421. Epub 2008/11/15. https://doi.org/10.1097/HCR.0b013e31818c3c9f. PubMed PMID: 19008699.

28. Feldman HI, Held PJ, Hutchinson JT, Stoiber E, Hartigan MF, Berlin JA. Hemodialysis vascular access morbidity in the United States. Kidney Int 1993;43(5):1091–1096. Epub 1993/05/01. PubMed PMID: 8510387.

29. Miller PE, Tolwani A, Luscy CP, Deierhoi MH, Bailey R, Redden DT, et al. Predictors of adequacy of arteriovenous fistulas in hemodialysis patients. Kidney Int 1999;56(1):275–280. Epub 1999/07/20. https://doi.org/10.1046/j.1523-1755.1999.00515.x. PubMed PMID: 10411703.

30. Gibbons CP. Primary vascular access. Eur J Vasc Endovasc Surg 2006;31(5):523–529. Epub 2005/11/22. https://doi.org/10.1016/j.ejvs.2005.10.006. PubMed PMID: 16298148.

31. Iyem H. Early follow-up results of arteriovenous fistulae created for hemodialysis. Vasc Health Risk Manag. 2011;7:321–325. Epub 2011/06/03. doi: https://doi.org/10.2147/vhrm.s14277. PubMed PMID: 21633522; PubMed Central PMCID: PMCPMC3104609.

32. Peterson WJ, Barker J, Allon M. Disparities in fistula maturation persist despite preoperative vascular mapping. Clin J Am Soc Nephrol. 2008;3(2):437–441. Epub 2008/02/01. https://doi.org/10.2215/cjn.03480807. PubMed PMID: 18235150; PubMed Central PMCID: PMCPMC2390953.

33. Ekicei Y, Karayalı FY, Yagmurdur FC. Snuff-box arteriovenous fistula for haemodialysis. Turkish VascSurg. 2008;17:73–9.
34. Palmes D, Kebschull L, Schaefer RM, Pelster F, Konner K. Perforating vein fistula is superior to forearm fistula in elderly haemodialysis patients with diabetes and arterial hypertension. Nephrol Dial Transplant 2011;26(10): 3309–3314. Epub 2011/02/18. https://doi.org/10.1093/ndt/gfr004. PubMed PMID: 21325347.
35. Cook NR. Use and misuse of the receiver operating characteristic curve in risk prediction. Circulation 2007;115(7):928–935. Epub 2007/02/21. https://doi.org/10.1161/circulationaha.106.672402. PubMed PMID: 17309939.
36. Mendelssohn DC, Ethier J, Elder SJ, Saran R, Port FK, Pisoni RL. Haemodialysis vascular access problems in Canada: results from the Dialysis Outcomes and Practice Patterns Study (DOPPS II). Nephrol Dial Transplant 2006;21(3):721–728. Epub 2005/11/29. https://doi.org/10.1093/ndt/gfi281. PubMed PMID: 16311264.
37. Pencina MJ, D'Agostino RB, Sr., D'Agostino RB, Jr., Vasan RS. Evaluating the added predictive ability of a new marker: from area under the ROC curve to reclassification and beyond. Stat Med 2008;27(2):157–172; discussion 207–12. Epub 2007/06/15. https://doi.org/10.1002/sim.2929. PubMed PMID: 17569110.
38. Obialo CI, Tagoe AT, Martin PC, Asche-Crowe PE. Adequacy and survival of autogenous arteriovenous fistula in African American hemodialysis patients. ASAIO J 2003;49(4):435–439. Epub 2003/08/16. PubMed PMID: 12918587.
39. Woods JD, Turenne MN, Strawderman RL, Young EW, Hirth RA, Port FK, et al. Vascular access survival among incident hemodialysis patients in the United States. Am J Kidney Dis 1997;30(1):50–57. Epub 1997/07/01. PubMed PMID: 9214401.
40. Chan MR, Young HN, Becker YT, Yevzlin AS. Obesity as a predictor of vascular access outcomes: analysis of the USRDS DMMS wave II study. Semin Dial 2008;21(3):274–279. Epub 2008/04/10. https://doi.org/10.1111/j.1525-139X.2008.00434.x. PubMed PMID: 18397205.
41. Lauvao LS, Ihnat DM, Goshima KR, Chavez L, Gruessner AC, Mills JL, Sr. Vein diameter is the major predictor of fistula maturation. J Vasc Surg 2009;49(6): 1499–1504. Epub 2009/06/06. https://doi.org/10.1016/j.jvs.2009.02.018. PubMed PMID: 19497513.
42. Khavanin Zadeh M, Gholipour F, Naderpour Z, Porfakharan M. Relationship between vessel diameter and time to maturation of arteriovenous fistula for hemodialysis access. Int J Nephrol. 2012;2012:942950. Epub 2011/12/22. https://doi.org/10.1155/2012/942950. PubMed PMID: 22187645; PubMed Central PMCID: PMCPMC3236464.
43. Brimble KS, RabbatCh G, Treleaven DJ. Utility of ultrasono-graphic venous assessment prior to forearm arteriovenous fistula creation. ClinNephrol. 2002;58:122–7.
44. Wong V, Ward R, Taylor J, Selvakumar S, How TV, Bakran A. Factors associated with early failure of arteriovenous fistulae for haemodialysis access. Eur J Vasc Endovasc Surg 1996;12(2):207–213. Epub 1996/08/01. PubMed PMID: 8760984.
45. Royston P, Moons KG, Altman DG, Vergouwe Y. Prognosis and prognostic research: developing a prognostic model. BMJ 2009;338:b604. Epub 2009/04/02. https://doi.org/10.1136/bmj.b604. PubMed PMID: 19336487.
46. Huijbregts HJ, Bots ML, Wittens CH, Schrama YC, Blankestijn PJ. Access blood flow and the risk of complications in mature forearm and upper arm arteriovenous fistulas. Blood Purif 2009;27(2):212–219. Epub 2009/01/30. https://doi.org/10.1159/000197561. PubMed PMID: 19176950.
47. Monroy-Cuadros M, Yilmaz S, Salazar-Banuelos A, Doig C. Risk factors associated with patency loss of hemodialysis vascular access within 6 months. Clin J Am Soc Nephrol. 2010;5(10):1787–1792. Epub 2010/06/26. https://doi.org/10.2215/cjn.09441209. PubMed PMID: 20576823; PubMed Central PMCID: PMCPMC2974378.
48. Pisoni RL, Young EW, Dykstra DM, Greenwood RN, Hecking E, Gillespie B, et al. Vascular access use in Europe and the United States: results from the DOPPS. Kidney Int 2002;61(1):305–316. Epub 2002/01/12. https://doi.org/10.1046/j.1523-1755.2002.00117.x. PubMed PMID: 11786113.

22

Nalfurafine hydrochloride for refractory pruritus in peritoneal dialysis patients: a phase III, multi-institutional, non-controlled, open-label trial

Hidetomo Nakamoto[1], Takanori Oh[2], Masahiro Shimamura[2], Eiji Iida[2*] and Sadanobu Moritake[3]

Abstract

Background: Nalfurafine hydrochloride ("nalfurafine"), the world's first selective oral κ-receptor agonist for improving pruritus, is approved in Japan for the treatment of pruritus resistant to existing treatments in hemodialysis (HD) or chronic liver disease patients. Peritoneal dialysis (PD) patients, like HD patients, suffer from end-stage renal disease (ESRD) and some experience refractory pruritus.

Methods: We investigated the efficacy and safety of nalfurafine in 37 ESRD patients who underwent PD and had refractory pruritus. Nalfurafine was given once daily for 4 weeks at 2.5 μg in weeks 1 and 2 of the treatment period and at 5 μg in weeks 3 and 4. The primary endpoint was visual analog scale (VAS) changes for pruritus (i.e., the value upon rising or before sleep in week 2, whichever larger).

Results: The mean VAS change from baseline in week 2 of the treatment period was 24.93 mm [18.67, 31.19] (the point estimate of the mean [90% confidence interval (CI)]); the lower limit of CI exceeded the point estimate of the mean VAS change (15.24 mm) of the placebo group at the evaluation point (week 2) in a preceding confirmatory trial suggesting that had demonstrated nalfurafine efficacy for refractory pruritus in HD patients. The observed VAS change was comparable to that of the 2.5-μg group (week 2) in the preceding confirmatory trial, demonstrating that nalfurafine is as effective for treating pruritus in PD patients as in HD patients. Nalfurafine 5 μg was associated with a mean VAS change of 32.13 mm at week 4, i.e., the full length of the trial treatment period suggesting efficacy at the dose of 5 μg. The incidence of adverse drug reactions (ADR) was 45.9% (1/37 patients) with no serious ADRs observed. ADRs occurring in ≥ 5% of patients included insomnia (13.5%), increased blood prolactin (13.5%), somnolence (8.1%), lower blood testosterone free (8.1%), and vomiting (5.4%), all of which were mild.

Conclusions: This trial demonstrated the efficacy and safety of nalfurafine against refractory pruritus in PD, suggesting clinical benefit for treating pruritus in PD patients.

Keywords: Nalfurafine, κ-receptor agonist, Peritoneal dialysis, Pruritus, Refractory, Visual analog scale, Phase III trial

* Correspondence: Eiji_Iida@nts.toray.co.jp
[2]Pharmaceutical Clinical Research Department, Toray Industries Inc., 1-1, Nihonbashi-muromachi 2-chome, Chuo-ku, Tokyo 103-8666, Japan
Full list of author information is available at the end of the article

Background

Peritoneal dialysis (PD) patients suffering from end-stage renal failure, as with hemodialysis (HD) patients, often experience pruritus manifesting as itch [1, 2]. Itch may accompany diseases such as skin diseases (urticaria, atopic dermatitis, etc.), liver diseases (primary biliary cholangitis, etc.), renal diseases (chronic renal failure, etc.), and endocrine disorders (diabetes, thyroid dysfunction, etc.) [3]. Skin itch in patients with urticaria, for which is largely induced by locally existing mediators such as histamine, can be controlled by antihistamines or other anti-allergy treatment. In contrast, renal disease-induced pruritus in PD patients (in common with HD patients) is often highly resistant to current treatments. The unmet medical need to establish a treatment with a useful agent for such patients is, therefore, pressing [1–3].

Nalfurafine hydrochloride (nalfurafine) is a novel selective κ-receptor agonist developed by the Pharmaceutical Research Laboratories of Toray Industries, Inc. In non-clinical studies, nalfurafine showed an antipruritic effect for an itch model in which antihistamine was not sufficiently effective [4, 5]. Based on this finding, clinical development of an oral agent was launched for the treatment of refractory pruritus in HD patients [6, 7]. Following confirmation of its clinical effectiveness, nalfurafine was approved for use in Japan in 2009 for the indication of improving refractory pruritus in HD patients. Nalfurafine efficacy for intractable pruritus in patients with chronic liver diseases (hepatitis, hepatic cirrhosis, primary biliary cholangitis, non-alcoholic steatohepatitis, etc.) was subsequently confirmed during clinical development of the agent [8]. Additional approval was consequently obtained in 2015 for the indication of improving refractory pruritus in patients with chronic liver disease.

In common with HD patients, pruritus in PD patients typically starts prior to the introduction of dialysis during the preservation period of chronic renal failure; no major differences have been observed in the incidence and severity of pruritus between these populations [1, 2, 9]. As the fundamental mechanism of PD is the same as that of HD (the exception being that PD is performed via the patient's peritoneum), pruritus may be attributed to chronic renal failure both in PD and HD patients, with endogenic opioids playing a role in its onset [10]. Given these features, it is hypothesized that nalfurafine could be as effective for refractory pruritus in PD patients as in HD patients.

The results of preceding clinical pharmacological studies indicated that there is no requirement for adjustment of the nalfurafine according to the different prescriptions of PD (unpublished observations). These earlier studies also suggest that the pharmacokinetics of nalfurafine is similar in PD and HD patients.

On the basis of these findings, the present trial was conducted to investigate the safety and efficacy (i.e., the ability to provide additional clinical benefit over the base treatment of pruritus) of nalfurafine administered to PD patients with refractory pruritus with the same dosage and regimen as in the preceding confirmatory trial in HD patients. This trial was registered on June 5, 2014 to Japan Pharmaceutical Information Center (JAPIC) as JapicCTI-142,565.

Methods

This open-label investigation of nalfurafine therapy added to a base treatment against pruritus was conducted at 25 institutions in Japan from August 2014 to June 2015. In consideration of the small number of PD patients in Japan with approximately 9300 patients [11], no control group was included. Instead, the observed results were compared to those of a preceding confirmatory trial in which nalfurafine was tested against pruritus resistant to existing treatments in HD patients [6]. Therefore, for the purpose of aligning patient characteristics as much as possible between the trials, virtually the same inclusion and exclusion criteria as the preceding confirmatory trial in HD patients were employed. The same evaluation criteria for efficacy were similarly adopted. The trial schedule consisted of a 2-week pretreatment period, a 4-week treatment period, and an 8-day follow-up period (Fig. 1).

During the pretreatment period, we observed the level of pruritus under base treatment alone to determine the baseline value. In weeks 1 and 2 of the treatment period, the additional clinical benefit of nalfurafine 2.5 μg over base treatment efficacy was determined. In weeks 3 and 4 of the treatment period, the dosage was increased from 2.5 μg to 5 μg and the added clinical benefit of nalfurafine was investigated.

This clinical trial obtained approval from each institutional review board of all the participating institutions. It was conducted in compliance with the ethical principles based on the Declaration of Helsinki, Pharmaceutical and Medical Device Act, and Ministerial Ordinance on Good Clinical Practice (J-GCP). Informed consent was obtained from all patients.

Trial population

Table 1 shows key inclusion criteria and exclusion criteria. Inclusion criteria 2 and 5 were set to ensure the time for patients to acclimatize to the PD manipulation and achieve a stable condition. Inclusion criteria 3 and 4 were set for the purpose of enrolling patients with pruritus refractory to existing treatments. The aim of inclusion criteria 6 and 8 were to confirm that the patient was not responding to the "supposedly most effective" base treatment, using the two pruritus endpoints (i.e.,

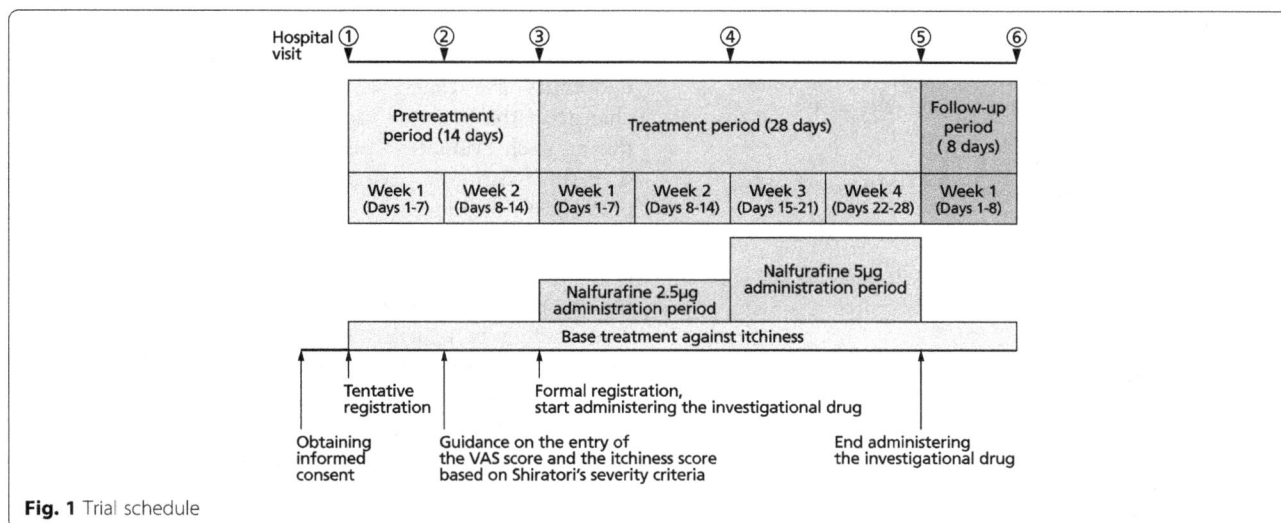

Fig. 1 Trial schedule

the VAS [12] and the Shiratori's criteria of pruritus severity [13]). In order to identify the severity and condition of pruritus, enrolled patients were required to have had the pruritus response endpoints recorded for five or more out of the 7 days during week 2 in the pretreatment period. Moreover, in order to enroll only those patients with severe pruritus and notable conditions sufficient for the assessment of pruritus, an inclusion criterion was established to require the severity and condition of pruritus in week 2 in the pretreatment period to be moderate or worse. Specifically, included patients had, on over half of the days, "the mean VAS of 50 mm or higher" and "the pruritus score of 3 or higher." Furthermore, inclusion criterion 7 was set to ensure the inclusion of patients with at least a certain level of constant pruritus. Exclusion criteria were established in order to eliminate any influence on the evaluation of efficacy and safety of nalfurafine.

Treatment

Previously used pruritus medical treatments were carried over as base treatment when a participant had either been treated prior to visit 1 with a prescription drug indicated for the treatment of pruritus, an over-the-counter (OTC) drug indicated for the treatment of pruritus, moisturizer, or an in-hospital preparation consisting of one or more of the above. In case a patient had received no pruritus medical treatment prior to visit 1, the most likely effective agent was chosen from the pruritus treatment drugs used within 1 year before the informed consent acquisition date. Enrolled patients received oral nalfurafine once daily after evening meals 2.5 μg [1 capsule] in weeks 1 and 2 in the treatment period and 5 μg [2 capsules] in weeks 3 and 4 in the treatment period. Use of opioid drugs was prohibited during clinical trial due to the concern that they might

enhance or reduce the effect of nalfurafine. The type, dosage, and regimen of prescription drugs and OTC drugs indicated for the treatment of pruritus remained unchanged, and newly initiating the use of the same drugs were prohibited to avoid their influence and allow adequate evaluation of pruritus during clinical trial. Specific designated drugs (i.e., hypnotics, antidepressants, antipsychotics, antiepileptics, anxiolytics, and non-prescription hypnotics) were also restricted due to the potential for increased adverse effects on the central nervous system when combined with nalfurafine.

Efficacy assessment

The severity and change of pruritus were evaluated by the VAS and the pruritus score based on Shiratori's criteria of pruritus severity (0 = no symptoms, 1 = slight, 2 = mild, 3 = moderate, 4 = severe) [13]. Both assessment methods had been used in a preceding confirmatory trial measuring pruritus in HD patients [6].

Participants recorded the severity and change of pruritus each day from the first day of the pretreatment period to the last day of the follow-up period; each patient recorded the severity of worst pruritus upon rising and before bed every day. The primary endpoint was mean VAS change (determined by using the larger value recorded either upon rising or before bed) in week 2 of the treatment period, with missing data imputed by the last observation carried forward (LOCF). A threshold was set at 15.24 mm, which derives from the point estimate of the mean change in the VAS (calculated using the larger value recorded either upon rising or before bed) of the placebo group in week 2 during the treatment period in the confirmatory trial enrolling HD patients. It was determined that nalfurafine was effective against refractory pruritus in PD patients when the lower limit of the 90% confidence interval (CI) of the

Table 1 Eligibility criteria

Key inclusion criteria
Included patients had to meet all of the conditions listed below,
all sexes and both inpatients and outpatients were eligible.

Upon obtaining informed consent
1. A patient of age 20 years or older
2. A patient undergoing peritoneal dialysis for three consecutive
   months or longer
3. A patient with a history within 1 year of drug treatment (a) and
   (b) against itch
   (a) systemic treatment (oral, injection, etc.) for two consecutive
       weeks or longer using antihistamine or antiallergic drugs
       indicated for the treatment of itch
   (b) topical treatment (external, etc.) using ointment indicated
       for the treatment of itch or moisturizer prescribed by a
       physician
4. A patient for whom neither of the treatment against itch listed
   in criteria 3 was evaluated sufficiently effective by the principal
   investigator or another investigator
Upon formal registration
5. A patient undergoing peritoneal dialysis continuously from the
   date of informed consent to the date of formal registration
6. A patient whose VAS score was recorded both on rising and
   before bed for five or more days in week 2 in pretreatment
   period, and the mean of the larger VAS score either upon
   rising or before bed was 50 mm or larger
7. A patient of whom the larger VAS score either upon rising or
   before bed was 20 mm or larger for five or more days in
   week 2 of the pretreatment period
8. A patient whose itch score based on Shiratori's severity criteria
   was recorded both on rising and before bed for 5 days or more
   in week 2 in the pretreatment period, and the itch score either
   upon rising or before bed, whichever was score of 3 or higher (i.e.,
   moderate or worse), for half of the days

Key exclusion criteria
Patients were excluded from the study if one or more of the
following conditions applied.
Upon obtaining informed consent
1. A patient who is concurrently undergoing hemodialysis
2. A patient who has been clinically diagnosed with the following
   complications
   (a) encapsulating peritoneal sclerosis
   (b) atopic dermatitis, chronic urticarial, or other skin disease
       that was determined to develop a systemic itch symptom
       that affects the evaluation of itch induced by renal disease
3. A patient who developed peritonitis within the last 4 weeks to
   make it difficult to continue peritoneal dialysis
4. A patient who received a phototherapy against itch in the
   last 1 month
5. A patient who has received nalfurafine in the past, who has
   participated in a clinical trial of nalfurafine and received it as
   the investigational drug, or who already participated as an
   eligible patient in this study
Upon formal registration
6. A patient who underwent hemodialysis between the date of
   informed consent and the date of formal registration
7. A patient who experienced onset of one of the following
   diseases between the date of informed consent and the date
   of formal registration
   (a) encapsulating peritoneal sclerosis
   (b) atopic dermatitis, chronic urticaria, or other skin disease
       that was determined to develop a systemic itch symptom
       that affects the evaluation of itch induced by renal disease
8. A patient who developed peritonitis between the date of
   informed consent and the date of formal registration, which
   made it difficult to continue peritoneal dialysis
9. A patient who received a phototherapy against itch between
   the date of informed consent and the date of formal registration

mean change in the VAS of a PD patient was larger than the threshold value. We also evaluated as secondary endpoints the mean change in the VAS, the mean change in the pruritus score, and the VAS improvement during each evaluation period (i.e., in weeks 1, 2, 3, and 4 in the treatment period and week 1 in the follow-up period); no imputation using LOCF was performed. The mean VAS change in each evaluation period was calculated by subtracting the mean VAS of each period from the mean VAS in week 2 of the pretreatment period. The change in pruritus score was calculated similarly. The VAS improvement was considered effective when the mean VAS change in each evaluation period was 20 mm or larger and considered ineffective if smaller than 20 mm [14]. We also assessed the mean VAS changes in week 2 (LOCF) of the treatment period in subgroups categorized according to demographic characteristics or other reference values.

Safety assessment
Adverse events (AEs) reported from the initiation of the treatment period to the end of the follow-up period were investigated. Incidents of adverse drug reactions (ADRs), which excluded AEs with no causal relations with the investigational drug, were also recorded. Laboratory values, vital signs, and incidents of ECG abnormalities were also included in the assessment. The data were aggregated for each of the following four periods: from the start of nalfurafine 2.5-µg administration to the end of the follow-up period (treatment period + follow-up period), from the start of 2.5-µg administration to its termination before switching to 5 µg (2.5-µg administration period), from the start of 5-µg administration to the first day of the follow-up period (5-µg administration period), and from the start of 5-µg administration to the end of the follow-up period (5-µg administration period + follow-up period). Once the 5-µg administration started, AEs were aggregated and analyzed only if the event had newly developed, or the severity had increased, after receiving 5 µg of nalfurafine. If the change from the value obtained before the start of the 5-µg administration was considered clinically abnormal, those changes in laboratory values and vital signs were considered to indicate AEs.

Statistical analysis
The efficacy analysis primarily targeted the full analysis set (FAS). The primary endpoint was represented by the point estimate and the two-sided 90% CI of the mean VAS change. Regarding secondary endpoints, the VAS change and the pruritus score change were shown by the fundamental statistics with two-sided 95% CIs; meanwhile, the VAS improvement was computed as the point estimate of the improvement rate with two-sided

95% CIs. The incidence of AEs and ADRs were counted in accordance with the MedDRA/J (version 18.0) preferred terms. The analyses were conducted by using SAS software version 9.3 (Cary, NC, USA).

Results

Patients

Informed consent was obtained from 44 patients, of whom 37 met the eligibility criteria and formally registered. In total, 37 patients received nalfurafine 2.5 µg. However, two patients dropped out due to AEs (one patient each for drug eruption and hypoaesthesia/hypoaesthesia oral/feeling hot/dizziness/vomiting); they did not receive nalfurafine 5 µg. The remaining 35 patients completed the entire course of nalfurafine 2.5 µg regimen followed by nalfurafine 5 µg. Table 2 shows the demographic characteristics of the formally registered patients. The residual "other primary diseases" category consisted of three for renal sclerosis, four for congenital cystic kidney disease, and one for benign prostatic hyperplasia (including patients with multiple diseases).

Efficacy

The FAS comprised all 37 patients enrolled in the trial. The FAS analysis showed the efficacy of nalfurafine 2.5 µg against pruritus resistant to existing treatments in PD patients as follows: the primary endpoint, that is, the mean VAS change in week 2 (LOCF) of the treatment period, was 24.93 mm [18.67, 31.19] (point estimate of the mean [90% CI]) and the lower limit of the CI was larger than the threshold (15.24 mm). Increased VAS changes were observed during the treatment period, while the VAS changes declined after administration was completed. The VAS change in each of the evaluation periods was 16.71 mm [10.11, 23.31] (point estimate of the mean [95% CI]), 24.02 mm [16.52, 31.53], 28.94 mm [21.38, 36.50], 32.13 mm [24.08, 40.18], and 19.48 mm [14.10, 24.85] in weeks 1, 2, 3, and 4 of the treatment period and in week 1 of the follow-up period, respectively (Fig. 2a). The course of the pruritus score change was similar to that of the VAS change. The pruritus score change in each of the evaluation periods was 0.61 [0.39, 0.83], 0.80 [0.52, 1.07], 0.97 [0.72, 1.22], 1.09 [0.80, 1.37], and 0.62 [0.40, 0.84] in weeks 1, 2, 3, and 4 of the treatment period and in week 1 of the follow-up period, respectively (Fig. 2b). The VAS improvement was continuously enhanced in weeks 1 through 3 and then sustained in weeks 3 and 4 of the treatment period and diminished after the end of administration (Table 3). No background factors were found to have influenced the efficacy of nalfurafine; none of the subgroups categorized by demographic characteristics or other reference values showed any specific tendencies in the subgroup analysis of the VAS change in week 2 in the treatment period.

The difference in PD prescriptions, including the type of dialysate solution and PD, had virtually no influence on the efficacy of the agent. The mean VAS change was 25.11 ± 20.65 mm (mean ± SD) in the subgroups that used dextrose plus icodextrin solutions, or icodextrin solution alone subgroup (subgroup of patients using icodextrin), 24.78 ± 24.60 mm in the dextrose solution subgroup (subgroup of patients not using icodextrin); 20.29 ± 19.72 mm in the continuous cycling peritoneal dialysis (CCPD) with automated peritoneal dialysis (APD) subgroup; and 27.45 ± 23.97 mm in the continuous ambulatory peritoneal dialysis (CAPD; without APD) subgroup. The effect of pruritus-related factors on efficacy was not evaluated.

Safety

All of the 37 patients were analyzed for safety. The incidence of AEs during clinical trial was 81.1% (30/37 patients), while that of ADRs was 45.9% (17/37 patients). The subgroup analysis of different evaluation periods found no increase in AEs or ADRs during the 5-µg administration period. The incidence of AEs and ADRs were, respectively, 51.4% (19/37 patients) and 35.1% (13/37 patients) in the 2.5-µg administration period and 48.6% (17/35 patients) and 17.1% (6/35 patients) in the 5-µg administration period. Among the ADRs listed in Table 4, the incident rate during treatment period + follow-up period was 5% or higher for insomnia, somnolence, vomiting, increased blood prolactin, and lower blood testosterone free; all of which were mild. The moderate ADRs occurred in one patient (2.7%) for drug eruption during the 2.5-µg administration period and none at all in the 5-µg administration period. None of the ADRs was severe. The difference in PD prescriptions seemed to have minimal effect on the frequency of ADRs. The incidence was 47.1% (8/17 patients) in the subgroup of patients using icodextrin, 45.0% (9/20 patients) in the subgroup of patients not using icodextrin, 46.2% (6/13 patients) in the CCPD subgroup, and 45.8% (11/24 patients) in the CAPD subgroup. Laboratory values showed no substantial changes over time. Neither did vital signs nor ECG abnormalities.

Discussion

Due to the technical need to compare the data obtained in this trial with those from a preceding confirmatory trial in HD patients, virtually the same inclusion and exclusion criteria were set at recruitment so that the characteristics of the patients in the two studies would be as similar as possible. As the equivalence of demographic characteristics was achieved, we decided that it was valid to compare and consider the results of the two studies against each other.

Table 2 Demographic characteristics and other reference values

Number of patients		PD patients with pruritus resistant to existing treatments (N = 37)
Sex	Male	27 (73.0%)
	Female	10 (27.0%)
Age (year)		63.5 ± 9.1
Weight(kg)		63.14 ± 11.03
Primary disease	Glomerulonephritis	15 (40.5%)
	Diabetic nephropathy	15 (40.5%)
	Renal failure, unspecified	1 (2.7%)
	Other	6 (16.2%)
Type of dialysis solution	Dextrose and icodextrin solutions, or icodextrin solution alone	17 (45.9%)
	Dextrose solution	20 (54.1%)
Type of peritoneal dialysis	CCPD (with APD)	13 (35.1%)
	CAPD (without APD)	24 (64.9%)
Duration of peritoneal dialysis (year)		2.30 ± 2.33
With anamnesis		20 (54.1%)
With complications		37 (100.0%)
Duration of itching (year)		1.76 ± 2.20
Mean VAS score in week 2 in the pretreatment period observation (mm) (the larger of the score upon rising or before bed)		77.22 ± 11.46
Mean itch score based on Shiratori's severity criteria in week 2 in the pretreatment period observation (the larger of the score upon rising or before bed)		3.11 ± 0.37
Pruritus treatments used within 1 year before the informed consent acquisition date		
Oral drug	Antihistamines or antiallergics	37 (100.0%)
	Steroid	0 (0.0%)
	Other	0 (0.0%)
	Total	37 (100.0%)
Topical product	Antihistamines or antiallergics	11 (29.7%)
	Steroid	12 (32.4%)
	Moisturizing agents	27 (73.0%)
	Other	11 (29.7%)
	Total	37 (100.0%)
Injection product	Antihistamines or antiallergics	0 (0.0%)
	Steroid	0 (0.0%)
	Stronger neo-minophagen C	0 (0.0%)
	Other	0 (0.0%)
	Total	0 (0.0%)
Pruritus treatments used during clinical trial		
Oral drug	Antihistamines or antiallergics	34 (91.9%)
	Steroid	0 (0.0%)
	Other	0 (0.0%)
	Total	34 (91.9%)
Topical product	Antihistamines or antiallergics	7 (18.9%)
	Steroid	11 (29.7%)

Table 2 Demographic characteristics and other reference values *(Continued)*

Number of patients		PD patients with pruritus resistant to existing treatments (N = 37)
	Moisturizing agents	24 (64.9%)
	Other	12 (32.4%)
	Total	37 (100.0%)
Injection product	Antihistamines or antiallergics	0 (0.0%)
	Steroid	0 (0.0%)
	Stronger neo-minophagen C	1 (2.7%)
	Other	0 (0.0%)
	Total	1 (2.7%)
Pruritus-related factors in CKD patients		
Complications (overlapping)	Hyperphosphatemia	28 (75.7%)
	Secondary hyperparathyroidism	27 (73.0%)
	Asteatosis	3 (8.1%)
	Hypocalcemia	1 (2.7%)
	Xeroderma	1 (2.7%)
	Immunodeficiency	1 (2.7%)
Laboratory value (pretreatment value)	Mean plasma hemoglobin (g/dL; ± SD)	10.58 ± 1.33
	Mean plasma eosinophils (%; ± SD)	7.43 ± 6.54
	Mean serum albumin (g/dL; ± SD)	3.49 ± 0.40
	Mean plasma hematocrit (%; ± SD)	31.98 ± 4.22
	Mean serum urea nitrogen (mg/dL; ± SD)	56.2 ± 14.1
	Mean serum creatinine (mg/dL; ± SD)	9.953 ± 3.179
	Mean serum phosphorus (mg/dL; ± SD)	5.18 ± 1.10
	Mean serum calcium (mg/dL; ± SD)	8.85 ± 0.89

Values are the number (percentage) of cases

CCPD continuous cycling peritoneal dialysis, *CAPD* continuous ambulatory peritoneal dialysis, *APD* automated peritoneal dialysis, *VAS* visual analog scale, *CKD* chronic kidney disease, *SD* standard deviation

The VAS change observed in this trial was equivalent to that in the preceding confirmatory trial; the VAS change (LOCF) in week 2 of the treatment period in this trial was 24.93 ± 22.56 mm (mean ± SD), compared to the primary endpoint (week 2 in the 2.5 µg group) of 24.52 ± 21.82 mm in the confirmatory trial in HD patients. Moreover, the present trial found the change over time in the mean VAS change, VAS improvement, and the course of changes in the mean pruritus score to be similar between the HD and PD patient groups. Thus, the present trial demonstrated the clinical effectiveness of nalfurafine 2.5 µg for the treatment of pruritus resistant to existing treatments in PD patients. Furthermore, subgroup analyses found no noticeable effect on efficacy of different prescriptions of PD. In terms of different methods of PD, the change in VAS was no difference between the subgroup with APD and without APD; additionally, the use of different dialysate solutions did not result in significantly different VAS changes. This trial also suggested that the efficacy of nalfurafine 5 µg in

PD patients was virtually the same as in HD patients. The VAS changes in weeks 3 and 4 in the treatment period of this trial, when participants received nalfurafine 5 µg (28.94 ± 22.01 mm in week 3, 32.13 ± 23.44 mm in week 4), were found to be equivalent to the 28.28 ± 23.14 mm VAS change observed in the 5 µg group in week 4 in the treatment period of a preceding long-term trial in HD patients [7].

Safety assessment showed that nalfurafine 2.5 µg or 5 µg in PD patients is well tolerated. No additional incidents of ADRs were observed in the 5-µg dosage period over the 2.5-µg dosage period. Most of the ADRs that did occur during this trial were mild; none was serious. The safety of nalfurafine according to different dialysis methods was also examined by comparing the incidents of ADRs in this trial with those in the preceding confirmatory trial in HD patients. Neither the incident rate of ADRs nor of serious drug reactions or moderate or worse drug reactions in PD patients was significantly higher than

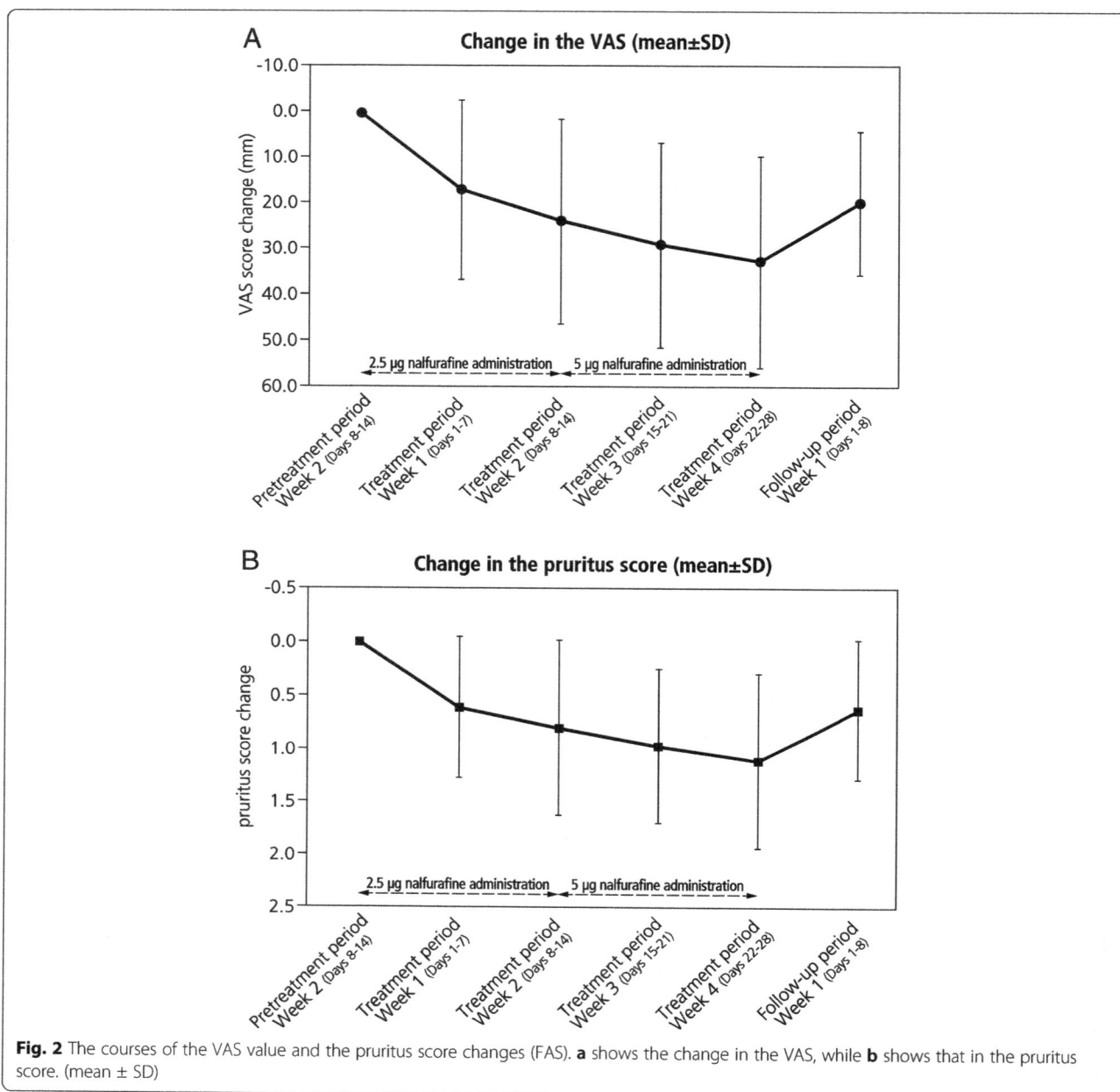

Fig. 2 The courses of the VAS value and the pruritus score changes (FAS). **a** shows the change in the VAS, while **b** shows that in the pruritus score. (mean ± SD)

in HD patients. Although PD patients reported relatively higher incidence of somnolence, vomiting, increased blood prolactin, and lower blood testosterone free than in HD patients, these ADRs were all mild and resolved without any treatment; none was serious. The effect of nalfurafine on the endocrine system has been confirmed in previous non-clinical and clinical trials. The agent appears to induce endocrinal changes by actions common to those of opioids, which are known to act on the central nervous system and may trigger endocrinal disorders [15]. Increased blood prolactin and lower blood

Table 3 VAS improvement (FAS)

	Treatment period week 1 (days 1–7) (N = 37)	Treatment period week 2 (days 8–14) (N = 36)	Treatment period week 3 (days 15–21) (N = 35)	Treatment period week 4 (days 22–28) (N = 35)	Follow-up period week 1 (days 1–8) (N = 36)
Improved patients (%) [95% CI]	11 (29.7) [15.9, 47.0]	18 (50.0) [32.9, 67.1]	22 (62.9) [44.9, 78.5]	22 (62.9) [44.9, 78.5]	19 (52.8) [35.5, 69.6]

Table 4 The list of adverse drug reactions

Adverse drug reactions	2.5-µg administration period N = 37	5-µg administration period N = 35	5-µg administration period + follow-up period N = 35	Treatment period + follow-up period N = 37
	Number of patients (%)	Number of patients (%)	Number of patients (%)	Number of patients (%)
Insomnia	3 (8.1)	2 (5.7)	2 (5.7)	5 (13.5)
Dizziness	1 (2.7)	0 (0.0)	0 (0.0)	1 (2.7)
Hypoaesthesia	1 (2.7)	0 (0.0)	0 (0.0)	1 (2.7)
Somnolence	3 (8.1)	0 (0.0)	0 (0.0)	3 (8.1)
Restless legs syndrome	0 (0.0)	1 (2.9)	1 (2.9)	1 (2.7)
Constipation	1 (2.7)	0 (0.0)	0 (0.0)	1 (2.7)
Gastrooesophageal reflux disease	0 (0.0)	1 (2.9)	1 (2.9)	1 (2.7)
Vomiting	1 (2.7)	1 (2.9)	1 (2.9)	2 (5.4)
Hypoaesthesia oral	1 (2.7)	0 (0.0)	0 (0.0)	1 (2.7)
Hepatic function abnormal	1 (2.7)	0 (0.0)	0 (0.0)	1 (2.7)
Drug eruption	1 (2.7)	0 (0.0)	0 (0.0)	1 (2.7)
Pruritus	1 (2.7)	0 (0.0)	0 (0.0)	1 (2.7)
Rash	1 (2.7)	0 (0.0)	0 (0.0)	1 (2.7)
Haematuria	1 (2.7)	0 (0.0)	0 (0.0)	1 (2.7)
Asthenia	1 (2.7)	0 (0.0)	0 (0.0)	1 (2.7)
Feeling hot	1 (2.7)	0 (0.0)	0 (0.0)	1 (2.7)
Aspartate aminotransferase increased	0 (0.0)	0 (0.0)	1 (2.9)	1 (2.7)
Blood prolactin increased	2 (5.4)	2 (5.7)	3 (8.6)	5 (13.5)
Blood testosterone free decreased	2 (5.4)	1 (2.9)	1 (2.9)	3 (8.1)

testosterone free observed in the present trial were only temporary changes. No endocrine-related clinical symptoms such as cardiovascular diseases or death were observed. These findings indicate that PD patients are very unlikely to experience clinically significant ADRs of nalfurafine, and that no special caution needs to be applied to those existing for use of nalfurafine in HD patients.

While HD is highly standardized, PD is diverse in terms of the choice and adjustment of the type of PD, the method of exchanging dialysate, and the dialysis dose which is tailored to each patient's physical status and lifestyle. After due consideration of adaptation to the specifically prescribed approach, it was decided that the results of a previous trial rejected the need for adjustment of the dosage and administration of nalfurafine according to different prescriptions of PD. In a preceding clinical pharmacology trial, 17 PD patients treated with a single oral dose of nalfurafine 2.5 µg or 5 µg had been examined for how different prescriptions of PD potentially affected nalfurafine pharmacokinetics. The trial found that neither the method of PD nor the type of dialysate affected nalfurafine pharmacokinetics (unpublished observations). The results were further reinforced by the present trial as detailed above in the efficacy and safety sections.

Overall, the available information suggests that PD is similar to HD in requiring no adjustment of dosage or administration. The pharmacokinetics of nalfurafine in the 17 PD patients in the preceding trial was compared with that in 16 HD patients who were enrolled in another clinical pharmacological trial. This comparison revealed the pharmacokinetics of nalfurafine in the two groups to be very similar.

Nalfurafine is approved in Japan and Korea for the treatment of intractable pruritus in HD patients, and two dosages of 2 µg and 5 µg have been in clinical use. In addition, Takahashi and others [16] have proposed a treatment algorithm of considering elevation to 5 µg if sufficient efficacy is not achieved after administering 2.5 µg for 2 to 4 weeks. Therefore, as in HD patients, the efficacy of nalfurafine for treating refractory pruritus in PD patients should be evaluated after administering 2.5 µg/day for 2 to 4 weeks. If the efficacy is insufficient without troublesome ADRs, elevation to 5 µg/day can be considered.

The limitations of this clinical trial include its open-label design, the use of short administration periods, and 2.5-µg and 5-µg nalfurafine dosage variation that did not allow adequate assessment of the effect of treatment for the pruritus of PD patients. Nevertheless, this trial is notable as the first study showing the efficacy and safety of nalfurafine in PD patients with pruritus resistant to existing treatments.

Conclusions

Nalfurafine at 2.5 μg and 5 μg may be effective for the treatment of refractory pruritus in patients undergoing PD as well as in HD patients. Since the safety profile of nalfurafine in PD patients was very similar to that in HD patients, we determined that the dosage and administration in PD patients can be the same as in HD patients; starting at 2.5 μg, the clinical dosage may be increased up to 5 μg according to prevailing symptoms. No adjustment of dosage and administration seems necessary relative to various PD prescriptions.

Abbreviations

ADR: Adverse drug reaction; APD: Automated peritoneal dialysis; CAPD: Continuous ambulatory peritoneal dialysis; CCPD: Continuous cycling peritoneal dialysis; CI: Confidence interval; ECG: Electrocardiogram; ESRD: End-stage renal disease; FAS: Full analysis set; IgA: Immunoglobulin A; J-GCP: Japanese Good Clinical Practice; LOCF: Last observation carried forward; OTC: Over-the-counter; SD: Standard deviation; VAS: Visual analog scale

Acknowledgements

We would like to express our gratitude to all patients registered in this clinical trial, all participating institutions, their principal and other investigators, and clinical research staff.

Funding

The financial cost to conduct this clinical trial was covered by its sponsor, Toray Industries, Inc. English translation was prepared by Jun Kishi of Medcore Associates, Inc. and Dr. Martin Guppy of Metamols Ltd.

Authors' contributions

HN provided medical advice in creating and amending the protocol. Receiving the information on safety, he provided medical advice when appropriate. He discussed each case and its handling in accordance with the GCPs with the sponsor. He read and signed the clinical study report and wrote this manuscript. TO, SM, and EI are responsible for the general administration and management of the clinical trial. They created and amended the protocol and responded to issues during the clinical trial. They gave instructions for the preparation of the clinical study report and assume responsibility for its content. MS analyzed the pharmacokinetics of the investigational drug in a peritoneal dialysis patient. All authors have read and approved the present paper and consented to its submission.

Competing interests

This clinical trial was funded by Toray Industries, Inc. HN received consulting fee from Toray Industries, Inc. TO, MS, EI, and SM are employees of Toray Industries, Inc. No other potential competing interest relevant to this article was reported.

Author details

[1]Department of General Internal Medicine, Saitama Medical University Hospital, 38 Morohongo, Moroyama-machi, Iruma-gun, Saitama 350-0495, Japan. [2]Pharmaceutical Clinical Research Department, Toray Industries Inc., 1-1, Nihonbashi-muromachi 2-chome, Chuo-ku, Tokyo 103-8666, Japan. [3]Pharmaceuticals Business Department, Toray International (China) Co., Ltd, 1601 West Nanjing Road, Jing An District, Shanghai 200040, China.

References

1. Tessari G, Dalle Vedove C, Loschiavo C, Tessitore N, Rugiu C, Lupo A, et al. The impact of pruritus on quality of life of patients undergoing dialysis: a single centre cohort study. J Nephrol. 2009;22:241–8.
2. Narita I, Iguchi S, Omori K, Gejyo F. Uremic pruritus in chronic hemodialysis patients. J Nephrol. 2008;21:161–5.
3. Krajnik M, Zylicz Z. Understanding pruritus in systemic disease. J Pain Symptom Manag. 2001;21:151–68.
4. Togashi Y, Umeuchi H, Okano K, Ando N, Yoshizawa Y, Honda T, et al. Antipruritic activity of the κ-opioid receptor agonist, TRK-820. Eur J Pharmacol. 2002;435:259–64.
5. Umeuchi H, Togashi Y, Honda T, Nakao K, Okano K, Tanaka T, et al. Involvement of central μ-opioid system in the scratching behavior in mice, and the suppression of it by the activation of κ-opioid system. Eur J Pharmacol. 2003;477:29–35.
6. Kumagai H, Ebata T, Takamori K, Muramatsu T, Nakamoto H, Suzuki H. Effect of a novel Kappa-receptor agonist, nalfurafine hydrochloride, on severe itch in 337 haemodialysis patients: a phase III, randomized, double-blind, placebo-controlled study. Nephrol Dial Transplant. 2010;25:1251–7.
7. Kumagai H, Ebata T, Takamori K, Miyasato K, Muramatsu T, Nakamoto H, et al. Efficacy and safety of a novel κ-agonist for managing intractable pruritus in dialysis patients. Am J Nephrol. 2012;36:175–83.
8. Kumada H, Miyakawa H, Muramatsu T, Ando N, Oh T, Takamori K, et al. Efficacy of nalfurafine hydrochloride in patients with chronic liver disease with refractory pruritus: a randomized, double-blind trial. Hepatol Res. 2017; 47:972–82.
9. Mistik S, Utas S, Ferahbas A, Tokgoz B, Unsal G, Sahan H, et al. An epidemiology study of patients with uremic pruritus. J Eur Acad Dermato. 2006;20:672–8.
10. Takamori K, et al. Role of the opioid system in systemic and peripheral itch. 20th World Congress of Dermatology. Paris, France 2002.
11. An overview of regular dialysis treatment in Japan as of Dec. 31, 2015. Japanese Society for Dialysis Therapy. http://docs.jsdt.or.jp/overview/pdf2016/p042.pdf. Accessed 1 Aug 2017.
12. Wahlgren CF, Ekblom A, Hägermark O. Some aspects of the experimental induction and measurement of itch. Acta Derm Venereol. 1989;69:185–9.
13. Kawashima M, Tango T, Noguchi T, Inagi M, Nakagawa H, Harada S. Addition of fexofenadine to a topical corticosteroid reduces the pruritus associated with atopic dermatitis in a 1-week randomized, multicentre, double-blind, placebo-controlled, parallel-group study. Br J Dermatol. 2003;148:1212–21.
14. Hiraga K, Ohashi Y. Efficacy evaluation of analgesic agents used for cancer pain management by visual analogue scale—a survey by questionnaire to physicians, nurses and patients. Pain Res. 1999;14:9–19.
15. Grossman A. Brain opiates and neuroendocrine function. Clin Endocrinol Metab. 1983;12:725–46.
16. Takahashi N, Yoshizawa T, Kumagai J, Kawanishi H, Moriishi M, Masaki T, et al. Response of patients with hemodialysis-associated pruritus to new treatment algorithm with nalfurafine hydrochloride: a retrospective survey-based study. Renal Replacement Therapy. 2016;2:27.

23

High prevalence of peripheral arterial disease (PAD) in incident hemodialysis patients: screening by ankle-brachial index (ABI) and skin perfusion pressure (SPP) measurement

Kunihiro Ishioka[*], Takayasu Ohtake, Hidekazu Moriya, Yasuhiro Mochida, Machiko Oka, Kyoko Maesato, Sumi Hidaka and Shuzo Kobayashi

Abstract

Background: Peripheral arterial disease (PAD) has much impact on mortality in hemodialysis (HD) patients. Ankle-brachial index (ABI) and skin perfusion pressure (SPP) are useful tools to detect PAD in HD patients. However, the prevalence of PAD in incident HD patients by ABI and SPP measurement has not been fully elucidated.

Methods: We examined both ABI and SPP in 185 consecutive patients with end-stage renal failure at the initiation of HD therapy. PAD was diagnosed by previous history, clinical symptoms, histories of endovascular peripheral intervention, bypass surgery, amputation due to PAD, and values of ABI and SPP. Cut-off value of ABI and SPP for diagnosing PAD was set at < 0.9 and < 50 mmHg, respectively.

Results: The percentage of limbs with ABI < 0.9 and SPP value < 50 mmHg among total limbs were 10.8 and 21.1%, respectively. Among 185 patients in incident HD patients, 45 patients were diagnosed as having PAD. ABI and SPP positively correlated ($r = 0.311$, $p = 0.006$). However, discrepancy between ABI and SPP values (normal or high ABI with low SPP, or low ABI with normal SPP) was also found. Among 45 incident HD patients with PAD, only 14 patients (31.1%) showed low ABI and low SPP values.

Conclusion: Measurement of both ABI and SPP might be necessary to improve the diagnostic accuracy of PAD. Prevalence of PAD in incident HD patients was proved to be very high.

Keywords: Peripheral artery disease (PAD), Hemodialysis (HD), Skin perfusion pressure (SPP), Ankle-brachial pressure index (ABI)

Background

Peripheral arterial disease (PAD) in lower extremities in hemodialysis (HD) patients has much impact on prognosis. Amputation rate of lower limbs in HD patients is reported to be 4.3/100 person year in USA [1]. Once PAD worsens to severe disease state, critical limb ischemia (CLI) which necessitates major amputation of lower limbs, the prognosis is severely poor, i.e., 1-year survival rate 30–50% [2, 3] and 5-year survival rate 14.4% [3].

Detecting early symptoms of PAD such as chillness and/or claudication are sometimes difficult and un-reliable in HD patients, and it is not unusual to find CLI as the first apparent symptom of PAD. Therefore, early detection of PAD would be extremely important to improve the prognosis of HD patients.

Ankle-brachial pressure index (ABI) is a useful screening test for detecting PAD. ABI value less than 0.9 is generally thought to have arterial stenosis or obstruction in lower limbs. However, we have previously reported that the sensitivity of ABI < 0.9 for detecting PAD in HD patients was only 29.9% (specificity was 100%) [4].

* Correspondence: kunihirock@hotmail.co.jp
Kidney Disease and Transplant Center, Shonan Kamakura General Hospital, 1370-1 Okamoto, Kamakura 247-8533, Japan

Accurate ABI values may not be obtained and pseudo-normalize in cases of high arterial calcification or incompressible arteries [5]. In this regard, skin perfusion pressure (SPP) might be a superior tool to ABI in order to detect microcirculatory impairment more accurately. SPP is also applicable to the patients with edema or severe blood vessel calcification cases as SPP detects circulation of the subcutaneous tissue, and SPP can detect the limb ischemia more accurately [6–9]. SPP values less than 50 mmHg could detect PAD in HD patients with high sensitivity of 84.9% and high specificity of 78.6% as we previously reported [4].

Most previous epidemiological reports concerning the prevalence of PAD in HD patients depended on the ABI value [4–6, 9–15], and reports concerning SPP as a diagnostic tool for PAD in HD patients are limited [4, 6, 7, 9, 16]. Furthermore, the prevalence of PAD at the initiation of HD therapy has not been so far elucidated. Therefore, we examined ABI and SPP in 185 consecutive incident HD patients to compare the results of two diagnostic methods, to evaluate the relationship between ABI and SPP, and to clarify the prevalence of PAD at the initiation of HD.

Methods

Patients

This study was performed in a single HD center in Shonan Kamakura General Hospital. Eligible subjects comprised all consecutive patients from December 2003 to November 2008 who newly started HD in our hospital. Patients who could not be evaluated by SPP due to involuntary movement were excluded. Patients who had history of previous major amputation of lower legs were registered as a subject, although they did not have SPP data.

Clinical information about age; sex; smoking history; comorbidity including hypertension, diabetes mellitus, dyslipidemia, ischemic heart disease (IHD), and stroke; and drug use including ARB, statin, medication of anti-platelet drugs including cilostazol, aspirin, sarpogrelate, and prostaglandin I_2 analogue was recorded by medical records and interviews to the patients. Laboratory data including hemoglobin, blood glucose, serum albumin, calcium, phosphate, total cholesterol, triglyceride, high-density lipoprotein, low-density lipoprotein, and C-reactive protein were evaluated using in-hospital laboratory in our hospital. All patients gave informed consent, and local ethical committee approved the study (ethical No. TGE00797-024) and was performed in accordance with the principles of the Declaration of Helsinki.

ABI/SPP

ABI was measured by ABI-form (Colin, Komaki, Japan) as previously reported [4, 5]. ABI-form simultaneously measures unilateral branchial pressure in the arm without an

arterio-venous fistula and ankle blood pressure by oscillometric method. ABI was calculated as the ratio of ankle systolic pressure divided by brachial systolic pressure.

SPP was measured by using a Laser Dopp PV3000® (Kaneka, Osaka, Japan) according to the method described by Castronuovo et al. [17]. Briefly, the laser Doppler skin perfusion pressure transducer consists of a laser Doppler probe secured within the bladder of a blood pressure cuff that contains a transparent polyvinylchloride window so that microcirculatory perfusion measurements can be made during cuff deflation. Two points were set to measure SPP in each patient, (a) a point between first and second metatarsal bones in instep and (b) a front middle point in sole. After inflating the cuff pressure at first to stop skin perfusion, then deflate the cuff pressure and measure the point of cuff pressure when skin perfusion restarted. SPP was expressed as pressure of restarting the skin perfusion. Each patient had four SPP data, i.e., right and left leg in instep and sole. SPP value less than 50 mmHg of at least one point among these 4 points was necessary to diagnose PAD. Measurement of SPP was performed within 1 h after an HD session, and ABI test was also performed on the same day after an HD session.

Validation of SPP measurement has been clearly reported [4]. We previously evaluated the diagnostic accuracy of ABI and SPP to detect PAD in HD patients using contrast-enhanced computed tomography as standard images. As a result, ABI value < 0.9 can detect PAD with 100% specificity and SPP value < 50 mmHg with specificity of 76.9%. Japanese Society for Dialysis Therapy Guideline suggested that ABI 1.0 might be used as cutoff value to detect PAD in maintenance HD patients because of high vascular calcification [18]. However, there is no evidence that ABI 1.0 could be also applied in incident HD patients. Therefore, we used ABI cutoff value 0.9, cutoff value in the general population and 100% specificity in maintenance HD patients for PAD, in this study.

Definition of PAD

Patients were interviewed about symptoms of PAD including chillness, numbness, claudication, and resting pain. Previous histories of intervention (percutaneous peripheral intervention or bypass surgery) or amputation due to PAD were also recorded. All patients then underwent physiological examination about skin color, warmth, pulse exam of femoral artery, popliteal artery, dorsal artery, posterior tibial artery, and skin lesion including ulcers and gangrenes. The symptomatic information, previous histories of intervention or amputation, and physiological examinations including ABI and SPP were used to assign a limb ischemia. When patients filled at least one criteria among (1) ABI < 0.9, (2) SPP < 50 mmHg, (3) apparent previous history of intervention or amputation of lower limbs due to PAD, and (4) apparent clinical symptoms including claudication, resting pain, or ulcer due to ischemia, they were defined as having PAD.

In patients who were diagnosed as having PAD, severity was categorized from I to IV by Fontaine's clinical severity classification [19].

Statistical analysis

All data are expressed as mean ± SD. Unpaired t test or Mann-Whitney U test were used for group comparisons. Categorical data were analyzed by means of chi-square test. Univariate analysis was performed using Spearman's rank correlation coefficient. Stepwise logistic regression analysis was performed based on a forward-backward procedure to define the independent variables related to PAD. Statistical analyses were done using statistical software (JMP 10: SAS Institute, JAPAN, and SPSS 10.0 software: SPSS Inc., Chicago, IL, USA) for Windows personal computer.

Results
Patients

There were 193 incident HD patients during 5-year study period in HD center in our hospital. Among them, 8 patients (4.1%) had involuntary movement of the legs and were excluded from this study due to inability to measure SPP. As a result, 185 patients were finally evaluated. History of amputations of lower extremities due to PAD at the start of HD was three patients in unilateral major amputation and one patient with minor amputation. There was no patient with bilateral major amputation.

Table 1 shows the basic characteristics of 185 patients (130 men, 55 women) with a median age of 70 years old [interquartile range (IQR) 61–78]. Almost half of the patients had diabetes (100/185: 54.5%), and 43.1% of the patients had ischemic heart disease. Median values of ABI and SPP among all patients were 1.18 (IQR 1.05–1.27) and 73 (IQR 52–85) mmHg, respectively.

Distribution of ABI and SPP value and the prevalence of PAD

Distribution of ABI and SPP in incident HD patients was shown in Fig. 1. While limbs with ABI value less than 0.9 were 10.8%, 21.1% of limbs showed SPP values less than 50 mmHg among total limbs. On the other hand, limbs with ABI value more than 1.3 were 19.6% among total limbs at the initiation of HD therapy (Fig. 1). If ABI value was set at 1.0, 19.6% of patients showed ABI < 1.0.

Prevalence of PAD at the initiation of HD assessed by ABI and SPP, histories of revascularization and amputation were 24.3% (45/185). Fontaine severity classification among incident HD patients with PAD is shown in Table 2. Among 45 patients with PAD, almost 70% of patients (31/45) were asymptomatic. The number of patients who have

Table 1 Baseline characteristics

	All patients (N = 185)
Age (years)	70 (61–78)
Male, n (%)	130 (70.2)
Hypertension, n (%)	148 (80.0)
Diabetes mellitus, n (%)	100 (54.1)
Dyslipidemia, n (%)	80 (43.2)
Ischemic heart disease, n (%)	74 (40.0)
Stroke, n (%)	27 (14.9)
ABI	1.18 (1.05–1.27)
SPP (mmHg)	73 (52–85)
Previous history of PAD, n (%)	13 (7.0)
Medications	
Cilostazol, n (%)	11 (5.9)
Sarpogrelate, n (%)	1 (0.5)
Aspirin, n (%)	48 (25.9)
Prostaglandin analogue, n (%)	17 (9.2)
Ticlopidine, n (%)	18 (9.7)
Clopidogrel, n (%)	1 (0.5)
Warfarin, n (%)	6 (3.2)
Dipyridamole, n (%)	10 (4.9)
Dilazep, n (%)	9 (5.4)
ARB, n (%)	74 (40.0)
Statin, n (%)	60 (32.4)

Data are presented as median (interquartile range)
ABI ankle brachial pressure index, *SPP* skin perfusion pressure, *PAD* peripheral arterial disease, *ARB* angiotensinII receptor blocker

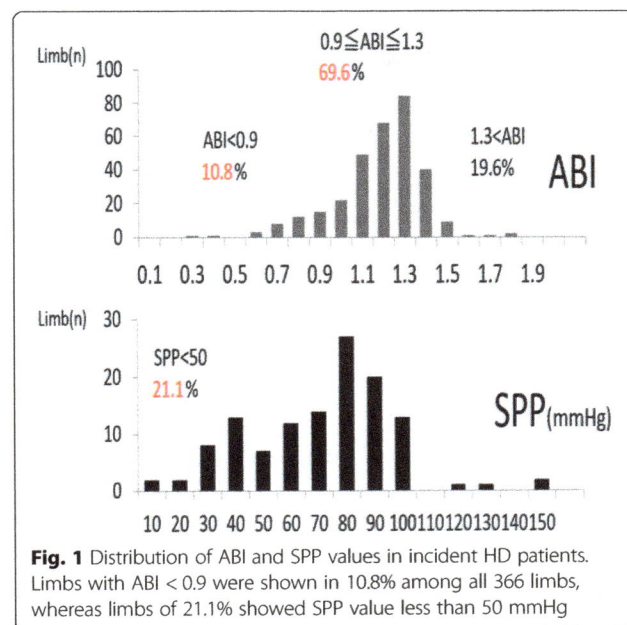

Fig. 1 Distribution of ABI and SPP values in incident HD patients. Limbs with ABI < 0.9 were shown in 10.8% among all 366 limbs, whereas limbs of 21.1% showed SPP value less than 50 mmHg

already been diagnosed as having PAD before starting HD was 29 patients (15.7%).

Relationship between ABI and SPP

SPP and ABI positively correlated ($r = 0.311$, $p = 0.006$; Fig. 2). Fourteen patients (7.6%) showed ABI < 0.9 and SPP < 50 mmHg, and 140 patients (75.6%) showed ABI ≥ 0.9 and SPP ≥ 50 mmHg, respectively. However, discrepancy between ABI and SPP values (normal or high ABI with low SPP, or low ABI with normal SPP) was also found. Six patients (3.2%) showed ABI < 0.9 and SPP ≥ 50 mmHg, and 25 patients (13.5%) showed ABI ≥ 0.9 and SPP < 50 mmHg, respectively.

Risk factors for PAD in incident HD patients

When patients were divided into two groups, i.e., PAD group and non-PAD group, there were significant differences in the prevalence of ischemic heart disease, total cholesterol, and LDL cholesterol between two groups. Ischemic heart disease was more prevalent in PAD patients compared with non-PAD patients (60 vs. 33.6%; $p < 0.001$) (Table 3). Multiple regression analysis, using significant variables in univariate analysis as independent variables, showed that only ischemic heart disease was an associating factor for PAD at the initiation of HD (Table 4). Both older age or diabetes mellitus were not independent associating factors for PAD in patients with end stage renal failure.

Discussion

We have clearly provided the evidence that the prevalence of PAD in incident HD patients was high (24.3%) by ABI and SPP measurements along with ischemic leg symptoms and histories of re-vascularization or amputation due to PAD. Previous epidemiological reports using ABI and SPP could not fully elucidate such high rate of PAD in incident HD patients. Risk factors for PAD include old age, male gender, smoking, diabetes mellitus, homocysteine, and C-reactive protein [20–23]. Furthermore, renal failure itself was an independent risk factor for PAD [23]. Patients at the initiation of HD have not only renal failure but also several risk factors as mentioned above. Therefore, it may be well appreciated that

Table 2 Fontaine's severity category in incident HD patients

PAD, n (% among total 185 pts)	45 (24.3)
Fontaine I	31 (16.8)
Fontaine II	2 (1.1)
Fontaine III	6 (3.2)
Fontaine IV	6 (3.2)
amputation	4 (2.2)

HD hemodialysis, *PAD* peripheral arterial disease

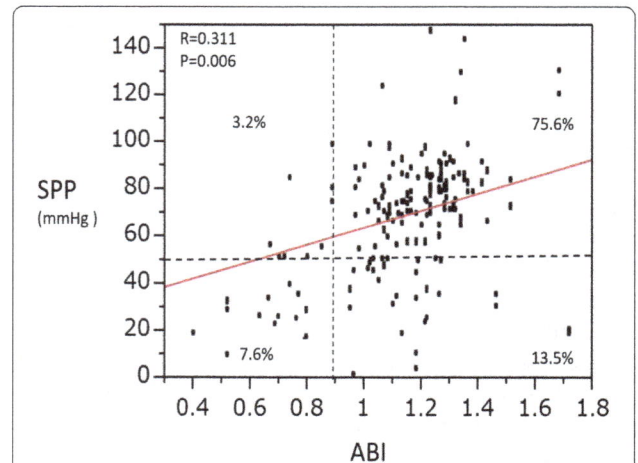

Fig. 2 Relationship between ABI and SPP. ABI and SPP significantly and positively correlated ($r = 0.311$, $p = 0.006$). Dotted lines indicate the cutoff values of ABI and SPP. Note that SPP varied from abnormally low levels to normal levels in normal ABI values

the prevalence of PAD is already very high at the initiation of HD.

The symptoms of PAD in its early stage are not so clinically prevalent or even might be asymptomatic so that patients do not complain of the symptoms related to PAD. Elderly HD patients might not walk long enough to complain of apparent intermittent claudication. Therefore, PAD might be missed when only judged by clinical symptoms. ABI has been widely used in previous reports as screening tool for PAD in HD patients. However, it has been well known that measurement of ABI might be strongly influenced in cases of highly calcified or incompressible arteries [5, 10].

SPP is a useful tool for PAD screening. SPP can evaluate the microcirculation of lower limbs. The importance of SPP was first reported in critical limb ischemia with intractable wound. SPP values more than 30 or 40 mmHg have been reported to predict healing of intractable wound [9, 17]. Thus, the significance of SPP measurement has, at first, established a consensus in evaluating severe limb ischemia and as a predictor of wound healing. Besides in the cases of critical limb ischemia (CLI), usefulness to measure SPP has recently been expanding its area as diagnosing tool of early stage of PAD.

As for discrepancy between ABI and SPP values, there might be some possible explanations. In cases with normal or high ABI value (≥ 0.9) and low SPP value (< 50 mmHg), high arterial calcification might pseudo-normalize or even elevate the ABI value to abnormally high levels. Another possibility is the existence of below-ankle arterial lesions. ABI was measured using ankle pressure, and SPP in this study examined microcirculation of below ankle lesions (instep and sole). If patient has PAD only in below ankle arteries, normal ABI and abnormally low SPP values might

Table 3 Characteristics of PAD patients and non-PAD patients

	Peripheral arterial disease		P
	+	−	
N	45	140	
Age (years)	72 (64–81)	69 (59–84)	0.055
Male n (%)	33 (73.3)	97 (69.3)	0.605
Smoking n (%)	17 (37.8)	58 (41.4)	0.694
Hypertension n (%)	40 (88.9)	108 (77.1)	0.087
Dyslipidemia n (%)	24 (53.3)	55 (39.3)	0.056
Diabetes mellitus n (%)	29 (64.4)	71 (50.7)	0.108
Ischemic heart disease n (%)	27 (60.0)	47 (33.6)	0.001
Stroke n (%)	10 (22.2)	17 (12.1)	0.095
ARB n (%)	19 (42.2)	55 (39.3)	0.646
Statin n (%)	19 (42.2)	41 (29.3)	0.086
Hemoglobin (g/dL)	8.7 (7.3–9.8)	8.3 (7.0–9.2)	0.079
ABI	0.92 (0.73–1.08)	1.22 (1.12–1.29)	< 0.0001
SPP	47 (34–71)	75 (69–86)	< 0.0001
Blood glucose (mg/dL)	124 (108–181)	127 (98–160)	0.406
Albumin (g/dL)	3.2 (2.8–3.6)	3.3 (2.8–3.6)	0.637
Ca (mg/dL)	7.8 (7.2–8.4)	7.7 (7.0–8.3)	0.486
P (mg/dL)	5.9 (4.7–7.1)	6.2 (5.0–7.4)	0.453
Total cholesterol (mg/dL)	176 (153–224)	158 (135–192)	0.015
Triglyceride (mg/dL)	98 (71–136)	101 (76–147)	0.821
HDL-C (mg/dL)	44.8 (34.6–55.2)	39.1 (31.0–48.6)	0.067
LDL-C (mg/dL)	106 (74–124)	83 (68.3–104.8)	0.025
CRP (mg/dL)	0.74 (0.615–2.815)	0.47 (0.120–3.730)	0.653
Cilstazol, n (%)	6 (13.3%)	5 (3.5%)	0.026
Sarpogrelate, n (%)	0 (0%)	1 (0.7%)	0.455
Aspirin, n (%)	26 (48.9%)	22 (22.6%)	0.0002
Prostaglandin analogue, n (%)	9 (20.5%)	8 (5.7%)	0.006

Data are presented as median (interquartile range)

PAD peripheral arterial disease, *ARB* angiotensin II receptor blocker, *Ca* calcium, *P* phosphate, *HDL-C* high-density lipoprotein cholesterol, *LDL-C* low-density lipoprotein cholesterol, *CRP* C-reactive protein

be accepted. In cases with low ABI and normal SPP values, below knee arterial lesions (above ankle) with well-developed collaterals in foot might explain the discrepancy of ABI and SPP. In anyway, sole ABI value below 0.9 might miss considerable number of PAD patients with normal or high ABI and low SPP values as shown in Fig. 2.

Table 4 Stepwise logistic regression analysis for independent determinants of PAD

	OR (95% CI)	P
Ischemic heart disease	2.76 (1.30–5.86)	0.008
Total cholesterol (mg/dL)	1.00 (0.98–1.01)	0.861
LDL-C (mg/dL)	1.01 (0.98–1.03)	0.347

Independent variables are ischemic heart disease, total cholesterol, and LDL-C(LDL-cholesterol)

Measurements of both ABI and SPP might improve the diagnostic accuracy of PAD.

In our study, previous history of ischemic heart disease was significantly associated with the prevalence of PAD (Table 3). Sixty percent of incident HD patients with PAD had the history of ischemic heart disease. Therefore, PAD might be presented as one of the systemic atherosclerotic disease as shown in REACH registry [24]. We should check other atherosclerotic diseases including ischemic heart disease or cerebrovascular disease when PAD was diagnosed at the initiation of HD. In this point, early diagnosis of PAD might contribute to improve the prognosis of HD patients.

The rate of prescription of anti-platelet drugs was significantly different between PAD group and non-PAD group in our study (Table 3). Aspirin was prescribed in

48.9% of incident HD patients with PAD whereas only 22.6% of patients without PAD took aspirin. However, aspirin was mainly prescribed for the purpose of secondary prevention of ischemia events in the heart and brain. In other words, aspirin prescription was only made in 48.9% of PAD patients. Far less HD patients with PAD took cilostazol, sarpogrelate, or prostaglandin analogue. Other antiplatelet drugs should be considered to be prescribed in terms of PAD [25–27]. The final purpose of medication for PAD is to increase walking distance, prevent CLI and amputation, and improve the prognosis. Early diagnosis using ABI and SPP might contribute to early prescription and improved quality of life and prognosis.

Recently, low values of ABI and/or SPP were reported to be a prognostic factor of cardiovascular disease (CVD) and mortality. Otani et al. reported that both low ABI and SPP values were independent risk factors for mortality among HD patients [28]. Ishi et al. reported that abnormal ABI (< 0.9 or > 1.4) predicted mortality due to CVD [29] in HD patients. Therefore, ABI and/or SPP might be used not only as diagnostic tools of PAD but also one of prognostic factors in HD patients.

Although this is a single center, cross-sectional observational study, we have provided that the prevalence of PAD in incident HD patients was surprisingly high and most of these patients were asymptomatic. Both ABI and SPP measurement might be useful for diagnosing PAD in incident HD patients. Further studies are needed to clarify whether early diagnosis of PAD might improve the outcome of incident HD patients.

Conclusion

Measurement of both ABI and SPP might be necessary to improve the diagnostic accuracy of PAD. Prevalence of PAD in incident HD patients was proved to be very high.

Authors' contributions

All authors read and approved the final manuscript.

Competing interests

The authors declare that they have no competing interests.

References

1. Eggers PW, Gohdes D, Pugh J. Nontraumatic lower extremity amputations in the Medicare end-stage renal disease population. Kidney Int. 1999;56:1524–33.
2. Dossa CD, Shepard AD, Amos AM, Kupin WL, Reddy DJ, Elliott JP, Wilczwski JM, Ernst CB. Results of lower extremity amputations in patients with end-stage renal disease. J Vasc Surg. 1994;20:14–9.
3. Aulivola B, Hile CN, Hamdan AD, Sheahan MG, Veraldi JR, Skillman JJ, Campbell DR, Scovell SD, LoGerfo FW, Pomposelli FB Jr. Major lower extremity amputation: outcome of a modern series. Arch Surg. 2004;139:395–9.
4. Okamoto K, Oka M, Maesato K, Ikee R, Mano T, Moriya H, Ohtake T, Kobayashi S. Peripheral arterial occlusive disease is more prevalent in patients with hemodialysis: comparison with the findings of multidetector-row computed tomography. Am J Kidney Dis. 2006;48:269–76.
5. Ohtake T, Oka M, Ikee R, Mochida Y, Ishioka K, Moriya H, Hidaka S, Kobayashi S. Impact of lower limbs' arterial calcification on the prevalence and severity of PAD in patients on hemodialysis. J Vasc Surg. 2011;53:676–83.
6. Shimazaki M, Matsuki T, Yamauchi K, Iwata M, Takahashi H, Genda S, Ohata J, Nakamura Y, Inaba Y, Yokouchi S, Kikuiri T, Ashie T. Assessment of lower limb ischemia with measurement of skin perfusion pressure in patients on hemodialysis. Ther Apher Dial. 2007;11:196–201.
7. Tsai FW, Tulsyan N, Jones DN, Abdel-Al N, Castronuovo JJ Jr, Carter SA. Skin perfusion pressure of the foot is a good substitute for toe pressure in the assessment of limb ischemia. J Vasc Surg. 2000;32:32–6.
8. Davis M, Rajagopalan S. Is skin perfusion pressure a useful screening tool for peripheral arterial disease in patients on hemodialysis? Nat Clin Pract Nephrol. 2007;3:598–9.
9. Yamada T, Ohta T, Ishibashi H, Sugimoto I, Iwata H, Takahashi M, Kawanishi J. Clinical reliability and utility of skin perfusion pressure measurement in ischemic limbs—comparison with other noninvasive diagnostic methods. J Vasc Surg. 2008;47:318–23.
10. Leskinen Y, Salenius JP, Lehtimäki T, Huhtala H, Saha H. The prevalence of peripheral arterial disease and medial arterial calcification in patients with chronic renal failure: requirements for diagnosis. Am J Kidney Dis. 2002;40:472–9.
11. Kitaura K, Kida M, Harima K. Assessment of peripheral arterial disease of lower limbs with ultrasonography and ankle brachial index at the initiation of hemodialysis. Renal Fail. 2009;31:785–90.
12. Morimoto S, Yurugi T, Aota Y, Sakuma T, Jo F, Nishikawa M, Iwasaka T, Maki K. Prognostic significance of ankle-brachial index, brachial-ankle pulse wave velocity, flow-mediated dilatation, and nitroglycerin-mediated dilation in end-stage renal failure. Am J Nephrol. 2009;30:55–63.
13. Ogata H, Kumata-Maeta C, Shishido K, Mizobuchi M, Yamamoto M, Koiwa F, Kinugasa E, Akizawa T. Detection of peripheral artery disease by duplex ultrasonography among hemodialysis patients. Clin J Am Soc Nephrol. 2010;5:2199–206.
14. Chen SC, Chang JM, Hwang SJ, Tsai JC, Liu WC, Wang CS, Lin TH, Su HM, Chen HC. Ankle brachial index as a predictor for mortality in patients with chronic kidney disease and undergoing haemodialysis. Nephrology. 2010;15:294–9.
15. Kato A, Takita T, Furuhashi M, Kumagai H, Hishida A. A small decrease in the ankle-brachial index is associated with increased mortality in patients on chronic hemodialysis. Nephron Clin Prac. 2010;114:c29–37.
16. Kondo Y, Muto A, Dardik A, Nishibe M, Nishibe T. Laser Doppler skin perfusion pressure in the diagnosis of limb ischemia in patients with diabetes mellitus and/or hemodialysis. Int Angiol. 2007;26:258–61.
17. Castronuovo JJ Jr, Adera HM, Smiell JM, Price RM. Skin perfusion pressure of the foot is valuable in the diagnosis of critical limb ischemia. J Vasc Surg. 1997;26:629–37.
18. Hirakata H, Nitta K, Inaba M, Shoji T, Fujii H, Kobayashi S, Tabei K, Joki N, Hase H, Nishimura M, Ozaki S, Ikari Y, Kumada Y, Tsuruya K, Fujimoto S, Inoue T, Yokoi H, Hirata S, Shimamoto K, Kugiyama K, Akiba T, Iseki K, Tsubakihara Y, Tomo T, Akizawa T; Japanese Society for Dialysis Therapy. Japanese Society for Dialysis Therapy guidelines for management of cardiovascular diseases in patients on chronic hemodialysis. Ther Apher Dial 2012; 16: 387–435.
19. Fontaine R, Kim M, Kieny R. Surgical treatment of peripheral circulation disorders. Helv Chir Acta. 1954;21:499–533.
20. Ridker PM, Stampfer MJ, Rifai N. Novel risk factors for systemic atherosclerosis: a comparison of C-reactive protein, fibrinogen, homocysteine, lipoprotein(a), and standard cholesterol screening as predictors of peripheral arterial disease. JAMA. 2001;285:2481–5.

21. Fowkes FG, Housley E, Riemersma RA, Macintyre CC, Cawood EH, Prescott RJ, Ruckley CV. Smoking, lipids, glucose intolerance, and blood pressure as risk factors for peripheral atherosclerosis compared with ischemic heart disease in the Edinburgh Artery Study. Am J Epidemiol. 1992;135:331–40.

22. Lowe GD, Fowkes FG, Dawes J, Donnan PT, Lennie SE, Housley E. Blood viscosity, fibrinogen, and activation of coagulation and leukocytes in peripheral arterial disease and the normal population in the Edinburgh Artery Study. Circulation. 1993;87:1915–20.

23. MacGregor AS, Price JF, Hau CM, Lee AJ, Carson MN, Fowkes FG. Role of systolic blood pressure and plasma triglycerides in diabetic peripheral arterial disease. The Edinburgh Artery Study. Diabetes Care. 1999;22:453–8.

24. Bhatt DL, Steg PG, Ohman EM, Hirsch AT, Ikeda Y, Mas JL, Goto S, Liau CS, Richard AJ, Röther J, Wilson PW; REACH Registry Investigators. International prevalence, recognition, and treatment of cardiovascular risk factors in outpatients with atherothrombosis. JAMA 2006; 11: 180–189.

25. Hidaka S, Kobayashi S, Iwagami M, Isshiki R, Tsutsumi D, Mochida Y, Ishioka K, Oka M, Maesato K, Moriya H, Ohtake T. Sarpogrelate hydrochloride, a selective 5-HT(2A) receptor antagonist, improves skin perfusion pressure of the lower extremities in hemodialysis patients with peripheral arterial disease. Ren Fail. 2013;35:43–8.

26. Ohtake T, Sato M, Nakazawa R, Kondoh M, Miyaji T, Moriya H, Hidaka S, Kobayashi S. Randomized pilot trial between prostaglandin I2 analog and anti-platelet drugs on peripheral arterial disease in hemodialysis patients. Ther Apher Dial. 2014;18:1–8.

27. Pande RL, Perlstein TS, Beckman JA, Creager MA. Secondary prevention and mortality in peripheral artery disease: National Health and Nutrition Examination Study, 1999 to 2004. Circulation. 2011;124:17–23.

28. Otani Y, Otsubo S, Kimata N, Takano M, Abe T, Okajima T, Miwa N, Tsuchiya K, Nitta K, Akiba T. Effects of the ankle-brachial blood pressure index and skin perfusion pressure on mortality in hemodialysis patients. Intern Med. 2013;52:2417–21.

29. Ishii H, Takahashi H, Ito Y, Aoyama T, Kamoi D, Sakakibara T, Umemoto N, Kumada Y, Suzuki S, Murohara T. The association of ankle brachial index, protein-energy wasting, and inflammation status with cardiovascular mortality in patients on chronic hemodialysis. Nutrients. 2017;9(4):416.

24

Cardiac hypertrophy in chronic kidney disease— role of Aldosterone and FGF23

Koichi Hayashi[1][*], Toshihiko Suzuki[2], Yusuke Sakamaki[1] and Shinsuke Ito[2]

Abstract

Cardiac hypertrophy is a life-threatening disorder and is frequently observed in patients with chronic kidney disease (CKD). Much attention has been focused on the derangement in hormonal factors, including aldosterone and FGF23, as novel causes of cardiac hypertrophy in CKD. Plasma aldosterone concentrations are elevated as renal function declines. Although aldosterone antagonists are available for the treatment of hypertension with cardiac hypertrophy, concern remains regarding the possible occurrence of serious hyperkalemia. Alternatively, certain types of calcium channel blockers suppress aldosterone synthesis or exert blocking action for mineralocorticoid receptors and could halt the progression of cardiac dysfunction. Recently, FGF23 is shown to be elevated as CKD progresses and may be responsible for the development of cardiac hypertrophy and heart failure. Furthermore, FGF23 not only inhibits the renal expression of angiotensin converting enzyme 2 but also enhances renin gene transcription, both of which could accelerate renin-angiotensin-aldosterone system. Although the increase in serum phosphate concentrations is a pivotal stimulus for FGF23 production, recent studies suggest that reduced iron status and elevated aldosterone levels, frequently seen in patients with CKD or on dialysis, might also contribute to the elevation in serum FGF23 levels. Conversely, phosphate binders and appropriate iron status could reduce serum FGF23, potentially leading to the alleviation of cardiac hypertrophy and heart failure. In conclusion, novel therapeutic strategies associated with aldosterone and FGF23 may confer a benefit in the management of cardiac disorders in CKD.

Keywords: Aldosterone, FGF23, Cardiac hypertrophy, Phosphate, Iron, Ca channel blockers, Mineralocorticoid receptor antagonists, Heart failure, Chronic kidney disease

Background

Chronic kidney disease (CKD) is a life-threatening disorder and relentlessly progresses to end-stage kidney disease requiring renal replacement therapy. A growing body of evidence has been accumulated that CKD is closely associated with increased risk of cardiovascular events and death. Go et al. [1] demonstrated that the event rate inversely parallels the level of renal function. Likewise, cardiovascular events are associated with the reduction in glomerular filtration rate (GFR) among Japanese population [2, 3]. Cardiovascular disease observed in CKD includes a variety of disorders such as heart failure and cardiac hypertrophy. Since cardiac hypertrophy per se is more prevalent as renal function deteriorates and reflects an ominous outcome

with increased mortality [4, 5], the alleviation of this disorder would offer improved survival to CKD patients.

Although hemodynamic derangement such as systemic hypertension and volume overload plays a major role in the development of cardiac hypertrophy, several lines of recent studies indicate that humoral factors also contribute to the development of cardiac hypertrophy. For example, angiotensin II is a well-known factor that exerts direct hypertrophic action on cardiomyocytes [6, 7]. Further evidence has accrued that aldosterone, a traditional hormone regulating serum electrolyte balance, not only induces renal glomerular hypertension [8] but also causes cardiac hypertrophy [9, 10] and heart failure [11]. Because such humoral factors are often elevated in CKD [12–15], the strategy to counter the action of these factors would improve various perturbed conditions in CKD and is currently proposed as a milestone treatment of CKD, particularly with the use of renin-angiotensin system (RAS) inhibitors [10, 11, 16, 17].

* Correspondence: khayashi@tdc.ac.jp
[1]Department of Internal Medicine, Tokyo Dental College Ichikawa General Hospital, 5-11-13 Sugano, Ichikawa, Chiba 272-8513, Japan
Full list of author information is available at the end of the article

It is well recognized that CKD is accompanied by a variety of disturbance of the internal milieu, including electrolyte disorders. Despite impaired ability of renal excretory function, serum phosphate levels remain relatively unchanged until GFR falls below half of the normal level. Recent studies disclose that fibroblast growth factor 23 (FGF23) contributes importantly to the regulation of the serum phosphate concentration by inhibiting the phosphate reabsorption in the proximal tubule, which mitigates the tendency toward phosphate retention in CKD [18, 19]. Although this mechanism teleologically serves to act as an adaptive regulatory factor to maintain serum phosphate levels constant, further deterioration of CKD causes the elevation in serum phosphate concentrations, which hence would stimulate FGF23 production. Furthermore, of importance is the finding that elevated serum FGF23 concentrations are associated with the development of cardiac disorders [20–23]. Thus, apparently homeostatic mechanism for phosphate metabolism may act to aggravate cardiac disease, leading to cardiac hypertrophy and heart failure.

In this review, we survey the role of aldosterone in the development of cardiac hypertrophy in CKD and evaluate the therapeutic strategy for aldosterone blockade. Furthermore, recent findings regarding the effect of FGF23 on cardiac hypertrophy as well as the modulatory factors or therapeutic tools affecting FGF23 production are also discussed.

Aldosterone in CKD

Canonical concept of aldosterone is typically referred to as the hormone regulating electrolyte metabolism in the epithelial cell, i.e., sodium and potassium balance in renal tubular cells, intestinal epithelial cells, and sweat glands. Among these, renal distal and collecting tubules are the major target sites of action of aldosterone, where aldosterone facilitates sodium reabsorption through epithelial sodium channels (ENaC) and concomitantly potassium excretion mainly through ROMK channels [24]. Furthermore, aldosterone upregulates Na/K/ATPase that extrudes sodium from the cell to interstitial spaces as well as augments the uptake of potassium into the cell [25]. The overall action of aldosterone comprises volume expansion, hypertension, and the decrease in serum potassium levels, as are evident in primary aldosteronism.

Plasma aldosterone levels are regulated by a couple of factors (Fig. 1). Angiotensin II and ACTH represent major regulatory hormones stimulating aldosterone synthesis. Furthermore, high serum potassium levels induce aldosterone release from adrenal cortical gland. In addition, previous studies demonstrated that plasma aldosterone concentrations were elevated in CKD [15, 26–30] and were correlated inversely with renal function [15] (Fig. 1). Although high potassium obviously constitutes a stimulus for aldosterone release in CKD, reduced aldosterone excretion is reported as a possible cause of elevated plasma aldosterone concentrations [31]. Alternatively, Wesson and Simoni [27] showed that acid retention during kidney failure induced aldosterone production and elevated plasma aldosterone concentrations. Furthermore, Hosoya et al. [15] have recently demonstrated that the expression of the aldosterone-producing enzyme CYP11B2 in the adipose tissue of 5/6-nephrectomized rats is upregulated, leading to increased tissue aldosterone content. Finally, aldosterone breakthrough phenomenon (i.e., an elevation in plasma aldosterone levels 3–6 months after the administration of RAS inhibitors) could be a possible mechanism for aldosterone dysregulation [32, 33]. Taken together, these mechanisms may act in concert to enhance aldosterone activity in CKD.

The kidney plays an important role in potassium homeostasis. In subjects with intact kidney function, approximately 90% of potassium is excreted from the kidney where aldosterone contributes importantly to potassium excretion, and only 10% of potassium is secreted from the intestine. In patients with end-stage kidney disease, including dialysis patients, however, potassium secretion from the large intestine is considerably increased [29, 34, 35], in which $K_{Ca}1.1$ (BK) channels are largely involved [36]. Whereas aldosterone is shown to enhance the colonic BK channel activity [37, 38] and contributes at least partly to the increased colonic potassium excretion [39], there are also reported several studies showing a modest role of aldosterone in colonic potassium secretion in both predialysis [29, 40] and dialysis CKD patients [35]. It requires further discussion whether aldosterone blockade causes perilous levels of hyperkalemia in dialysis patients with end-stage kidney disease (see below).

Non-epithelial action of aldosterone

In addition to conventional action in epithelial cells, aldosterone is demonstrated to exert non-epithelial action in various organs. In the study evaluating the role of aldosterone in patients with heart failure, treatment with a mineralocorticoid receptor blocker (spironolactone) on top of conventional therapies (i.e., ACE inhibitors plus diuretics) conferred a profound benefit in terms of survival rate [11]. Since this clinical trial (i.e., RALES), a novel idea has emerged that aldosterone constitutes a critical determinant of cardiac function in patients with heart failure. Similarly, Zannad et al. [41] showed that a more selective aldosterone blocker, eplerenone, reduced the risk of death and hospitalization among patients with systolic heart failure and mild symptoms. It has also been demonstrated that aldosterone causes detrimental effects on vascular tension (enhanced vascular tone) [42] and glucose metabolism (insulin resistance) [15], both of which could influence mortality and morbidity.

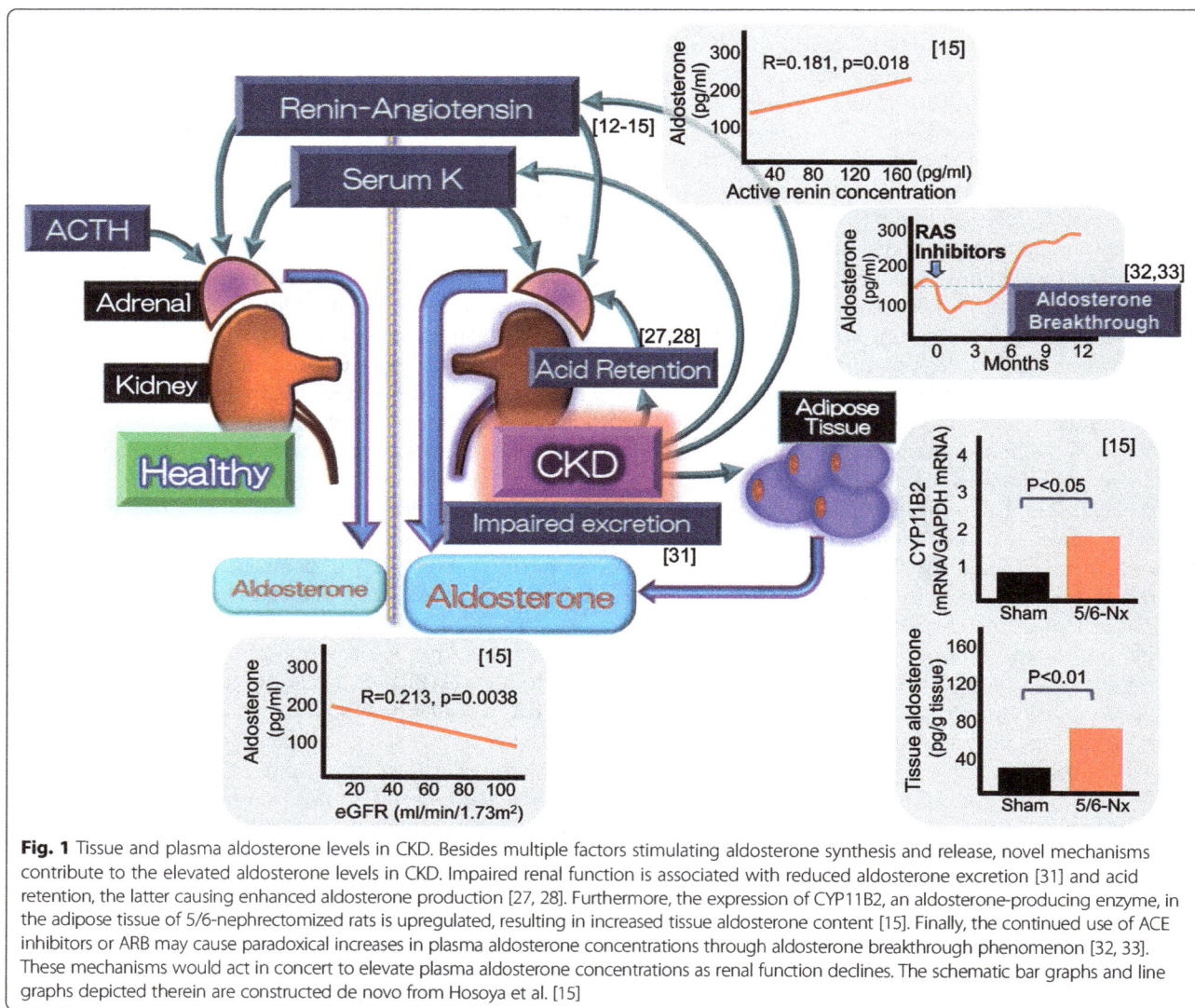

Fig. 1 Tissue and plasma aldosterone levels in CKD. Besides multiple factors stimulating aldosterone synthesis and release, novel mechanisms contribute to the elevated aldosterone levels in CKD. Impaired renal function is associated with reduced aldosterone excretion [31] and acid retention, the latter causing enhanced aldosterone production [27, 28]. Furthermore, the expression of CYP11B2, an aldosterone-producing enzyme, in the adipose tissue of 5/6-nephrectomized rats is upregulated, resulting in increased tissue aldosterone content [15]. Finally, the continued use of ACE inhibitors or ARB may cause paradoxical increases in plasma aldosterone concentrations through aldosterone breakthrough phenomenon [32, 33]. These mechanisms would act in concert to elevate plasma aldosterone concentrations as renal function declines. The schematic bar graphs and line graphs depicted therein are constructed de novo from Hosoya et al. [15]

Besides the critical role of aldosterone in survival rates in heart failure [11, 41], accumulating evidence indicates that aldosterone is responsible for the development of cardiac hypertrophy and impaired cardiac function. In primary aldosteronism in which overproduction of aldosterone causes hypertension, left ventricular (LV) hypertrophy can be induced independently of systemic hypertension [43, 44]. Furthermore, in patients with CKD, plasma aldosterone concentrations are inversely associated with GFR [15, 30] and parallel LV mass index [30]. Alternatively, aldosterone blockade with spironolactone elicited a regression of LV hypertrophy despite no changes in systemic blood pressure in diabetic patients with microalbuminuria [10] (Table 1). Furthermore, spironolactone treatment significantly ameliorated LV mass index and/or cardiac function not only in patients with early stage CKD [45, 46] but also in patients with advanced CKD on hemodialysis [47–49] or peritoneal

dialysis [50–52]. More importantly, Matsumoto et al. [53] elegantly demonstrated that 3-year treatment with spironolactone reduced the death rate from cardiovascular or cerebrovascular events in patients on hemodialysis in Dialysis Outcomes Heart Failure Aldactone Study (DOHAS). In concert, these observations suggest that aldosterone is responsible substantially for the development of cardiac hypertrophy and remodeling in humans.

Although aldosterone has a great impact on cardiovascular organs, multiple signal transduction systems appear to be involved in the non-epithelial action of aldosterone. Several lines of experimental studies show that aldosterone promotes the signal transduction of ERK pathways [54, 55] and generates reactive oxygen species [56] and inflammation [57], all of which cause cardiac hypertrophy and remodeling. Very recently, it has been demonstrated that aldosterone upregulates TNF receptor-associated factor 3 interacting protein 2

Table 1 Aldosterone blockers for LV hypertrophy in CKD

	Authors	Study duration	LV mass index	LV function	Hyperkalemia vs placebo	Ref
CKD						
DM nephropathy	Sato A. et al.	24 weeks	Decreased		(No change)	[10]
Stage 2~3 CKD	Edwards NC et al.	40 weeks	Decreased	Improved	No difference	[45, 46]
Hemodialysis						
	Feniman-De-Ste fano GM et al.	6 months	Decreased	No change	No difference	[47]
	Taheri S et al.	6 months	Decreased	Improved	No difference	[48]
	Lin C. et al.	2 years	Decreased	Improved	No difference	[49]
	Matsumoto Y et al.	3 years	Reduced death from cardiovascular events		3 of 157 patients discontinued	[53]
Peritoneal dialysis						
	Ito Y. et al.	2 years	Decreased	Improved	No difference	[50]
	Taheri S. et al.	6 months		Improved	No difference	[51]
	Hausmann MJ et al.	10 months		Improved	(No change)	[52]

(TRAF3IP2), which serves as an upstream regulator of multiple signaling components, including I kappa B kinase, JNK and c-Jun, and then stimulates the production of IL-18, IL-6, and CTGF [58, 59]. These results hence indicate a pivotal role of TRAF3IP2 and the multiple subordinate signal transduction pathways described above in mediating the aldosterone-induced adverse cardiac effects. Of interest, the mineralocorticoid receptor pathway is also stimulated by Rac1 activation through salt loading [60] and obesity [61] as a ligand-independent modulator without alterations in systemic aldosterone status. Furthermore, the Rac1-mediated activation of the mineralocorticoid receptor in the myocardium is responsible for the development of heart failure [62]. It follows therefore that mineralocorticoid receptor activation, whether a ligand-dependent or not, stimulates the downstream signaling pathways associated with growth and inflammation and induces cardiac hypertrophy and impaired contractility.

Aldosterone blockade in CKD

As indicated above, aldosterone blockade reduces cardiac hypertrophy and improves cardiac function in patients on hemodialysis [47–49] and peritoneal dialysis [50–52] (Table 1). Furthermore, DOHAS trial clearly demonstrates that aldosterone blockade by spironolactone prevents cardiovascular events and ameliorates the survival rate in hemodialysis patients [53]. Caveat is in order, however, because of the potential risk for hyperkalemia when the blockers are given to CKD patients. Thus, potassium secretion from the intestine is increased in patients with advanced CKD or on dialysis therapy [29, 34, 35], and mineralocorticoid receptor blockers are reported to suppress this mechanism [38]. Indeed, several studies have

reported that the administration of spironolactone is associated with increased incidence of hyperkalemia in patients on maintenance hemodialysis therapy [63–65] although pronounced hyperkalemia (serum potassium ≥ 6 mEq/L) does not occur commonly [66]. Notably, there are also reported a substantial number of studies showing that spironolactone does not cause significantly higher levels of serum potassium in patients on hemodialysis [47–49] or peritoneal dialysis therapy [50, 51, 67, 68], when compared with placebo (Table 1). Taken together, the use of aldosterone blockers is teleologically reasonable in terms of cardiovascular protection, although the adverse effect of these blockers might hamper the wide-spread use of this type of agents in patients with CKD.

Alternatively, there exist several types of antihypertensive agents that act to inhibit aldosterone synthesis and/or release (Table 2) [69]. It is now well established that certain types of calcium channel blockers, including efonidipine [70], benidipine [71], azelnidipine [72], and cilnidipine [73], inhibit aldosterone synthesis in adrenocortical cells. Furthermore, clinical studies show that these agents decrease serum aldosterone levels in hypertensive patients [74–79]. Of interest, these calcium channel blockers are endowed with the ability to inhibit not only L-type but also T-type (efonidipine, benidipine, azelnidipine) or N-type calcium channels (benidipine, cilnidipine), whereas conventional calcium channel blockers such as nifedipine and amlodipine exert inhibitory action solely on L-type calcium channels [80–82]. Additionally, several calcium channel blockers, including nifedipine and benidipine, are shown to compete with aldosterone for mineralocorticoid receptor binding and block aldosterone activity [83, 84] (Table 2). Thus, divergent inhibitory action on calcium channel subtypes (i.e., L-, T-, and N-type calcium channels) and

Table 2 Calcium channel blockers affecting aldosterone synthesis

Ca channel blockers	Inhibition of Ca channel subtypes			Inhibition of aldosterone production		Mineralocorticoid receptor blockade
	L-type	T-type	N-type	Adrenal cells	Human plasma concentrations	
Nifedipine	+					+ [83]
Amlodipine	+					
Efonidipine	+	+		+ [70]	+ [74, 75]	
Nilvadipine	+	+				
Azelnidipine	+	+		+ [72]	+ [77]	
Cilnidipine	+		+	+ [73]	+ [78, 79]	
Benidipine	+	+	+	+ [71]	+ [76]	+ [84]

distinct antagonistic action on mineralocorticoid receptors inherent in certain calcium channel blockers could provide additive cardiovascular benefits in CKD patients. Indeed, in our preliminary study, we found that T-type calcium channel blockers (efonidipine, benidipine, azelnidipine) and nifedipine reduced LV mass index more markedly than other calcium channel blockers in hemodialysis patients (unpublished observation). This presumption, however, requires further investigations showing that these calcium channel blockers could contribute to the prevention of cardiac hypertrophy.

FGF23 and phosphate in CKD

FGF23 is identified as a glycoprotein hormone that has been discovered as a member of the FGF family [85]. The subsequent investigations have unveiled an important role of FGF23 in the homeostatic mechanism of serum phosphate levels [18, 19]. The conventional hypothesis, i.e., "trade-off theory" [86, 87], where secondary hyperparathyroidism is assumed to play a central role in phosphate metabolism in CKD, therefore, has been updated by the introduction of FGF23 to the concept of the phosphate metabolism in CKD.

Serum FGF23 levels have been shown to rise at early stages of CKD. Several studies demonstrate that serum FGF23 is elevated even prior to the stage when serum parathyroid hormone rises [19, 88]. Although the precise cellular mechanisms for the release and synthesis of FGF23 remain fully undetermined, the elevation in serum phosphate and parathyroid hormone constitute determinants that trigger the release of FGF23 from osteocytes and osteoblasts (Fig. 2). Because FGF23 is a potent phosphaturic hormone that inhibits phosphate reabsorption through Na/P cotransporter 2a/c in the proximal tubule [18, 86, 89], FGF23 would serve to mitigate hyperphosphatemia entailing impaired renal function. FGF23 also suppresses vitamin D activity by inhibiting renal 1α-hydroxylase (the enzyme that converts 25-hydroxyvitamin D3 to its active form) and stimulating 24-hydroxylase (the enzyme degrading to inactive form) [90], leading to the decrease in phosphate

and calcium absorption from the intestine. Although FGF23 can inhibit parathyroid hormone production [88, 91], the effects of suppressed vitamin D activity along with decreased Ca levels would govern the serum parathyroid hormone level more robustly in CKD, which results in elevated parathyroid hormone levels characteristics of the hormonal profiles seen in CKD patients [92, 93].

FGF23 and sodium in CKD

In addition to the phosphaturic action in renal proximal tubules, FGF23 is found to exert sodium retaining action in distal tubular segments. Thus, Andrukhova et al. [94] have recently demonstrated that FGF23 upregulates the sodium chloride cotransporter (NCC) in distal tubules, which conceivably results in systemic volume expansion and hypertension (Fig. 2). This finding encompasses an important issue because FGF23 could cause the suppression of RAS due to systemic volume expansion and subsequently decrease plasma aldosterone levels [95]. In contrast, a positive correlation between FGF23 and aldosterone concentrations is also reported in patients with CKD and heart failure [96]. In this regard, CKD is demonstrated to be associated with decreased renal expression of Klotho [97, 98]. Since the action of FGF23 on NCC requires the integrity of the FGF receptor/Klotho complex [94], the ability of FGF23 to promote sodium retention and the subsequent development of hypertension may depend on intact FGF receptor/Klotho complex activity. Indeed, the observation that plasma aldosterone levels are elevated in advanced CKD [12–15, 26, 27, 29] suggests the diminished ability of elevated FGF23 to induce volume expansion, possibly due to reduced Klotho expression in the kidney.

FGF23 and RAS/aldosterone

Recent investigations reveal a cross talk between FGF23 and RAS/aldosterone [99] (Fig. 2). Dai et al. [100] demonstrated that FGF23 suppressed the renal expression of angiotensin converting enzyme 2 (ACE2), the enzyme mediating the conversion mainly from angiotensin II to angiotensin-(1-7), in FGF23-transgenic mice. The

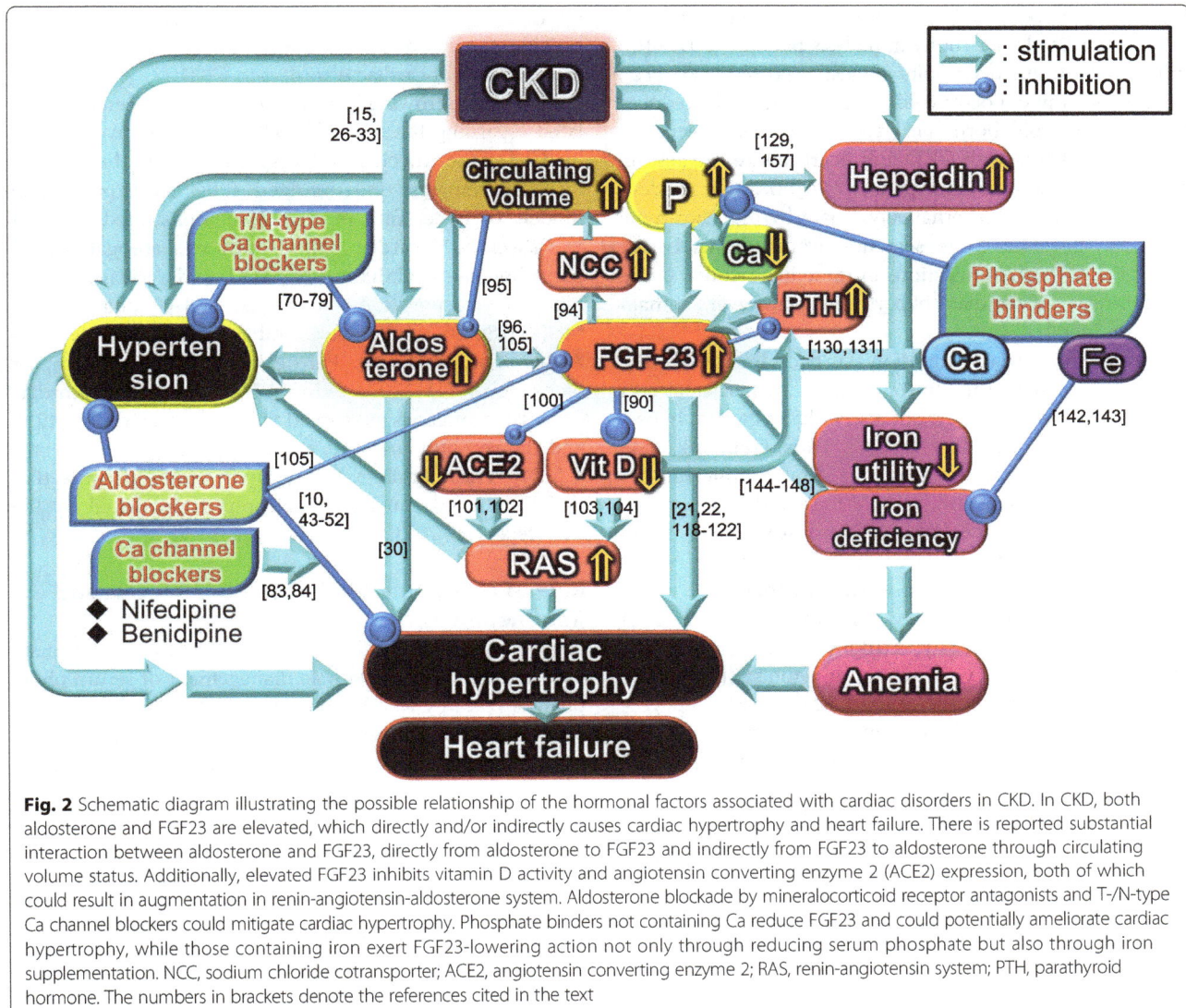

Fig. 2 Schematic diagram illustrating the possible relationship of the hormonal factors associated with cardiac disorders in CKD. In CKD, both aldosterone and FGF23 are elevated, which directly and/or indirectly causes cardiac hypertrophy and heart failure. There is reported substantial interaction between aldosterone and FGF23, directly from aldosterone to FGF23 and indirectly from FGF23 to aldosterone through circulating volume status. Additionally, elevated FGF23 inhibits vitamin D activity and angiotensin converting enzyme 2 (ACE2) expression, both of which could result in augmentation in renin-angiotensin-aldosterone system. Aldosterone blockade by mineralocorticoid receptor antagonists and T-/N-type Ca channel blockers could mitigate cardiac hypertrophy. Phosphate binders not containing Ca reduce FGF23 and could potentially ameliorate cardiac hypertrophy, while those containing iron exert FGF23-lowering action not only through reducing serum phosphate but also through iron supplementation. NCC, sodium chloride cotransporter; ACE2, angiotensin converting enzyme 2; RAS, renin-angiotensin system; PTH, parathyroid hormone. The numbers in brackets denote the references cited in the text

suppression of ACE2 activity results in the decrease in vasodilatory angiotensin-(1-7) and the increase in angiotensin II [101, 102]. It is inferred therefore that in CKD, where plasma FGF23 is elevated, altered balance between angiotensin II and angiotensin-(1-7) might play a part in hypertension and volume retention. Furthermore, accumulating evidence indicates that vitamin D inhibits RAS by downregulating renin gene transcription [99, 103, 104]. Because FGF23 suppresses vitamin D activity, elevated plasma FGF23 would augment RAS and possibly aldosterone as well and may play a role in the development of hypertension in CKD.

Finally, the interaction between FGF23 and aldosterone merits comment. Imazu et al. [96] showed that serum FGF23 levels correlated with plasma aldosterone concentrations in patients with CKD and heart failure. An in vitro study also demonstrates that FGF23

transcription is upregulated by aldosterone and is inhibited by an aldosterone receptor blocker (eplerenone) in cultured osteoblasts [105]. Although clinical evidence endorsing a causative role of aldosterone in FGF23 production remains insufficient, these findings are consistent with the notion that aldosterone contributes to the enhanced FGF23 production in CKD (Fig. 2).

FGF23 and cardiac hypertrophy

Cardiac hypertrophy is a critical complication that is frequently observed in CKD [106, 107]. Cardiac hypertrophy develops beginning at early stages of CKD and is quite common in patients on dialysis therapy. In addition to the traditional determinants causing cardiac hypertrophy, including hypertension, renin-angiotensin system [6, 7], and chronic anemia [108], aldosterone is also established as a crucial factor for cardiac hypertrophy [9, 10, 15, 30,

43]. Furthermore, parathyroid hormone is suggested as a cause of cardiac hypertrophy in dialysis patients [109, 110], although contradictory results are also reported [111, 112]. Of interest, mineralocorticoid receptor blockade reduces serum parathyroid hormone levels in normal subjects as well as in patients with CKD and heart failure, suggesting that aldosterone stimulates parathyroid hormone production [113, 114]. Alternatively, parathyroid hormone enhances the aldosterone secretion from adrenal cortex [115, 116]. Clinical implications of these interactions in the development of cardiac hypertrophy, however, remain undetermined [117].

More recently, much attention has been focused on the role of FGF23 since this substance not only participates in the phosphate homeostasis but also induces cardiac hypertrophy (Table 3) [21, 22, 118–122]. Thus, Gutierrez et al. [21] discovered that there existed a close relationship between serum FGF23 levels and LV mass index in patients with CKD. Faul et al. [22] also demonstrated that LV mass index was increased as serum FGF23 levels were elevated. This relationship was also observed in patients on maintenance hemodialysis. Finally, intravenous injection of FGF23 caused cardiac hypertrophy in mice, and the administration of an FGF receptor antagonist (PD173074) prevented the development of the CKD (i.e., 5/6 nephrectomy)-induced cardiac hypertrophy. Of importance, elevated serum FGF23 levels are causally linked to reduced

ejection fraction [22]. Collectively, these observations provide conclusive evidence for the role of FGF23 in the development of cardiac disorders in CKD.

Although a growing body of evidence has been accumulated regarding the role of FGF23 in cardiac hypertrophy in CKD, the mechanism responsible for the cardiac disorder remains undetermined fully. In experimental models of mice, Faul et al. [22] demonstrated that the FGF23-induced cardiac hypertrophy was abrogated by a phospholipase Cγ inhibitor (U73122) and a calcineurin inhibitor (cyclosporine A), but not by a MAP kinase inhibitor (PD98059), a PI3 kinase inhibitor (wartmannin), or an Akt inhibitor (A6730). Furthermore, pan FGF receptor blockade by PD173074 reduced LV mass and the cardiac expression of genes associated with LV hypertrophy [123], and the receptor involved was identified as FGF receptor 4 [124]. These findings lend support to the premise that FGF23-induced cardiac hypertrophy is mediated by the FGF receptor 4/PLCγ/calcineurin pathway.

Role of phosphate binders in FGF23 levels and iron metabolism

Great progress in the therapeutic modalities for phosphate binders offers more favorable management of serum phosphate levels in CKD. Following the established use of Ca carbonate, new (i.e., second generation) phosphate binders, including sevelamer, bixalomer, and lanthanum carbonate,

Table 3 FGF23 and cardiac hypertrophy in CKD

Authors	n	Effects of FGF23 on cardiac hypertrophy	Ref.
Humans			
Gutierrez OM et al.	162 CKD	Incidence of LVH (%), FGF23 < 75 RU/ml; 7%, 75–150 RU/ml, 21%, > 150 RU/ml; 25%	[21]
Faul C et al.	3070 CKD	Incidence of LVH (eccentric+concentric)%, FGF23 quarfile 1; 38%, quarfile 2; 45%, quartile 3; 54%, quarfile 4; 70%	[22]
Hsu HJ et al.	124 hemodialysis	Serum FGF23 level is independently associated with LVH in hemodialysis patients	[118]
Seifert Me et al.	31 CKD stage 3	The change in FGF23/klotho ratio was strongly correlated with changes in LV mass index.	[119]
Sarmento-Dias M et al.	48 peritoneal dialysis	In multivariate adjusted analysis, FGF23was associated with LVMI ($\beta = 0.298$, $p = 0.041$),	[120]
Javanovich A et al.	2255 elderly CKD	Higher FGF23 concentrations were associated with greater LVM in adjusted analyses ($\beta = 6.71$ [95% CI 4.35–9.01] g per doubling of FGF23).	[121]
Tanaka S. et al	903 CKD stage 1 to 5	The correlation between FGF23 and LVMI was significant among those with CKD stage G1/G2, G3a, and G4.	[122]
Chue CD. et al	120 CKD stage 3	Sevelamer carbonate reduced FGF23 but failed to improve LV mass	[134]
Animals			
Maizel J et al.	CKD mice	Sevelamer reduced serum phosphate and LV hypertrophy but not FGF23.	[135]
Yamazaki-Nakazawa A et al.	CKD rats	Lanthanum carbonate reduced LV weight but failed to decrease FGF23 levels.	[136]

have come into common use. Because of the physiological interaction between serum phosphate and FGF23, it is judiciously anticipated that phosphate binders should reduce serum FGF23 levels [125–129]. In this regard, Ca load is reported to be associated with an elevation in serum FGF23 levels [130, 131] (Fig. 2). Furthermore, a cross-sectional study shows that FGF23 levels correlate with serum Ca ion concentrations and Ca-phosphate product [132]. Thus, phosphate binders containing Ca (e.g., Ca carbonate) may have less ameliorating impact on serum FGF23 levels than those without Ca (e.g., sevelamer, lanthanum) in both pre-dialysis [133] and dialysis patients [125, 128, 129].

Although FGF23 constitutes an important determinant inducing cardiac hypertrophy, whether the improvement in serum FGF23 levels by phosphate binders exerts beneficial action on cardiac hypertrophy is a matter of controversy (Table 3). Thus, it has been reported that 40-week treatment with sevelamer decreases serum FGF23 levels but fails to reduce LV mass in patients with stage 3 CKD, though the inability to ameliorate LV mass might be attributable to the insufficient treatment period [134]. Furthermore, sevelamer and lanthanum are shown to reduce serum phosphate concentrations and ameliorate LV hypertrophy without changes in FGF23 levels in experimental animals [135, 136]. Of interest, a strong association between serum phosphate concentrations and

LV mass is demonstrated in humans [137, 138] and animals [139], and hyperphosphatemia per se could be a potential risk factor causing cardiac hypertrophy [140, 141]. Accordingly, the ability of phosphate binders to alleviate cardiac hypertrophy may vary, depending on the responsiveness of serum FGF23 and/or phosphate to these drugs. Further investigations are required to clarify this important issue.

Recently, iron-containing phosphate binders, including ferric citrate hydrate and sucroferric oxyhydroxide, have been developed and are actually available in clinical practice [142, 143]. Because of the nature of iron loss during hemodialysis sessions, the use of this type of phosphate binders appears reasonable in such condition since iron is dissociated from the binders and then absorbed in part from the intestine. Of note, iron deficiency and the subsequent anemia are associated with the elevation in plasma FGF23 concentrations [95, 144–147] and the upregulation of bone FGF23 mRNA expression (Table 4) [147, 148]. An in vitro study also shows that osteocytes in the medium containing low iron produce greater FGF23 mRNA expression [149]. Conversely, oral [146, 150, 151], but not intravenous [152, 153], iron supplementation is associated with a decrease in serum FGF23 levels. Additionally, switching from sevelamer to ferric citrate hydrate has recently been shown to replenish iron status and reduce

Table 4 Iron status and FGF23

Authors	Subjects/animals, n	Iron deficiency and FGF23	Ref.
Humans			
Bozentowics-Wikarek M et al.	3780 elderly	Low iron levels are associated with increased FGF23 levels. FGF23 levels were nearly linearly increased by 0.285 pg/mL for each unit of serum iron decrease in patients with serum iron levels < 59 ng/mL,	[144]
Lewerin C et al.	1010 elderly	FGF 47.4 μmol/L (transferrin saturation (TS) < 15%) vs 41.9 μmol/L (TS > 15%)	[145]
Braithwaite V. et al.	79 children non-CKD	Iron status is a negative predictor of plasma FGF23 concentration. Improvements in iron status following iron supplementation are associated with a significant decrease in FGF23 concentration.	[146]
Deger SM et al.	73 hemodialysis	There was a negative relationship between iron administration and serum iFGF23 level in a dialysis population	[150]
Yamashita K et al.	31 hemodialysis	Serum FGF23 was reduced from 1820 pg/mL (342-4370) to 1240 pg/mL (214-2840) after 3-month treatment with sodium ferrous citrate.	[151]
Takeda Y, et al	27 hemodialysis	Intravenous saccharated ferric oxide induces further increase in FGF23 levels.	[152]
Iguchi A et al	124 hemodialysis	Serum FGF23 level decreased from 2000 pg/mL (1300-3471.4) to 1771.4 pg/mL (1142.9-2342.9) after switching from sevelamer to ferric citrate hydrate.	[154]
Animals			
David V et al	Mice	Three-week low iron diet intake resulted in significantly increased levels of bone FGF23 mRNA. Functional iron deficiency with hepcidin injection caused increased bone expression of FGF23 mRNA.	[147]
Hanudel MR et al	Adenin-induced CKD mice	Eight-week adenine-containing and low iron diet intake increased the bone FGF23 mRNA levels.	[148]
Farrow EG et al.	Mice	Mice receiving low-iron diet had significantly elevated bone Fgf23 mRNA.	[149]
Gravesen E et al.	Non-iron depleted uremic rats	Intravenous iron isomaltoside and ferric carboxymaltose had no effect on plasma levels of FGF23 and phosphate.	[153]

circulating FGF23 levels independently of serum phosphate concentrations in hemodialysis patients [154]. In concert, an appropriate level of iron status is required to suppress serum FGF23 levels and potentially to prevent the development of cardiac hypertrophy.

In this regard, hepcidin, a regulatory molecule that inhibits iron absorption in the duodenum and iron recruitment from the liver and the reticuloendothelial system, is elevated in CKD [155, 156]. Furthermore, serum hepcidin levels are tightly associated with serum phosphate concentrations [157], and the reduction in serum phosphate by lanthanum is causally correlated with the decrement in serum hepcidin levels [129]. These observations therefore suggest complex interaction between phosphate-FGF23 pathways and iron metabolism (Fig. 2).

Conclusions

Cardiac hypertrophy is a serious complication observed frequently in patients with CKD. Among multiple factors involved in cardiac disease, humoral factors, including aldosterone and FGF23, are gaining much attention as critical components responsible substantially for the development of cardiac hypertrophy and heart failure that lead to increased morbidity and mortality. Recent progresses in the therapeutic strategies using novel tools facilitate the management of CKD. Novel approaches from the standpoint of hormonal (aldosterone and FGF23) and mineral/electrolyte factors (phosphate) as well as iron status appear to be a promising strategy and could constitute a mainstay in the treatment of cardiovascular disorders in CKD.

Abbreviations
ACE2: Angiotensin converting enzyme 2; ACTH: Adrenocortical stimulating hormone; CKD: Chronic kidney disease; FGF23: Fibroblast growth factor 23; GFR: Glomerular filtration rate; LV: Left ventricle; NCC: Sodium chloride cotransporter; RAS: Renin-angiotensin system; ROMK: Renal outer medullary potassium channels

Acknowledgements
Not applicable

Funding
There is no funding to be disclosed.

Authors' contributions
KH and TS designed and wrote the manuscript. YS and SI collected the literature and discussed the contents of the manuscript with TS and KH. All authors read and approved the final version of the manuscript.

Competing interests
The authors declare that they have no competing interests.

Author details
[1]Department of Internal Medicine, Tokyo Dental College Ichikawa General Hospital, 5-11-13 Sugano, Ichikawa, Chiba 272-8513, Japan. [2]Department of Internal Medicine, Tokyo Bay Urayasu Ichikawa Medical Center, 3-4-32 Todaijima, Urayasu, Chiba 279-0001, Japan.

References
1. Go AS, Chertow GM, Fan D, et al. Cheonic kidney disease and the cardiovascular events, and hospitalization. N Engl J Med. 2004;351:1296–305.
2. Ninomiya T, Kiyohara Y, Tokuda Y, et al. Japan arteriosclerosis longitudinal Study Group. Impact of kidney disease and blood pressure on the development of cardiovascular disease: an overview from the Japanese Longitudinal Study. Circulation 2008; 118: 2694-2701.
3. Tanaka K, Watanabe T, Takeuchi A, et al. CKD-JAC Investigators. Cardiovascular events and death in Japanese patients with chronic kidney disease. Kidney Int 2017; 91:227-234.
4. Zoccali C, Benedetto FA, Mallamaci F, et al. Left ventricular mass monitoring in the follow-up of dialysis patients: prognostic value of left ventricular hypertrophy progression. Kidney Int. 2004;65:1492–8.
5. Dubin RF, Deo R, Bansal N, et al. Associations of conventional echocardiographic measures with incident heart failure and mortality: the chronic renal insufficiency cohort. Clin J Am Soc Nephrol. 2017;12:60–8.
6. Nishida M, Tanabe S, Maruyama Y, et al. $G\alpha_{12/13}$- and reactive oxygen species-dependent activation of c-Jun NH_2-terminal kinase and p38 MAPK by angiotensin receptor stimulation in rat neonatal cardiomyocytes. J Biol Chem. 20015;280:18434–41.
7. Yamazaki T, Komuro I, Shiojima I, et al. The renin-angiotensin system and cardiac hypertrophy. Heart. 1996;76(3 Suppl 3):33–5.
8. Arima S, Kohagura K, Xu HL, et al. Nongenomic vascular action of aldosterone in the glomerular microcirculation. J Am Soc Nephrol. 2003;14: 2253–1163.
9. Brilla CG, Pick R, Tan LB, et al. Remodeling of the rat right and left ventricles in experimental hypertension. Circ Res. 1990;67:1355–64.
10. Sato A, Hayashi K, Naruse M, et al. Effectiveness of aldosterone blockade in patients with diabetic nephropathy. Hypertension. 2003;41:64–8.
11. Pitt B, Zannad F, Remme WJ, et al. The effect of spironolactone on morbidity and mortality in patients with severe heart failure. N Engl J Med. 1999;341:709–17.
12. Reubi FC, Weidmann P. Relationships between sodium clearance, plasma renin activity, plasma aldosterone, renal hemodynamics and blood pressure in essential hypertension. Clin Exp Hypertens. 1980;2:593–612.
13. Berle T, Katz FH, Henrich WL, et al. Role of aldosterone in the control of sodium excretion in patients with advanced chronic renal failure. Kidney Int. 1978;14:228–35.
14. Hene RJ, Boer P, Koomans HA, et al. Plasma aldosterone concentrations in chronic renal disease. Kidney Int. 1982;21:98–101.
15. Hosoya K, Minakuchi H, Wakino S, et al. Insulin resistance in chronic kidney disease is ameliorated by spironolactone in rats and humans. Kidney Int. 2015;87:749–60.
16. Sarafidis PA, Khosla N, Bakris GL. Antihypertensive therapy in the presence of proteinuria. Am J Kidney Dis. 2007;49:12–26.
17. Saruta T, Hayashi K, Ogihara T, et al. Effects of candesartan and amlodipine on cardiovascular events in hypertensive patients with chronic kidney disease: subanalysis of the CASE-J study. Hypertens Res. 2009;32:505–12.
18. Bowe AE, Finnegan R, Jan de Beur SM, et al. FGF-23 inhibits renal tubular phosphate transporter and is a PHEX substrate. Biochem Biophys Res Commun. 2001;284:977–81.
19. Evenepoel P, Meijers B, ViaeneL, et al. Fibroblast growth factor-23 in early chronic kidney disease: additional support in favor of a phosphate-centric paradigm for the pathogenesis of secondary hyperparathyroidism. Clin J Am Soc Nephrol. 2010;5:1268–76.
20. Holden RM, Beseau D, Booth SL, et al. FGF-23 is associated with cardiac troponin T and mortality in hemodialysis patients. Hemodial Int. 2012;16:53–8.

21. Gutierrez OM, Januzzi JL, Isakova T, et al. Fibroblast growth factor 23 and left ventricular hypertrophy in chronic kidney disease. Circulation. 2009;119:2545–52.

22. Faul C, Amaral AP, Oskouei B, et al. FGF-23 induces left ventricular hypertrophy. J Clin Invest. 2011;121:4393–408.

23. Hamano T, Sakaguchi Y, Fujii N, et al. Clinical features of CKD-MBD in Japan: cohort studies and registry. Clin Exp Nephrol. 2017;21(Suppl 1):9–20.

24. Wang WH, Giebisch G. Regulation of potassium (K) handling in the renal collecting duct. Pflugers Arch. 2009;458:157–68.

25. O'Neil RG. Aldosterone regulation of sodium and potassium transport in the cortical collecting duct. Semin Nephrol. 1990;10:365–74.

26. Gant CM, Laverman GD, Vogt L, et al. Renoprotective RAAS inhibition does not affect the association between worse renal function and higher plasma aldosterone levels. BMC Nephrol. 2017;18:370. https://doi.org/10.1186/s12882-017-0789-x.

27. Wesson DE, Simoni J. Acid retention during kidney failure induces endothelin and aldosterone production which lead to progressive GFR decline, a situation ameliorated by alkali diet. Kidney Int. 2010;78:1128–35.

28. Wesson DE, Simoni J, Broglio K, et al. Acid retention accompanies reduced GFR in humans and increases plasma levels of endothelin and aldosterone. Am J Phys. 2011;300:F830–7.

29. Martin RS, Panese S, Virginillo M, et al. Increased secretion of potassium in the rectum of humans with chronic renal failure. Am J Kidney Dis. 1986;8:105–10.

30. Mulè G, Nardi E, Guarino L, et al. Plasma aldosterone and its relationship with left ventricular mass in hypertensive patients with early-stage chronic kidney disease. Hypertens Res. 2015;38:276–83.

31. Williams GH, Bailey GL, Hamper GL, et al. Studies on the metabolism of aldosterone on chronic renal failure and anephric man. Kidney Int. 1973;4:280–8.

32. Otani H, Otsuka F, Inagaki K, et al. Aldosterone breakthrough caused by chronic blockade of angiotensin type 1 receptors in human adrenocortical cells: possible involvement of bone morphogenetic protein-6 actions. Endocrinology. 2008;149:2816–25.

33. Moranne O, Bakris G, Fafin C, et al. Determinants and changes associated with aldosterone breakthrough after angiotensin II receptor blockade in patients with type 2 diabetes with overt nephropathy. Clin J Am Soc Nephrol. 2013;8:1694–701.

34. Bastl C, Hayslett JP, Binder HJ. Increased large intestinal secretion of potassium in renal insufficiency. Kidney Int. 1977;12:9–16.

35. Sandle GI, Gaiger E, Tapster S, et al. Evidence for large intestinal control of potassium homeostasis in uraemic patients undergoing long-term dialysis. Clin Sci. 1987;73:247–52.

36. Mathialahan T, Maclennan KA, Sandle LN, et al. Enhanced large intestinal potassium permeability in end-stage renal disease. J Pathol. 2005;206:46–51.

37. Sorensen MV, Leipziger J. The essential role of luminal BK channels in distal colonic K+ secretion. J Med Investig. 2009;56(Suppl):301.

38. Sorensen MV, Matos JE, Sausbier M, et al. Aldosterone increases KCa1.1 (BK) channel-mediated colonic K+ secretion. J Physiol. 2008;586:4251–64.

39. Wilson DR, Ing TS, Metcafe-Gibson A, et al. The chemical composition of faeces in uraemia, as revealed by in vivo faecal dialysis. Clin Sci. 1968;35:197–209.

40. Sandle GI, Gaiger E, Tapster S, et al. Enhanced rectal potassium secretion in chronic renal insufficiency: evidence for large intestinal potassium adaptation in man. Clin Sci. 1986;71:393–401.

41. Zannad F, McMurray JJ, Krum H, et al. Eplerenone in patients with systolic heart failure and mild symptoms. N Engl J Med. 2011;364:11–21.

42. Leopold JA, Dam A, Maron BA, et al. Aldosterone impairs vascular reactivity by decreasing glucose-6-phosphate dehydrogenase activity. Nat Med. 2007;13:189–97.

43. Ori Y, Chagnac A, Korzets A, et al. Regression of left ventricular hypertrophy in patients with primary aldosteronism/low-renin hypertension on low-dose spironolactone. Nephrol Dial Transplant. 2013;28:1787–93.

44. Catena C, Colussi G, Nait F, et al. Aldosterone and the heart: still an unresolved issue? Front Endocrinol. 2014;5:168. https://doi.org/10.3389/fendo.2014.00168.eCollection 2014.

45. Edwards NC, Steeds RP, Stewart PM, et al. Effect of spironolactone on left ventricular mass and aortic stiffness in early-stage chronic kidney disease: a randomized controlled trial. J Am Coll Cardiol. 2009;54:505–12.

46. Edwards NC, Ferro CJ, Kirkwood H, et al. Effect of spironolactone on left ventricular systolic and diastolic function in patients with early stage chronic kidney disease. Am J Cardiol. 2010;106:1505–11.

47. Feniman-De-Stefano GM, Zanati-Basan SG, De Stefano LM, et al. Spironolactone is secure and reduces left ventricular hypertrophy in hemodialysis patients. Ther Adv Cardiovasc Dis. 2015;9:158–67.

48. Taheri S, Mortazavi M, Shahidi S, et al. Spironolactone in chronic hemodialysis patients improves cardiac function. Saudi J Kidney Dis Transpl. 2009;20:392–7.

49. Lin C, Zhang Q, Zhang H, et al. Long-term effects of low-dose spironolactone on chronic dialysis patients: a randomized placebo-controlled study. J Clin Hypertens (Greenwich). 2016;18:121–8.

50. Ito Y, Mizuno M, Suzuki Y, et al. Long-term effects of spironolactone in peritoneal dialysis patients. J Am Soc Nephrol. 2014;25:1094–102.

51. Taheri S, Mortazavi M, Pourmoghadas A, et al. A prospective double-blind randomized placebo-controlled clinical trial to evaluate the safety and efficacy of spironolactone in patients with advanced congestive heart failure on continuous ambulatory peritoneal dialysis. Saudi J Kidney Dis Transpl. 2012;23:507–12.

52. Hausmann MJ, Liel-Cohen N. Aldactone therapy in a peritoneal dialysis patients with decreased left ventricular function. Nephrol Dial Tranplant. 2002;17:2035–6.

53. Matsumoto Y, Mori Y, Kageyama S, et al. Spironolactone reduces cardiovascular and cerebrovascular morbidity and mortality in hemodialysis patients. J Am Coll Cardiol. 2014;63:528–36.

54. Fiebeler A, Haller H. Participation of the mineralocorticoid receptor in cardiac and vascular remodeling. Nephron Physiol. 2003;94:47–50.

55. Okoshi MP, Yan X, Okoshi K, et al. Aldosterone directly stimulates cardiac hypertrophy. J Card Fail. 2004;10:511–8.

56. Park YM, Park MY, Suh YL, et al. NAD(P)H oxidase inhibitor prevents blood pressure elevation and cardiovascular hypertrophy in aldosterone-infused rats. Biochem Biol Res Commun. 2004;313:812–7.

57. Brown NJ. Contribution of aldosterone to cardiovascular and renal inflammation and fibrosis. Nat Rev Nephrol. 2013;9:459–69.

58. Somanna NK, Yariswamy M, Garagliano JM, et al. Aldosterone-induced cardiomyocyte growth, and fibroblast migration and proliferation are mediated by TRAF2IP2. Cell Signal. 2015;27:1928–38. https://doi.org/10.1016/j.cellsig.2015.07.001.

59. Sakamuri SS, Valente AJ, Siddesha JM, et al. TRAF3IP2 mediates aldosterone/salt-induced cardiac hypertrophy and fibrosis. Mol Cell Endocrinol. 2016;429:84–92.

60. Shibata S, Nagase M, Yoshida S, et al. Modification of mineralocorticoid receptor function by Rac1 GTPase: implication in proteinuric kidney function. Nat Med. 2008;14:1370–6.

61. Nagase M, Fujita T. Mineralocorticoid receptor activation in obesity hypertension. Hypertens Res. 2009;32:649–57.

62. Ayuzawa N, Nagase M, Ueda K, et al. Rac1-mediated activation of mineralocorticoid receptor in pressure overload-induced cardiac injury. Hypertension. 2016;67:99–106.

63. Papadimitriou V, Vyzantiadis A, Milionis A, et al. The effect of spironolactone in hypertensive patients on regular haemodialysis and after renal allotransplantation. Life Support Syst. 1983;1:197–205.

64. Flevari P, Kalogeropoulou S, Drakou A, et al. Spironolactone improves endothelial and cardiac autonomic function in non heart failure hemodialysis patients. J Hypertens. 2013;31:1239–44.

65. Walsh M, Manns B, Garg AX, et al. The safety of eplerenone in hemodialysis patients: a noninferiority randomized controlled trial. Clin J Am Soc Nephrol. 2015;10:1602–8.

66. Tawada M, Suzuki Y, Sakata F, et al. Mineralocorticoid receptor antagonists in dialysis patients. Ren Replace Ther. 2016;2:64. https://doi.org/10.1186/s41100-016-0077-4, 2016.

67. Yelken B, Gorgulu N, Gursu M, et al. Effects of spironolactone on residual renal function and peritoneal function in peritoneal dialysis patients. Adv Perit Dial. 2014;30:5–10.

68. Vazquez-Rangel A, Soto V, Escalona M, et al. Spironolactone to prevent peritoneal fibrosis in peritoneal dialysis patients: a randomized controlled trial. Am J Kidney Dis. 2014;63:1072–4.

69. Homma K, Hayashi K, Yamaguchi S, et al. Renal microcirculation and calcium channel subtypes. Cur Hypertens Rev. 2013;9:182–6.

70. Imagawa K, Okayama S, Takaoka M, et al. Inhibitory effect of efonidipine on aldosterone synthesis and secretion in human adrenocarinoma (H295R) cells. J Cardiovasc Pharmacol. 2006;47:133–8.

71. Akizuki O, Inayoshi A, Kitayama T, et al. Blockade of T-type voltage-dependent Ca2+ channels by benidipine, a dihydropyridine calcium channel blocker, inhibits aldosterone production in human adrenocortical cell line NCI-H295R. Eur J Pharmacol. 2008;584:424–34.

72. Isaka T, Ikeda K, Takada Y, et al. Azelnidipine inhibits aldosterone synthesis and secretion in human adrenocortical cell line NCI-H295R. Eur J Pharmacol. 2009;605:49–52.

73. Aritomi S, Wagatsuma H, Numata T, et al. Expression of N-type calcium channels in human adrenocortical cells and their contribution to corticosteroid synthesis. Hypertens Res. 2011;34:193–201.

74. Tsutamoto T, Tanaka T, Nishiyama K, et al. Long-term effect of efonidipine therapy on plasma aldosterone and left ventricular mass index in patients with essential hypertension. Hypertens Res. 2009;32:670–4.

75. Nakano N, Ishimitsu T, Takahashi T, et al. Effects of efonidipine, an L- and T-type calcium channel blocker, on the renin-angiotensin-aldosterone system in chronic hemodialysis patients. Int Heart J. 2010;51:188–92.

76. Abe M, Okada K, Maruyama N, et al. Benidipine reduces albuminuria and plasma aldosterone in mild-to-moderate stage chronic kidney disease with albuminuria. Hypertens Res. 2011;34:268–73.

77. Nakamura T, SugayaT KY, et al. Azelnidipine reduces urinary protein excretion and urinary liver-type fatty acid binding protein in patients with hypertensive chronic kidney disease. Am J Med Sci. 2007;333:321–6.

78. Konoshita T, Makino Y, Kimura T, et al. A new-generation N/L-type calcium channel blocker leads to less activation of the renin-angiotensin system compared with conventional L type calcium channel blocker. J Hypertens. 2010;28:2156–60.

79. Abe M, Maruyama N, Suzuki H, et al. L/N-type calcium channel blocker cilnidipine reduces plasma aldosterone, albuminuria, and urinary liver-type fatty acid binding protein in patients with chronic kidney disease. Heart Vessel. 2012;28:480–9.

80. Furukawa T, Nukada T, Namiki Y, et al. Five different profiles of dihydrppyridines in blocking T-type Ca(2+) channel subtypes (Ca(v)3.1(alfa(1G)), Ca(v)3.2(alfa(1H)), and Ca(v)3.3(alfa(1I))) expressed in Xenopus oocytes. Eur J Pharmacol. 2009;613:100–7.

81. Hayashi K, Wakino S, Sugano N, et al. Ca^{2+} channel subtypes and pharmacology in the kidney. Circ Res. 2007;100:342–53.

82. Hayashi K, Ozawa Y, Saruta T, Epstein M. Renal hemodynamic effects of calcium antagonists. In: Epstein M, editor. Calcium Antagonists in Clinical Medicine. 3rd ed. Philadelphia: Hanley & Belfus; 2002. p. 559–78.

83. Dietz JD, Du S, Bolten CW, et al. A number of marketed dihydropyridine calcium channel blockers have mineralocorticoid receptor antagonist activity. Hypertension. 2008;51:742–8.

84. Kosaka H, Hirayama K, Yoda N, et al. The L-, N-, and T-type triple calcium channel blocker benidipine acts as an antagonist of mineralocorticoid receptor, a member of nuclear receptor family. Eur J Pharmacol. 2010;635:49–55.

85. Shimada T, Mizutani S, Muto T, et al. Cloning and characterization of FGF 23 as a causative factor of tumor-induced osteomalacia. Proc Natl Acad Sci U S A. 2001;98:6500–5.

86. Felsenfeld AJ, Levine BS, Rodriguez M. Pathophysiology of calcium, phosphorus, and magnesium dysregulation in chronic kidney disease. Semin Dial. 2015;28:564–77.

87. Bricker NS. On the pathogenesis of the uremic state. An exposition of the "trade-off hypothesis". N Engl J Med. 1972;286:1093–9.

88. Isakova T, Wahl P, Vargas GS, et al. Fibroblast growth factor 23 is elevated before parathyroid hormone and phosphate in chronic kidney disease. Kidney Int. 2011;79:1370–8.

89. Tomoe Y, Segawa H, Shiozawa K, et al. Phosphaturic action of fibroblast growth factor 23 in Npt2 null mice. Am J Physiol. 2010;298:F1341-50.

90. Schiavi SC, Kumar R. The phosphatonin pathway: new insights in phosphate homeostasis. Kidney Int. 2004;65:1–14.

91. Ben-Dov IZ, Galitzer H, Lavi-Moshayoff V, et al. The parathyroid is a target organ for FGF23 in rats. J Clin Invest. 2007;117:4003–8.

92. Kovesdy CP, Quarles LD. FGF23 from bench to bedside. Am J Phys. 2016; 310:F1168–74.

93. Ritter CS, Slatopolsky E. Phosphate toxicity in CHD: the killer among UA. Clin J Am Soc Nephrolo. 2016;11:1088–100.

94. Andrukhova O, Slavic S, Smorodchenko A, et al. FGF23 regulates renal sodium handling and blood pressure. EMBO Mol Med. 2014;6:744–59.

95. Tsai MH, Leu JG, Fang YW, et al. High fibroblast growth factor 23 levels associated with low hemoglobin levels in patients with chronic kidney disease stages 3 and 4. Medicine. 2016;95:e3049. https://doi.org/10.1097/MD. 0000000000003049.

96. Imazu M, Takahama H, Asanuma H, et al. Pathophysiological impact of serum fibroblast growth factor 23 in patients with non-ischemic cardiac disease and early chronic kidney disease. Am J Phys. 2014;307:H1504–11.

97. Hu MC, Kuro-o M, Moe OW. Klotho and chronic kidney disease. Contrib Nephrol. 2013;180:47–63.

98. de Seigneux S, Courbebaisse M, Rutkowski JM, Wilhelm-Bals A, et al. Proteinuria increases plasma phosphate by altering its tubular handling. J Am Soc Nephrol. 2015;26:1608–18.

99. De Borst MH, Vervloet MG, ter Wee PM, et al. Cross talk between the renin-angiotensin-aldosterone system and vitamin D-FGF23-klotho in chronic kidney disease. J Am Soc Nephrol. 2011;22:1603–9.

100. Dai B, David V, Martin A, et al. A comparative transcriptome analysis identifying FGF23 regulated genes in the kidney of a mouse CKD model. PLoS One. 2012;7:e44161. https://doi.org/10.1371/journal.pone.0044161.

101. Santos RA, Rerreira AJ. Angiotensin-(1-7) and the renin-angiotensin system. Curr Opin Nephrol Hypertens. 2007;16:122–8.

102. Varaqic J, Ahmad S, Nagata S, Ferrario CM. ACE2: angiotensin II/angiotensin-(1-7) balance in cardiac and renal injury. Curr Hypertens Rep. 2014;16:420. https://doi.org/10.1007/s11906-014-0420-5.

103. Li YC, Kong J, Wei M, et al. 1,25-Dihydroxyvitamin D(3) is a negative endocrine regulator of the renin-angiotensin system. J Clin Invest. 2002; 110:229–38.

104. Freundlich M, Quiroz Y, Zhang Z, et al. Suppression of renin-angiotensin gene expression in the kidney by paricalcitol. Kidney Int. 2008 Dec;74(11): 1394–402. https://doi.org/10.1038/ki.2008.408.

105. Zhang B, Umbach AT, Chen H, et al. Up-regulation of FGF23 release by aldosterone. Biochem Biophy Res Commun. 2016;470:384–90.

106. Di Lullo L, Gorini A, Russo D, et al. Left ventricular hypertrophy in chronic kidney disease patients: from pathophysiology to treatment. Cardiorenal Med. 2015;5:254–66.

107. Nardi E, Palermo A, Mule G, et al. Left ventricular hypertrophy and geometry in hypertensive patients with chronic kidney disease. J Hypertens. 2009;27: 633–41.

108. Hayashi T, Joki N, Tanaka Y, et al. Anaemia and early phase cardiovascular events on haemodialysis. Nephrology (Carlton). 2015;20(Suppl 4):1–6.

109. Randon RB, Rohde LE, Comerlato L, et al. The role of secondary hyperparathyroidism in left ventricular hypertrophy of patients under chronic hemodialysis. Braz J Med & Biol Res. 2005;38:1409–16.

110. Strozecki P, Adamowicz A, Nartowicz E, et al. Parathormone, calcium, phosphorus and left ventricular structure and function in normotensive hemodialysis patients. Ren Fail. 2001;23:115–26.

111. London GM, De Vernejoul MC, Fabiani F, et al. Secondary hyperparathyroidism and cardiac hypertrophy in hemodialysis patients. Kidney Int. 1997;32:900–7.

112. Wang AY, Fang F, Chan J, et al. Effect of paricalcitol on left ventricular mass and function in CKD-the OPERA trial. J Am Soc Nephrol. 2014;25:175–86.

113. Hassan M, Qureshi W, Sroujieh LS, et al. Interplay of parathyroid hormone and aldosterone antagonist in prevention of heart failure hospitalizations in chronic kidney disease. J Renin-Angiotensin-Aldosterone Syst. 2014;15:278–85.

114. Brown JM, Williams JS, Luther JM, et al. Human interventions to characterize novel relationships between the renin-angiotensin-aldosterone system and parathyroid hormone. Hypertension. 2014;63:273–80.

115. Olgaard K, Lewin E, Bro S, et al. Enhancement of the stimulatory effect of calcium on aldosterone secretion by parathyroid hormone. Miner Electrolyte Metab. 1994;20:309–14.

116. Mazzocchi G, Aragona F, Malendowicz LK, et al. PTH and PTH-related peptide enhance steroid secretion from human adrenocortical cells. Am J Physiol Endocrinol Metab. 2001;280:E209–13.

117. Tomaschitz A, Ritz E, Pieske B, et al. Aldosterone and parathyroid hormone interactions as mediators of metabolic and cardiovascular disease. Metabolism Clin & Exp. 2014;63:20–31.

118. Hsu HJ, Wu MS. Fibroblast growth factor 23: a possible cause of left ventricular hypertrophy in hemodialysis patients. Am J Med Sci. 2009; 337:116–22.

119. Seifert ME, de Las FL, Ginsberg C, et al. Left ventricular mass progression despite stable blood pressure and kidney function in stage 3 chronic kidney disease. Am J Nephrol. 2014;39:392–9.

120. Sarmento-Dias M, Santos-Araújo C, Poínhos R, Oliveira B, et al. Fibroblast growth factor 23 is associated with left ventricular hypertrophy, not with uremic vasculopathy in peritoneal dialysis patients. Clin Nephrol. 2016;85:135–41.

121. Jovanovich A, Ix JH, Gottdiener J, et al. Fibroblast growth factor 23, left ventricular mass, and left ventricular hypertrophy in community-dwelling older adults. Atherosclerosis. 2013;231:114–9.

122. Tanaka S, Fujita S, Kizawa S, et al. Association between FGF23, α-Klotho, and cardiac abnormalities among patients with various chronic kidney disease stages. PLoS One. 2016;11(7):e0156860. https://doi.org/10.1371/journal.pone.0156860. eCollection 2016

123. Di Marco GS, Reuter S, Kentrup D, et al. Treatment of established left ventricular hypertrophy with fibroblast growth factor receptor blockade in an animal model of CKD. Nephrol Dial Transplant. 2014;29:2028-35.

124. Grabner A, Amaral AP, Schramm K, et al. Activation of cardiac fibroblast growth factor receptor 4 causes left ventricular hypertrophy. Cell Metab. 2015;22:1020-32.

125. Koiwa F, Kazawa JJ, Tokumoto A, et al. Sevelamer hydrochloride and calcium bicarbonate reduce serum fibroblast growth factor 23 levels in dialysis patients. Ther Apher Dial. 2005;9:336-9.

126. Gonzalez-Parra E, Gonzalez-Casaus ML, Galan A, et al. Lanthanum carbonate reduces FGF23 in chronic kidney disease stage 3 patients. Nephrol Dial Transplant. 2011;26:2567-71.

127. Shigematsu T, Negi S, for the COLC Research Group. Combined therapy with lanthanum carbonate and calcium carbonate for hyperphosphatemia decreases serum FGF-23 independently of calcium and PTH (COLC Study). Nephrol Dial Transpant. 2012;27:1050-4.

128. Lin HH, Liou HH, Wu MS, et al. Long-term sevelamer treatment lowers serum fibroblast growth factor 23 accompanied with increasing serum Klotho levels in chronic haemodialysis patients. Nephrology (Carlton). 2014;19:672-8.

129. Chang YM, Tsai SC, Shiao CC, et al. Effects of lanthanum carbonate and calcium carbonate on fibroblast growth factor 23 and hepcidin levels in chronic hemodialysis patients. Clin Exp Nephrol. 2016; https://doi.org/10.1007/s10157-016-1362-9.

130. Rodriguez-Ortiz ME, Lopez I, Munoz-Castaneda JR, et al. Calcium deficiency reduces circulating levels of FGF23. J Am Soc Nephrol. 2012;23:1190-7.

131. David V, Dai B, Martin A, et al. Calcium regulates FGF-23 expression in bone. Endocrinology. 2013;154:4469-82.

132. Yasin A, Liu D, Chau L, et al. Fibroblast growth factor-23 and calcium phosphate product in young chronic kidney disease patients: a cross-sectional study. BMC Nephrol. 2013;14:39. https://doi.org/10.1186/1471-2369-14-39.

133. Siriano S, Ojeda R, Rodriguez M, et al. The effect of phosphate binders, calcium and lanthanum carbonate on FGF23 levels in chronic kidney disease patients. Clin Nephrol. 2013;80:17-22.

134. Chue CD, Townend JN, Moody WE, et al. Cardiovascular effects of sevelamer in stage 3 CKD. J Am Soc Nephrol. 2013;24:842-52.

135. Maizel J, Six I, Dupont S, et al. Effects of sevelamer treatment on cardiovascular abnormalities in mice with chronic renal failure. Kidney Int. 2013;84:491-500.

136. Yamazaki-Nakazawa A, Mizobuchi M, Ogata H, et al. Correction of hyperphosphatemia suppresses cardiac remodeling in uremic rats. Clin Exp Nephrol. 2014;18:56-64.

137. Chue CD, Edwards NC, Moody WE, et al. Serum phosphate is associated with left ventricular mass in patients with chronic kidney disease: a cardiac magnetic resonance study. Heart. 2012;98:219-24.

138. Dhingra R, Gona P, Benjamin EJ, et al. Relations of serum phosphorus levels to echocardiographic left ventricular mass and incidence of heart failure in the community. Eur Heart Fail. 2010;12:812-8.

139. Nakamura H, Tokumoto M, Mizobuchi M, et al. Novel markers of left ventricular hypertrophy in uremia. Am J Nephrol. 2010;31:292-302.

140. Achinger SG, Ayus JC. Left ventricular hypertrophy: is hyperphosphatemia among dialysis patients a risk factor? J Am Soc Nephrol. 2006;17(12 Suppl 3):S255-61.

141. Liu YL, Huang CC, Chang CC, et al. Hyperphosphate-induced myocardial hypertrophy through the GATA-4/NFAT-3 signaling pathway is attenuated by ERK inhibitor treatment. Cardiorenal Med. 2015;5:79-88. https://doi.org/10.1159/000371454.

142. Yagil Y, Fadem SZ, Kant KS, et al. Managing hyperphosphatemia in patients with chronic kidney disease on dialysis with ferric citrate: latest evidence and clinical usefulness. Ther Adv Chronic Dis. 2015;6:252-63.

143. Floege J, Covic AC, Ketteler M, et al. Long-term effects of the iron-based phosphate binder, sucrferric oxyhydroxide, in dialysis patients. Nephrol Dial Transplant. 2015;30:1037-46.

144. Bozentowicz-Wikarek M, Kocelak P, Owczarek A, et al. Plasma fibroblast growth factor 23 concentration and iron status. Does the relationship exist in the early elderly population? Clin Biochem. 2015;48:431-6.

145. Lewerin C, Ljunggren O, Nilsson-Ehle H, et al. Low serum iron is associated with high serum intact FGF23 in elderly men. The Swedish MrOS study. Bone. 2017;98:1-8.

146. Braithwaite V, Prentice AM, Doherty C, et al. FGF23 is correlated with iron status but not with inflammation and decreases after iron supplementation: a supplementation study. Int J Pediatr Endocrinol. 2012;2012(1):27. https://doi.org/10.1186/1687-9856-2012-27.

147. David V, Martin A, Isakova T, et al. Inflammation and functional iron deficiency regulate fibroblast growth factor 23 production. Kidney Int. 2016;89:135-46.

148. Hanudel MR, Chua K, Rappaport M, et al. Effects of dietary iron intake and chronic kidney disease on fibroblast growth factor 23 metabolism in wild-type and hepcidin knockout mice. Am J Phys. 2016;311:F1369-77.

149. Farrow EG, Yu X, Summers LJ, et al. Iron deficiency drives an autosomal dominant hypophosphatemic ricket (ADHR) phenotype in fibroblast growth factor-23 knock-in mice. Proc Natl Acad Sci U S A. 2011;108:E1146-55.

150. Deger SM, Erten Y, Pasaoglu OT, et al. The effects of iron on FGF23-mediated Ca-P metabolism in CKD patients. Clin Exp Nephrol. 2013;17:416-23. https://doi.org/10.1007/s10157-012-0725-0.

151. Yamashita K, Mizuiri S, Nishizawa Y, et al. Oral iron supplementation with sodium ferrous citrate reduces the serum intact and c-terminal FGF23 levels of maintenance hemodialysis patients. Nephrology (Carlton). 2016. https://doi.org/10.1111/nep.12909.

152. Takeda Y, Komaba H, Goto S, et al. Effect of intravenous saccharated ferric oxide on serum FGF23 and mineral metabolism in hemodialysis patients. Am J Nephrol. 2011;33:421-6. https://doi.org/10.1159/000327019. Epub 2011 Apr 19.

153. Gravesen E, Hofman-Bang J, Mace ML, et al. High dose intravenous iron, mineral homeostasis and intact FGF23 in normal and uremic rats. BMC Nephrol. 2013;27(14):281. https://doi.org/10.1186/1471-2369-14-281.

154. Iguchi A, Kazama JJ, Yamamoto S, et al. Administration of ferric citrate hydrate decreases circulating FGF23 levels independently of serum phosphate levels in hemodialysis patients with iron deficiency. Nephron. 2015;131:161-6.

155. Babitt JL, Lin HY. Mechanisms of anemia in CKD. J Am Soc Nephrol. 2012;23:1631-4.

156. Tsuchiya K, Nitta K. Hepcidin is a potential regulator of iron status in chronic kidney disease. Ther Apher Dial. 2013;17:1-8. https://doi.org/10.1111/1744-9987.12001.

157. Carvalho C, Isakova T, Collerone G, et al. Hepcidin and disordered mineral metabolism in chronic kidney disease. Clin Nephrol. 2011;76:90-8.

25

Serum uric acid is an independent predictor of new-onset diabetes after living-donor kidney transplantation

Kentaro Tanaka[1,2*], Ken Sakai[1], Akifumi Kushiyama[2], Shigeko Hara[2], Masakazu Hattori[3], Yasushi Ohashi[1], Masaki Muramatsu[1], Takeshi Kawamura[1], Seiichiro Shishido[1] and Atsushi Aikawa[1]

Abstract

Background: We investigated whether serum uric acid (SUA) levels before kidney transplantation predict new-onset diabetes after kidney transplantation (NODAT) and compared SUA levels with known risk factors for NODAT by prospective cohort study.

Methods: A total of 151 adult kidney recipients without diabetes (84 men, 67 women) who underwent living-donor kidney transplantation between 2001 and 2011 were followed in this study. The Cox proportional hazards model was used to analyse the risk of NODAT.

Results: During the follow-up period (median 3.3 years, range 0–10 years), 32 (21.2%) adult kidney recipients without diabetes developed NODAT, and an incidence rate was 5.6 per 100 person-years and a 10-year cumulative incidence of 26.9%. When subjects were stratified by SUA levels into tertiles, the patients in the highest tertile (> 8.6 mg/dl for men, > 7.7 mg/dl for women) had a significantly higher risk of NODAT than the patients in the lower 2 tertiles (log-rank test, $P = 0.03$). In the univariate analysis, increased level of SUA was associated with NODAT (hazard ratio 1.27 [95% CI 1.04–1.55], $P = 0.01$). In the multivariate analysis, increased level of SUA was significantly associated with NODAT after correction by any factors, e.g. (age, sex, family history of diabetes, BMI, HbA1c, serum creatinine, tacrolimus, HCV) factors directly affecting the SUA value (1.26 [1.02–1.56], $P = 0.03$), risk factors for T2DM onset (1.34 [1.10–1.64], $P = 0.03$), and factors previously reported risk factors for NODAT (1.36 [1.11–1.66], $P = 0.003$).

Conclusion: SUA independently predicts NODAT in living-donor kidney transplantation patients.

Keywords: Diabetes, Living-donor kidney transplantation, Uric acid

Background

New-onset diabetes after kidney transplantation (NODAT) is a serious metabolic complication of kidney transplantation that predisposes patients to graft dysfunction, infectious complications, cardiovascular disease, and death [1, 2]. The reported incidence of NODAT in kidney transplantation varies between 2 and 53% [1, 3, 4]. The lack of uniformity in the reported NODAT incidence rates is thought to be caused by variations in the studied populations, varying immunosuppressive regimens, and different definitions of diabetes [3]. To improve the outcome of kidney transplantation and patient prognosis, precise knowledge of the risk factors that contribute to NODAT development and maintenance are of great importance. Several risk factors have been shown to be independent predictors of NODAT. These include older age, higher body mass index (BMI), risk factors for type 2 diabetes mellitus (T2DM) onset, ethnicity, hepatitis C virus (HCV)-positive status, and the use of tacrolimus [1, 5]. The risk factors for T2DM onset are relatively well investigated and include age, family history of diabetes, BMI, haemoglobin A1c (HbA1c), such indexes as the insulinogenic index, and the homeostasis model assessment of insulin resistance (HOMA-IR) [6, 7].

* Correspondence: kentarot@oak.ocn.ne.jp
[1]Department of Nephrology, School of Medicine, Faculty of Medicine, Toho University, 6-11-1 Omori-Nishi, Ota-ku, Tokyo 143-0015, Japan
[2]Division of Diabetes and Metabolism, Institute for Adult Diseases, Asahi Life Foundation, Tokyo, Japan
Full list of author information is available at the end of the article

The serum uric acid (SUA) level has also been suggested to be associated with a risk of T2DM onset [8]. SUA concentration is significantly correlated with risk factors for metabolic syndrome, and SUA levels affect insulin resistance [9]. Pre-transplant metabolic syndrome is an independent predictor of NODAT [10]. The mechanism of NODAT is not yet known, and whether SUA and/or risk factors for the onset of T2DM are applicable to NODAT has not been well established. Herein, we aim to provide the first evidence that the pre-transplant SUA level is a predictor of NODAT among kidney allograft recipients.

Methods

This was an observational cohort study on the development of NODAT in kidney transplant recipients who underwent living-donor kidney transplantation at the Department of Nephrology, Toho University Omori Medical Center, Tokyo, Japan. For this study, we initially enrolled all recipients who underwent kidney transplantation at our hospital between January 2001 and June 2011 ($n = 296$). We excluded recipients who were diagnosed with diabetes before transplantation ($n = 34$), had received cadaveric kidney transplantation ($n = 14$), were

< 20 years old ($n = 57$), had experienced post-transplant allograft loss due to acute rejection ($n = 1$), or did not undergo a pre-transplant oral glucose tolerance test ($n = 39$). Thus, our study included all non-diabetic adult (> 20 years old) kidney allograft recipients who successfully underwent living-donor kidney transplantation between January 2001 and April 2011 ($n = 151$; Fig. 1). All of the remaining 151 transplant patients (87 men and 64 women, 20–69 years old, pre-transplant dialysis modality: 119 haemodialysis (HD) patients, 20 peritoneal dialysis patients, 12 preemptive) were followed until October 2011. NODAT was defined as fasting plasma glucose ≥ 126 mg/dL, random plasma glucose ≥ 200 mg/dL confirmed by repeated testing on a different day, and/or starting oral hypoglycaemic agents or insulin for diabetes treatment after the first 2 weeks post-transplant [11], as defined by the American Diabetes Association and the Japanese diabetes criteria described in 1999 by the Japan Diabetes Society guidelines. The following data were collected from electronic medical records and transplant charts: recipient age and sex, BMI, family history of diabetes, duration of dialysis, blood pressure, serum albumin, serum creatinine, HbA1c, insulinogenic index, HOMA-IR, total cholesterol, triglycerides, HCV

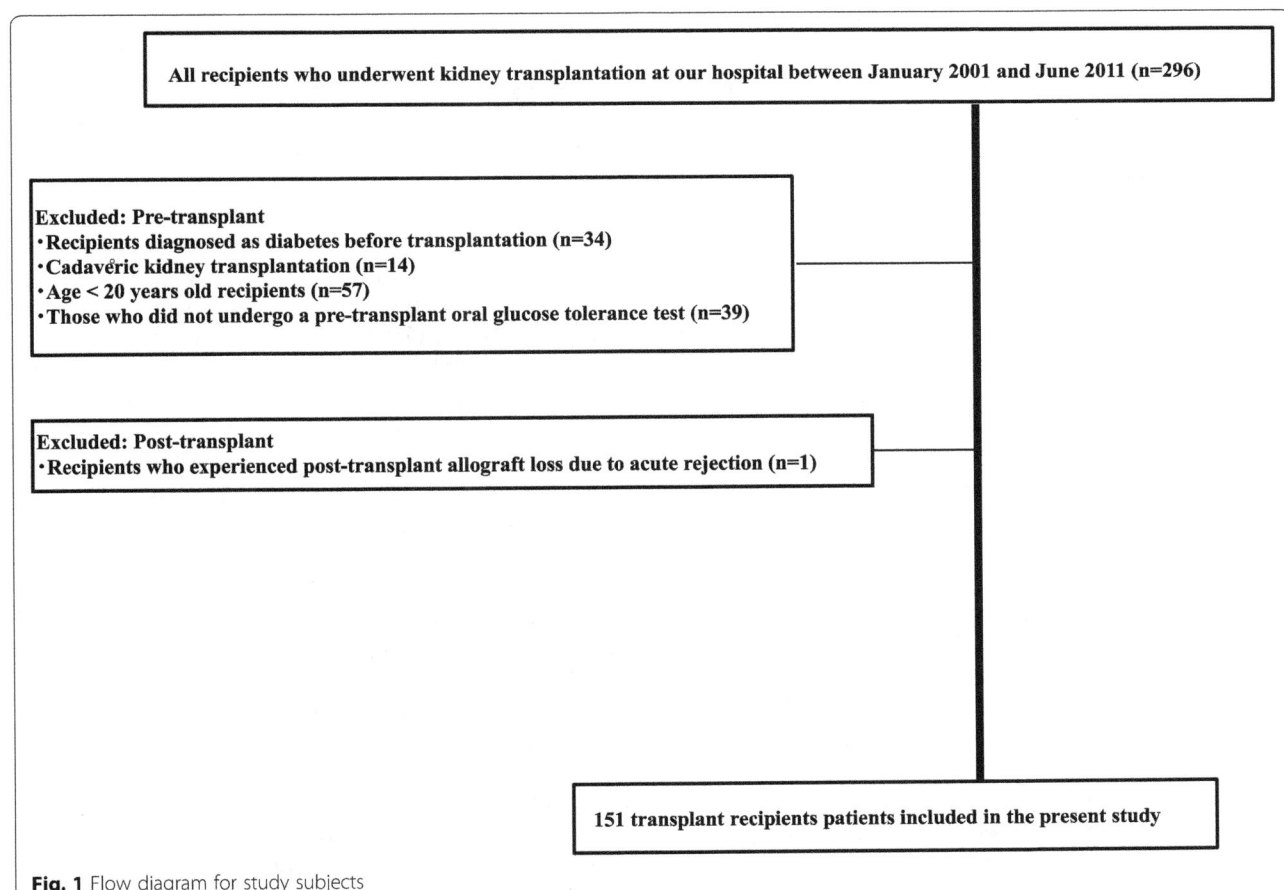

Fig. 1 Flow diagram for study subjects

infection status, and medication use (anti-hyperuricae-mics, diuretics, and induction immunosuppressive agents). All of the anti-hyperuricaemic agents used were allopurinol. The SUA value is measured according to the protocol for transplantation, at the time of hospitalization just prior to transplantation. SUA levels and other laboratory data were obtained at fasting and pre-dialysis, on the first dialysis day after hospitalization. The SUA levels after transplantation were measured approximately 2 months later with renal function stabilized. The present study was performed with the approval of the Clinical Research Ethics Committee of the Toho Omori Medical Center (approval number 24-103).

All patients were on maintenance immunosuppressive therapy, which included methylprednisolone and calcineurin inhibitors (e.g. tacrolimus or cyclosporine) and anti-proliferative agents (mycophenolate mofetil, mizoribin, or azathioprine) before transplant. Methylprednisolone was administered at a starting dose of 12 mg/day. The starting doses of cyclosporine and tacrolimus were 5 and 0.2 mg/kg/day, respectively. Both agents were administered in two divided doses and were adjusted to maintain levels at 200 to 300 ng/mL up to 1 week after operation and 8 to 12 ng/mL up to 1 month after operation, respectively. Mycophenolate mofetil was administered at a dose of 25–30 mg/kg/day in two divided doses. The estimated glomerular filtration rate (eGFR) was calculated using the estimation formula advocated by the Japanese Society of Nephrology [12]: eGFR (mL/min/1.73 m2) = 194 × Cr − 1.094 × age − 0.287 (× 0.739 for women).

Statistical analysis
The data are expressed as the mean ± standard deviation or as frequency. The differences among the three groups were assessed using a one-way analysis of variance and Fisher's exact test. To investigate the relationship between SUA levels and the onset of NODAT, the SUA levels were stratified into tertiles, which were calculated separately for men (lower tertile < 429 μmol/L [7.2 mg/dL]; middle 429–511 μmol/L [7.2–8.6 mg/dL]; upper > 511 μmol/L [8.6 mg/dL]) and women (lower < 387 μmol/L [6.5 mg/dL]; middle 387–457 μmol/L [6.5–7.7 mg/dL]; upper > 457 μmol/L [7.7 mg/dL]), because SUA levels in women tend to be lower than those in men [13]. The onset of NODAT was analysed using the Kaplan-Meier method, and the significance was calculated using the log-rank test. The Cox proportional hazards regression model was used to assess the independent predictors of NODAT. Three multivariate regression models were performed. The first was adjusted for the factors that directly affect the SUA value: serum creatinine, diuretics (yes/no), and allopurinol therapy (yes/no). A second regression model was adjusted for risk factors for the onset of T2DM: age (years), sex

(male vs. female), family history of diabetes (yes/no), BMI, HbA1c, I-I, and HOMA-IR. A third model was adjusted for the significant factors used in the first and second models and previously reported risk factors for the onset of NODAT: HCV infection (yes/no) and immunosuppressive agents (tacrolimus vs. cyclosporine). The results are presented as hazard ratios with 95% confidence intervals (CI). P values < 0.05 were considered to indicate statistically significant differences. The analyses were performed using JMP software (version 13.0; SAS Institute, Cary, NC, USA).

Power calculation
We are planning a study with 50 experimental participants, 100 control participants, an accrual interval of 0.5 year, and additional median follow-up after the accrual interval of approximately 3 years. If the true hazard ratio of control participants relative to experimental participants is 2.5 in the end of follow-up, we will be able to reject the null hypothesis that the experimental and control survival curves are equal with probability (power) 0.878. The type I error probability associated with this test of this null hypothesis is 0.05.

Results
In the study population, the median baseline SUA value was 7.4 mg/dL, with a range of 1.7 to 12.2 mg/dL. The baseline clinical and biochemical characteristics of the recipients, grouped by sex-specific SUA tertiles, are shown in Table 1.

There were no differences between the groups in sex, age, family history of diabetes, BMI, HbA1c, HOMA-IR, I-I, HCV infection status, or the frequency of medication use, including diuretics, lipid-lowering agents, antihypertensive agents, antiplatelet agents, and immunosuppressive agents (Table 1). Serum creatinine and eGFR differed between the groups and were associated with elevated SUA values. Figure 2 shows the results of the Kaplan-Meier survival analysis for NODAT incidence. Thirty-two of the 151 recipients developed NODAT during the follow-up period (median 3.3 years, range 0–10 years) with an incidence rate of 5.6 per 100 person-years and a total cumulative incidence of 26.9% as of 10 years of follow-up. Analysis according to the tertiles of SUA at baseline revealed a cumulative incidence of NODAT of 13.8% in the lowest SUA tertile, 19.0% in the middle tertile, and 44.1% in the highest tertile as of 10 years of follow-up (log-rank test, $P = 0.03$).

Recipients in the highest tertile of SUA levels had a significantly higher risk of NODAT than those in the lower 2 tertiles. In a univariate analysis using the Cox proportional hazards model (Table 2), SUA (hazard ratio 1.27 [95% CI 1.04–1.55], $P = 0.01$), age (1.04 [1.01–1.07],

Table 1 Characteristics of renal transplant recipients stratified into sex-specific tertiles of serum uric acid levels

	Tertile 1	Tertile 2	Tertile 3	P value
Type of renal failure (haemodialysis/peritoneal dialysis/preemptive)	(36/9/3)	(38/6/6)	(38/9/6)	0.7
Sex (men/women)	27/21	26/24	31/22	0.79
Age (years)	43.3 ± 10.6	41.9 ± 13.7	38.1 ± 10.5	0.07
Family history of diabetes (%)	10.4	16.0	13.2	0.71
Smoking history (%)	66.6	44.0	54.7	0.07
Duration of dialysis (years)	3.4 ± 4.7	2.4 ± 3.4	3.0 ± 5.4	0.56
BMI (kg/m^2)	20.3 ± 2.9	20.1 ± 2.8	21.3 ± 3.5	0.14
Systolic BP (mmHg)	149.3 ± 22.9	149.3 ± 21.3	154.0 ± 21.2	0.45
Diastolic BP (mmHg)	85.7 ± 13.1	84.6 ± 12.2	87.5 ± 13.9	0.51
Albumin (g/dL)	4.1 ± 0.5	3.9 ± 0.4	3.9 ± 0.4	0.17
Total cholesterol (mg/dL)	176.4 ± 37.4	171.3 ± 40.1	165.0 ± 38.5	0.33
Triglycerides (mg/dL)	171.0 ± 11.5	158.4 ± 7.4	171.0 ± 11.5	0.76
SUA (mg/dL)	5.7 ± 1.1	7.3 ± 0.4	9.4 ± 1.0	NA
SUA after transplantation(mg/dL)	6.4 ± 0.2	6.2 ± 0.2	7.2 ± 0.2	0.003
Creatinine (mg/dL)	10.2 ± 2.9	12.0 ± 2.8	12.2 ± 3.1	0.001
eGFR (mL/min/1.73 m^2)	5.2 ± 2.6	4.1 ± 1.2	4.2 ± 1.5	0.01
Haemoglobin (g/dL)	10.7 ± 0.2	10.4 ± 0.1	10.3 ± 0.1	0.36
HbA1c (%)	5.3 ± 0.4	5.2 ± 0.4	5.3 ± 0.5	0.67
HOMA-IR	1.0 ± 0.5	1.2 ± 1.0	1.4 ± 0.9	0.06
Insulinogenic index	0.7 ± 0.4	1.0 ± 0.9	1.4 ± 2.6	0.08
Diuretics (%)	41.6	38.0	30.1	0.46
Allopurinol therapy (%)	22.9	34.0	26.4	0.45
Statin (%)	10.4	8.0	13.2	0.69
Antiplatelet agents (%)	14.5	26.0	11.3	0.12
RAS inhibitor (%)	47.9	48.0	50.9	0.94
CCB agents (%)	62.5	62.0	54.7	0.66
β-Blockers (%)	16.6	14.0	20.7	0.65
Calcineurin inhibitor (tacrolimus/cyclosporin A) (%)	52.0:47.9	56.0:44.0	52.8:47.1	0.91
HCV-positive (%)	2.0	2.0	9.4	0.11

Cohort size $n = 151$ (84 men and 67 women). The statistical significance was estimated with a one-way analysis of variance and Fisher's exact text ($P < 0.05$). Data are expressed as mean ± standard deviation or percent
BMI body mass index, *BP* blood pressure, *CCB* calcium channel blocker, *eGFR* estimated glomerular filtration rate, *HbA1c* haemoglobin A1c, *HCV* hepatitis C virus, *HOMA-IR* homeostasis model assessment of insulin resistance, *NA* not applicable, *RAS* renin-angiotensin system, *SUA* serum uric acid

$P = 0.02$), and HbA1c (2.39 [1.07–5.34], $P = 0.03$) were associated with a higher risk of NODAT. SUA (1.26 [1.02–1.56], $P = 0.03$) was associated with an increased risk of NODAT when the model was adjusted for the factors that directly affected the SUA level (Table 2, multivariate model 1). Age (1.04 [1.01–1.07], $P = 0.008$) and SUA (1.34 [1.10–1.64], $P = 0.003$) were associated after correcting for risk factors for the onset of T2DM (Table 2, multivariate model 2). Age (1.05 [1.02–1.08], $P = 0.0007$) and SUA (1.36 [1.11–1.66], $P = 0.003$) remained significantly associated after correcting for previously reported risk factors for the onset of

NODAT and the significant factors adjusted for in models 1 and 2 (Table 2, multivariate model 3).

The SUA level before transplantation correlated with the SUA level after transplantation with renal function stabilized ($\rho = 0.17$, $P = 0.03$ by Spearman's correlation analysis).

Discussion

In this cohort study of kidney transplant recipients over a 10-year period, NODAT was found in 21.2% of the patients and the 10-year cumulative incidence was 26.9%. In the tertile stratification, a high SUA level (> 511 μmol/L [8.6 mg/dL] for men and >457 μmol/L

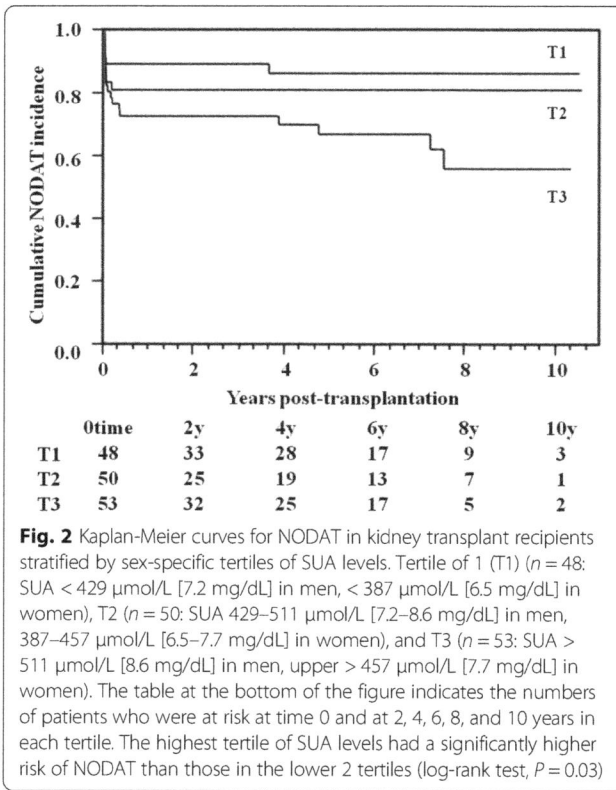

Fig. 2 Kaplan-Meier curves for NODAT in kidney transplant recipients stratified by sex-specific tertiles of SUA levels. Tertile of 1 (T1) ($n = 48$: SUA < 429 µmol/L [7.2 mg/dL] in men, < 387 µmol/L [6.5 mg/dL] in women), T2 ($n = 50$: SUA 429–511 µmol/L [7.2–8.6 mg/dL] in men, 387–457 µmol/L [6.5–7.7 mg/dL] in women), and T3 ($n = 53$: SUA > 511 µmol/L [8.6 mg/dL] in men, upper > 457 µmol/L [7.7 mg/dL] in women). The table at the bottom of the figure indicates the numbers of patients who were at risk at time 0 and at 2, 4, 6, 8, and 10 years in each tertile. The highest tertile of SUA levels had a significantly higher risk of NODAT than those in the lower 2 tertiles (log-rank test, $P = 0.03$)

[7.7 mg/dL] for women) was an independent and strong predictor of NODAT in our study. We constructed three Cox hazard regression models that indicated a significant association between SUA and NODAT after adjusting for known risk factors for T2DM onset, NODAT,

and factors that directly affect the SUA level. We demonstrated for the first time that a high SUA level is a strong and independent predictor of NODAT.

A previous report did not reveal an association between SUA and NODAT; however, pre-transplant anti-hyperuricaemic medication was associated with NODAT [14]. Conversely, allopurinol therapy did not predict NODAT in our study, but SUA did. SUA level is reportedly affected by the variables in model 1, related to uric acid excretion [15]. We confirm SUA is independent of factors from renal function, and correlation of SUA levels between before and after transplantation with renal function stabilized. Therefore, SUA is suggested to reflect elevated production, predisposed by xanthine oxidoreductase (XOR) activity, in a manner independent of renal function. Uric acid has thought to have diabetogenic action since 1950 [16], by exacerbating insulin resistance [17]. Moreover, uric acid production via XOR promotion, associated with oxidative stress and inflammation such as macrophage activation [18], is suggested to induce a vulnerability to NODAT development. The role of uric acid metabolism-related inflammation in pathogenesis of diabetes, non-alcoholic steatohepatitis, and arteriosclerosis has been reported in several studies in many countries [19–22]. To the best of our knowledge, our study is the first to clarify the association between increased SUA production and development of NODAT.

Many risk factors have been proposed for the development of NODAT: age, race, family history of diabetes, BMI, glucose intolerance, metabolic syndrome, acute

Table 2 Predictors of NODAT as assessed with multivariate Cox proportional hazards models

Variable	Univariate model	P value	Multivariate models					
			Model 1	P value	Model 2	P value	Model 3	P value
SUA, per 1 mg/dL	1.27 (1.04–1.55)	0.01	1.26 (1.02–1.56)	0.03	1.34 (1.10–1.64)	0.003	1.36 (1.11–1.66)	0.003
Use of diuretics (yes/no)	1.05 (0.48–2.16)	0.88	1.08 (0.50–2.63)	0.82				
Use of allopurinol therapy (yes/no)	0.67 (0.25–1.45)	0.36	0.66 (0.24–1.53)	0.36				
Creatinine, per 1 mg/dL	0.77 (0.55–1.01)	0.06	1.07 (0.95–1.21)	0.23				
Sex (men)	0.77 (0.37–1.58)	0.47			0.73 (0.32–1.65)	0.41		
Age, per 1 year	1.04 (1.01–1.07)	0.006			1.04 (1.01–1.07)	0.008	1.05 (1.02–1.08)	0.0007
BMI, per 1 kg/m²	1.00 (089–1.11)	0.88			0.99 (0.86–1.13)	0.94		
Family history of diabetes (yes/no)	0.49 (0.07–1.63)	0.28			0.57 (0.09–1.93)	0.38		
HbA1c, per 1%	2.39 (1.07–5.34)	0.03			2.06 (0.85–5.02)	0.10		
Insulinogenic index, per 1 change	0.82 (0.47–1.09)	0.27			0.81 (0.43–1.18)	0.38		
HOMA-IR, per 1 unit	1.05 (0.69–1.45)	0.76			0.95 (0.54–1.46)	0.84		
Calcineurin inhibitor (tacrolimus/cyclosporin A)	1.73 (0.85–3.57)	0.12					1.99 (0.97–4.17)	0.05
HCV-positive (yes/no)	1.49 (0.24–4.97)	0.60					1.11 (0.17–3.88)	0.88

Results are expressed as hazard ratios (95% confidence intervals). Cohort size $n = 151$ (84 men and 67 women)
BMI body mass index, *HbA1c* haemoglobin A1c, *HCV* hepatitis C virus, *HOMA-IR* homeostasis model assessment of insulin resistance

rejection, cadaveric kidney transplantation, chronic infection with HCV, and the type of immunosuppression used [1, 3, 5]. Furthermore, SUA is correlated with metabolic syndrome and T2DM [8, 9, 23–25]. Another T2DM risk might also be a NODAT risk; therefore, we included known T2DM risks in model 2 for multivariate analysis. HOMA-IR and I-I tended to be higher in patients in the highest tertile for SUA values than for those in the lower 2 tertiles. However, after adjusting for both factors, they were not associated with NODAT. Known risk factors for NODAT relating to transplantation are included in model 3. Older age has consistently been an important contributing factor to the development of T2DM and NODAT [1, 2, 26] and is an important determinant of β-cell dysfunction after renal transplantation [27]. Our recipients represent a relatively young population for T2DM onset, with median ages of 39 and 47 years in non-NODAT and NODAT patients, respectively.

Evidence suggests that immunosuppressive drugs account for the risk for NODAT development [3]. The association between corticosteroids and NODAT is clearly established and is related to cumulative dosages and therapy duration [4]. The avoidance of steroids is associated with a significant reduction in the likelihood of developing NODAT [28]. However, to date, there has been no steroid-free maintenance regimen in Japan, and our protocol is based on pre-transplant induction therapy and does not include post-transplant therapy.

This study has several limitations. First, all donors and recipients were Japanese, and it was not revealed whether the risk of high SUA for NODAT is applicable to other ethnicities. Second, this is a single-institution study; therefore, the magnitude of SUA significance might vary according to unknown factors resulting from intra-institutional differences. Third, it is unknown whether uric acid reduction therapy prevents NODAT because of the observational nature of this study. Fourth, although the results of kidney transplantation in Japan are as good as those observed in European countries and the USA, the number of transplantations performed in Japan is extremely small compared with these countries. An interventional study with a large number of patients is needed to verify the usefulness of pre-transplant uric acid-lowering therapy. Despite these limitations, this is the first long-term follow-up study to report a novel predictor and potential target for NODAT. Certain care for recipients with preoperative hyperuricemia of living-donor kidney transplantation is probably important in clinical situation. From now on, frequent check of the glycemic control and uric acid level are recommended for both clinical practice and future research field.

Conclusions

In summary, we conclude that the pre-transplant SUA level is an independent predictor of NODAT, particularly when it falls into the upper range (> 8.6 mg/dL for men, > 7.7 mg/dL for women). Patients with a high pre-transplant SUA level should be carefully followed up.

Abbreviations
BMI: Body mass index; CI: Confidence intervals; eGFR: Estimated glomerular filtration rate; HbA1c: Haemoglobin A1c; HCV: Hepatitis C virus; HD: Haemodialysis; NODAT: New-onset diabetes after kidney transplantation; SUA: Serum uric acid; T2DM: Type 2 diabetes mellitus; XOR: Xanthine oxidoreductase

Acknowledgements
The authors thank Takashi Ozawa and Yoko Yoshida for their kind help, Toshihiko Oota for his programming efforts, and Takefumi Kitazawa and Kunichika Matsumoto for the assistance with the statistical analysis.

Authors' contributions
KT designed this study. KS summarized Tables 1 and 2. AK performed the statistical analysis and created Figs. 1 and 2. Other co-authors summarized and wrote the "Discussion" section. All authors have contributed significantly, have read, and approved the manuscript.

Competing interests
The authors declare that they have no competing interests.

Author details
[1]Department of Nephrology, School of Medicine, Faculty of Medicine, Toho University, 6-11-1 Omori-Nishi, Ota-ku, Tokyo 143-0015, Japan. [2]Division of Diabetes and Metabolism, Institute for Adult Diseases, Asahi Life Foundation, Tokyo, Japan. [3]Division of Diabetes, Clinical Research Center for Endocrinology and Metabolic Diseases, National Hospital Organization Kyoto Medical Center, Kyoto, Japan.

References
1. Kasiske BL, Snyder JJ, Gilbertson D. Diabetes mellitus after kidney transplantation in the United States. Am J Transplant. 2003;3:178–85.
2. Cosio FG, Kudva Y, van der Velde M, Larson TS, Textor SC, GriffinMD et al. New onset hyperglycemia and diabetes are associated with increased cardiovascular risk after kidney transplantation. Kidney Int. 2005; 67: 2415–2421.
3. Montori VM, Basu A, Erwin PJ, Velosa JA, Gabriel SE, Kudva YC. Posttransplantationdiabetes: a systematic review of the literature. Diabetes Care. 2002;25:583–92.
4. Davidson JA, Wilkinson A. New-onset diabetes after transplantation 2003 international consensus guidelines: an endocrinologist's view. Diabetes Care. 2004;27:805.
5. Lv C, Chen M, Xu M, Xu G, Zhang Y, He S, et al. Influencing factors of new-onset diabetes after a renal transplant and their effects on complications and survival rate. PLoS One. 2014;9(6):e99406.

6. Yoshinaga H, Kosaka K. Heterogeneous relationship of early insulin response and fasting insulin level with development of non-insulin-dependent diabetes mellitus in non-diabetic Japanese subjects with or without obesity. Diabetes Res Clin Pract. 1999;44:129–36.

7. Nguyen QM, Xu JH, Chen W, Srinivasan SR, Berenson GS. Correlates of age-onset of type 2 diabetes among relatively young black and white adults in a community: the Bogalusa Heart Study. Diabetes Care. 2012;35(6):1341–6.

8. Kodama S, Saito K, Yachi Y, Asumi M, Sugawara A, Totsuka K, et al. Association between serum uric acid and development of type 2 diabetes. Diabetes Care. 2009;32:1737–42.

9. Yoo TW, Sung KC, Shin HS, Kim BJ, Kim BS, Kang JH, et al. Relationship between serum uric acid concentration and insulin resistance and metabolic syndrome. Circ J. 2005;69:928–33.

10. Bayer ND, Cochetti PT, Anil Kumar MS, Teal V, Huan Y, Doria C, et al. Association of metabolic syndrome with development of new-onsetdiabetes after transplantation. Transplantation. 2010;90(8):861–6.

11. Bee YM, Tan HC, Tay TL, Kee TY, Goh SY, Kek PC. Incidence and risk factors for development of new-onset diabetes after kidney transplantation. Ann Acad Med Singapore. 2011; 40(4): 160–168.

12. Matsuo S, Imai E, Horio M, Yasuda Y, Tomita K, Nitta K, et al. Revised equations for estimated GFR from serum creatinine in Japan. Am J Kidney Dis. 2009;53:982–92.

13. Akizuki S. Serum uric acid levels among thirty-four thousand people in Japan. Ann Rheum Dis. 1982;41:272–4.

14. Chakkera HA, Weil EJ, Swanson CM, Dueck AC, Heilman RL, Reddy KS, et al. Pretransplant risk score for new-onset diabetes after kidney transplantation. Diabetes Care. 2011;34(10):2141–5.

15. Rieselbach RE, Steele TH. Intrinsic renal disease leading to abnormal urate excretion. Nephron. 1975;14(1):81–7.

16. Griffiths M. The mechanism of the diabetogenic action of uric acid. J BiolChem. 1950;184(1):289–98.

17. Facchini F, Chen YD, Hollenbeck CB, Reaven GM. Relationship between resistance to insulin-mediated glucose uptake, urinary uric acid clearance, and plasma uric acid concentration. JAMA. 1991;266:3008–11.

18. Kushiyama A, Okubo H, Sakoda H, Kikuchi T, Fujishiro M, Sato H, et al. Xanthine oxidoreductase is involved in macrophage foam cell formation and atherosclerosis development. ArteriosclerThrombVascBiol. 2012;32(2):291–8.

19. Bhole V, Choi JW, Kim SW, de Vera M, Choi H. Serum uric acid levels and the risk of type 2 diabetes: a prospective study. Am J Med. 2010;123(10):957–61.

20. Jia Z, Zhang X, Kang S, Wu Y. Serum uric acid levels and incidence of impaired fasting glucose and type 2 diabetes mellitus: a meta-analysis of cohort studies. Diabetes Res Clin Pract. 2013;101(1):88–96.

21. Lv Q, Meng X-F, He F-F, Chen S, Su H, Xiong J, et al. High serum uric acid and increased risk of type 2 diabetes: a systemic review and metaanalysis of prospective cohort studies. PLoS One. 2013;8(2):e5686.

22. Kushiyama A, Nakatsu Y, Matsunaga Y, Yamamotoya T, Mori K, Ueda K, et al. Role of uric acid metabolism-related inflammation in the pathogenesis of metabolic syndrome components such as atherosclerosis and nonalcoholic steatohepatitis. Mediat Inflamm. 2016;2016:8603164.

23. Klein BE, Klein R, Lee KE. Components of the metabolic syndrome and risk of cardiovascular disease and diabetes in Beaver Dam. Diabetes Care. 2002;25:1790–4.

24. Tsouli SG, Liberopoulos EN, MikhailidisDP AVG, Elisaf MS. Elevated serum uric acid levels in metabolic syndrome: an active component or an innocent bystander? Metabolism. 2006;55:1293–301.

25. Hara S, Tsuji H, Ohmoto Y, Amakawa K, Hsieh SD, Arase Y, et al. High serum uric acid level and low urine pH as predictors of metabolic syndrome: a retrospective cohort study in a Japanese urban population. Metabolism. 2012;61(2):281–8.

26. Fletcher B, Gulanick M, Lamendola C. Risk factors for type 2 diabetes mellitus. J Cardiovasc Nurs. 2002;16:17–23.

27. Hjelmesaeth J, Jenssen T, Hagen M, Egeland T, Hartmann A. Determinants of insulin secretion after renal transplantation. Metabolism. 2003;52:573–8.

28. Luan FL, Steffick DE, Ojo AO. New-onset diabetes mellitus in kidney transplant recipients discharged on steroid-free immunosuppression. Transplantation. 2011;91(3):334–41.

26

Effects of hydrophilic polymer-coated polysulfone membrane dialyzers on intradialytic hypotension in diabetic hemodialysis patients (ATHRITE BP Study): a pilot study

Kenji Tsuchida[1*], Hirofumi Hashimoto[2], Kazuhiko Kawahara[3], Ikuro Hayashi[4], Yoshio Fukata[5], Munenori Kashiwagi[6], Akihiro C. Yamashita[7], Michio Mineshima[8], Tadashi Tomo[9], Ikuto Masakane[10], Yoshiaki Takemoto[11], Hideki Kawanishi[12], Kojiro Nagai[13] and Jun Minakuchi[13]

Abstract

Background: Intradialytic hypotension (IDH) is a common clinical manifestation associated with poor prognosis in hemodialysis (HD) patients. HD patients who suffer from diabetic nephropathy (DN) are increasing and diabetes is a major cause of IDH. Effective interventional treatments for IDH have yet to be fully evaluated. The aim of this multicenter prospective study is to clarify the effect of biocompatible hydrophilic polymer-coated polysulfone (PS) membrane, TORAYLIGHT® NV (NV) dialyzers on IDH.

Methods: This is a prospective stratified-randomized multicenter trial. Forty DN patients undergoing HD and receiving two or more times of treatments for IDH per month were enrolled in this study. They were stratified by the number of treatments for IDH and divided to two groups using NV or conventional PS/polyethersulfone (PES) dialyzers. The number of treatments for IDH and changes in systolic blood pressure (SBP) were monitored for 6 months. Patients' demographic and clinical characteristics were also collected at enrollment and the last month of the observation period. In order to clarify the patient characteristics that induced preferable effects by using NV dialyzers, responders were defined as the patients whose average SBP falls in 1 month improved from over 30 mmHg to no more than 30 mmHg.

Results: The total number of treatments for IDH decreased significantly in NV group, even though pre-dialysis body weight and ultrafiltration volume were similar. In addition, patients using NV had significantly higher post-dialysis SBP and the lowest SBP during HD at sixth month compared as those in PS/PES group. NV responders had valuables suggesting malnutrition and microinflammation, and better lipid profiles than non-responders. However, the representative markers related to nutritional status, arteriosclerosis, and inflammation were not improved by NV treatment.

Conclusions: NV had preferable effects on IDH in DN HD patients. Our results suggest the usefulness of NV as a possible method to deal with IDH. Further studies are needed to clarify the mechanism of NV effects on hemodynamic status.

Keywords: Diabetic nephropathy, Hemodialysis, Intradialytic hypotension, Multicenter prospective study

* Correspondence: tuchiken52@yahoo.co.jp
[1]Tsuchida Dialysis Access Clinic, 2-10-18, Fujiidera DH building 4F, Oka, Fujiidera-shi, Osaka 583-0027, Japan
Full list of author information is available at the end of the article

Background

Intradialytic hypotension (IDH) is a common side effect in hemodialysis (HD) patients and occurs in approximately 30% of all HD sessions [1]. IDH is caused by failure in the compensation of reduced circulating blood volume, and is associated with increased mortality [2–4]. Several patient-related characteristics and comorbidities increase the risk of IDH, mainly through impairment of the counter-regulatory cardiovascular hemodynamic and neuro-hormonal mechanisms, such as age and diabetes [5]. HD patients are getting older, and diabetes nephropathy (DN) is the major primary disease of HD in Japan [6]. Therefore, IDH-prone patients are also increasing. Several studies of the interventional effects on IDH include comparison of the dialysate components such as sodium and acetic acid [7, 8], and difference of treatment methods [9]. However, few studies investigated the advantage of new dialyzer over conventional dialyzers to deal with IDH [10].

Recently, the state of water molecules in the vicinity of a membrane was reported to play an important role in the biocompatibility of synthetic polymer membranes [11]. A new polysulfone (PS) membrane dialyzer, TOR-AYLIGHT® NV (NV) (Toray Industries Inc., Tokyo, Japan), was developed by focusing on the state of water molecules on the membrane surface [12]. Yamaka et al. confirmed that platelet adhesion to the membrane surface of NV after HD was less than that of conventional PS dialyzers [13]. Ronco et al. showed that more patients in NV group reached heparin-free dialysis without clotting events during the heparin reduction test, suggesting anti-thrombogenic effects of the NV dialyzers as compared to conventional dialyzers [14]. Hidaka et al. reported that 3-month use of NV reduced the level of platelet-derived microparticles (PDMPs) in HD patients [15]. PDMPs are significantly increased in many prothrombotic diseases, including diabetes, cardiovascular disease and uremia [16, 17], which contribute to the development and progression of atherosclerosis [18]. In summary, improved biocompatibility provides some preferable effects on the maintenance of blood vessels, especially in patients with atherosclerosis.

Therefore, in this study, we investigated whether "biocompatible" hydrophilic polymer-coated PS dialyzers improve IDH in HD patients with DN compared as conventional PS/polyethersulfone (PES) dialyzers. In addition, to analyze the effects of "biocompatible" dialyzers on IDH, we also evaluated clinical and serological parameters of anemia, mineral-bone disorder, nutritional status, lipid profile, arteriosclerosis, and inflammation.

Methods

Study design and subjects

This study was designed as a prospective stratified-randomized multicenter trial. Six dialysis centers participated in this study. IDH was defined as systolic blood pressure (SBP) fall over 20 mmHg from baseline, or presentation of symptoms such as unconsciousness, nausea, chest discomfort, and muscle cramps associated with hypotension requiring any medical interventions [19]. We performed the following treatments for IDH: (1) saline administration, over 100 mL at one time; (2) decrease of ultrafiltration rate; (3) interruption of ultrafiltration; (4) extracorporeal ultrafiltration method; (5) dialysis discontinuation; (6) leg elevation; and (7) vasopressor administration [20].

Study flow diagram is shown in Fig. 1. The subjects enrolled in this study were DN patients aged between 20 and 80 years with more than 1-year HD vintage using PS, PES, or polyester-polymer alloy (PEPA) dialyzers, who received two or more times of treatments for IDH in 1 month. Exclusion criteria were as follows: (i) treatment by the other renal insufficiency therapies, such as continuous ambulatory peritoneal dialysis and hemodiafiltration; (ii) enrollment in the other clinical study; (iii) anamnestic cardiovascular diseases (heart attack, stroke) within less than 3 months; and (iv) pregnancy, infectious disease, cancer, or acute inflammation. First, in "patient-selection period," the number of IDH treatments for each enrolled patient was counted. Then, they were stratified by the number of IDH treatments and allocated to two groups, called NV and PS/PES group. Second, in "pre-observation period" (zero month), the patients' demographic and clinical characteristics were collected. The values of ejection fraction, comorbidities, and antiplatelet/anticoagulant medications in six cases were unavailable because of lack of recent echocardiography data and uncertainty of patient's statements. The number of IDH treatments was counted continuously. Third, in "comparative period" (first to sixth month), dialyzers in NV group were changed to NV and both groups were observed for 6 months. The dialyzers used are shown in Additional files 1 and 2.

There were no differences in dialysis conditions (blood flow rate, dialysate flow rate, dialysis time) including sodium concentration of dialysis fluid between NV and PS/PES groups during the whole study period (from zero to sixth month) (data not shown).

Primary outcome

Primary outcome was the average of the total number of IDH treatments performed in 1 month, expressed as "total number (times/month/patient)" in each group. Besides, pre-dialysis SBP, post-dialysis SBP, the lowest SBP during HD, SBP fall, pre-dialysis body weight, and ultrafiltration volume were measured in each dialysis session for 1 month and the average value was analyzed. In addition, in order to analyze the characteristics of responders to the dialyzer treatment, we sought the references to find out the cutoff value of average SBP fall

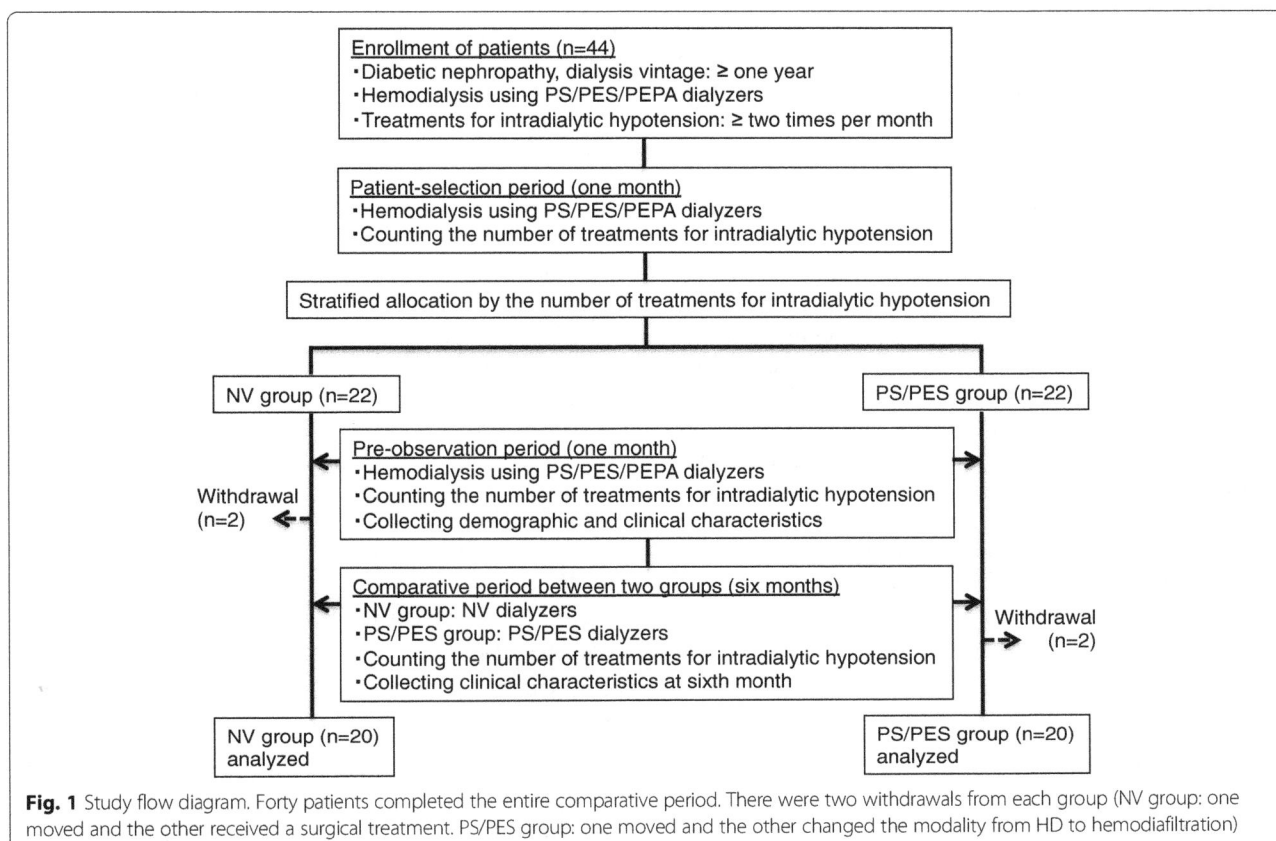

Fig. 1 Study flow diagram. Forty patients completed the entire comparative period. There were two withdrawals from each group (NV group: one moved and the other received a surgical treatment. PS/PES group: one moved and the other changed the modality from HD to hemodiafiltration)

in 1 month that was related to prognosis. However, there is no consensus, evidence-based medical definition for IDH which is related to prognosis [21]. Therefore, we referred to a previous paper investigating the relationship of IDH with mortality in Japanese HD patients reported by Shoji et al. [2]. Shoji et al. described that a greater fall in SBP was associated with increased mortality. This relationship was most clearly demonstrated when the cutoff point for the fall in SBP was set at 40 mmHg (greater fall: 40 mmHg or greater, smaller fall: less than 39 mmHg). The impact of the intradialytic fall in SBP on mortality was independent of the pre-dialysis SBP. However, Shoji et al. recorded SBP within a single HD session that was the first session of the week, which was different from average SBP fall in 1 month evaluated in our analysis. Shoji et al. also reported that the mean intradialytic falls in SBP in the patients who died and those who survived were about 28 and 32 mmHg, respectively. Therefore, the cutoff point for average SBP fall in 1 month at 30 mmHg is reasonable considering the results reported by Shoji et al. Moreover, Chou et al. reported that intradialytic SBP change of less than 15 mmHg and more than 50 mmHg had poor prognosis compared with intradialytic SBP change of 21 to 30 mmHg by analyzing a US-based cohort of 112,013

incident patients over a 5-year period [22]. Consequently, another outcome was defined as the improvement of average SBP fall in 1 month from over 30 mmHg at zero month to no more than 30 mmHg at sixth month. The parameters that strongly associate with IDH such as cardiothoracic ratio (CTR) and the number of antihypertensive drug users were also examined. Blood pressure was measured by oscillometric method.

Secondary outcome

The following items were evaluated in the beginning of pre--observation period (zero month) and sixth month to clarify the effects of dialyzers: "Nutritional status" (body mass index, albumin); "blood cell count" (white blood cell, platelet); "anemia management" (hemoglobin, the number of erythropoiesis-stimulating agent users, ferritin); "mineral-bone disorder control" (phosphate, calcium, intact-parathyroid hormone); "lipid" (total cholesterol, triglyceride, high-density lipoprotein cholesterol); "arteriosclerosis and inflammation" (ankle brachial index, homocysteine, pentosidine, high-sensitivity C-reactive protein (hsCRP), pentraxin 3 (PTX3)); and "catecholamine" (adrenaline, noradrenaline, dopamine). Serum homocysteine and pentosidine levels were measured by HPLC assay. hsCRP and PTX3 was measured by latex enhanced immunoturbidimetric assay and ELISA, respectively. The analyses of homocysteine, pentosidine, hsCRP, PTX3, and catecholamine were entrusted to LSI Medience Corporation (Tokyo, Japan). Ankle brachial index was measured by oscillometric method.

Statistical analysis

All values are expressed as mean ± SD. Statistical analysis was performed using SPSS for Windows version 13.0 (SPSS, Inc., Chicago, IL, USA). Variables such as SBP, the number of treatments for IDH between NV and PS/PES groups were compared using Student's t test or Welch's t test, if data were normally distributed. Non-normally distributed data were analyzed by Man-Whitney's U test. Prevalence data were analyzed by means of chi-square or Fisher's exact probability test. The changes of serological and clinical parameters in the time course of treatment were analyzed using paired t test or Wilcoxon signed-ranks test, as appropriate. Time-dependent changes of the parameters were compared using repeated-measures analysis of variance or Friedman's test, followed by a post hoc test. Significance was defined by P less than 0.05.

Results

Subject characteristics

Of the 44 enrolled patients in six dialysis centers, 40 patients ($n = 20$ each for NV and PS/PES groups) completed the entire comparative period. There were two withdrawals from each group (NV group: one moved and the other received a surgical treatment. PS/PES group: one moved and the other changed the modality from HD to hemodiafiltration.). There were no significant differences in the demographic and clinical characteristics of the patients between two groups, except the number of antihypertensive drug users and the value of ejection fraction. Patients in NV group had more difficulty to control blood pressure and better ejection fraction values than ones in PS/PES group (Table 1). There was one patient who took a vasopressor drug in NV group (data not shown).

Changes in the number of treatments for IDH

As shown in Fig. 2a, the total number of treatments was not statistically different between NV and PS/PES groups during the whole study period. However, in NV group, it decreased significantly at fifth and sixth month, compared with that in pre-observation period. In contrast, in PS/PES group, the total number of treatments did not decrease significantly.

The number of each treatment is shown in Fig. 2b–h. In NV group, the number of every treatment decreased at sixth month compared to that in pre-observation period. Especially, the number of dialysis discontinuation and leg elevation decreased significantly at fifth and

Table 1 Demographic and clinical characteristics of the patients enrolled

	NV group	PS/PES group	P
Patients (n)	20	20	
Age (years)	62.3 ± 9.1	61.5 ± 10.1	0.78
Female (%)	7 (35%)	6 (30%)	0.74
Dialysis vintage (years)	9.2 ± 4.8	6.7 ± 4.5	0.11
Antihypertensive drug users (%)	16 (80%)	9 (45%)	0.02
Antiplatelet/anticoagulant users (%)[a]	14 (82%)	17 (100%)	0.23
Ejection fraction (%)[a]	70.4 ± 5.2	60.7 ± 8.0	< 0.01
Comorbidities			
Ischemic heart disease (%)[a]	7 (41%)	12 (71%)	0.17
Heart failure (%)[a]	6 (35%)	5 (29%)	1.00
Cerebral infarction (%)[a]	3 (18%)	2 (12%)	1.00
Cerebral hemorrhage (%)[a]	0 (0%)	1 (6%)	1.00
BMI (kg/m^2)	24.0 ± 5.0	24.9 ± 4.3	0.57
White blood cell count (×10^3/μL)	6.3 ± 1.8	6.6 ± 2.7	0.53
Hemoglobin (g/dL)	11.2 ± 0.8	11.0 ± 2.6	0.66
Platelet (×10^4/μL)	20.0 ± 5.2	18.5 ± 4.9	0.35
ESA user (%)	13 (65%)	10 (50%)	0.34
Ferritin (ng/mL)	122.4 ± 141.4	94.2 ± 53.8	0.41
Phosphate (mg/dL)	5.6 ± 1.5	5.4 ± 1.6	0.72
Calcium (mg/dL)	9.1 ± 0.7	8.8 ± 0.6	0.20
Intact PTH (ng/mL)	122 ± 98	162 ± 163	0.34
Albumin (g/dL)	3.5 ± 0.3	3.5 ± 0.3	0.78
Total-cholesterol (mg/dL)	171 ± 36	154 ± 28	0.10
Triglyceride (mg/dL)	124 ± 70	142 ± 86	0.49
HDL-cholesterol (mg/dL)	44 ± 14	44 ± 15	0.96
Ankle brachial index (right)	1.03 ± 0.25	1.09 ± 0.28	0.51
Ankle brachial index (left)	1.11 ± 0.19	1.12 ± 0.26	0.91
Homocysteine (nmol/mL)	35.8 ± 25.1	34.7 ± 18.5	0.87
Pentosidine (μg/mL)	0.415 ± 0.218	0.326 ± 0.108	0.11
hsCRP (mg/dL)	0.221 ± 0.174	0.187 ± 0.196	0.57
Pentraxin 3 (ng/mL)	4.04 ± 1.68	4.55 ± 3.76	0.58
Adrenaline (ng/mL)	0.02 ± 0.01	0.02 ± 0.01	0.10
Noradrenaline(ng/mL)	0.33 ± 0.19	0.38 ± 0.19	0.46
Dopamine (ng/mL)	0.04 ± 0.02	0.05 ± 0.02	0.13

BMI body mass index, *ESA* erythropoiesis-stimulating agent, *HDL* high-density lipoprotein, *hsCRP* high-sensitivity C-reactive protein
[a]$n = 17$ in both NV and PS/PES groups

sixth month. Conversely, in PS/PES group, the numbers of some treatments such as decrease of ultrafiltration rate and dialysis discontinuation increased and the others such as saline administration and leg elevation decreased. In addition, one patient who took a vasopressor drug in NV group could stop the medication during the study period.

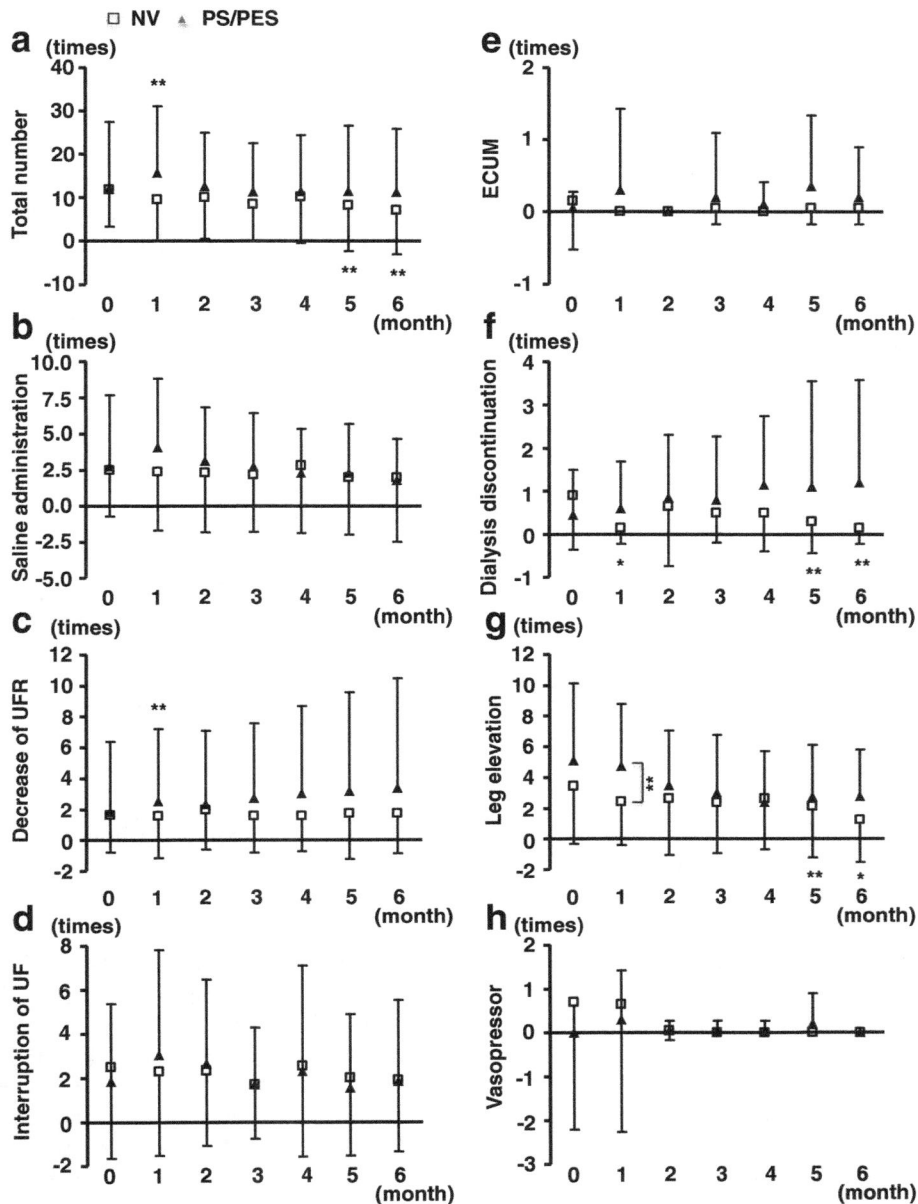

Fig. 2 The number of treatments for intradialytic hypotension in NV and PS/PES groups. **a** The total number of treatments was not significantly different between NV and PS/PES groups during the whole study period. However, in NV group, it decreased significantly compared with that in pre-observation period. In contrast, in PS/PES group, the total number of treatments did not decrease significantly. **b–h** In NV group, the number of every treatment decreased at sixth month compared as that in pre-observation period. Especially, the number of dialysis discontinuation and leg elevation decreased significantly at fifth and sixth month. Conversely, in PS/PES group, the number of some treatments such as decrease of ultrafiltration rate and dialysis discontinuation increased and the others such as saline administration and leg elevation decreased. UFR: ultrafiltration rate. UF: ultrafiltration. ECUM: extracorporeal ultrafiltration method. All values are expressed as mean ± SD. *$P < 0.01$. **$P < 0.05$

Changes in SBP

Pre-dialysis SBP, post-dialysis SBP, the lowest SBP and SBP fall were also monitored continuously (Fig. 3). In pre-observation period, there were no differences in pre-dialysis, post-dialysis, the lowest SBP and SBP fall between NV and PS/PES groups. However, in NV group, post-dialysis and the lowest SBP were significantly higher at sixth month compared as those in PS/PES group. As for SBP fall, the average value was significantly relieved in NV group at sixth month compared as that in pre-observation period, while SBP fall was not improved in PS/PES group. Besides, the number of patients whose average SBP fall over 30 mmHg in 1 month also decreased significantly in NV group at

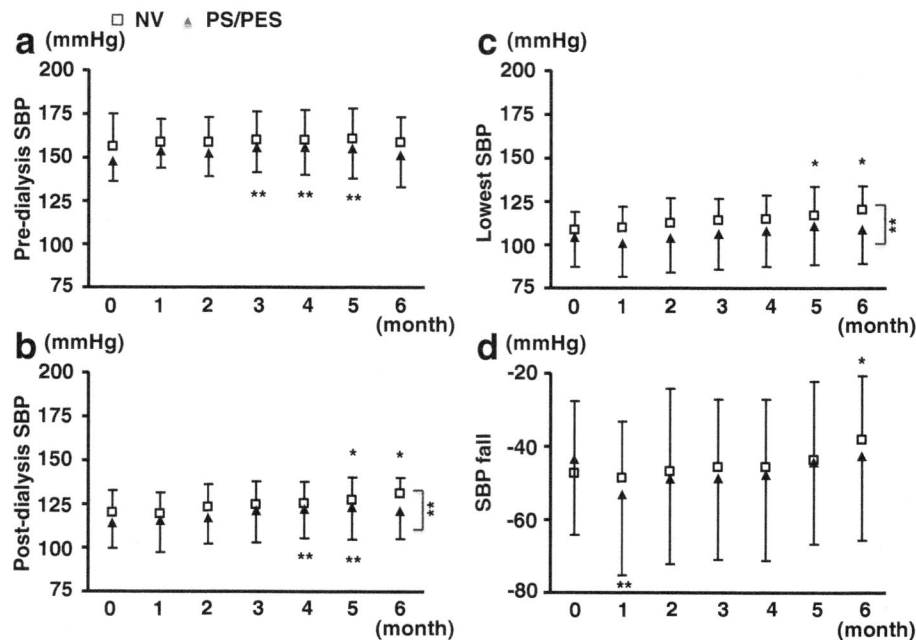

Fig. 3 Systolic blood pressure in NV and PS/PES groups. **a–c** In pre-observation period, there were no differences in pre-dialysis, post-dialysis, and lowest systolic blood pressure (SBP) between NV and PS/PES groups. However, in NV group, post-dialysis and the lowest SBP were significantly higher at sixth month compared to those in PS/PES group. **d** The average value of SBP fall during hemodialysis was significantly relieved in NV group at sixth month compared as that in pre-observation period, while SBP fall was not improved in PS/PES group. All values are expressed as mean ± SD. *$P < 0.01$. **$P < 0.05$

sixth month (from 18 to 12 patients), but showing no statistical difference from PS/PES group (Table 2).

Of note, there were no significant differences in pre--dialysis body weight, ultrafiltration volume, CTR between both groups and no changes in the number of patients who used antihypertensive drugs or antiplatelet/anticoagulant drugs in both groups during the whole study period (Table 3).

Patients' clinical characteristics at sixth month

Table 4 shows the data including the markers of nutritional states, mineral-bone disorder, anemia, lipid, arteriosclerosis, inflammation, and catecholamine at sixth month (the end of comparative period). There were no significant differences between two groups. These results indicated that nutritional status was similar between both groups and the therapy targets for anemia and mineral-bone disorder were commonly recognized in every dialysis center. NV group did not receive advantageous effects on arteriosclerosis and inflammation markers compared to PS/PES group at sixth month.

Differences between NV non-responders and responders

From the 18 patients in NV group with average SBP fall over 30 mmHg in 1 month in pre-observation period, we divided 12 patients as NV non-responders whose SBP falls remained over 30 mmHg at sixth month and 6

patients as NV responders whose SBP falls decreased no more than 30 mmHg at sixth month (Table 2). Between the two groups, we examined the statistical difference of various parameters at zero month. Then, NV responders had significantly longer dialysis vintages, lower body weights, lower potassium and higher HDL cholesterol levels than NV non-responders. NV responders also had lower body mass indexes, higher ferritin and hsCRP levels, but not reaching significant difference (Table 5).

Regarding PS group, we were not able to analyze the difference between non-responders and responders statistically, because PS responders included only one case.

Table 2 The number of patients with average systolic blood pressure fall over 30 mmHg in 1 month

		Pre-observation period (zero month)	Sixth month	
NV group	> 30 mmHg	18	> 30 mmHg	12[a]
			≤ 30 mmHg	6[b]
	≤ 30 mmHg	2	> 30 mmHg	0
			≤ 30 mmHg	2
PS/PES group	> 30 mmHg	14	> 30 mmHg	13
			≤ 30 mmHg	1
	≤ 30 mmHg	6	> 30 mmHg	1
			≤ 30 mmHg	5

[a]NV non-responders
[b]NV responders

Table 3 Changes in parameters related to IDH

	NV group	PS/PES group	P
Pre-dialysis body weight (kg)			
Pre-observation period (zero month)	66.7 ± 17.5	67.7 ± 12.4	0.84
First month	66.7 ± 17.4	67.9 ± 12.4	0.81
Second month	66.7 ± 17.5	67.8 ± 12.4	0.83
Third month	66.9 ± 17.6	68.1 ± 12.6	0.80
Fourth month	66.8 ± 17.6	68.0 ± 12.5	0.81
Fifth month	66.6 ± 17.6	67.8 ± 12.7	0.81
Sixth month	66.6 ± 17.5	68.1 ± 13.1	0.76
Ultrafiltration volume (ml/session)			
Pre-observation period (zero month)	3071 ± 1134	3163 ± 996	0.79
First month	3014 ± 1173	3066 ± 985	0.88
Second month	2939 ± 1168	2988 ± 964	0.89
Third month	2949 ± 1201	3129 ± 1015	0.61
Fourth month	2995 ± 1171	3015 ± 1005	0.95
Fifth month	3023 ± 1305	2956 ± 1020	0.86
Sixth month	3028 ± 1202	3134 ± 1018	0.77
Cardiothoracic ratio (%)			
Pre-observation period (zero month)	50.1 ± 4.9	50.7 ± 5.3	0.72
Sixth month	51.4 ± 4.5	52.1 ± 5.6	0.69
Antihypertensive drug users (%)			
Pre-observation period (zero month)	16 (80%)	9 (45%)	0.02
	ARB (8)	ARB (5)	
	Ca antag. (13)	Ca antag. (4)	
	β blocker (3)	β blocker (3)	
	α blocker (1)	α blocker (1)	
	αβ blocker (1)	αβ blocker (2)	
Sixth month	17 (85%)	10 (50%)	0.02
	ARB (7)	ARB (6)	
	Ca antag. (13)	Ca antag. (5)	
	β blocker (1)	β blocker (4)	
	α blocker (3)	α blocker (1)	
	αβ blocker (1)	αβ blocker (2)	
Antiplatelet/anticoagulant users (%)[a]			
Pre-observation period (zero month)	14 (82%)	17 (100%)	0.23
	Aspirin (12)	Aspirin (15)	
	Clopidogrel (1)	Clopidogrel (2)	
	Warfarin (0)	Warfarin (3)	
	EPA (0)	EPA (0)	
	O3FAE (0)	O3FAE (0)	
	Other (3)	Other (6)	
	Statin (1)	Statin (3)	
Sixth month	14 (82%)	17 (100%)	0.23
	Aspirin (12)	Aspirin (15)	
	Clopidogrel (3)	Clopidogrel (3)	
	Warfarin (1)	Warfarin (2)	
	EPA (0)	EPA (0)	
	O3FAE (0)	O3FAE (0)	
	Other (3)	Other (7)	
	Statin (1)	Statin (3)	

ARB angiotensin receptor blocker, Ca antag. calcium antagonist, EPA Epadel, O3FAE, Omega-3-fatty acid ethyl esters, Other Other antiplatelet/anticoagulant
[a]n = 17 in both NV and PS/PES groups

Table 4 Patients' clinical characteristics at sixth month

	NV group	PS/PES group	P
BMI (kg/m^2)	24.0 ± 5.0	24.8 ± 4.2	0.57
White blood cell count (×10^3/μL)	6.1 ± 2.0	6.7 ± 2.3	0.37
Hemoglobin (g/dL)	10.6 ± 2.5	10.8 ± 0.9	0.75
Platelet (×10^4/μL)	18.6 ± 5.0	18.2 ± 4.7	0.84
ESA user (%)	16 (80%)	15 (75%)	0.71
Ferritin (ng/mL)	104.6 ± 88.1	88.3 ± 55.6	0.50
Phosphate (mg/dL)	5.8 ± 1.1	5.2 ± 0.9	0.10
Calcium (mg/dL)	8.9 ± 0.7	8.9 ± 0.6	1.00
Intact PTH (ng/mL)	154 ± 121	161 ± 152	0.87
Albumin (g/dL)	3.5 ± 0.3	3.5 ± 0.2	0.96
Total-cholesterol (mg/dL)	169 ± 31	157 ± 29	0.20
Triglyceride (mg/dL)	119 ± 60	155 ± 115	0.22
HDL-cholesterol (mg/dL)	45 ± 12	45 ± 13	0.92
Ankle brachial index (right)	1.00 ± 0.28	1.11 ± 0.25	0.33
Ankle brachial index (left)	1.00 ± 0.28	1.08 ± 0.23	0.33
Homocysteine (nmol/mL)	34.5 ± 17.6	29.6 ± 12.0	0.31
Pentosidine (μg/mL)	0.399 ± 0.177	0.351 ± 0.184	0.40
hsCRP (mg/dL)	0.179 ± 0.191	0.212 ± 0.201	0.60
Pentraxin 3 (ng/mL)	4.47 ± 2.12	3.71 ± 2.51	0.31
Adrenaline (ng/mL)	0.02 ± 0.01	0.02 ± 0.01	0.81
Noradrenaline (ng/mL)	0.44 ± 0.24	0.41 ± 0.19	0.73
Dopamine (ng/mL)	0.04 ± 0.02	0.06 ± 0.04	0.15

BMI body mass index, ESA erythropoiesis-stimulating agent, HDL high-density lipoprotein, hsCRP high-sensitivity C-reactive protein

Discussion

In this study, we demonstrated that NV dialyzers increased post-dialysis and the lowest SBP compared as conventional PS/PES dialyzers, even though the total number of treatments for IDH decreased. The reduction of intervention for IDH correlated with the increase of SBP during HD. It gives validity to the results and supports the usefulness of NV as a possible method to deal with IDH.

Intradialytic blood pressure was controlled by complex mechanisms. Many factors including dry weight setting, ultrafiltration rate, nutritional status, anemia, and inflammation are involved in the maintenance of blood pressure during HD. Therefore, it is really difficult to estimate the effects of new equipment on the improvement of IDH. We intervened IDH by using hydrophilic polymer-coated PS membrane NV dialyzers. NV could reduce the number of treatments for IDH and improve intradialytic SBP (Figs. 2 and 3), even though representative influential factors on IDH such as pre-dialysis body weight, ultrafiltration rate were similar during the whole study period (Table 3). In addition, the number of patients with average SBP fall over 30 mmHg in 1 month

Table 5 Demographic and clinical characteristics of NV non-responders and responders

	NV non-responders	NV responders	P
Patients (n)	12	6	
Age (years)	60.8 ± 11.6	64.7 ± 1.8	0.43
Female (%)	3 (25%)	3 (50%)	0.31
Dialysis vintage (years)	7.0 ± 4.1	14.0 ± 3.5	< 0.01
Antihypertensive drug users (%)	10 (83%)	5 (83%)	1
	ARB (3)	ARB (3)	
	Ca antag. (8)	Ca antag. (3)	
	β blocker (1)	β blocker (2)	
	α blocker (0)	α blocker (1)	
	αβ blocker (1)	αβ blocker (0)	
Antiplatelet/anticoagulant users (%)[a]	7 (70%)	5 (100%)	0.49
	Aspirin (6)	Aspirin (4)	
	Clopidogrel (1)	Clopidogrel (0)	
	Warfarin (0)	Warfarin (0)	
	EPA (0)	EPA (0)	
	O3FAE (0)	O3FAE (0)	
	Other (1)	Other (2)	
	Statin (0)	Statin (1)	
Ejection fraction (%)[a]	70.2 ± 5.5	71.5 ± 5.4	0.69
Comorbidities			
Ischemic heart disease (%)[a]	2 (20%)	3 (60%)	0.33
Heart failure (%)[a]	3 (30%)	2 (40%)	0.85
Cerebral infarction (%)[a]	1 (10%)	2 (40%)	0.49
Cerebral hemorrhage (%)[a]	0 (0%)	0 (0%)	1
BMI (kg/m²)	25.8 ± 5.1	20.7 ± 4.1	0.05
White blood cell count (×10³/μL)	6.43 ± 1.73	6.47 ± 2.16	0.91
Hemoglobin (g/dL)	11.5 ± 0.9	11.0 ± 0.3	0.33
Platelet (×10⁴/μL)	20.5 ± 5.9	20.0 ± 4.3	0.93
ESA user (%)	67%	50%	0.86
Ferritin (ng/mL)	77 ± 68	205 ± 227	0.08
Sodium (mEq/L)	138 ± 2	139 ± 2	0.37
Potassium (mEq/L)	5.5 ± 0.8	4.5 ± 0.9	0.02
Phosphate (mg/dL)	6.1 ± 1.6	5.3 ± 1.0	0.24
Calcium (mg/dL)	9.0 ± 0.7	9.4 ± 0.8	0.29
Intact PTH (ng/mL)	148 ± 105	77 ± 80	0.17
Albumin (g/dL)	3.6 ± 0.3	3.5 ± 0.2	0.55
Total-cholesterol (mg/dL)	168 ± 38	175 ± 39	0.71
Triglyceride (mg/dL)	127 ± 73	95 ± 53	0.53
HDL-cholesterol (mg/dL)	38 ± 10	56 ± 13	

Table 5 Demographic and clinical characteristics of NV non-responders and responders *(Continued)*

	NV non-responders	NV responders	P
			< 0.01
Ankle brachial index (right)	1.06 ± 0.25	0.94 ± 0.27	0.40
Ankle brachial index (left)	1.12 ± 0.17	1.10 ± 0.26	0.85
Homocysteine (nmol/mL)	32.6 ± 16.0	46.4 ± 39.8	0.30
Pentosidine (μg/mL)	0.46 ± 0.23	0.39 ± 0.19	0.54
hsCRP (mg/dL)	0.17 ± 0.17	0.34 ± 0.17	0.06
Pentraxin 3 (ng/mL)	3.77 ± 1.40	5.00 ± 2.08	0.15
Adrenaline (ng/mL)	0.018 ± 0.009	0.022 ± 0.012	0.40
Noradrenaline (ng/mL)	0.34 ± 0.21	0.38 ± 0.11	0.69
Dopamine (ng/mL)	0.033 ± 0.018	0.043 ± 0.021	0.26
Pre-dialysis body weight (kg)	74.4 ± 17.1	54.0 ± 8.6	0.02
Post-dialysis body weight (kg)	71.1 ± 16.1	51.2 ± 8.8	0.01
Ultrafiltration volume (ml/session)	3604 ± 1234	2693 ± 607	0.11
Cardiothoracic ratio (%)	51.4 ± 5.1	48.3 ± 4.7	0.24

ARB angiotensin receptor blocker, *Ca antag.* calcium antagonist, *EPA* epadel, *O3FAE* omega-3-fatty acid ethyl esters, *Other* other antiplatelet/anticoagulant, *BMI* body mass index, *ESA* erythropoiesis-stimulating agent, *HDL* high-density lipoprotein, *hsCRP* high-sensitivity C-reactive protein
[a] $n = 10$ in NV non-responders and $n = 5$ in NV responders

decreased significantly at sixth month in NV group (Table 2). However, we could not find the significant difference of clinical characteristics that can be related to blood pressure control between NV and PS/PES groups (Table 4). Therefore, NV could show preferable effects to manage IDH compared to conventional PS/PES dialyzers, even though the mechanism of advantageous effects on IDH by NV has not been clarified yet.

The reason why NV showed several advantages over PS/PES dialyzers is still unknown. The values of ejection fraction were significantly higher in NV group than those in PS/PES group (Table 1), though it was not sufficient to explain NV advantage in avoiding hypotension because pulse rates in NV group were not increased after HD and not different from those in PS/PES groups at sixth month (data not shown). In addition, there was no difference of ejection fraction values between NV non-responders and responders (Table 5). In our study, the improvement of IDH by NV dialyzers appeared at later time points in comparative period. In addition to pre-dialysis body weight and ultrafiltration volume, nutritional status was similar during the whole study period. Therefore, we guess that NV played some indirect roles to improve peripheral vascular response to volume depletion during HD. Hidaka et al. showed that three-month HD using NV increased flow-mediated dilatation of the brachial artery, which suggested the improvement of endothelial dysfunction [15]. The continuous use of NV could improve the dysfunction of vascular endothelial cells and reduce the number of IDH. Recently, Kakuta et al. demonstrated that NV dialyzer induces less IL-6 than the conventional dialyzers, but pre-dialysis IL-6 values did not change during 1-year observation period [23]. Plasma IL-6 levels were reported to influence the severity of arterial wall stiffness in chronic kidney disease patients [24]. Therefore, the long-term use of NV might suppress the progression of arteriosclerosis, resulted in decrease in the number of IDH. NV responders had significantly longer dialysis vintages, lower body weights, lower potassium, and higher HDL cholesterol levels than non-responders. NV responders also had lower body mass indexes, higher ferritin and hsCRP levels, but not reaching significant difference. Thus, NV responders possessed valuables suggesting malnutrition and microinflammation, and better lipid profiles (Table 5). NV responders had similar characteristics including low ankle brachial index as the dialysis patients with peripheral artery disease do [25, 26], which can evoke better response to NV treatment.

Consequently, our hypothesis about the role of "biocompatibility" of NV is as follows. Dialysis membrane surface is made hydrophilic. The activations of platelets and white blood cells during HD are suppressed, followed by decreased production of microparticles derived from activated platelets [15] and inflammatory cytokines [23]. Thus, microinflammation and oxidative stress production during HD are relieved. Endothelial cell function is improved and the vasoconstriction response to hypotention is recovered during HD. However, relevant factors should be investigated to clarify the mechanism of NV effects on hemodynamic status.

In our study, we failed to find significant alterations of inflammation markers such as hsCRP and PTX3 in NV group and significant differences of them compared to PS/PES group. As Kakuta et al. did, we may have to focus on the alteration of these parameters during HD. We also should have monitored the vascular response such as flow-mediated dilatation of the brachial artery, orthostatic hypotension, or skin perfusion pressure, more sensitive marker to detect peripheral artery disease than ankle brachial index, to clarify the NV effects on IDH [27].

Kakuta et al. also reported that NV dialyzer would reduce the risk of erythropoiesis-stimulating agent hypo-responsiveness by inducing less IL-6 production during HD in patients with high IL-6 concentrations than the conventional dialyzers. NV group in our study did not have an improvement of anemia management (Tables 1 and 4). Our enrolled subjects did not have high values of hsCRP and PTX3. NV effects on the improvement of anemia control would be limited to the patients with inflammation-related erythropoiesis-stimulating agent hypo-responsiveness.

A weakness of this study is its relatively small sample size that could cause unknown source of bias in the findings. The other limitation is that dialyzers for control patients were not limited to PS only, to avoid too much interference to hypotension-prone patients.

Conclusions

In summary, this prospective stratified-randomized multicenter study compared the number of treatments for IDH in DN HD patients between NV and PS/PES dialysis users. Post-dialysis SBP and the lowest SBP during HD became significantly higher in NV group than those in PS/PES group. In addition, the total number of treatments for IDH was significantly decreased in NV group. Thus, NV prevented IDH in DN patients undergoing HD. NV responders possessed valuables suggesting malnutrition and microinflammation. Further studies are needed to clarify the NV effect on IDH.

Acknowledgements
The authors thank all the participants and our collaborators: Hiroyuki Michiwaki and Daisuke Hirose at Kawashima Dialysis Clinic and Kouji Mizuta, Hideki Hayashi, and Tadanobu Hosokawa at Yoshinogawa Medical Center. We also thank Michael Hann (Naval Medical Center San Diego) for English-language editing.

Funding
This study was funded in part by Toray Industries Inc.

Authors' contributions
KT designed and promoted the study. HH, KK, IH, YF, MK, and YT acquired data and informed consent. MM and ACY statistically analyzed the data. TT, IM, and HK gave critical revision of article. KN analyzed the results and wrote the manuscript. JM conceived and designed the study. All authors read and approved the final manuscript.

Competing interests
Kenji Tsuchida, Akihiro C Yamashita, Michio Mineshima, Tadashi Tomo, Ikuto Masakane, Yoshiaki Takemoto, Hideki Kawanishi, and Jun Minakuchi have received honoraria and travel expenses for speaking at events organized by Toray Industries Inc. Kenji Tsuchida, Akihiro C Yamashita, Michio Mineshima, Tadashi Tomo, Ikuto Masakane, and Jun Minakuchi have received research funds from Toray Industries Inc. for other research projects. The other authors declare that they have no competing interests.

Author details
[1]Tsuchida Dialysis Access Clinic, 2-10-18, Fujiidera DH building 4F, Oka, Fujiidera-shi, Osaka 583-0027, Japan. [2]Yoshinogawa Medical Center, Nishichiejima 120, Kamojimachochiejima, Yoshinogawa-shi, Tokushima 776-8511, Japan. [3]Kamojima Kawashima Clinic, Fukui 396-3, Kamojimacho-inoo, Yoshinogawa-shi, Tokushima 776-0033, Japan. [4]Naruto Kawashima Clinic, Nishi 68-5, Otsuchodanzeki, Naruto-shi, Tokushima 772-0043, Japan. [5]Wakimachi Kawashima Clinic, Tatejinja-shimominami 39-2, Ooaza-Inoshiri, Wakimachi, Mima-shi, Tokushima 779-3602, Japan. [6]Seijukai Clinic, 4-5-16, Honcho, Chuo-ku, Osaka 541-0053, Japan. [7]Department of Chemical Science and Technology, Faculty of Bioscience and Applied Chemistry, Hosei University, 3-7-2, Kajinocho, Koganei-shi, Tokyo 184-8584, Japan. [8]Department of Clinical Engineering, Tokyo Women's Medical University, 8-1, Kawadacho, Shinjuku-ku, Tokyo 162-8666, Japan. [9]Oita University Hospital Blood Purification Center, Idai-gaoka, 1-1, Hasama-machi, Yufu-shi, Oita 879-5593, Japan. [10]Yabuki Hospital, 4-5-5, Shimakita, Yamagata 990-0885, Japan. [11]Department of Urology, Osaka City University, 1-4-3, Asahimachi, Abeno-ku, Osaka 545-0051, Japan. [12]Tsuchiya General Hospital, 3-30, Nakajimacho, Naka-ku, Hiroshima 730-8655, Japan. [13]Kawashima Hospital, 1-39, Kitasakoichibancho, Tokushima-shi, Tokushima 770-0011, Japan.

References
1. Daugirdas JT. Pathophysiology of dialysis hypotension: an update. Am J Kidney Dis. 2001;38(4 Suppl 4):S11–7.
2. Shoji T, Tsubakihara Y, Fujii M, Imai E. Hemodialysis-associated hypotension as an independent risk factor for two-year mortality in hemodialysis patients. Kidney Int. 2004;66:1212–20.
3. Santoro A, Mancini E, Basile C, Amoroso L, Di Giulio S, Usberti M, et al. Blood volume controlled hemodialysis in hypotension-prone patients: a randomized, multicenter controlled trial. Kidney Int. 2002;62:1034–45.
4. Tislér A, Akócsi K, Borbás B, Fazakas L, Ferenczi S, Görögh S, et al. The effect of frequent or occasional dialysis-associated hypotension on survival of patients on maintenance haemodialysis. Nephrol Dial Transplant. 2003;18:2601–5.
5. Dasselaar JJ, Huisman RM, de Jong PE, Franssen CF. Measurement of relative blood volume changes during haemodialysis: merits and limitations. Nephrol Dial Transplant. 2005;20:2043–9.
6. Nakai S, Iseki K, Itami N, Ogata S, Kazama JJ, Kimata N, et al. An overview of regular dialysis treatment in Japan (as of 31 December 2010). Ther Apher Dial. 2012;16:483–521.
7. Zhou YL, Liu HL, Duan XF, Yao Y, Sun Y, Liu Q. Impact of sodium and ultrafiltration profiling on haemodialysis-related hypotension. Nephrol Dial Transplant. 2006;21:3231–7.
8. Spongano M, Santoro A, Ferrari G, Badiali F, Rossi M, Parrino A, et al. Continuous computerized monitoring of hemodynamic parameters during acetate dialysis, bicarbonate dialysis, and acetate-free biofiltration. Artif Organs. 1988;12:476–81.
9. Muñoz R, Gallardo I, Valladares E, Saracho R, Martínez I, Ocharan J, Montenegro J. Online hemodiafiltration: 4 years of clinical experience. Hemodial Int. 2006;10(Suppl 1):S28–32.
10. Koremoto M, Takahara N, Takahashi M, Okada Y, Satoh K, Kimura T, et al. Improvement of intradialytic hypotension in diabetic hemodialysis patients using vitamin E-bonded polysulfone membrane dialyzers. Artif Organs. 2012;36:901–10.
11. Tanaka M, Hayashi T, Morita S. The roles of water molecules at the biointerface of medical polymers. Polym J. 2013;45:701–10.
12. Oshihara W, Ueno Y, Fujieda H. A new polysulfone membrane dialyzer, NV, with low-fouling and antithrombotic properties. Contrib Nephrol. 2017;189:222–9.
13. Yamaka T, Ichikawa K, Saito M, Watanabe K, Nakai A, Higuchi N, et al. Biocompatibility of the new anticoagulant dialyzer TORAYLIGHT® NV. Sci Postprint. 2014;1:e00020.
14. Ronco C, Brendolan A, Nalesso F, Zanella M, De Cal M, Corradi V, et al. Prospective, randomized, multicenter, controlled trial (TRIATHRON 1) on a new antithrombogenic hydrophilic dialysis membrane. Int J Artif Organs. 2017;40:234–9.
15. Hidaka S, Kobayashi S, Maesato K, Mochida Y, Ishioka K, Oka M, et al. Hydrophilic polymer-coated polysulfone membrane improves endothelial function of hemodialysis patients: a pilot study. J Clin Nephrol Res. 2015;2:1020.
16. Daniel L, Fakhouri F, Joly D, Mouthon L, Nusbaum P, Grunfeld JP, et al. Increase of circulating neutrophil and platelet microparticles during acute vasculitis and hemodialysis. Kidney Int. 2006;69:1416–23.
17. Tan KT, Tayebjee MH, Lynd C, Blann AD, Lip GY. Platelet microparticles and soluble P selectin in peripheral artery disease: relationship to extent of disease and platelet activation markers. Ann Med. 2005;37:61–6.
18. Namba M, Tanaka A, Shimada K, Ozeki Y, Uehata S, Sakamoto T, et al. Circulating platelet-derived microparticles are associated with atherothrombotic events: a marker for vulnerable blood. Arterioscreler Thromb Vasc Biol. 2007;27:255–6.
19. Kooman J, Basci A, Pizzarelli F, Canaud B, Haage P, Fouque D, et al. EBPG guideline on haemodynamic instability. Nephrol Dial Transplant. 2007; 22(Suppl 2):ii22–44.
20. Koda Y, Aoike I, Hasegawa S, Osawa Y, Nakagawa Y, Iwabuchi F, et al. Feasibility of intermittent back-filtrate infusion hemodiafiltration to reduce intradialytic hypotension in patients with cardiovascular instability: a pilot study. Clin Exp Nephrol. 2017;21:324–32.
21. Assimon MM, Flythe JE. Definitions of intradialytic hypotension. Semin Dial. 2017;30:464–72.
22. Chou JA, Streja E, Nguyen DV, Rhee CM, Obi Y, Inrig JK, et al. Intradialytic hypotension, blood pressure changes and mortality risk in incident hemodialysis patients. Nephrol Dial Transplant. 2017. doi:10.1093/ndt/gfx037.
23. Kakuta T, Komaba H, Takagi N, Takahashi Y, Suzuki H, Hyodo T, et al. A prospective multicenter randomized controlled study on interleukin-6 removal and induction by a new hemodialyzer with improved biocompatibility in hemodialysis patients—a pilot study. Ther Apher Dial. 2016;20:569–78.
24. Krzanowski M, Janda K, Dumnicka P, Dubiel M, Stompór M, Kuśnierz-Cabala B, et al. Relationship between aortic pulse wave velocity, selected proinflammatory cytokines, and vascular calcification parameters in peritoneal dialysis patients. J Hypertens. 2014;32:142–8.
25. Takahara M, Iida O, Soga Y, Kodama A, Azuma N, SPINACH study investigators. Absence of preceding intermittent claudication and its associated clinical features in patients with critical limb ischemia. J Atheroscler Thromb. 2015;22:718–25.
26. Shiraki T, Iida O, Takahara M, Okamoto S, Kitano I, Tsuji Y, et al. Predictive scoring model of mortality after surgical or endovascular evascularization in patients with critical limb ischemia. J Vasc Surg. 2014;60:383–9.
27. Okamoto K, Oka M, Maesato K, Ikee R, Mano T, Moriya H, et al. Peripheral arterial occlusive disease is more prevalent in patients with hemodialysis: comparison with the findings of multidetector-row computed tomography. Am J Kidney Dis. 2006;48:269–76.

27

Effects of preoperative cinacalcet hydrochloride treatment on the operative course of parathyroidectomy and pathological changes in resected parathyroid glands

Akiko Takeshima[1], Hiroaki Ogata[1]*, Yoshiyuki Kadokura[2], Yoshihiro Yamada[2], Kei Asakura[1], Tadashi Kato[1], Yoshinori Saito[1], Kantaro Matsuzaka[1], Go Takahashi[1], Masanori Kato[1], Masahiro Yamamoto[1], Hidetoshi Ito[1] and Eriko Kinugasa[1]

Abstract

Background: Secondary hyperparathyroidism (SHPT) is associated with higher cardiovascular risk and mortality in patients undergoing dialysis. Cinacalcet hydrochloride (CH), which has been clinically available in Japan since 2008, could effectively reduce parathyroid hormone (PTH) levels even in patients with severe SHPT. However, parathyroidectomy (PTx) is performed in patients with severe SHPT refractory to CH. This study investigated the effects of preoperative CH treatment on the operative course and pathological findings of resected parathyroid glands (PTGs) in patients undergoing PTx.

Methods: We retrospectively analyzed 194 PTx cases for SHPT in long-term hemodialysis patients at Showa University Northern Yokohama Hospital from April 2002 to March 2014.

Results: A total of 45 patients were administered CH before PTx (CH group), and 149 patients never received CH (non-CH group). No significant difference was seen in intact PTH levels, the number of resected PTGs, or operative time between the two groups. However, the total volume of all PTGs and the volume of the largest PTG were significantly lower in the CH than in the non-CH group. Patients with PTG adhesion to surrounding tissues were significantly more prevalent in the CH than in the non-CH group. In addition, cystic changes or hemorrhagic necrosis in the resected PTGs was observed more frequently in the CH group than in the non-CH group.

Conclusions: The results of the present study suggest that preoperative CH treatment might introduce pathological changes in resected PTGs in PTx for severe SHPT, but it does not affect the operative time.

Keywords: Parathyroidectomy, Secondary hyperparathyroidism, Cinacalcet hydrochloride, Hemodialysis

* Correspondence: ogatah@med.showa-u.ac.jp
[1]Department of Internal Medicine, Showa University Northern Yokohama Hospital, 35-1 Chigasaki-chuo, Tsuzuki, Yokohama 2248503, Japan
Full list of author information is available at the end of the article

Background

Secondary hyperparathyroidism (SHPT) frequently develops in dialysis patients and is associated with various complications in end-stage kidney disease [1–4]. In fact, treatment of SHPT contributes to improved clinical outcomes, including fracture, vascular calcification, cardiovascular events, and mortality. The prevention and treatment of SHPT remain challenging for nephrologists. Phosphate (P) management with dietary P restriction and P binders, as well as vitamin D receptor activator (VDRA) administration, is useful in the prevention and management of SHPT [1–4]. However, severe SHPT refractory to medical management may develop, leading to the necessity of parathyroidectomy (PTx) for considerable numbers of dialysis patients [5–7].

In 2008, cinacalcet hydrochloride (CH), a calcimimetic compound, became clinically available in Japan. CH is effective in reducing serum parathyroid hormone (PTH) levels even in patients with SHPT refractory to VDRA. In fact, the incidence of PTx has dramatically decreased in Japan since 2008 [5]. However, because of its adverse gastrointestinal effects, the efficacy of CH in patients with more severe SHPT or in those who cannot be administered larger doses of CH is limited. CH has been reported to reduce the size of hypertrophic parathyroid glands (PTGs) in experimental and clinical studies [8–14]. Interestingly, CH may evoke cystic formation and hemorrhagic necrosis in hypertrophic PTGs. Thus, CH treatment might induce PTG adhesion to surrounding tissues, which might then affect the PTx procedure [14]. Accordingly, this study investigated whether preoperative CH treatment affects the pathological findings of resected PTGs and the PTx procedure in hemodialysis (HD) patients with refractory SHPT.

Methods

We performed a retrospective observational study to evaluate the effects of preoperative CH treatment on the pathological findings of resected hypertrophic PTGs and the intraoperative course in HD patients with refractory SHPT who had undergone PTx between April 2002 and March 2014. PTx was performed in cases refractory to medical treatment. In general, refractory SHPT is defined as intact PTH (iPTH) > 500 pg/mL or whole PTH > 300 pg/mL, respectively, regardless of VDRA and/or CH administration. It is also reasonable to consider surgical PTx at lower PTH levels if it is difficult to manage hyperphosphatemia or hypercalcemia with medical treatment [15]. In the clinical guidelines published by the Japanese Society for Dialysis Therapy (JSDT), the target ranges for serum P, corrected calcium (Ca), and iPTH concentrations are 3.5–6.0, 8.4–10.0, and 60–240 pg/mL, respectively [15]. Patients who had previously undergone PTx or percutaneous ethanol injection

therapy were excluded. The indications for PTx for SHPT were based on clinical and laboratory data according to the JSDT guidelines [15]. All operative procedures were performed by one surgeon (Y.K.) at Showa University Northern Yokohama Hospital.

The patients were divided into CH and non-CH groups. Patients who had been administered CH for at least 4 weeks within 6 months before PTx were placed in the CH group, while those who had never received CH before PTx were placed in the non-CH group. We compared preoperative data such as age, sex, HD vintage, primary disease, and preoperative therapy with CH, VDRA, and P binders. All blood samples for biochemical measurements were collected within 1 week before PTx. White blood cells (WBC), hemoglobin (Hb), platelets (Plt), total protein (TP), albumin (Alb), serum urea nitrogen (UN), creatinine (Cr), alkaline phosphatase (ALP), Ca, P, and iPTH were measured using standard methods. The measured serum Ca concentrations were adjusted to Alb levels using the following equation: corrected Ca = measured serum Ca concentration – serum Alb concentration + 4.0.

We then compared the number of resected PTGs, their estimated volume, their pathological findings (cyst formation [cystic lesions] and intraglandular hemorrhagic lesion [hemorrhagic necrosis]), and operative course (operation time, total intraoperative hemorrhage volume, and PTG adhesion to surrounding tissues). PTG adhesion to surrounding tissues was evaluated based on the operation record written by the surgeons. All PTGs were gauged intraoperatively immediately after resection. We calculated the estimated PTG volume using the following formula: estimated PTG volume = $\pi/6 \times a \times b \times c$ (where a, b, and c are the dimensions of the gland in centimeters). All specimens were fixed in 10% formalin and embedded in paraffin, and then, 4-μm-thick sections were stained with hematoxylin-eosin. Histopathological studies of the PTGs using light microscopy were performed in a blinded fashion by a single investigator (A.T.). Hyperplasia was classified as either diffuse or nodular. Diffuse hyperplasia was defined as an increased number of parenchymal cells with normal lobular structures, while nodular hyperplasia was defined as at least one well-circumscribed, encapsulated, and virtually fat-cell-free accumulation of parenchymal cells. Next, the presence of hemorrhagic necrosis and cystic lesions was evaluated. Hemorrhagic necrosis was defined as a hemorrhage filled with red blood cells and observed inside the parenchyma of the hypertrophic nodules. This study was approved by our institutional ethics committee (no. 1507-09) and was performed in accordance with the principles of the Declaration of Helsinki.

Continuous variables were expressed as means ± standard deviation and categorical variables as frequencies, unless noted otherwise. Statistical significances were determined by the χ^2 test for categorical data. Differences between groups were analyzed by Fisher's exact test and t test for categorical data and continuous variables, respectively.

Results

Study patients

A total of 194 patients were enrolled in the present study, 45 of whom had received CH for SHPT treatment (CH group) before PTx (Fig. 1). Table 1 shows the clinical characteristics of the study patients. The mean age of the enrolled patients was 55.3 ± 11.7 years, with women representing 44.3% of the population (86 patients). The average HD vintage was 13.0 ± 6.3 years. Although no significant differences were observed in age, sex, or underlying diseases between the CH and non-CH groups, the HD vintage in the CH group was significantly shorter than that in the non-CH group (11.1 ± 5.7 vs. 13.6 ± 6.4 years, respectively; $P = 0.020$). The preoperative laboratory data are shown in Table 1. The WBC count was significantly higher in the CH than in the non-CH group (5285 ± 1326 vs. 4805 ± 1253/μL, respectively; $P = 0.027$), and the serum-corrected Ca concentration was significantly lower in the CH than that in the non-CH group (9.7 ± 1.0 vs. 10.2 ± 0.8 mg/dL, respectively; $P < 0.001$). The Hb level, Plt count, and serum concentrations of TP, Alb, UN, Cr, ALP, P, and iPTH were comparable between the two groups. The medication for chronic kidney disease-mineral bone disorder (CKD-MBD) management included P binders and VDRA. Although calcium carbonate ($CaCO_3$) was administered to 55.6% of the patients in the CH and 45.0% of the patients in the non-CH group, respectively, the difference was not statistically significant. The mean $CaCO_3$ dosage was similar in both groups. Non-Ca-containing P binders were similarly administered

in the two groups. No significant differences were observed between groups in the VDRA administration patterns. The mean dosage of CH was 56.6 ± 25.5 mg/day in the CH group on admission.

Resected PTGs

Although 761 PTGs were obtained from the 194 patients, we histologically evaluated 743 glands. Fourteen glands could not be evaluated pathologically because they were too small for pathological examination. The number and estimated volume of all PTGs resected from each patient were determined immediately after PTx in the operating room. The numbers of resected PTGs did not significantly differ between the two groups (Table 2). The estimated volumes of all PTGs and the largest PTGs were significantly lower in the CH than in the non-CH group (1930.2 ± 1157.1 vs. 2526.9 ± 2524.7 mm^3, $P = 0.028$; and 1021.2 ± 737.7 vs. 1557.7 ± 2036.9 mm^3, $P = 0.010$, respectively) (Table 2). The ratio of nodular hyperplasia and diffuse hyperplasia in resected PTGs was similar in both groups ($P = 0.168$) (Table 3). Cystic lesions and hemorrhagic necrosis of the resected PTGs were observed significantly more frequently in the CH than in the non-CH group (cystic lesions 30.2 vs. 22.8%, $P = 0.046$; and hemorrhagic necrosis 23.8 vs. 13.1%, $P < 0.001$, respectively). Semiquantitative analysis revealed a significantly higher percentage of oxyphil cell area relative to total area in the CH than in the non-CH group (55.1% [95% confidence interval (CI) 51.3–59.8%] vs. 38.2% [95% CI 33.7–48.8%], respectively; $P = 0.011$).

Next, we evaluated the relationship between resected PTG volume and each histological change, including nodular hyperplasia, hemorrhagic necrosis, and cystic lesions (Fig. 2a–d). For each histological change, the PTG was significantly smaller in the CH than in the non-CH group (Fig. 2b–d). In the CH group, the PTG volumes were similar in nodular and diffuse hyperplasia (Fig. 2b). Regardless of CH treatment, PTG with hemorrhagic necrosis or cystic lesions was significantly larger than that without (Fig. 2c, d).

In addition, we assessed the effect of the iPTH level during the preoperative period on histological changes in the PTGs. No difference was observed in cystic lesions or hemorrhagic necrosis of the resected PTGs between patients with low PTH (minimum to median, 221–673 pg/mL in the non-CH group and 83–476 pg/mL in the CH group) and those with high PTH (median to maximum, 673–2616 and 476–2596 pg/mL, respectively), regardless of CH treatment (Fig. 3a, b). However, CH treatment was significantly associated with both cystic lesions and hemorrhagic necrosis in patients with low PTH levels. Interestingly, the prevalence of both pathologic changes was comparable in patients with high PTH levels, regardless of CH treatment. No significant difference was

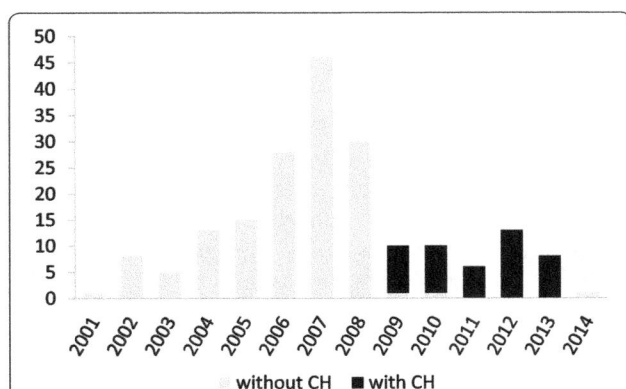

Fig. 1 Changes in the annual number of PTx procedures performed for SHPT in Showa University Northern Yokohama Hospital. Since the introduction of CH, the annual number of PTx procedures has decreased. CH has been clinically available since 2008 in Japan. After 2009, most patients were previously treated with CH before PTx. *PTx* parathyroidectomy, *SHPT* secondary hyperparathyroidism, *CH* cinacalcet hydrochloride

Table 1 Clinical, biochemical, and therapeutic characteristics of the study patients

	All ($n = 194$)	Non-CH group ($n = 149$)	CH group ($n = 45$)	P value
Age, years	55.3 ± 11.7	55.9 ± 11.7	53.3 ± 11.7	0.186
Female (%)	44.3	46.3	37.8	0.313
Dialysis vintage, years	13.0 ± 6.3	13.6 ± 6.4	11.1 ± 5.7	0.020
Underlying diseases (%)				
CGN	54.1	55.0	51.1	0.747
DMn	8.8	7.4	13.3	
Nephrosclerosis	6.7	6.7	6.7	
PCK	8.8	8.1	11.1	
Others	3.6	3.4	44.4	
Unknown	18.0	19.5	13.3	
WBC (/μL)	4916.6 ± 1283.2	4805.4 ± 1253.4	5284.9 ± 1325.9	0.027
Hb (g/dL)	10.6 ± 1.4	10.5 ± 1.4	10.8 ± 1.5	0.265
Plt (× 104/μL)	18. 2 ± 5.3	18.0 ± 5.1	18.8 ± 5.8	0.360
TP (g/dL)	6.3 ± 0.5	6.3 ± 0.5	6.3 ± 0.4	0.385
Alb (g/dL)	3.7 ± 0.3	3.7 ± 0.3	3.7 ± 0.3	0.183
SUN (mg/dL)	64.2 ± 16.5	64.9 ± 16.9	61.8 ± 14.9	0.286
Cr (mg/dL)	12.5 ± 3.0	12.5 ± 3.0	12.6 ± 2.9	0.841
ALP(U/L)	398.5 ± 284.3	386.1 ± 230.7	483.7 ± 413.5	0.419
corrected Ca (mg/dL)	10.1 ± 0.9	10.2 ± 0.8	9.7 ± 1.0	< 0.001
P (mg/dL)	6.3 ± 1.3	6.3 ± 1.3	6.0 ± 1.5	0.168
Intact PTH (pg/mL)	740.1 ± 408.1	764.6 ± 373.9	662.4 ± 498.5	0.210
CaCO$_3$ (%)	47.4	45.0	55.6	0.213
(Dose g/day)	2.7 ± 1.9	2.6 ± 1.9	3.1 ± 1.7	0.252
Non-Ca containing P binders (%)	79.4	83.9	86.7	0.139
Oral VDRA (%)	4.1	4.0	4.4	0.902
Intravenous VDRA (%)	59.8	57.7	66.7	0.283
CH (%)	23.2	0	100	–

Data are presented as percentage or mean ± standard deviation

CGN chronic glomerulonephritis, *DMn* diabeteic nephropathy, *PCK* polycystic kidney disease, *WBC* white blood cell, *Hb* hemoglobin, *Plt.* Platelets, *TP* total protein, *Alb* albumin, *SUN* serum urea nitrogen, *Cr* creatinine, *ALP* alkaline phosphatase, *Ca* calcium, *P* phosphate, *PTH* parathyroid hormone, *VDRA* vitamin D receptor activator, *CH* cinacalcet hydrochloride

observed in PTG adhesion to surrounding tissues between patients with low and high PTH levels, regardless of CH treatment (Fig. 3c). However, CH treatment significantly increased the prevalence of PTG adhesion to surrounding tissues, regardless of serum PTH level.

An analysis to assess the effect of CH dose immediately before PTx on pathologic changes in the resected PTGs revealed no differences in cystic lesions or hemorrhagic necrosis between patients administered ≤ 50 or > 50 mg/day CH ($P = 0.9988$ and $P = 0.3729$, respectively) (Fig. 4). In addition, no significant difference was found in the

Table 2 Macroscopic characteristics of resected PTGs

	All ($n = 194$)	Non-CH group ($n = 149$)	CH group ($n = 45$)	P value
Number of resected PTGs	3.9 ± 0.4	3.9 ± 0.4	3.9 ± 0.4	0.854
Total volume of resected PTGs (mm³)	2388.5 ± 2292.8	2526.9 ± 2524.7	1930.2 ± 1157.1	0.028
Volume of the largest PTG (mm³)	1431.7 ± 1917.5	1557.7 ± 2036.9	1021.2 ± 737.7	0.010
Cases with adhesions (%)	8.8	4.7	22.2	< 0.001

Data are presented as percentage or mean ± standard deviation

PTG parathyroid gland, *CH* cinacalcet hydrochloride

Table 3 Histopathological changes of resected PTGs

	All	Non-CH group	CH group	P value
Total number of PTGs	743	571	172	0.417
Nodular hyperplasia	567 (76.3)	429 (75.1)	138 (80.2)	0.168
Diffuse hyperplasia	176 (23.7)	142 (24.9)	34 (19.8)	
Cystic lesions	182 (24.5)	130 (22.8)	52 (30.2)	0.046
Hemorrhagic necrosis	116 (15.6)	75 (13.1)	41 (23.8)	< 0.001
Oxyphil cell area, %	49.1 (43.4–50.4)	38.2 (33.7–48.8)	55.1 (51.3–59.8)	0.011

Data are expressed as the number (%) or median (95% confidential interval)
PTG parathyroid gland, *CH* cinacalcet hydrochloride

prevalence of PTG adhesion to surrounding tissues between these CH dosages ($P = 0.4764$) (Fig. 4).

We also assessed factors contributing to PTG adhesion. Among the patient characteristics, only CH use was significantly associated with adhesion in the resected PTGs (Additional file 1: Table S1).

PTx procedure
Although the operative time did not significantly differ between the two groups (non-CH group, median 112 min [95% CI 108–117] vs. CH group 103 min [95% CI 95–112], $P = 0.062$), the volume of intraoperative bleeding was significantly lower in the CH than in the non-CH group (median 17.3 mL [95% CI 6.9–27.7] vs. 29.7 mL [95% CI 24.0–35.5], $P = 0.040$) (Fig. 5). Recurrent nerve palsy is the most common complication of PTx. No significant difference was observed in the prevalence of transient recurrent nerve palsy in the postoperative period between groups (nine vs. four patients in the non-CH and CH groups, respectively; $P = 0.072$).

Discussion
PTx has been demonstrated to significantly improve clinical outcomes, including fracture, cardiovascular disease, and all-cause mortality [16–19] in patients with severe SHPT. After CH became clinically available, the rate of PTx for SHPT was greatly reduced [5–7]. This study showed that the incidence of PTx for SHPT has dramatically decreased in our hospital (Fig. 1). CH effectively decreases serum PTH levels, even in patients with SHPT refractory to VDRA [8, 20]. However, a considerable number of patients with severe SHPT cannot be managed with medical treatment including CH and VDRA, and PTx is therefore necessary for such patients. In addition, PTx is superior to CH in terms of medical economics. CH not only decreases serum PTH levels but also suppresses PTG proliferation [9, 10]. CH treatment has been demonstrated to reduce the volume of hypertrophic PTGs in patients with SHPT [8, 11, 20]. The results of experimental studies suggest that calcimimetic compounds have the potential to provoke apoptosis in hypertrophic PTGs [21–23]. Thus, CH is likely

to induce pathological changes in hypertrophic PTGs, including cystic changes, hemorrhagic lesions, or adhesion to surrounding tissues. In this study, we assessed whether CH treatment before PTx affected the pathological findings of resected PTGs and PTx procedures in HD patients with severe SHPT. The results revealed that the number of resected PTGs was similar between the two groups, but both the total volume of resected PTGs and the volume of the largest gland were lower in patients with CH than in those without (Table 2). Microscopic examination revealed that hemorrhagic necrosis and cystic lesions were more prevalent in PTGs resected from patients with CH than from those without (Table 3). As previously reported [14], the oxyphil cell area of the PTGs was significantly larger in the CH than in the non-CH group. In nodular hyperplastic PTGs or PTGs with hemorrhagic necrosis or cystic lesions, PTG volume was significantly smaller in the CH than in the non-CH group (Fig. 2). These results suggest that a reduction in PTG volume was associated with CH-induced histopathological changes. In this study, we assessed the effect of the preoperative PTH level on histopathological changes in resected PTGs. PTH levels did not affect the prevalence of cystic lesions or hemorrhagic necrosis in resected PTGs, regardless of CH treatment (Fig. 3). The prevalence of adhesion was comparable between patients with low and high PTH levels. In addition, the daily dose of CH did not affect the prevalence of any histopathological changes in the resected PTGs (Fig. 4).

Although the mean operative time was comparable between the two groups, the total volume of intraoperative hemorrhage was significantly smaller in the CH than in the non-CH group (Fig. 5). However, cases with PTG adhesion to surrounding tissues were significantly more frequent in the CH than in the non-CH group. This result was unexpected because CH-induced pathologic changes in hypertrophic PTGs, including adhesion to surrounding tissues, can complicate PTG removal. The total volume of resected PTGs and the volume of the largest PTG were significantly greater in the non-CH than in the CH group. Therefore, a larger PTG size

A Representative photographs of hemorrhagic necrosis and cystic lesion

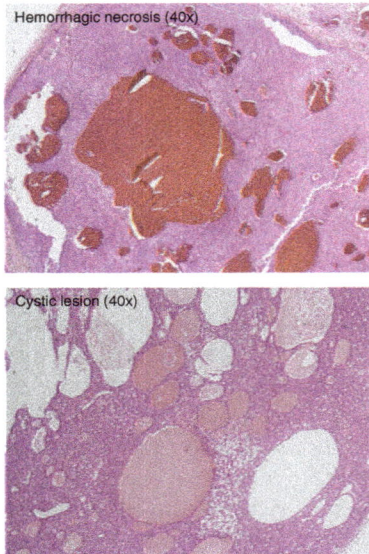

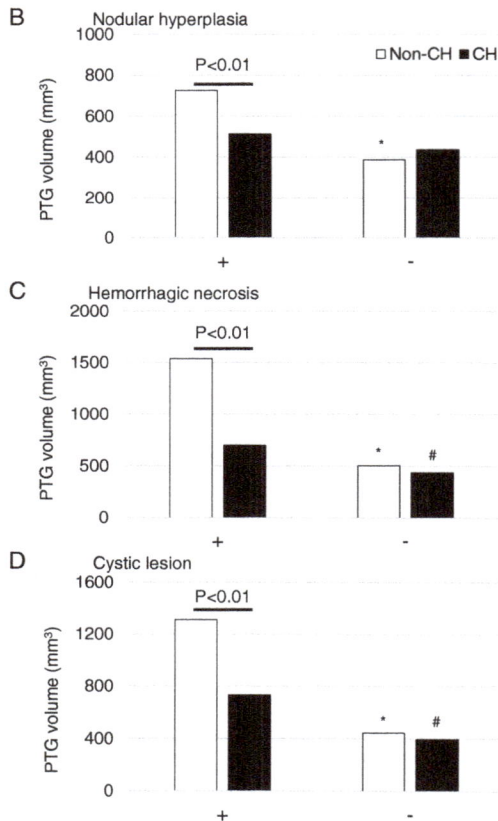

Hemorrhagic necrosis (40x)

Cystic lesion (40x)

B Nodular hyperplasia

C Hemorrhagic necrosis

D Cystic lesion

Fig. 2 Representative photographs of hemorrhagic necrosis and cystic lesions (**a**). The relationship between PTG volume and histological changes, including nodular hyperplasia (**b**), hemorrhagic necrosis (**c**), and cystic lesions (**d**), in samples resected from patients with or without CH treatment. *$P < 0.05$ vs. PTG with each histological change, nodular hyperplasia (**b**), hemorrhagic necrosis (**c**), or cystic lesion (**d**), not treated with CH. #$P < 0.05$ vs. PTG with each histological change, nodular hyperplasia (**b**), hemorrhagic necrosis (**c**), or cystic lesion (**d**), treated with CH. *PTG* parathyroid gland, *CH* cinacalcet hydrochloride

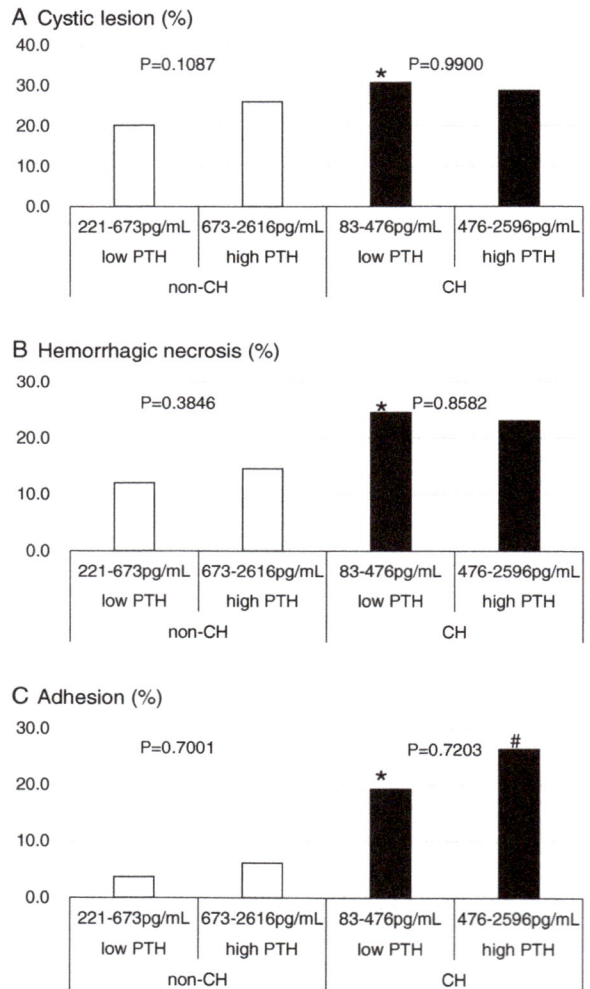

A Cystic lesion (%)

B Hemorrhagic necrosis (%)

C Adhesion (%)

Fig. 3 Preoperative intact PTH levels and the prevalence of histological changes, including cystic lesions (**a**), hemorrhagic necrosis (**b**), and adhesion (**c**), in samples resected from patients with or without CH treatment. Each PTH group was divided according to the median value of intact PTH. *$P < 0.05$ vs. low PTH group without CH treatment. #$P < 0.05$ vs. high PTH group without CH treatment. *PTH* parathyroid hormone, *CH* cinacalcet hydrochloride

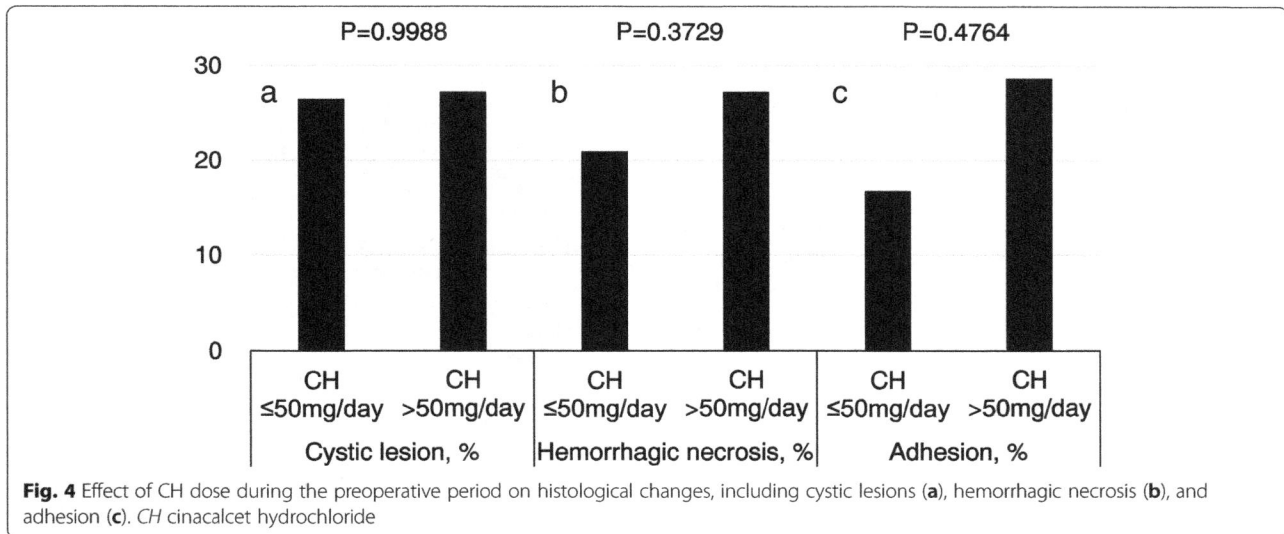

Fig. 4 Effect of CH dose during the preoperative period on histological changes, including cystic lesions (**a**), hemorrhagic necrosis (**b**), and adhesion (**c**). *CH* cinacalcet hydrochloride

might make resection more difficult. Consequently, the total volume of intraoperative bleeding was significantly greater in the non-CH than in the CH group, regardless of PTG adhesion to surrounding tissues. All PTx procedures were performed by a single surgeon (Y.K.) who would have become more skillful over time. Most PTx procedures in the non-CH group were performed between 2002 and 2008 (Fig. 1); however, all PTx procedures in the CH group were performed after 2009. This result might be attributed to differences in the timing of PTx between the two groups. The results reported by relatively small studies lack consistency. Sumida et al. reported that total PTG weight was comparable between patients with and without CH treatment before PTx, but the maximal PTG weight was significantly greater in patients with CH than in those without [14]. However, another study showed that PTG weights were similar between patients with and without CH treatment [24].

Factors other than preoperative CH treatment, including disease duration of SHPT, P and Ca management, and VDRA treatment, might affect PTG size. Vulpio et al. reported that intraglandular hemorrhagic lesions were more prevalent in patients with CH than in those without [24]. Sumida et al. reported that the hemorrhagic score of resected PTGs was comparable, but the hemosiderosis score was significantly higher in patients with CH than in those without [14]. CH treatment is likely to cause hemorrhagic changes in the hypertrophic PTGs of SHPT. Doppler ultrasonographic studies have shown that CH treatment induces reduced intraglandular vasculature and blood flow [12, 13].

This study did have some limitations. First, this was a retrospective observational study; therefore, no causal explanations are provided for the observed results. Second, unselected variables might have affected the results. Serum fibroblast growth factor-23 level, adherence to

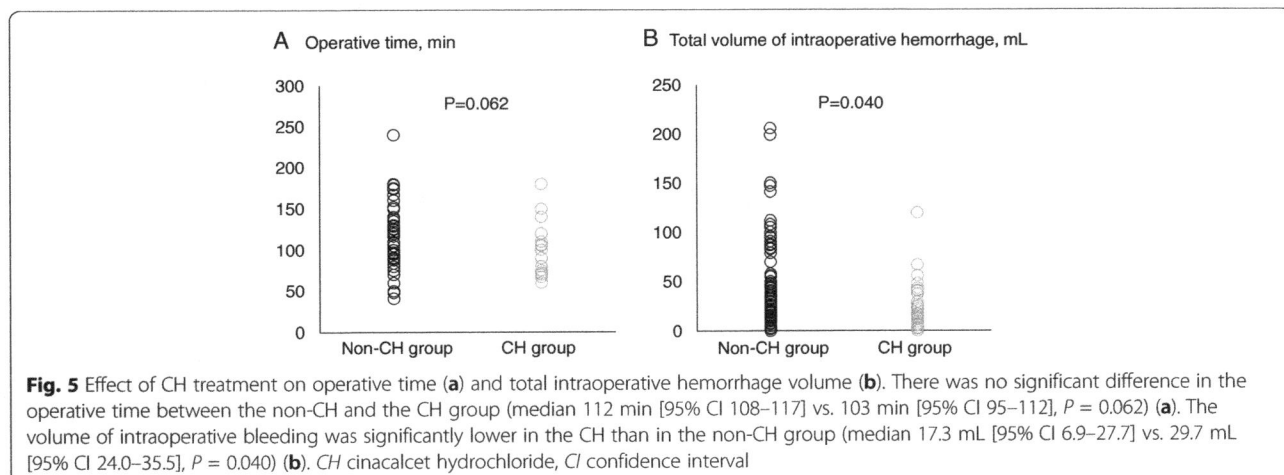

Fig. 5 Effect of CH treatment on operative time (**a**) and total intraoperative hemorrhage volume (**b**). There was no significant difference in the operative time between the non-CH and the CH group (median 112 min [95% CI 108–117] vs. 103 min [95% CI 95–112], *P* = 0.062) (**a**). The volume of intraoperative bleeding was significantly lower in the CH than in the non-CH group (median 17.3 mL [95% CI 6.9–27.7] vs. 29.7 mL [95% CI 24.0–35.5], *P* = 0.040) (**b**). *CH* cinacalcet hydrochloride, *CI* confidence interval

CH, differences in VDRA formulations (calcitriol or its analogs), and individual anatomical structures of the neck might be associated with the clinical cause of SHPT, responsiveness to medical treatment, and the PTx procedure. Third, as mentioned above, there were evident differences in the timing of PTx procedures between patients with and without CH. These differences might have affected the results, including operative time and operative hemorrhage volume. Fourth, we did not have detailed data on the CH administration period before PTx because the CH-treated patients in this study were defined as patients who had been administered CH for at least 4 weeks within 6 months before PTx. The administration period of CH might affect the histological changes in hypertrophic PTGs in patients with SHPT.

Recently, a new calcimimetic compound, etelcalcetide, has become clinically available in the USA and Japan. Etelcalcetide is expected to be administrated in patients who cannot be administered CH because of gastrointestinal symptoms. Therefore, greater numbers of patients with SHPT are expected to be treated with calcimimetic compounds. It will be of interest to investigate whether etelcalcetide provokes any histological changes in hypertrophic PTGs in patients with SHPT.

Conclusions

The results of this study suggest that both the total volume of resected PTGs and the volume of the largest PTG were significantly smaller in patients with than in patients without CH treatment before PTx. Pathological examinations revealed that CH treatment was significantly associated with hemorrhagic necrosis and cystic lesions of the resected PTGs. Although operative time was comparable between patients with and without CH treatment, the volume of intraoperative hemorrhage was significantly smaller in the CH than in the non-CH group.

Abbreviations

Alb: Albumin; ALP: Alkaline phosphatase; Ca: Calcium; CaCO₃: Calcium carbonate; CH: Cinacalcet hydrochloride; CI: Confidence interval; Cr: Creatinine; Hb: Hemoglobin; HD: Hemodialysis; JSDT: Japanese Society for Dialysis Therapy; P: Phosphate; Plt: Platelets; PTG: Parathyroid gland; PTH: Parathyroid hormone; PTx: Parathyroidectomy; SHPT: Secondary hyperparathyroidism; TP: Total protein; UN: Urea nitrogen; VDRA: Vitamin D receptor activator; WBC: White blood cells

Acknowledgements
The authors thank the medical staff at Showa University Northern Yokohama Hospital for supporting this study.

Funding
The authors have no specific sources to disclose.

Authors' contributions
AT, HO, KA, TK, YS, KM, GT, and EK contributed to the conception and design of the research. YK performed PTx as the surgeon. YY assisted in the PTx procedure and processed the resected PTG samples for pathological examination. AT, MK, MY, HI, and HO analyzed the data. AT performed the pathological examinations. HO and AT interpreted the results of the study. HO and AT prepared the figure and drafted the manuscript. All authors read and approved the final manuscript.

Competing interests
The authors declare that they have no competing interests.

Author details
¹Department of Internal Medicine, Showa University Northern Yokohama Hospital, 35-1 Chigasaki-chuo, Tsuzuki, Yokohama 2248503, Japan. ²Department of Otorhinolaryngology, Showa University Northern Yokohama Hospital, 35-1 Chigasaki-chuo, Tsuzuki, Yokohama 2248503, Japan.

References
1. Akizawa T, Kamimura M, Mizobuchi M, et al. Management of secondary hyperparathyroidism of dialysis patients. Nephrology (Carlton). 2003;8(Suppl):S53–7.
2. Fukagawa M, Komaba H, Kakuta T. Hyperparathyroidism in chronic kidney disease patients: an update on current pharmacotherapy. Expert Opin Pharmacother. 2013;14(7):863–71.
3. Ogata H, Koiwa F, Kinugasa E, et al. CKD-MBD: impact on management of kidney disease. Clin Exp Nephrol. 2007;11(4):261–8.
4. Mizobuchi M, Ogata H, Koiwa F, et al. Research on kidney and mineral metabolism in Japan: past, present, and future. Clin Exp Nephrol. 2017;21(Suppl 1):4–8.
5. Tominaga Y, Kakuta T, Yasunaga C, et al. Evaluation of parathyroidectomy for secondary and tertiary hyperparathyroidism by the Parathyroid Surgeons' Society of Japan. Ther Apher Dial. 2016;20(1):6–11.
6. Li S, Chen YW, Peng Y, et al. Trends in parathyroidectomy rates in US hemodialysis patients from 1992 to 2007. Am J Kidney Dis. 2011;57(4):602–11.
7. Lafrance JP, Cardinal H, Leblanc M, et al. Effect of cinacalcet availability and formulary listing on parathyroidectomy rate trends. BMC Nephrol. 2013;14:100.
8. Komaba H, Nakanishi S, Fujimori A, et al. Cinacalcet effectively reduces parathyroid hormone secretion and gland volume regardless of pretreatment gland size in patients with secondary hyperparathyroidism. Clin J Am Soc Nephrol. 2010;5(12):2305–14.
9. Colloton M, Shatzen E, Miller G, et al. Cinacalcet HCl attenuates parathyroid hyperplasia in a rat model of secondary hyperparathyroidism. Kidney Int. 2005;67(2):467–76.
10. Imanishi Y, Kawata T, Kenko T, et al. Cinacalcet HCl suppresses Cyclin D1 oncogene-derived parathyroid cell proliferation in a murine model for primary hyperparathyroidism. Calcif Tissue Int. 2011;89(1):29–35.
11. Ichii M, Ishimura E, Okuno S, et al. Decreases in parathyroid gland volume after cinacalcet treatment in hemodialysis patients with secondary hyperparathyroidism. Nephron Clin Pract. 2010;115(3):c195–202.
12. Meola M, Petrucci I, Barsotti G. Long-term treatment with cinacalcet and conventional therapy reduces parathyroid hyperplasia in severe secondary hyperparathyroidism. Nephrol Dial Transplant. 2009;24(3):982–9.
13. Meola M, Petrucci I, Colombini E, et al. Use of ultrasound to assess the response to therapy for secondary hyperparathyroidism. Am J Kidney Dis. 2011;58(3):485–91.
14. Sumida K, Nakamura M, Ubara Y, et al. Histopathological alterations of the parathyroid glands in haemodialysis patients with secondary hyperparathyroidism refractory to cinacalcet hydrochloride. J Clin Pathol. 2011;64(9):756–60.
15. Fukagawa M, Yokoyama K, Koiwa F, et al. Clinical practice guideline for the management of chronic kidney disease-mineral and bone disorder. Ther Apher Dial. 2013;17(3):247–88.
16. Komaba H, Taniguchi M, Wada A, et al. Parathyroidectomy and survival among Japanese hemodialysis patients with secondary hyperparathyroidism. Kidney Int. 2015;88(2):350–9.

17. Li W, Zhang M, Du S, et al. Impact of parathyroidectomy on survival among haemodialysis patients: a prospective cohort study. Nephrology (Carlton). 2016;21(2):133–8.
18. Ivarsson KM, Akaberi S, Isaksson E, et al. The effect of parathyroidectomy on patient survival in secondary hyperparathyroidism. Nephrol Dial Transplant. 2015;30(12):2027–33.
19. Iwamoto N, Sato N, Nishida M, et al. Low parathyroid hormone levels after parathyroidectomy reduce cardiovascular mortality in chronic hemodialysis patients. Clin Exp Nephrol. 2016;20(5):808–14.
20. Yamamoto M, Ogata H, Mizobuchi M, et al. Number of enlarged parathyroid glands might be a predictor of cinacalcet response in advanced secondary hyperparathyroidism. Clin Exp Nephrol. 2012;16(2):292–9.
21. Mizobuchi M, Ogata H, Hatamura I, et al. Activation of calcium-sensing receptor accelerates apoptosis in hyperplastic parathyroid cells. Biochem Biophys Res Commun. 2007;362(1):11–6.
22. Mizobuchi M, Hatamura I, Ogata H, et al. Calcimimetic compound upregulates decreased calcium-sensing receptor expression level in parathyroid glands of rats with chronic renal insufficiency. J Am Soc Nephrol. 2004;15(10):2579–87.
23. Tatsumi R, Komaba H, Kanai G, et al. Cinacalcet induces apoptosis in parathyroid cells in patients with secondary hyperparathyroidism: histological and cytological analyses. Nephron Clin Pract. 2013;124(3–4):224–31.
24. Vulpio C, Bossola M, Di Stasio E, et al. Histology and immunohistochemistry of the parathyroid glands in renal secondary hyperparathyroidism refractory to vitamin D or cinacalcet therapy. Eur J Endocrinol. 2013;168(6):811–9.

28

Patency with antiplatelet treatment after vascular access intervention therapy: a retrospective observational study

Tomohito Mizuno[1], Motonobu Nakamura[1*], Nobuhiko Satoh[1], Hiroyuki Tsukada[1], Akihiko Matsumoto[2,3], Yoshifumi Hamasaki[1,3], Haruki Kume[2] and Masaomi Nangaku[1,3]

Abstract

Background: Vascular access (VA) intervention therapy (VAIVT) has been increasingly used for treating VA failure (VAF) in patients undergoing hemodialysis; however, clinical evidence demonstrating the efficacy of prevention of VAF after VAIVT is limited. Therefore, we aimed to assess characteristics of patients developing VAF after VAIVT and analyze risk factors for VAF after VAIVT.

Methods: This retrospective study included 96 patients with VAF who underwent ultrasound-guided VAIVT by interventional nephrologists between January 2013 and March 2018 at the Department of Nephrology, University of Tokyo Hospital, Japan. Patient information included age, sex, medication history, and comorbidities that could potentially affect VAF onset. Patients were categorized into two groups based on antiplatelet treatment. Multivariate Cox regression analysis was performed for evaluating effect of various factors on VAF after VAIVT.

Results: Median age of patients at the time of VAIVT was 71 years (interquartile range 63–79); the most prevalent etiology underlying end-stage renal disease was diabetic nephropathy (40.7%). Comparison between the antiplatelet and non-antiplatelet groups revealed that the incidence of VAF was significantly lower in the antiplatelet group. Multivariate analysis revealed that antiplatelet treatment was associated with a lower risk of VAF after VAIVT.

Conclusion: Administration of antiplatelet agents was associated with a significant reduction in VAF risk after VAIVT.

Keywords: Vascular access failure, Vascular access intervention therapy, Hemodialysis, Antiplatelet

Background

Vascular access (VA) is a lifeline for patients undergoing hemodialysis (HD). According to the Japanese Society for Dialysis Therapy (JSDT) guidelines, complications, such as stenosis and thrombosis, cannot be avoided because of prolonged VA use [1]. Moreover, VA failure (VAF) due to stenosis or thrombosis of the VA site hinders dialysis continuation, with a serious impact on patients undergoing HD and increase in medical expenses that are incurred during restoring VA. Therefore, VA stability is critical for maintaining the quality of life of patients undergoing HD and for reducing their medical expenses. For instance, the annual expenditure associated with VA is more than one billion US dollars in the USA [2, 3]. Therefore, several studies investigating approaches for preventing VAF that often occurs after VA construction reported that treatment with antiplatelet agents reduced the risk of stenosis and improved the duration of primary unassisted patency of newly created VA [4, 5].

Recently, vascular access intervention therapy (VAIVT) has become one of the established therapy options for resolving VAF [1, 6–11]. Although VAIVT is less invasive than surgical reconstruction [7, 12–14], information on prevention of VAF after VAIVT is limited.

To clarify these issues, we conducted a retrospective analysis of 96 patients with VAF at a single institute, with the definition of VAF based on the JSDT guidelines

* Correspondence: nakamura-stm@umin.ac.jp
[1]Division of Nephrology and Endocrinology, The University of Tokyo Hospital, 7-3-1 Hongo, Bunkyo-ku, Tokyo 113-8655, Japan
Full list of author information is available at the end of the article

[1]. Our findings indicated that antiplatelet treatment might prevent VAF due to frequent restenosis after VAIVT.

Methods

Study design

This retrospective study included data from 96 patients with VAF who underwent ultrasound-guided VAIVT by intervention nephrologists at the University of Tokyo Hospital between January 2013 and March 2018. These enrolled patients were hospitalized. All procedures during this study were performed by the same team.

Indications for VAIVT were defined according to the JSDT guidelines [1] and included a stenosis rate of $\geq 50\%$ in addition to ≥ 1 of the following clinical medical abnormalities: (i) decreased blood flow, (ii) increased venous pressure, (iii) an abnormally high blood urea nitrogen level, and (iv) unexplained reduction in dialysis efficiency [1].

Among the 96 adults who underwent ultrasound-guided VAIVT included in this study, six with primary failure of intervention and 31 with VA construction within 180 days before intervention were excluded. Therefore, 59 patients with a primary VAF episode were eligible for the final analysis (Fig. 1).

The primary outcome was 1-year VA patency after VAIVT; the secondary outcome was frequency of any complication after VAIVT.

Definitions

Primary success was defined according to the reporting standards of the American Society of Interventional Radiology [15]. Clinical success was defined as recovery of palpable continuous thrill perception, loss of initial clinical abnormalities associated with VAF, or at least one successfully performed dialysis session. According to the JSDT guidelines, VAF was defined as HD discontinuation because of stenosis or acute thrombus occlusion [1].

Patients who continuously received any of the antiplatelet agents, such as aspirin, clopidogrel, and cilostazol, before VAIVT were categorized in the antiplatelet group, whereas those who did not receive any antiplatelet agent were categorized in the non-antiplatelet group. The antiplatelet group was further divided into two groups according to the type of antiplatelet agent as monotherapy (aspirin or clopidogrel) and dual antiplatelet therapy (DAPT).

Older age has been reported as an independent risk factor for VAF after VA construction. Therefore, to examine the influence of age on vascular access outcome, we defined individuals age older than the median age in this study group as "the older age" [16, 17].

Ultrasound-guided VAIVT

VA was accessed with a single-entry needle under ultrasound guidance using a diagnostic Noblus ultrasound scanner (Hitachi Healthcare, Tokyo, Japan). All procedures were completed via a 4- or 5-Fr sheath introducer, with a 0.018–0.035-in. curved or straight-tip guidewire (Radifocus guidewire M, GT wire angle, or straight type; Terumo, Tokyo, Japan) and a balloon with a diameter ranging from 4 to 6 mm and a length of 40 mm (SABER®, Cardinal Health Japan, Japan, Mustang™ and Sterling™ Boston Scientific, USA). Brachial artery blood flow volume was measured by using ultrasound scanner before and after VAIVT.

Statistical analysis

All data were presented as means ± standard deviation or median (interquartile range). Categorical variables,

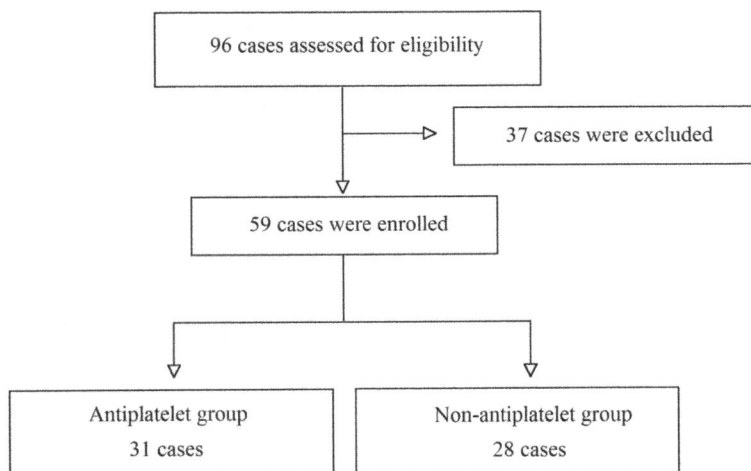

Fig. 1 The flowchart of the enrolled patients. Antiplatelet agents included aspirin, clopidogrel, and cilostazol

Table 1 Baseline clinical characteristics

Characteristic	
Number	59
Age	71 (63–79)
Older age (%)	49.2
Sex (male, %)	76.3
Etiology of ESRD (%)	
DN	40.7
NS	23.7
CGN	15.3
ADPKD	1.7
IgAN	5.1
Other or unknown	13.6
Smoking history (%)	64.4
DM (%)	57.6
Dyslipidemia (%)	57.6
Major CVD (%)	54.2
IHD	35.6
CHF	13.6
Stroke	8.5
PAD (%)	13.6
RASI (%)	52.5
Statin (%)	49.1
Antiplatelet agents (%)	52.5
Aspirin	47.5
Clopidogrel	23.7
Cilostazol	1.7
DAPT	20.3
Warfarin (%)	8.4
ESA	
Epoetin α or β (IU/week)	3204.5 ± 2326.0
Darbepoetin α (μg/week)	40.4 ± 41.2
CERA (μg/2 week)	62.5 ± 17.7
Hb (g/dl)	10.4 ± 1.4
Platelet ($\times 10^3/\mu l$)	18.9 ± 6.7
PT-INR	1.0 ± 0.4
CRP (mg/dl)	0.7 ± 1.4
Dialysis duration (month)	28.6 ± 30.9
AVF anastomosis type (%)	
Radiocephalic	81.4
Brachiocephalic	16.9
Radiobasilic	1.7
Quantity of blood flow (ml/min)	192.3 ± 33.6
Flow volume (ml/min)	
Before VAIVT	418.7 ± 362.5
After VAIVT	843.3 ± 723.2

Table 1 Baseline clinical characteristics (Continued)

Characteristic	
VAF (%)	
Stenosis/thrombosis	15.3/84.7
Adverse event (%)	
Serious bleeding event	
Intracranial	0
Gastrointestinal	0
CVD event after VAIVT	
IHD	11.9
CHF	5.1
Stroke	1.7

We defined individuals aged > 71 years as "the older age"
ESRD end-stage renal disease, *DN* diabetic nephropathy, *NS* nephrosclerosis, *CGN* chronic glomerulonephritis, *ADPKD* autosomal dominant polycystic kidney disease, *IgAN* IgA nephropathy, *DM* diabetes mellitus, *CVD* cardiovascular disease, *IHD* ischemic heart disease, *CHF* congestive heart failure, *PAD* peripheral artery disease, *RASI* renin–angiotensin–aldosterone system inhibitor, *DAPT* dual antiplatelet therapy, *ESA* erythropoiesis-stimulating agent, *CERA* continuous erythropoietin receptor activator, *AVF* arteriovenous fistula, *VAIVT* vascular access intervention therapy, *VAF* vascular access failure

including age, sex, medical history, and etiology of chronic kidney disease G5D (CKDG5D), were compared using Pearson's chi-squared or Fisher's exact test. Significance of associations among categorical variables was assessed using the chi-squared test and Spearman's rank correlation coefficient, and, to evaluate the relative risk to VA patency after VAIVT, univariate and multivariate Cox regression analyses were performed; results were reported as hazard ratios and 95% confidence intervals. Before performing Cox regression analysis, we tested the proportional hazards assumption using the Schoenfeld residual test. Covariates assessed in univariate analyses included the older age; sex; prevalence of smoking history; prevalence of diabetes mellitus (DM); prevalence of diabetic nephropathy (DN); cardiovascular disease (CVD); dyslipidemia; peripheral artery disease (PAD); medications, including renin–angiotensin–aldosterone system (RAAS) inhibitors, statins, and antiplatelet agents; and arteriovenous fistula (AVF) anastomosis type. According to the Japan Atherosclerosis Society 2012 guidelines, dyslipidemia was defined as low-density lipoprotein cholesterol level ≥ 140 mg/dl, high-density lipoprotein cholesterol level < 40 mg/dl, or triglyceride level ≥ 150 mg/dl [18]. Dyslipidemia also included patients who received statin or ezetimibe. The primary patency rate after VAIVT was analyzed using the Kaplan–Meier test; patency curves were compared using the log-rank and Wilcoxon tests.

Statistical significance was defined as a p value < 0.05. Statistical analyses were performed using JMP® software (version 8.0; SAS Institute, Cary, NC, USA) or EZR software (version 1.37; Saitama Medical Center, Jichi Medical University, Saitama, Japan).

This study was approved by the institutional review board of the University of Tokyo [IRB number 2879-(6)] and was conducted in accordance with guidelines of the Declaration of Helsinki. Informed consent was obtained from all patients at the time of hospital admission for VAIVT.

Results
Patient characteristics
Patient characteristics are shown in Table 1. The study group comprised 59 patients (45 men and 14 women) who were followed up for 266.6 ± 326.2 days. Median age was 71 years; therefore, we defined individuals aged > 71 years as "the older age" (Additional file 1: Figure S1). The most prevalent etiology underlying CKDG5D in the current study was DN (40.7%). The median duration of dialysis was approximately 28.6 months. The most common AVF type was radiocephalic fistula (n = 48), followed by brachiocephalic (n = 10) and radiobasilic (n = 1) fistula. The median flow volume before VAIVT was 418.7 ml/min. More than half of the patients received any of antiplatelet agents; aspirin, clopidogrel, and cilostazol were administered to 28 (47.5%), 14 (23.7%), and 1 (1.7%) patients, respectively. Of these, 20 patients received DAPT. Antiplatelet agents were administrated in 31 patients. At the end of the observation period, although the administration conditions were unknown without data in three (9.7%) patients, 28 (90.3%) had continuously received these antiplatelet agents.

Initial success and primary patency rates
During the entire study period, the initial VAIVT success rate was 93.8%, similar to that reported by previous studies [19–25]. In addition, the 1-year patency rate was 39.7% (Fig. 2).

Characterization of patients in the antiplatelet and non-antiplatelet group
Clinical characteristics of patients in the antiplatelet and non-antiplatelet group are summarized in Table 2. Rates of patients with smoking history (p = 0.008), dyslipidemia (p = 0.009), and CVD (p < 0.001) were significantly higher in the antiplatelet group than in the non-antiplatelet group. However, there were no statistical differences in rates of DN, DM, or PAD between the two groups. Adverse events were similar between the two study groups. There were no serious bleeding events, such as intracranial or gastrointestinal hemorrhage, and no significant differences in CVD events occurred during the follow-up period.

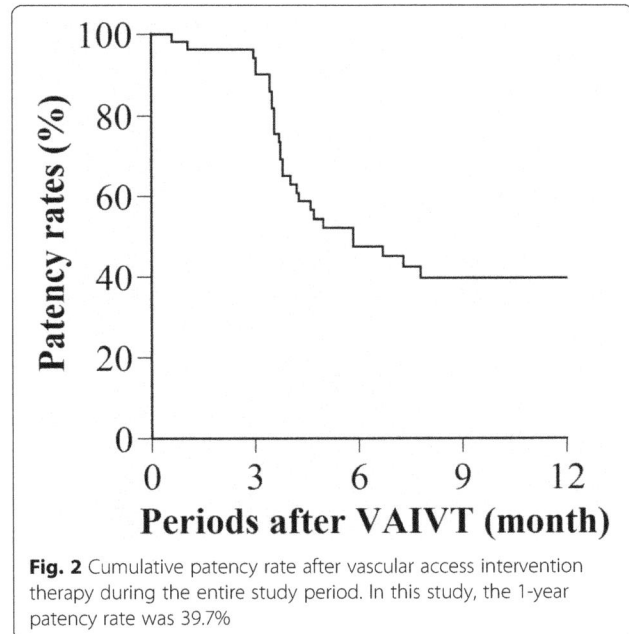

Fig. 2 Cumulative patency rate after vascular access intervention therapy during the entire study period. In this study, the 1-year patency rate was 39.7%

Primary patency in the antiplatelet group
Next, we assessed the association between antiplatelet agent treatment and cumulative primary patency rates by the Kaplan–Meier test (Fig. 3). The 1-year patency rate after VAIVT was significantly higher in the antiplatelet group than in the non-antiplatelet group (p = 0.035). We also assessed the number of antiplatelet agents used to examine whether there was a difference in 1-year patency rate between monotherapy and DAPT (Fig. 4). There was a significant difference in the 1-year patency rate after VAIVT among the three groups (p = 0.048). However, we did not find a significant difference between monotherapy and DAPT.

Analysis of independent risk factor for VAF
To identify variables that were significantly associated with VAF after VAIVT, we conducted a univariate Cox regression analysis after confirming the proportional hazards assumption using a Schoenfeld residuals test. The result of the proportional hazards assumption is shown in Additional file 2: Table S1 and Additional file 3: Figure S2. We excluded age from covariates because the proportional assumption of age was violated. As shown in Table 3, only treatment with antiplatelet agents was significantly associated with VAF. Conversely, the older age, sex, DN, DM, dyslipidemia, CVD, PAD, smoking history, or AVF anastomosis type were not found to be risk factors for primary patency.

In several studies, old age, female sex, smoking history, dyslipidemia, and CVD were reported as independent risk factors for VAF after VA construction [12, 16, 17, 26–29]. Therefore, we conducted a multivariate Cox regression

Table 2 Clinical characteristics of patients who did or did not receive antiplatelet agents

	Antiplatelet group	Non-antiplatelet group	p value
Number	31	28	
Age	73 (68–78)	71 (58.5–80)	0.27
Older age (%)	54.8	42.9	0.44
Sex (male, %)	80.7	64.3	0.22
Etiology of ESRD (%)			
DN	48.4	32.1	0.20
NS	25.8	21.4	0.69
CGN	9.7	21.4	0.21
ADPKD	3.2	0	0.34
IgAN	6.5	3.6	0.62
Other or unknown	6.5	21.4	0.093
Smoking history (%)	80.7	46.4	0.008
DM (%)	61.3	53.6	0.60
Dyslipidemia (%)	74.2	39.3	0.009
CVD (%)	80.7	25.0	< 0.001
IHD	58.1	10.7	< 0.001
CHF	16.1	10.7	0.54
Stroke	22.6	0	0.007
PAD (%)	22.6	3.6	0.55
RASI (%)	45.2	60.7	0.30
Statin (%)	29.0	75.0	< 0.001
Warfarin (%)	6.5	10.7	0.67
ESA			
Epoetin α or β (IU/week)	3750.0 ± 1068.5	2750.0 ± 975.4	0.51
Darbepoetin α (μg/week)	33.1 ± 9.7	47.4 ± 9.4	0.29
CERA (μg/2 week)	50	75	–
Hb (g/dl)	10.6 ± 0.3	10.1 ± 0.29	0.28
Platelet ($\times 10^3$/μl)	19.8 ± 1.2	17.9 ± 1.3	0.28
PT-INR	1.0 ± 0.1	1.1 ± 0.1	0.50
CRP (mg/dl)	0.6 ± 0.3	0.8 ± 0.3	0.71
Dialysis duration (month)	31.8 ± 33.2	20.8 ± 27.0	0.42
AVF anastomosis type (%)			
Radiocephalic	71.0	92.9	0.031
Brachiocephalic	25.8	7.1	0.056
Radiobasilic	3.2	0	0.34
Quantity of blood flow (ml/min)	194.1 ± 6.5	190 ± 7.6	0.69
Flow volume (ml/min)			
Before VAIVT	461.8 ± 86.1	373.1 ± 88.5	0.47
After VAIVT	816.2 ± 172.9	872.1 ± 177.9	0.82
VAF			
Thrombosis (%)	19.4	10.7	0.48
Adverse event (%)			
Serious bleeding event			
Intracranial	0	0	–

Table 2 Clinical characteristics of patients who did or did not receive antiplatelet agents *(Continued)*

	Antiplatelet group	Non-antiplatelet group	*p* value
Gastrointestinal	0	0	–
CVD event after VAIVT			
IHD	19.4	3.6	0.061
CHF	6.5	3.6	0.62
Stroke	3.2	0	0.34

We defined individuals aged > 71 years as "the older age"
ESRD end-stage renal disease, *DN* diabetic nephropathy, *NS* nephrosclerosis, *CGN* chronic glomerulonephritis, *ADPKD* autosomal dominant polycystic kidney disease, *IgAN* IgA nephropathy, *DM* diabetes mellitus, *CVD* cardiovascular disease, *IHD* ischemic heart disease, *CHF* congestive heart failure, *PAD* peripheral artery disease, *RASI* renin–angiotensin–aldosterone system inhibitor, *ESA* erythropoiesis-stimulating agent, *CERA* continuous erythropoietin receptor activator, *AVF* arteriovenous fistula, *VAIVT* vascular access intervention therapy, *VAF* vascular access failure

analysis using these factors to determine if they were independent risk factors for VAF after VAIVT (Table 4). Treatment with antiplatelet agents was found to be independently associated with patency after VAIVT (hazard ratio, 0.28; 95% confidence interval, 0.09–0.82; $p = 0.02$).

Overall, these findings supported an association between antiplatelet agent treatment and primary patency.

Discussion

The current study investigating the association between primary patency after VAIVT and antiplatelet agent treatment using a medical record review determined that the long-term patency rate was good, with a cumulative patency rate of 39.7% for 1 year after VAIVT (Fig. 2), and that the cumulative patency rate was higher in patients treated with antiplatelet agents than in those not treated with an antiplatelet agent. The frequency of bleeding or other serious adverse events was not higher in the antiplatelet group. Our results showed that administration of antiplatelet agents may contribute to the improvement of 1-year patency rate after VAIVT (Table 4). To the best of our knowledge, this is the first study to demonstrate the protective effect of antiplatelet agents against VAF after VAIVT.

Previous studies and systematic reviews have reported that antiplatelet agents are effective in preventing VAF,

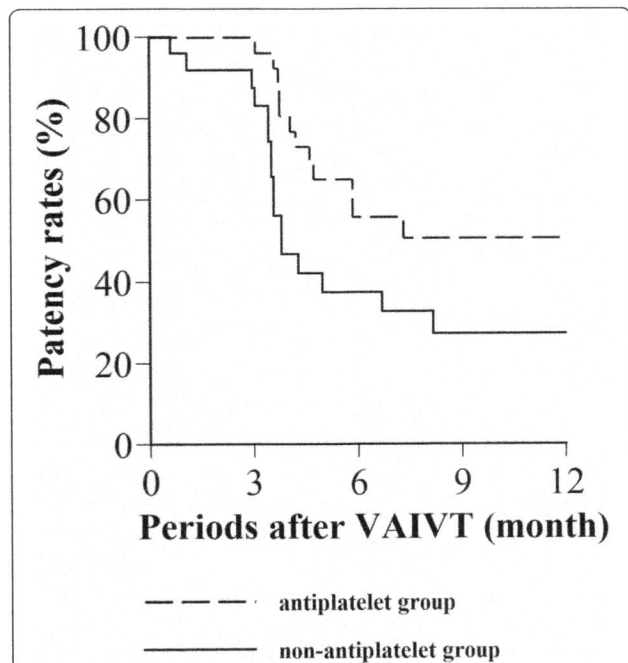

Fig. 3 Kaplan–Meier curves for vascular access patency rate. Patency rate after VAIVT was significantly lower in the non-antiplatelet group (50.8% vs. 27.3%; *p* = 0.035)

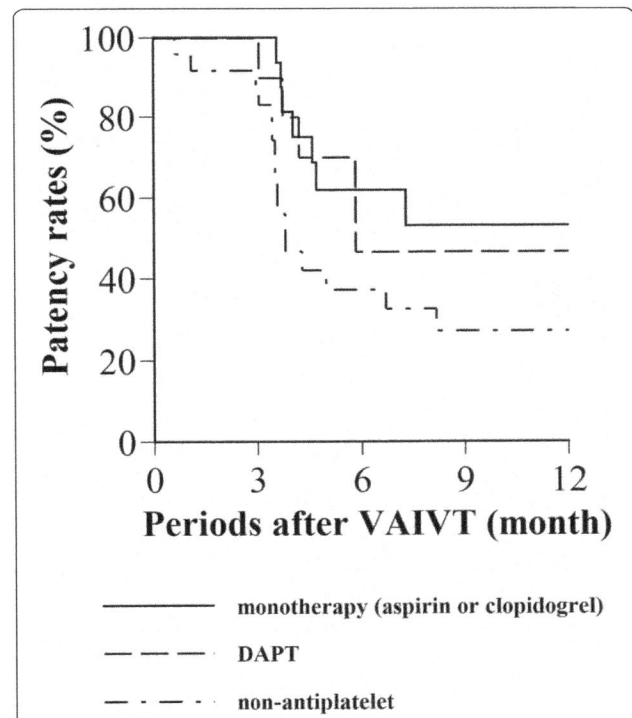

Fig. 4 Kaplan–Meier curves of the cumulative patency rate after vascular access intervention therapy. The 1-year patency rate was 53.0%, 46.7%, and 27.3% in the monotherapy group, the DAPT group, and the non-antiplatelet group, respectively (*p* = 0.048)

Table 3 Factors associated with VA failure after VAIVT in univariate Cox regression model

	HR	95% CI	p value
Older age	0.78	0.35–1.65	0.52
Sex (male)	1.95	0.75–6.64	0.18
Etiology of ESRD			
DN	1.30	0.61–2.74	0.50
NS	0.58	0.17–1.50	0.28
CGN	0.96	0.32–2.34	0.94
ADPKD	–	–	–
IgAN	0.81	0.20–4.15	0.78
Other or unknown	1.13	0.27–3.23	0.85
Smoking history	0.83	0.38–1.92	0.64
DM	1.95	0.87–4.95	0.11
Dyslipidemia	1.46	0.69–3.31	0.33
CVD	0.75	0.35–1.58	0.45
IHD	0.74	0.22–1.93	0.57
CHF	1.25	0.20–4.20	0.77
Stroke	0.27	0.02–1.29	0.12
PAD	0.56	0.13–1.60	0.31
RASI	1.69	0.80–3.71	0.17
Statin	1.41	0.67–3.10	0.37
Warfarin	0.61	0.10–2.03	0.46
Antiplatelet agents	0.45	0.21–0.95	0.036
AVF anastomosis type (%)			
Radiocephalic	3.22	0.96–20.0	0.060
Brachiocephalic	0.36	0.06–1.21	0.11

We defined individuals aged > 71 years as "the older age"
VA vascular access, *VAIVT* vascular access intervention therapy, *HR* hazard ratio, *CI* confidence interval, *ESRD* end-stage renal disease, *DN* diabetic nephropathy, *NS* nephrosclerosis, *CGN* chronic glomerulonephritis, *ADPKD* autosomal dominant polycystic kidney disease, *IgAN* IgA nephropathy, *DM* diabetes mellitus, *CVD* cardiovascular disease, *IHD* ischemic heart disease, *CHF* congestive heart failure, *PAD* peripheral artery disease, *RASI* renin–angiotensin–aldosterone system inhibitor, *AVF* arteriovenous fistula

Table 4 Factors associated with VA failure after VAIVT in multivariate Cox regression model

	HR	95% CI	p value
Antiplatelet agents	0.28	0.09–0.82	0.020
Older age	0.95	0.38–2.29	0.91
Sex (male)	2.14	0.75–7.67	0.16
Dyslipidemia	1.89	0.81–4.69	0.14
CVD	1.29	0.51–3.37	0.59
Smoking history	1.07	0.39–3.13	0.89

We defined individuals aged > 71 years as "the older age"
VA vascular access, *VAIVT* vascular access intervention therapy, *HR* hazard ratio, *CI* confidence interval, *CVD* cardiovascular disease

including those resulting from thrombosis [4, 30–33]. For example, a randomized control study showed that VAF risk after arteriovenous graft construction was reduced by 5% following administration of antiplatelet agents [4]. A recent systematic review demonstrated that antiplatelet agents were effective in preventing AVF and central venous thrombosis [32]. The same systematic review also reported that VAF was significantly reduced by 57% in the antiplatelet group compared with that in the placebo or non-treatment groups (relative risk, 0.43; 95% confidence interval, 0.26–0.73; I^2 = 25%) [31]. However, these studies investigated the efficacy of antiplatelet agents against primary patency after VA construction. Conversely, results of the current study suggest that antiplatelet agents are useful for VA patency after VAIVT. Based on a previous study [34], we excluded patients with VA construction within 180 days before intervention because our study aim was to examine the effect of antiplatelet agents on secondary patency and not primary patency.

This study showed that the cumulative VA patency after VAIVT was significantly higher in patients treated with antiplatelet agents than in those who were not treated with antiplatelet agents. This outcome is biologically plausible because several recent reports have suggested that high levels of local oxidative stress or inflammatory mediators are involved in development of VAF [35–39]. Several recent studies showed that some mediators such as heme oxygenase-1 and heme oxygenase-2, monocyte chemoattractant protein-1, Kruppel-like factor-2, and TGF-b1 play an important role in AVF dysfunction in mouse model [40, 41]. Antiplatelet agents, such as aspirin, clopidogrel, and cilostazol, have been reported to reduce oxidative stress and inflammation [42, 43]. For example, these agents have a great effect on suppression of the onset or progression of vascular disease after invasive treatment for major CVD and PAD [44–51]. In addition, our results are consistent with those of a recent systematic review showing that antiplatelet agents reduced VAF incidence in AVFs [32].

In the present study, there were no serious bleeding events related to antiplatelet agent treatment; this finding is consistent with that of a recent meta-analysis that showed that antiplatelet agents are not associated with serious adverse events [32].

A recent study has shown that protein-bound uremic toxins, such as indoxyl sulfate, resulted from the metabolism of dietary tryptophan were associated with vascular access patency after VAIVT [52]. Uremic toxins were not measured in the present study, which may have influenced vascular access outcomes between the two groups. However, no participant had dysphagia and all participants were educated regarding the medical nutrition therapy for chronic kidney disease.

Our study has several limitations. First, this retrospective cohort study at a single institution included a small number of patients. Because the proportional assumption of age was violated, selection bias related to age may have influenced the analysis result. Second, cause-specific risk of VAF after VAIVT could not be analyzed. Third, the rate of patients with radiocephalic fistula was significantly higher in the non-antiplatelet group than in the antiplatelet group. Although there might be selection bias such as technical problem and selection bias involving surgeon skill, AVF anastomosis type was not significantly associated with VAF. Finally, because all study subjects were hospitalized, their overall condition was worse than the general dialysis population, which might have led to a selection bias.

In Japan, antiplatelet therapy for the treatment or prevention of VAF has not been covered by the Japanese health insurance system. Therefore, in the present state, it is not possible to administer antiplatelet agents against VAF to patients with VAF.

Conclusions

This retrospective study on a cohort of patients with VAF at a single institution revealed that administration of antiplatelet agents was associated with a reduced VAF rate after VAIVT and that there was no significant difference in serious adverse event rates between the two groups. Overall, these results suggest that antiplatelet agents are useful in reducing the development of VAF after VAIVT. We, interventional nephrologists, believe that some vascular access failure pathology may be implicated in platelet and inflammation, but there is little existing evidence. Therefore, progress of research in this field is expected in future.

Additional files

Additional file 1: Figure S1. Box plot showing the age distribution of the patients in this study. People over 71 years old was defined as the older age. Box plot explanation: upper horizontal line of box, 75th percentile; lower horizontal line of box, 25th percentile; horizontal bar within box, median; upper horizontal bar outside box, maximum; lower horizontal bar outside box, minimum.

Additional file 2: Table S1. Results of the proportional hazards assumption by a Schoenfeld residuals test.

Additional file 3: Figure S2. Scaled Schoenfeld residuals for each factor. The residual was estimated as the time-dependent coefficient beta (t) vs. transformed time. The proportional hazards assumption of age was violated ($p < 0.001$), but that of the other factors was fitted ($p > 0.05$) (Additional file 2: Table S1). a Age, b Older age, c Sex, d DN, e NS, f CGN, g IgAN, h Other or unknown, i Smoking history, j DM, k Dyslipidemia, l CVD, m IHD, n CHF, o Stroke, p PAD, q RASI, r Statin, s Warfarin, t Antiplatelet agents, u Radiocephalic, v Brachiocephalic

Abbreviations
AVF: Arteriovenous fistula; CHF: Congestive heart failure; CKD: Chronic kidney disease; CVD: Cardiovascular disease; DAPT: Dual antiplatelet therapy; DM: Diabetes mellitus; DN: Diabetic nephropathy; HD: Hemodialysis; IHD: Ischemic heart disease; JSDT: Japanese Society for Dialysis Therapy;

PAD: Peripheral artery disease; RAAS: Rennin–angiotensin–aldosterone system; VA: Vascular access; VAF: Vascular access failure; VAIVT: Vascular access intervention therapy

Acknowledgements
The authors are grateful to all investigators and contributors of our study.

Funding
The study was supported by JSPS KAKENHI (Grant Number JP17K16071).

Authors' contributions
All authors have read and approved the final manuscript.

Authors' information
TM, MN, NS, HT, YH, and MN are members of the Division of Nephrology and Endocrinology at the University of Tokyo Hospital, and AM and HK are members of the Department of Urology at the University of Tokyo Hospital.

Competing interests
The authors declare that they have no competing interests.

Author details
[1]Division of Nephrology and Endocrinology, The University of Tokyo Hospital, 7-3-1 Hongo, Bunkyo-ku, Tokyo 113-8655, Japan. [2]Department of Urology, The University of Tokyo Hospital, 7-3-1 Hongo, Bunkyo-ku, Tokyo 113-8655, Japan. [3]Department of Hemodialysis and Apheresis, The University of Tokyo Hospital, 7-3-1 Hongo, Bunkyo-ku, Tokyo 113-8655, Japan.

References
1. Kukita K, Ohira S, Amano I, Naito H, Azuma N, Ikeda K, et al. 2011 update Japanese Society for Dialysis Therapy Guidelines of vascular access construction and repair for chronic hemodialysis. Ther Apher Dial. 2015; 19(Suppl 1):1–39.
2. Feldman HI, Kobrin S, Wasserstein A. Hemodialysis vascular access morbidity. J Am Soc Nephrol. 1996;7(4):523–35.
3. Manns B, Tonelli M, Yilmaz S, Lee H, Laupland K, Klarenbach S, et al. Establishment and maintenance of vascular access in incident hemodialysis patients: a prospective cost analysis. J Am Soc Nephrol. 2005;16(1):201–9.
4. Dixon BS, Beck GJ, Vazquez MA, Greenberg A, Delmez JA, Allon M, et al. Effect of dipyridamole plus aspirin on hemodialysis graft patency. N Engl J Med. 2009;360(21):2191–201.
5. Tanner NC, Da Silva A. Medical adjuvant treatment to increase patency of arteriovenous fistulae and grafts. Cochrane Database Syst Rev. 2015;7: CD002786.
6. Group VAW. Clinical practice guidelines for vascular access. Am J Kidney Dis. 2006;48(Suppl 1):S176–247.
7. Forauer AR, Hoffer EK, Homa K. Dialysis access venous stenoses: treatment with balloon angioplasty--1- versus 3-minute inflation times. Radiology. 2008;249(1):375–81.
8. Safa AA, Valji K, Roberts AC, Ziegler TW, Hye RJ, Oglevie SB. Detection and treatment of dysfunctional hemodialysis access grafts: effect of a surveillance program on graft patency and the incidence of thrombosis. Radiology. 1996;199(3):653–7.

9. Leskovar B, Furlan T, PozniÄ S, Potisek M, Adamlje A, KljuÄevÅ¡ek T. Ultrasound-guided percutaneous endovascular treatment of arteriovenous fistula/graft. Clin Nephrol. 2017;88(13):61â€“4.

10. Wakabayashi M, Hanada S, Nakano H, Wakabayashi T. Ultrasound-guided endovascular treatment for vascular access malfunction: results in 4896 cases. J Vasc Access. 2013;14(3):225â€“30.

11. Gray RJ. Percutaneous intervention for permanent hemodialysis access: a review. J Vasc Interv Radiol. 1997;8(3):313â€“27.

12. Kim SM, Ko HK, Noh M, Ko GY, Kim MJ, Kwon TW, et al. Factors affecting patency following successful percutaneous intervention for dysfunctional hemodialysis vascular access. Ann Vasc Surg. 2018;47:54â€“61.

13. Cho S, Lee YJ, Kim SR. Clinical experience with ultrasound guided angioplasty for vascular access. Kidney Res Clin Pract. 2017;36(1):79â€“85.

14. Tordoir JHM, Zonnebeld N, van Loon MM, Gallieni M, Hollenbeck M. Surgical and endovascular intervention for dialysis access maturation failure during and after arteriovenous fistula surgery: review of the evidence. Eur J Vasc Endovasc Surg. 2018;55(2):240â€“8.

15. Gray RJ, Sacks D, Martin LG, Trerotola SO. Committee SoIRTA. Reporting standards for percutaneous interventions in dialysis access. J Vasc Interv Radiol. 2003;14(9 Pt 2):S433â€“42.

16. Lazarides MK, Georgiadis GS, Antoniou GA, Staramos DN. A meta-analysis of dialysis access outcome in elderly patients. J Vasc Surg. 2007;45(2):420â€“6.

17. Miller PE, Tolwani A, Luscy CP, Deierhoi MH, Bailey R, Redden DT, et al. Predictors of adequacy of arteriovenous fistulas in hemodialysis patients. Kidney Int. 1999;56(1):275â€“80.

18. Teramoto T, Sasaki J, Ishibashi S, Birou S, Daida H, Dohi S, et al. Executive summary of the Japan Atherosclerosis Society (JAS) guidelines for the diagnosis and prevention of atherosclerotic cardiovascular diseases in Japan - 2012 version. J Atheroscler Thromb. 2013;20(6):517â€“23.

19. Sadaghianloo N, Declemy S, Jean-Baptiste E, Haudebourg P, Robino C, Islam MS, et al. Radial artery deviation and reimplantation inhibits venous juxta-anastomotic stenosis and increases primary patency of radial-cephalic fistulas for hemodialysis. J Vasc Surg. 2016;64(3):698â€“706.e1.

20. Turmel-Rodrigues L, Mouton A, BirmelÃ© B, Billaux L, Ammar N, GrÃ©zard O, et al. Salvage of immature forearm fistulas for haemodialysis by interventional radiology. Nephrol Dial Transplant. 2001;16(12):2365â€“71.

21. Beathard GA, Arnold P, Jackson J, Litchfield T, Lifeline POFR. Aggressive treatment of early fistula failure. Kidney Int. 2003;64(4):1487â€“94.

22. NatÃ¡rio A, Turmel-Rodrigues L, Fodil-Cherif M, Brillet G, Girault-Lataste A, Dumont G, et al. Endovascular treatment of immature, dysfunctional and thrombosed forearm autogenous ulnar-basilic and radial-basilic fistulas for haemodialysis. Nephrol Dial Transplant. 2010;25(2):532â€“8.

23. Park JY, Yoo CH. On postoperative day balloon angioplasty for salvage of newly-placed, flow-limiting native arteriovenous fistula. Vasc Specialist Int. 2015;31(1):20â€“4.

24. Jeon EY, Cho YK, Cho SB, Yoon DY, Suh SO. Predicting factors for successful maturation of autogenous haemodialysis fistulas after salvage percutaneous transluminal angioplasty in diabetic nephropathy: a study on follow-up Doppler ultrasonography. Iran J Radiol. 2016;13(1):e32559.

25. Park HS, Lee YH, Kim HW, Baik JH, Won YS, Park CW, et al. Usefulness of assisted procedures for arteriovenous fistula maturation without compromising access patency. Hemodial Int. 2017;21(3):335â€“42.

26. Woods JD, Turenne MN, Strawderman RL, Young EW, Hirth RA, Port FK, et al. Vascular access survival among incident hemodialysis patients in the United States. Am J Kidney Dis. 1997;30(1):50â€“7.

27. Astor BC, Coresh J, Powe NR, Eustace JA, Klag MJ. Relation between gender and vascular access complications in hemodialysis patients. Am J Kidney Dis. 2000;36(6):1126â€“34.

28. Ravani P, Marcelli D, Malberti F. Vascular access surgery managed by renal physicians: the choice of native arteriovenous fistulas for hemodialysis. Am J Kidney Dis. 2002;40(6):1264â€“76.

29. Shin DH, Rhee SY, Jeon HJ, Park JY, Kang SW, Oh J. An increase in mean platelet volume/platelet count ratio is associated with vascular access failure in hemodialysis patients. PLoS One. 2017;12(1):e0170357.

30. Kaufman JS, O'Connor TZ, Zhang JH, Cronin RE, Fiore LD, Ganz MB, et al. Randomized controlled trial of clopidogrel plus aspirin to prevent hemodialysis access graft thrombosis. J Am Soc Nephrol. 2003;14(9):2313â€“21.

31. Trimarchi H, Young P, Forrester M, Schropp J, Pereyra H, Freixas E. Clopidogrel diminishes hemodialysis access graft thrombosis. J Vasc Access. 2005;6(1):29â€“33.

32. Palmer SC, Di Micco L, Razavian M, Craig JC, Ravani P, Perkovic V, et al. Antiplatelet therapy to prevent hemodialysis vascular access failure: systematic review and meta-analysis. Am J Kidney Dis. 2013;61(1):112â€“22.

33. Hiremath S, Holden RM, Fergusson D, Zimmerman DL. Antiplatelet medications in hemodialysis patients: a systematic review of bleeding rates. Clin J Am Soc Nephrol. 2009;4(8):1347â€“55.

34. Hu H, Patel S, Hanisch JJ, Santana JM, Hashimoto T, Bai H, et al. Future research directions to improve fistula maturation and reduce access failure. Semin Vasc Surg. 2016;29(4):153â€“71.

35. Kang L, Grande JP, Farrugia G, Croatt AJ, Katusic ZS, Nath KA. Functioning of an arteriovenous fistula requires heme oxygenase-2. Am J Physiol Renal Physiol. 2013;305(4):F545â€“52.

36. Juncos JP, Grande JP, Kang L, Ackerman AW, Croatt AJ, Katusic ZS, et al. MCP-1 contributes to arteriovenous fistula failure. J Am Soc Nephrol. 2011; 22(1):43â€“8.

37. Kang L, Hillestad ML, Grande JP, Croatt AJ, Barry MA, Farrugia G, et al. Induction and functional significance of the heme oxygenase system in pathological shear stress in vivo. Am J Physiol Heart Circ Physiol. 2015; 308(11):H1402â€“13.

38. Juncos JP, Tracz MJ, Croatt AJ, Grande JP, Ackerman AW, Katusic ZS, et al. Genetic deficiency of heme oxygenase-1 impairs functionality and form of an arteriovenous fistula in the mouse. Kidney Int. 2008;74(1):47â€“51.

39. Lee T, Misra S. New insights into dialysis vascular access: molecular targets in arteriovenous fistula and arteriovenous graft failure and their potential to improve vascular access outcomes. Clin J Am Soc Nephrol. 2016;11(8):1504â€“12.

40. Janardhanan R, Yang B, Vohra P, Roy B, Withers S, Bhattacharya S, et al. Simvastatin reduces venous stenosis formation in a murine hemodialysis vascular access model. Kidney Int. 2013;84(2):338â€“52.

41. Kang L, Grande JP, Hillestad ML, Croatt AJ, Barry MA, Katusic ZS, et al. A new model of an arteriovenous fistula in chronic kidney disease in the mouse: beneficial effects of upregulated heme oxygenase-1. Am J Physiol Renal Physiol. 2016;310(6):F466â€“76.

42. Kambayashi J, Liu Y, Sun B, Shakur Y, Yoshitake M, Czerwiec F. Cilostazol as a unique antithrombotic agent. Curr Pharm Des. 2003;9(28):2289â€“302.

43. Kattoor AJ, Pothineni NVK, Palagiri D, Mehta JL. Oxidative stress in atherosclerosis. Curr Atheroscler Rep. 2017;19(11):42.

44. Kakkos SK, Nicolaides A, Griffin M, Sabetai M, Dhanjil S, Thomas DJ, et al. Factors associated with mortality in patients with asymptomatic carotid stenosis: results from the ACSRS study. Int Angiol. 2005;24(3):221â€“30.

45. Hobson RW, Krupski WC, Weiss DG. Influence of aspirin in the management of asymptomatic carotid artery stenosis. VA Cooperative Study Group on Asymptomatic Carotid Stenosis. J Vasc Surg. 1993;17(2):257â€“63 discussion 63-5.

46. Kernan WN, Ovbiagele B, Black HR, Bravata DM, Chimowitz MI, Ezekowitz MD, et al. Guidelines for the prevention of stroke in patients with stroke and transient ischemic attack: a guideline for healthcare professionals from the American Heart Association/American Stroke Association. Stroke. 2014; 45(7):2160â€“236.

47. Chimowitz MI, Lynn MJ, Howlett-Smith H, Stern BJ, Hertzberg VS, Frankel MR, et al. Comparison of warfarin and aspirin for symptomatic intracranial arterial stenosis. N Engl J Med. 2005;352(13):1305â€“16.

48. Conte MS, Pomposelli FB, Clair DG, Geraghty PJ, McKinsey JF, Mills JL, et al. Society for Vascular Surgery practice guidelines for atherosclerotic occlusive disease of the lower extremities: management of asymptomatic disease and claudication. J Vasc Surg. 2015;61(3 Suppl):2Sâ€“41S.

49. Dember LM, Beck GJ, Allon M, Delmez JA, Dixon BS, Greenberg A, et al. Effect of clopidogrel on early failure of arteriovenous fistulas for hemodialysis: a randomized controlled trial. JAMA. 2008;299(18):2164â€“71.

50. Iida O, Yokoi H, Soga Y, Inoue N, Suzuki K, Yokoi Y, et al. Cilostazol reduces angiographic restenosis after endovascular therapy for femoropopliteal lesions in the Sufficient Treatment of Peripheral Intervention by Cilostazol study. Circulation. 2013;127(23):2307â€“15.

51. Romiti M, Albers M, Brochado-Neto FC, Durazzo AE, Pereira CA, De Luccia N. Meta-analysis of infrapopliteal angioplasty for chronic critical limb ischemia. J Vasc Surg. 2008;47(5):975â€“81.

52. Wu CC, Hsieh MY, Hung SC, Kuo KL, Tsai TH, Lai CL, et al. Serum indoxyl sulfate associates with postangioplasty thrombosis of dialysis grafts. J Am Soc Nephrol. 2016;27(4):1254â€“64.

29

Associations between fluid removal and number of B-lines, peak early mitral inflow wave velocity, and inferior vena cava dimensions in hemodialysis patients

Kazuo Kimura[1,2], Katsuya Kajimoto[3], Shigeru Otsubo[1,4*], Takashi Akiba[2] and Kosaku Nitta[1]

Abstract

Background: The inferior vena cava (IVC) dimensions represent the right ventricular preload, whereas the peak early mitral inflow wave velocity (peak E-velocity) represents the left ventricular preload. On the other hand, B-lines represent extravascular lung water. The aim of this study was to evaluate possible acute changes in the IVC dimensions, peak E-velocity, and number of B-lines during hemodialysis therapy.

Methods: A total of 55 consecutive patients receiving maintenance hemodialysis were enrolled in this study. We performed echo-graphic examinations at three time points (just after the start, during the middle, and just before the end of the hemodialysis therapy). We then investigated the changes in the IVC dimensions, peak E-velocity, and number of B-lines.

Results: The peak E-velocity decreased from 80 ± 26 cm/s at the start of the therapy to 58 ± 22 cm/s during the middle and 51 ± 21 cm/s at the end of the therapy. The IVC dimensions also decreased from 15 ± 4 mm at the start of the therapy to 12 ± 3 mm during the middle and 11 ± 3 mm at the end of the therapy. The number of B-lines also decreased from 12 ± 5 at the start of the therapy to 9 ± 4 during the middle and 5 ± 3 at the end of the therapy. The changes in the peak E-velocity and IVC dimensions were significantly greater during the first half of the dialysis period than during the second half of the dialysis period ($P < 0.0001$ and $P < 0.0001$, respectively). On the other hand, the changes in the number of B-lines during these periods were significantly smaller during the first half of the dialysis period than during the second half of the dialysis period ($P = 0.0016$).

Conclusions: We showed that the peak E-velocity and the IVC dimensions were reduced mainly during the first half of the dialysis period, while the number of B-lines showed a significant decrease mainly during the last half of the dialysis period. Even if the IVC dimensions are reduced sufficiently, caution is needed as lung congestion may still exist.

Keywords: B-lines, Early diastolic filling velocity, Early diastolic filling wave, Hemodialysis, Inferior vena cava, Lung ultrasound

* Correspondence: sotsubo@hb.tp1.jp
[1]Department of Medicine, Kidney Center, Tokyo Women's Medical University, Tokyo, Japan
[4]Department of Blood Purification, Tohto Sangenjaya Clinic, 2-13-2 Taishido, Setagaya-ku, Tokyo 154-0004, Japan
Full list of author information is available at the end of the article

Background

Chronic fluid overloading frequently occurs in hemodialysis patients, so volume assessment during hemodialysis is a primary, and often challenging, goal of nephrologists. Volume overload is directly associated with hypertension, increased arterial stiffness, left ventricular hypertrophy, heart failure, and ultimately higher rates of mortality and morbidity [1].

Lung ultrasound has recently been shown to be a useful, noninvasive technique for the assessment of extravascular lung water [2]. The most commonly observed finding was a comet tail artifact fanning out from the lung-wall interface and spreading upwards to the edge of the screen, previously named a "B-line" [3]. In patients with heart failure, the number of B-lines was correlated with the degree of extravascular lung water [4, 5]. Lung ultrasound is also reportedly useful for the accurate evaluation of dry weight and fluid status in hemodialysis patients [2, 6, 7].

The inferior vena cava (IVC) dimensions represent the right ventricular preload [8], whereas the peak early mitral inflow wave velocity (peak E-velocity) represents the left ventricular preload [9, 10]. On the other hand, B-lines represent extravascular lung water. The aim of this study was to evaluate possible acute changes in IVC dimensions, peak E-velocity, and B-lines during hemodialysis therapy.

Methods

A total of 55 patients receiving maintenance hemodialysis at Sekikawa Hospital and in whom more than 1 kg was removed during hemodialysis were enrolled in this study. Patients with lung disease or chest injury were excluded from this study.

Clinical data including age, sex, duration of hemodialysis therapy, presence of diabetes mellitus and/or hypertension and/or dyslipidemia complications, and the results of biological examinations were collected from the patients' clinical records. Hypertension was defined as a systolic blood pressure of 140 mmHg or higher, a diastolic blood pressure of 90 mmHg or higher, and/or the current use of antihypertensive drugs. Diabetes mellitus was defined as a fasting glucose level ≥ 126 mg/dL, a nonfasting glucose level ≥ 200 mg/dL, or the use of medication. Dyslipidemia was defined as a low-density lipoprotein cholesterol level ≥ 140 mg/dL, a high-density lipoprotein cholesterol level < 40 mg/dL, a triglyceride level ≥ 150 mg/dL, or the use of medication.

A peripheral blood sample was obtained before hemodialysis during the first session of the week. The serum N-terminal pro-brain natriuretic peptide (NT-proBNP) level in the pre-dialysis blood sample was measured using an electrochemiluminescence immunoassay on an Elecsys platform (Roche, Basel, Switzerland).

A lung ultrasound examination was performed during the first session of the week (at the same time as the peripheral blood sample preparation) using Vscan® (GE Healthcare, Japan), which is a hand-held ultrasound device with a wide-bandwidth phased-array probe (1.7–3.5 MHz) [11, 12]. Bilateral scanning of the anterior and lateral chest walls was performed with the patient in a supine position. An intercostal scan with a maximum extension of the visual pleural line was performed. The chest wall was divided into eight areas (two anterior and two lateral areas per side), and one scan was obtained for each area [13]. The anterior zone of the chest wall was designated from the sternum to the anterior axillary line and was then divided into upper and lower halves (from the clavicle to the third intercostal spaces and from the third space to the diaphragm). The lateral zone was positioned from the anterior axillary line to the posterior axillary line and was also divided into the upper and lower halves. The investigators attempted to detect comet tail artifacts fanning out from the lung-wall interface and spreading to the edge of the screen, which were previously named as B-lines (Fig. 1) [5, 6]. The total number of B-lines was estimated. Echocardiographic measurements were obtained at the same time, and the IVC dimensions and peak E-velocity were estimated. We performed echographic examinations three times (just after the start, just in the middle (for example, 2 h after the start of hemodialysis therapy if the treatment time is 4 h), and just before the end of the hemodialysis therapy). We then investigated the changes in the IVC dimensions, peak E-velocity, and B-lines. This study was conducted in accordance with the principles of the Declaration of Helsinki and was permitted by the research ethics committee of Sekikawa Hospital (Approved No. H2705). The data were expressed as the means ± SD or median (interquartile range, IQR). Paired t tests were used to examine changes in the variables.

All the statistical calculations were performed using JMP 5.1 software. P values less than 0.05 were considered statistically significant.

Results

The patient background characteristics are shown in Table 1. The mean age was 75 ± 11 years. Elderly patients were common in this study. Diabetic nephropathy was the major cause of end-stage kidney disease. Hypertension, diabetes mellitus, and dyslipidemia were present in 89.1, 47.3, and 16.4% of the study participants, respectively. The results of the biochemistry analyses,

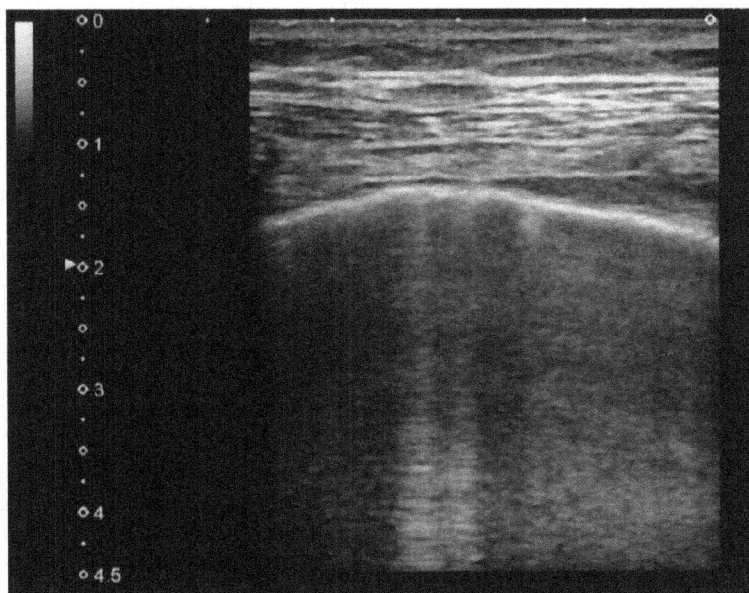

Fig. 1 B-lines—comet tail artifacts fanning out from the lung-wall interface and spreading upwards to the edge of the screen

including the NT-proBNP level, are shown in Table 2. The serum albumin level was relatively low (3.1 ± 0.5 g/dL), and the serum NT-proBNP level was relatively high (13,650 [4901–35,825] pg/mL) among the study participants. Table 3 shows the background characteristics of the echocardiographic indices. The mean ejection fraction was 60% $\pm$ 12%.

The treatment time was 3.7 ± 0.4 h, and 2.1 ± 0.9 kg water was removed. The blood pressure and pulse rate were $146 \pm 25/74 \pm 15$ mmHg and 75 ± 13 beats/min at the first echo examination, $134 \pm 24/72 \pm 14$ mmHg and 72 ± 16 beats/min at the second, $132 \pm 27/73 \pm 16$ mmHg and 73 ± 15 beats/min at the final examination. Table 4 shows the changes in the echocardiographic indices. The peak E-velocity decreased from 80 ± 26 cm/s at the start of the therapy to 58 ± 22 cm/s during the middle and 51 ± 21 cm/s at the end of the therapy. The IVC dimensions also decreased from 15 ± 4 mm at the start of the

Table 1 Background characteristics of the study participants

Characteristic	Quantity
Gender (M/F)	26/29
Age (year)	75 ± 11
Duration of HD (year)	6.5 ± 8.8
Primary cause of ESKD, n (%)	
Chronic glomerulonephritis	8 (14.5)
Diabetic nephropathy	26 (47.3)
Nephrosclerosis	13 (23.6)
Unknown and others	8 (14.5)
Hypertention, n (%)	49 (89.1)
Diabetes mellitus, n (%)	26 (47.3)
Dyslipidemia, n (%)	9 (16.4)
Atrial fibrillation, n (%)	8 (14.5)
History of PCI or CABG	8 (14.5)
History of valve replacement	2 (3.6)[a]
Body weight (kg)	52.0 ± 10.9
Systolic blood pressure (mmHg)	147 ± 25
Diastolic blood pressure (mmHg)	74 ± 15
Heart rate (beat/min)	75 ± 13

Mean ± SD, median (interquartile range)
HD hemodialysis, *ESKD* end-stage kidney disease, *PCI* percutaneous coronary intervention, *CABG* coronary artery bypass graft
[a]Both patients underwent aortic valve replacement therapy

Table 2 Background characteristics of laboratory data

Characteristic	Quantity
Albumin (g/dL)	3.1 ± 0.5
Urea nitrogen (mg/dL)	50.2 ± 18.3
Creatinine (mg/dL)	7.36 ± 2.56
Sodium (mEq/L)	137 ± 4
C-reactive protein (mg/dL)	0.27 (0.10–0.86)
Hemoglobin (g/dL)	10.4 ± 1.2
NT-proBNP (pg/mL)	13,650 (4901–35,825)

Mean ± SD, median (interquartile range)
NT-proBNP N-terminal pro-brain natriuretic peptide

Table 3 Background characteristics of the echocardiographic indices

Parameter	Value
LVDd (mm)	46 ± 6
LVDs (mm)	31 ± 7
EF (%)	60 ± 14
Max WT (mm)	12 ± 2

Mean ± SD

LVDd left ventricular diastolic diameter, *LVDs* left ventricular systolic diameter, *EF* ejection fraction, *WT* wall thickness

therapy to 12 ± 3 mm during the middle and 11 ± 3 mm at the end of the therapy. The number of B-lines also decreased from 12 ± 5 at the start of the therapy to 9 ± 4 during the middle and 5 ± 3 at the end of the therapy (also shown in Fig. 2).

Table 5 shows a comparison of the changes in values between the middle to pre-dialysis periods and the post-dialysis to middle periods. The changes in the peak E-velocity and the IVC dimensions were significantly greater during the first half of the dialysis period than during the second half of the dialysis period ($P < 0.0001$ and $P < 0.0001$, respectively). On the other hand, the changes in the B-lines between these periods was significantly smaller during the first half of the dialysis period than during the second half of the dialysis period ($P = 0.0016$).

Figure 3 shows a representative case in this study. The peak E-velocity and IVC dimensions decreased mainly during the first half of the dialysis period, while the number of B-lines decreased steadily throughout the dialysis period.

Discussion

We found that the peak E-velocity and IVC dimensions decreased significantly mainly during the first half of the dialysis period, while the number of B-lines decreased significantly mainly during the last half of the dialysis period.

Lung ultrasound is a novel, well-validated technique that allows reliable estimates of lung water in clinical practice [14]. B-lines can be evaluated anywhere (including extreme environmental conditions using pocket-sized instruments to detect high-altitude pulmonary edema), anytime (during dialysis), by anyone (even a novice sonographer after 1 h of training), and on anybody (since the chest acoustic window usually remains patent even when an echocardiography is not feasible) [15].

The peak E-velocity represents the flow to the left ventricle, which occurs after the left ventricle diastole, reflecting the preload status [9, 10]. Ultrafiltration during hemodialysis results in a marked reduction in the circulating blood volume with a concomitant reduction in the left atrial pressure. Acharya et al. examined the parameters of left ventricular diastolic function among hemodialysis patients [16]. A comparison of the pre- and post-hemodialysis peak mitral E and A velocities showed a decrease in E-velocity, whereas the change in A velocity was not significant. Ultrafiltration during hemodialysis causes a rapid reduction in the preload, resulting in decreased early left ventricular diastolic filling without a change in the atrial phase of filling, thereby reducing the calculated E/A ratio [16]. We confirmed the change in the peak E-velocity and revealed a greater reduction during the first half of the dialysis period than during the second half of the dialysis period. We also confirmed that E/A ratio was declined during the hemodialysis therapy.

The IVC dimensions are strongly associated with the right atrial pressure and blood volume and therefore reflect the intravascular volume accurately.

Table 4 Changes in echocardiographic indices

Parameter	Just after the start (1st)	Middle (2nd)	Just before the end (3rd)	P (1st vs 2nd)	P (2nd vs 3rd)
E (cm/s)	80 ± 26	58 ± 22	51 ± 21	< 0.0001	< 0.0001
A (cm/s)[a]	87 ± 30	77 ± 22	72 ± 20	0.0006	0.0039
E/A	0.95 ± 0.39	0.72 ± 0.26	0.68 ± 0.26	< 0.0001	0.0083
Dct (msec)	255 ± 97	271 ± 92	281 ± 94	Ns	Ns
Ea (cm/s)	5.3 ± 1.7	5.4 ± 1.6	5.6 ± 1.6	0.0459	Ns
TRPG (mmHg)	4.5 ± 12.4	2.8 ± 9.5	2.4 ± 9.0	0.0237	Ns
IVC-ex (mm)	15 ± 4	12 ± 3	11 ± 3	< 0.0001	< 0.0001
IVC-in (mm)	11 ± 5	5 ± 3	3 ± 3	< 0.0001	< 0.0001
IVC collapsibility (%)	31 ± 19	61 ± 18	74 ± 20	< 0.0001	< 0.0001
B-lines	12 ± 5	9 ± 4	5 ± 3	< 0.0001	< 0.0001

Mean ± SD

E peak early diastolic filling velocity, *A* peak Atrial filling velocity, *Dct* deceleration time, *Ea* lateral early diastolic mitral annular velocities, *TRPG* tricuspid regurgitation pressure gradient, *IVC* inferior vena cava dimensions, *ex* exhalation, *in* inspiration

[a]Exclude eight atrial fibrillation

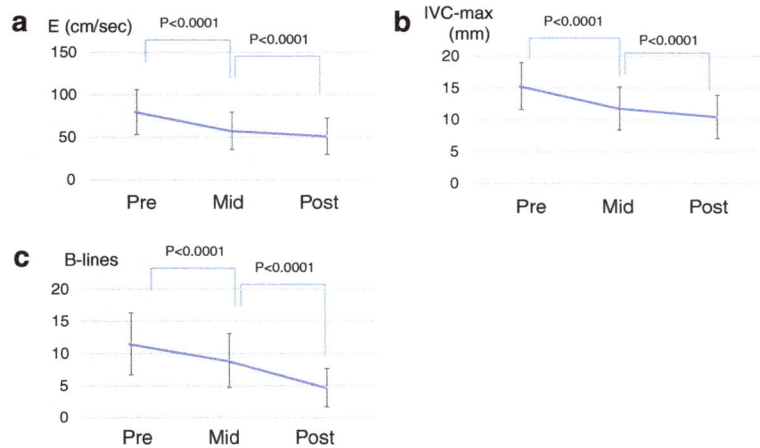

Fig. 2 Changes in echocardiographic indices. **a** Changes of peak E-velocity. **b** Changes of IVC dimensions. **c** Changes of B-lines. *Peak E-velocity* peak early mitral inflow wave velocity, *IVC* inferior vena cava

However, a major limitation of IVC dimension measurements is that ultrasound might not be sensitive enough to detect rapid volume decreases in HD patients because it reflects the intravascular filling grade [17, 18]. Indeed, similar to the change in the peak E-velocity, we showed that the IVC dimensions decreased mainly during the first half of the dialysis period, while the B-lines, which represent lung congestion, decreased significantly mainly during the last half of the dialysis period. This finding may be largely dependent on the time lag in plasma refilling. Alexiadis et al. reported that the number of B-lines has better discriminative power for predicting over- and underhydration, as determined by the IVC dimensions [2]. Mallamaci et al. suggested that the detection of extracellular water in the lung compartment constitutes a reliable tool for the prognosis of overhydration and is thus amenable to intervention [19]. So, we should be careful that even if the IVC dimensions are sufficiently reduced, lung congestion may still exist and should be treated.

Our study had some limitations. The sample size was relatively small, and the study was performed at a single institution. Activities of daily living of some patients

Table 5 Comparison of the changes in values between the middle to pre-dialysis periods and the post-dialysis to middle periods

	2nd–1st	3rd–2nd	P value
ΔE (cm/s)	− 23 ± 14	− 7 ± 6	< 0.0001
ΔIVC-ex (mm)	− 4 ± 3	− 1 ± 2	< 0.0001
ΔB-lines	− 3 ± 3	− 4 ± 2	0.0016

Mean ± SD

1st just after the start, *2nd* middle, *3rd* just before the end, *E* peak early diastolic filling velocity, *IVC* inferior vena cava dimensions, *ex* exhalation

were poor, so we could not examine height of patients. In addition, the limitations of lung ultrasound are essentially patient-dependent. Obese patients may be more difficult to examine because of the thickness of their ribcages and soft tissues. Furthermore, in this analysis, we performed ultrasound examinations only at the end of the hemodialysis therapy. However, it has been suggested that post-dialysis assessments should ideally occur 2 h after hemodialysis because of the re-equilibration of interstitial and intravascular compartments [20, 21]. Accordingly, further study is needed to evaluate the relationship between fluid removal and the timing of post-dialysis assessments in hemodialysis patients. Factors which could affect the change of the number of B-lines are important for the clinician. The change of B-lines was negatively related to the number of B-lines at the start of the hemodialysis therapy (r^2 = 0.609, $P < 0.0001$, data not shown). We should examine the association between the change of the number of B-lines and various factor under the same number of B-lines at the start of hemodialysis therapy, but we could not because of the small number of study participant. Even though ultrasound of extravascular lung water is reported as a new standard for pulmonary congestion [15], there is still no gold standard of examination to evaluate excess body water. In this study, we could not show other possible parameters such as chest X-ray or bioimpedance spectroscopy. Accordingly, further study will be needed to clarify this finding. Another limitation of this study is that we could not show the optimal number of B-lines after hemodialysis therapy. B-lines within physiological range may be present. We have previously reported that B-lines are associated with low serum level of albumin and low body weight [6]. So, optimal number of B-lines may be different among hemodialysis patients.

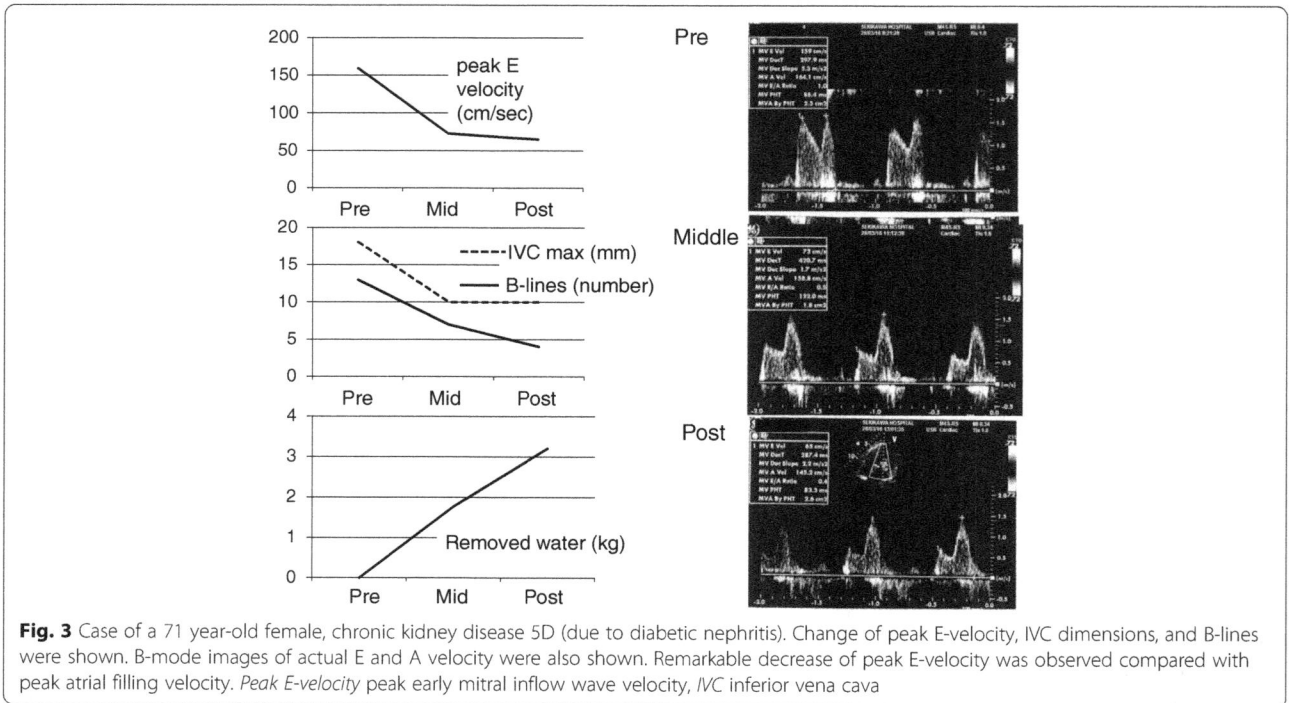

Fig. 3 Case of a 71 year-old female, chronic kidney disease 5D (due to diabetic nephritis). Change of peak E-velocity, IVC dimensions, and B-lines were shown. B-mode images of actual E and A velocity were also shown. Remarkable decrease of peak E-velocity was observed compared with peak atrial filling velocity. *Peak E-velocity* peak early mitral inflow wave velocity, *IVC* inferior vena cava

Conclusions

We showed that the peak E-velocity and IVC dimensions were reduced mainly during the first half of the dialysis period, while the number of B-lines decreased significantly mainly during the last half of the dialysis period. Even if the IVC dimensions are sufficiently reduced, caution is required as lung congestion may still exist.

Abbreviations

E-velocity: Peak early mitral inflow wave velocity; IVC: Inferior vena cava peak; NT-proBNP: N-terminal pro-brain natriuretic peptide

Acknowledgements

The authors are very grateful to the dialysis staff who understood the clinical importance of this study and who provided high-quality data in Sekikawa Hospital.

Funding

This study was not supported by any grants or funding.

Authors' contributions

KK planned the study, searched the literature, assessed the studies, extracted the data, analyzed the data, and prepared the article. KK and SO searched the literature, assessed the studies, and assisted in the article preparation. KK performed the lung echo. KN and TA assisted in the article preparation. All authors read and approved the final manuscript.

Competing interests

The authors declare that they have no competing interests.

Author details

[1]Department of Medicine, Kidney Center, Tokyo Women's Medical University, Tokyo, Japan. [2]Department of Nephrology, Sekikawa Hospital, Tokyo, Japan. [3]Department of Cardiology, Sekikawa Hospital, Tokyo, Japan. [4]Department of Blood Purification, Tohto Sangenjaya Clinic, 2-13-2 Taishido, Setagaya-ku, Tokyo 154-0004, Japan.

References

1. Tonelli M, Wiebe N, Culleton B, et al. Chronic kidney disease and mortality risk: a systematic review. J Am Soc Nephrol. 2006;17:2034–47.
2. Alexiadis G, Panagoutsos S, Roumeliotis S, Stibiris I, Markos A, Kantartzi K, et al. Comparison of multiple fluid status assessment methods in patients on chronic hemodialysis. Int Urol Nephrol. 2017;49:525–32.
3. Lichtenstein D. Pneumothorax and introduction to ultrasound signs in the lung. In: Heilmann U, Wilbertz H, Gosling A, editors. General ultrasound in the critically ill. 1st ed. Heidelberg: Springer-Verlag; 2005. p. 105–15.
4. Agricola E, Bove T, Oppizzi M, Marino G, Zangrillo A, Margonato A, et al. "Ultrasound comet-tail images": a marker of pulmonary edema: a comparative study with wedge pressure and extravascular lung water. Chest. 2005;127:1690–5.
5. Kajimoto K, Madeen K, Nakayama T, Tsudo H, Kuroda T, Abe T. Rapid evaluation by lung-cardiac-inferior vena cava (LCI) integrated ultrasound for differentiating heart failure from pulmonary disease as the cause of acute dyspnea in the emergency setting. Cardiovasc Ultrasound. 2012;10:49–51.
6. Kuzuhara S, Otsubo S, Kajimoto K, Akiba T, Nitta K. Association between B-lines detected during lung ultrasound and various factors in hemodialysis patients. Ren Replace Ther. 2017;3:17.
7. Noble VE, Murray AF, Capp R, Sylvia-Reardon MH, Steele DJ, Liteplo A. Ultrasound assessment for extravascular lung water in patients undergoing hemodialysis: time course for resolution. Chest. 2009;135:1433–9.

8. Simonson JS, Schiller NB. Sonospirometry: a new method for noninvasive estimation of mean right atrial pressure based on two-dimensional echographic measurements of the inferior vena cava during measured inspiration. J Am Coll Cardiol. 1988;11:557–64.

9. Triulzi MO, Castini D, Ornaghi M, Vitolo E. Effects of preload reduction on mitral flow velocity pattern in normal subjects. Am J Cardiol. 1990; 66:995–1001.

10. Sztajzel J, Ruedin P, Monin C, Stoermann C, Leski M, Rutishauser W, et al. Effect of altered loading conditions during haemodialysis on left ventricular filling pattern. Eur Heart J. 1993;14:655–61.

11. Cardim N, Fernandez Golfin C, Ferreira D, Aubele A, Toste J, Cobos MA, et al. Usefulness of a new miniaturized echocardiographic system in outpatient cardiology consultations as an extension of physical examination. J Am Soc Echocardiogr. 2011;24:117–24.

12. Liebo MJ, Israel RL, Lillie EO, Smith MR, Rubenson DS, Topol EJ. Is pocket mobile echocardiography the next-generation stethoscope? A cross-sectional comparison of rapidly acquired images with standard transthoracic echocardiography. Ann Intern Med. 2011;155:33–8.

13. Volpicelli G, Elbarbary M, Blaivas M, Lichtenstein DA, Mathis G, Kirkpatrick AW, et al. International liaison committee on lung ultrasound (ILC-LUS) for international consensus conference on lung ultrasound (ICC-LUS). International evidence-based recommendations for point-of-care lung ultrasound. Intensive Care Med. 2012;38:577–91.

14. Zoccali C. Lung ultrasound in the management of fluid volume in dialysis patients: potential usefulness. Semin Dial. 2017;30:6–9.

15. Picano E, Pellikka PA. Ultrasound of extravascular lung water: a new standard for pulmonary congestion. Eur Heart J. 2016;37:2097–104.

16. Acharya P, Ranabhat K, Trikhatri Y, Manandhar DN, Sharma SK, Karki P. Effect of preload reduction by haemodialysis on doppler indices of diastolic function in patients with end-stage renal disease. Kathmandu Univ Med J (KUMJ). 2008;6:98–101.

17. Feissel M, Michard F, Faller JP, Teboul JL. The respiratory variation in inferior vena cava diameter as a guide to fluid therapy. Intensive Care Med. 2004;30:1834–7.

18. Brennan JM, Ronan A, Goonewardena S, Blair JE, Hammes M, Shah D, et al. Handcarried ultrasound measurement of the inferior vena cava for assessment of intravascular volume status in the outpatient hemodialysis clinic. Clin J Am Soc Nephrol. 2006;1:749–53.

19. Mallamaci F, Benedetto FA, Tripepi R, Rastelli S, Castellino P, Tripepi G, et al. Detection of pulmonary congestion by chest ultrasound in dialysis patients. JACC Cardiovasc Imaging. 2010;3:586–94.

20. Katzarski KS, Nisell J, Randmaa I, Danielsson A, Freyschuss U, Bergstrom J. A critical evaluation of ultrasound measurement of inferior vena cava diameter in assessing dry weight in normotensive and hypertensive hemodialysis patients. Am J Kidney Dis. 1997;30:459–65.

21. Kouw PM, Kooman JP, Cheriex EC, Olthof CG, de Vries PM, Leunissen KM. Assessment of postdialysis dry weight: a comparison of techniques. J Am Soc Nephrol. 1993;4:98–104.

30

Decreased level of serum carnitine might lead to arteriosclerosis progression via the accumulation of advanced glycation end products in maintenance hemodialysis patients

Yumi Kamada[1,2], Takashi Masuda[2*], Kazuhiko Kotani[4], Shinya Tanaka[2], Takeshi Nakamura[1,3], Nobuaki Hamazaki[2], Yoko Itoh[1], Ibuki Moriguchi[1], Naoyuki Kobayashi[1], Michihito Okubo[1], Kazuhiro Takeuchi[5], Shokichi Naito[5] and Yasuo Takeuchi[5]

Abstract

Background: Carnitine is reported to improve insulin resistance and reduce oxidative stress. Hyperglycemia and increased oxidative stress are well known to promote the production of advanced glycation end products (AGEs) that can lead to arteriosclerosis in patients with maintenance hemodialysis (HD). In the present study, we aimed to determine whether decreased level of serum carnitine accelerated arteriosclerosis and to clarify the relationships between carnitine, AGEs, and arteriosclerosis in HD patients.

Methods: We recruited 116 patients (65 men and 51 women, 62 ± 13 years) undergoing HD three times a week. We measured pre-HD serum free carnitine prior to the first weekly session. AGE level was quantitatively evaluated by measuring skin autofluorescence (SAF) with AGE reader. Arteriosclerosis was evaluated by measuring carotid intima-media thickness (cIMT). Relationships between free carnitine, SAF, and cIMT were analyzed, and significant limiting factors for arteriosclerosis were identified using univariate and multivariate regression analyses.

Results: Free carnitine ranged from 14.9 to 53.3 μmol/L (mean, 28.6 ± 8.1 μmol/L). Free carnitine was negatively correlated with SAF ($r = -0.223$, $P = 0.017$) and cIMT ($r = -0.252$, $P = 0.006$). SAF was positively correlated with cIMT ($r = 0.263$, $P = 0.005$). Free carnitine was identified as a significant independent limiting factor for cIMT ($\beta = -0.194$, $P = 0.037$).

Conclusions: Decreased level of serum carnitine might lead to the progression of arteriosclerosis via the AGE accumulation in HD patients.

Keywords: Advanced glycation end products, Arteriosclerosis, Carnitine, Hemodialysis

---

* Correspondence: tak9999@med.kitasato-u.ac.jp
[2]Department of Angiology and Cardiology, Kitasato University Graduate School of Medical Sciences, 1-15-1 Kitasato, Minami-ku, Sagamihara, Kanagawa, Japan
Full list of author information is available at the end of the article

Background

In maintenance hemodialysis (HD) patients, oxidative stress and hyperglycemia are known to contribute to the formation of advanced glycation end products (AGEs) that are formed by non-enzymatic glycation reactions between reduced sugars and biological macromolecules such as proteins [1, 2]. In addition, AGEs are slowly metabolized in HD patients, given the role of the kidney in their degradation and excretion [3]. Consequently, AGE accumulation accelerates in the tissues and organs of HD patients [4]. AGEs, binding to AGE receptors on vascular endothelial cells, generate reactive oxygen species and induce vascular inflammation, which can accelerate the progression of arteriosclerosis [5]. Indeed, a number of studies have found that the progression of arteriosclerosis is more accelerated in HD patients due to the high accumulation of AGEs relative to age- and sex-matched healthy individuals [4].

Carnitine is an essential cofactor for the transport of long-chain fatty acids and β-oxidation in mitochondria [6]. It enhances the oxidative utilization of glucose through the acceleration of pyruvate uptake in mitochondria [7]. Moreover, it improves insulin sensitivity in skeletal muscles by promoting glucose utilization [8]. Carnitine also suppresses oxidative stress by chelating free Fe^{2+} ion and activating antioxidants [9]. The antioxidant efficacy of carnitine treatment has been reported in various conditions such as hypertension, hypercholesterolemia, atherosclerosis, or aging that increase systemic oxidative stress [10–13]. Thus, carnitine can prevent AGE accumulation in tissues and organs by reducing oxidative stress and improving glucose metabolism. The muscle content of carnitine is substantially reduced in HD patients due to decreased carnitine synthesis in kidney, removal from blood during HD, and insufficient dietary intake, which is reflected in serum carnitine level [14]. Based on this, we hypothesized that decreased level of serum carnitine would enhance AGE accumulation by exacerbating glucose metabolism and increasing oxidative stress, thereby promoting the progression of arteriosclerosis. However, it remains unclear whether decreased level of serum carnitine has this effect in HD patients. To this end, this study aimed to determine whether decreased level of serum carnitine serves as a factor that accelerates arteriosclerosis and to clarify the relationships between carnitine, AGEs, and arteriosclerosis in HD patients.

Methods

This study was approved by the Bioethics Committee for Clinical Research A of Jichi Medical University Hospital. Written informed consent was obtained from all patients after they received a detailed explanation of the study protocol.

One hundred and thirty patients with end-stage renal disease who received outpatient care for regular maintenance HD three times a week at Sohbudai Nieren Clinic in August 2015 were recruited. Exclusion criteria were as follows: patients with malignancy or dementia or those regularly taking a carnitine-based drug. That is, 8, 3, and 3 patients were excluded for malignancy, dementia, and taking a carnitine-based drug, respectively. Consequently, the final study population consisted of 116 patients on maintenance HD.

Study design

After clinical characteristics of the patients were obtained from medical records or by interview, we performed blood examinations and AGE measurements and assessed carotid intima-media thickness (cIMT) as an indicator of arteriosclerosis.

Clinical characteristics and blood examination

The following clinical characteristics were assessed: gender, age, height, dry body weight, body mass index, systolic and diastolic blood pressure, heart rate, duration of HD, prevalence of diabetes mellitus, treatment, and left ventricular ejection fraction. Body mass index was calculated as dry body weight in kilograms divided by height in meters squared. Systolic and diastolic blood pressure and heart rate were measured in the supine position using a vascular profile device (BP-203RPE, Omron Colin, Kyoto, Japan) before the HD session. Left ventricular ejection fraction was measured with an echocardiogram (SSD-5500 system, Aloka, Tokyo, Japan) as an indicator of left ventricular function when patients had stable hemodynamic condition under the optimal dry weight after the HD session.

Blood samples were collected just before the HD session after a 2-day HD interval to measure blood hemoglobin A1c and serum levels of glycated albumin (GA), triglyceride, total cholesterol, low-density lipoprotein cholesterol, and high-density lipoprotein cholesterol as indicators of glycolipid metabolism. We also measured serum levels of albumin, creatinine, uric acid, urea nitrogen, β2-microglobumin, C-reactive protein, corrected calcium [15], and phosphate. Serum levels of free carnitine, acyl carnitine, and total carnitine were measured with the enzyme cycling method [16].

Fractional clearance of urea (Kt/V) was used to evaluate the HD adequacy, which was given by urea clearance (K, mL/min), HD treatment time (t, min), and urea distribution volume (V, mL) [17].

Advanced glycation end products

We measured skin autofluorescence (SAF) as an indicator of AGEs. SAF was determined using an AGE reader with an ultraviolet source of specific wavelengths (DiagOptics

BV, Groningen, The Netherlands), which was reported to reflect AGE accumulation in biopsied skin [18]. The forearm was placed on the AGE reader to measure SAF at three sites, 1 cm away from each other, where neither bruises nor obvious pigmentation was present. SAF was automatically analyzed with a device connected to a computer that had analysis software installed [19].

Arteriosclerosis

The carotid intima-media thickness (cIMT) was measured in the supine position with an ultrasonogram (SSD-5500 system, Aloka) by a skilled technician who had no prior knowledge of patients' clinical characteristics. The far and near walls of the right and left common carotid arteries, carotid bulbs, and internal carotid arteries were scanned in both short-axis and long-axis views using a 11-MHz linear probe. The thickest site of the intima-media complex including plaque lesions was measured as the maximum cIMT in increments of 0.1 mm to assess the severity of arteriosclerosis.

Statistical analysis

All data are expressed as mean ± standard deviation. We analyzed relationships between free carnitine, GA, SAF, and cIMT using Spearman's correlation coefficient. $P < 0.050$ was considered statistically significant. Univariate and multivariate regression analyses were performed to clarify the relationship between free carnitine and cIMT. In the analyses, we used cIMT as a dependent variable, and factors related to arteriosclerosis progression as independent variables, after assessing the multicollinearity among independent variables [20]. All statistical analyses were performed using the Statistical Package for Social Sciences, version 23.0 for Windows (IBM Corporation, NY, USA).

Results

Clinical characteristics of the patients are summarized in Table 1. The mean age of patients was 62 ± 13 years, and 54.9% were male. Patients with a history of type 2 diabetes mellitus comprised 41.4% of the study population. Serum level of free carnitine ranged from 14.9 to 53.3 μmol/L (mean, 28.6 ± 8.1 μmol/L), and cIMT from 0.6 to 3.3 mm (mean, 1.6 ± 0.6 mm).

Relationships between free carnitine, GA, and SAF are shown in Fig. 1. No significant relationship was found between free carnitine and GA. SAF was negatively correlated with free carnitine ($r = -0.223$, $P = 0.017$).

Relationships between free carnitine, SAF, and cIMT are shown in Fig. 2. The cIMT was negatively correlated with free carnitine ($r = -0.252$, $P = 0.006$) and positively correlated with SAF ($r = 0.263$, $P = 0.005$).

Table 1 Clinical characteristics

Number of patients (male/female) (n)	116 (65/51)
Age (years)	62 ± 13
Body mass index (kg/m^2)	21.3 ± 3.3
Type 2 diabetes mellitus (+/−)(n)	48/68
Treatment (%)	
ARB/ACE inhibitor	31.0
Iron therapy	37.1
Systolic blood pressure (mmHg)	149 ± 24
Diastolic blood pressure (mmHg)	88 ± 16
Heart rate (/min)	77 ± 12
Duration of hemodialysis (years)	7.6 ± .2
Kt/V (range)	1.10 ± 0.31
Hemoglobin A1c (%)	5.4 ± 0.7
Glycated albumin (%)	16.7 ± 3.8
Triglyceride (mg/dL)	139 ± 110
Total cholesterol (mg/dL)	169 ± 32
Low-density lipoprotein cholesterol (mg/dL)	94 ± 26
High-density lipoprotein cholesterol (mg/dL)	51 ± 19
Albumin (g/dL)	3.8 ± 0.3
Creatinine (mg/dL)	11.26 ± 3.08
Uric acid (mg/dL)	6.9 ± 1.4
Urea nitrogen (mg/dL)	62.9 ± 13.5
Corrected calcium (mg/dL)	9.0 ± 0.8
Phosphate (mg/dL)	5.7 ± 1.3
C-reactive protein (mg/dL)	0.27 ± 0.79
β2-microglobumin (mg/L)	24.9 ± 5.4
Total carnitine (μmol/L)	44.5 ± 11.7
Free carnitine (μmol/L)	28.6 ± 8.1
Acyl carnitine (μmol/L)	15.9 ± 4.7
Acyl carnitine/free carnitine	0.6 ± 0.1
Skin autofluorescence (arbitrary unit)	3.4 ± 0.7
Left ventricular ejection fraction (%)	66.9 ± 8.9

Data are presented as mean ± standard deviation. Kt/V is used to evaluate the hemodialysis adequacy
ARB angiotensin II receptor blocker, *ACE inhibitor* angiotensin-converting enzyme inhibitor

The results of univariate and multivariate regression analyses for cIMT are shown in Table 2. There was no significant multicollinearity in independent variables. Age, prevalence of diabetes mellitus, creatinine, albumin, and free carnitine were significantly correlated with cIMT ($\beta = 0.548$, $P = 0.001$; $\beta = 0.225$, $P = 0.015$; $\beta = -0.364$, $P = 0.001$; $\beta = -0.336$, $P = 0.001$; $\beta = -0.252$, $P = 0.006$, respectively). Age, albumin, and free carnitine were identified as significant independent limiting factors for cIMT ($\beta = 0.310$, $P = 0.006$; $\beta = -0.176$, $P = 0.044$; $\beta = -0.194$, $P = 0.037$, respectively).

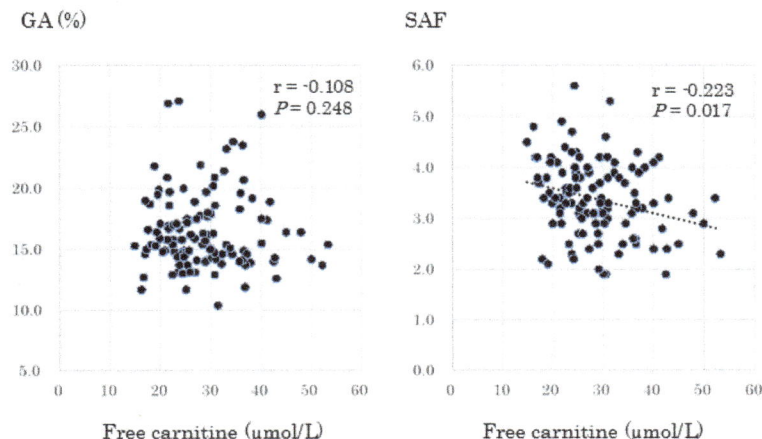

Fig. 1 Relationships between free carnitine, GA, and SAF. GA glycated albumin, SAF skin autoflourescence

Discussion

In the present study, we found that a decreased level of serum carnitine was a significant independent determinant of the arteriosclerosis progression in HD patients. That is, multivariate regression analysis revealed that free carnitine was identified as one of significant factors increasing cIMT. In addition, we found that free carnitine was negatively correlated with SAF and that SAF was positively correlated with cIMT.

A previous study showed that decreased serum level of carnitine was independently correlated with increased tissue accumulation of AGEs in HD patients [21]. It has been also reported that AGE accumulation accelerates the progression of arteriosclerosis in HD patients [4]. Therefore, our findings showed that decreased level of serum carnitine might enhance AGE accumulation, thereby promoting the progression of arteriosclerosis in them.

Carnitine has been known to reduce AGE accumulation in tissues and organs by reducing oxidative stress

and activating glucose metabolism [22]. However, the present study showed no significant relationship between free carnitine and GA. Because we recruited HD patients whose glucose metabolism was well controlled, most of their GA values were under the target value for glycemic control [23]. That may be the reason why we could not find the significant relationship between them.

Systolic blood pressure and low-density lipoprotein cholesterol are generally known to accelerate arteriosclerosis [24]. However, there were no significant relationships between systolic blood pressure or low-density lipoprotein cholesterol and cIMT in the present study. Savage et al. reported that no significant relationship between systolic blood pressure and cIMT was found in HD patients [25]. As the reason, they stated that the values of systolic blood pressure well controlled with antihypertensives were used for the data analysis. Furthermore, it was reported that hypertension or dyslipidemia was correlated with the progression of arteriosclerosis,

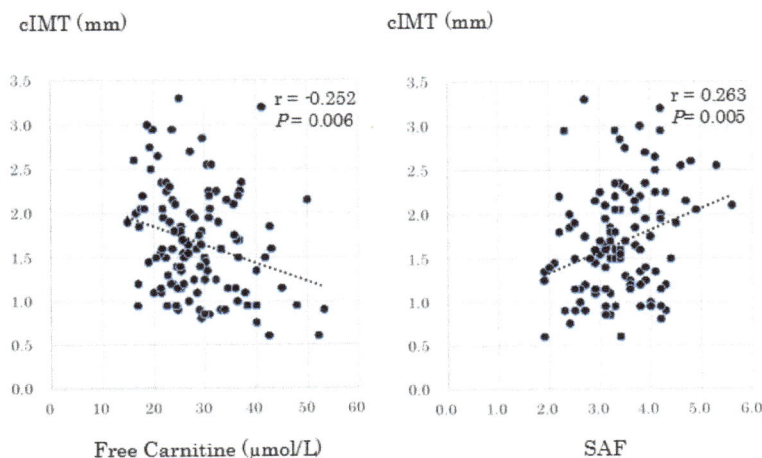

Fig. 2 Relationships between free carnitine, SAF, and cIMT. SAF skin autoflourescence, cIMT carotid intima-media thickness

Table 2 Results of univariate and multivariate regression analyses for carotid intima-media thickness

	Univariate regression		Multivariate regression	
	β	P	β	P
Gender	0.132	0.158	0.159	0.108
Age (years)	0.548	0.001	0.310	0.006
Type 2 diabetes mellitus	0.225	0.015	0.106	0.235
Body mass index (kg/m^2)	− 0.162	0.082	− 0.037	0.685
Systolic blood pressure (mmHg)	− 0.089	0.344	− 0.065	0.432
Low-density lipoprotein cholesterol (mg/dL)	− 0.143	0.124	− 0.017	0.833
Creatinine (mg/dL)	− 0.364	0.001	− 0.091	0.411
Albumin (g/dL)	− 0.336	0.001	− 0.176	0.044
Corrected calcium (mg/dL)	0.055	0.556	0.040	0.628
Phosphorus (mg/dL)	− 0.092	0.327	0.063	0.480
Free carnitine (μmol/mL)	− 0.252	0.006	− 0.194	0.037

when arteriosclerosis was assessed by the mean cIMT that reflected the arterial wall thickness [26]. However, the maximum cIMT was used to assess arteriosclerosis in the present study, which was known to reflect the arterial wall thickness and atheroma formation [26]. The reason why no significant relationships were found between them is to adopt the values of systolic blood pressure and low-density lipoprotein cholesterol that were well controlled with medications and also to adopt the maximum cIMT for data analysis.

There are some limitations worth noting. First, although we speculated that reduced oxidative stress was an underlying mechanism by which carnitine reduces AGEs, we did not evaluate the relationship between carnitine and oxidative stress. In future studies, free radical and lipid peroxide production should be assessed in order to examine the relationship between carnitine and oxidative stress. Second, we could not demonstrate the significant relationship between carnitine and glucose metabolism in the present study. In order to clarify whether carnitine reduces AGEs through the improvement of glucose metabolism, we should perform the re-analysis using large sample sizes in diabetic HD patients and non-diabetic HD patients taking into consideration their condition such as diabetes treatment. Finally, the study design was cross-sectional, and we did not directly examine the effects of carnitine on the progression of arteriosclerosis. Future prospective clinical studies should be planned to elucidate the relationship between carnitine administration, AGEs, and arteriosclerosis.

Because arteriosclerosis is the primary cause of death in HD patients [27], there is a need for promising strategies to prevent its progression. Previous studies showed that carnitine administration attenuated the progression of atherosclerosis and improved cardiovascular dysfunction in HD patients [28, 29]. Given that serum level of carnitine is significantly reduced in most HD patients

[14], administering carnitine to this population could potentially prevent the progression of arteriosclerosis and improve prognosis.

Conclusions

Decreased level of serum carnitine might lead to the progression of arteriosclerosis via the AGE accumulation in maintenance HD patients.

Abbreviations
AGEs: Advanced glycation end products; cIMT: Carotid intima-media thickness; GA: Glycated albumin; HD: Hemodialysis; SAF: Skin autofluorescence

Acknowledgements
We thank Mr. Makoto Takenaka and Ms. Hitomi Noda for the carotid artery ultrasound examination.

Funding
This study was not supported by any grants or funding.

Authors' contributions
YK designed the study, collected the clinical data, performed the data analysis, and wrote the manuscript. TM designed the study and wrote the manuscript. KK designed the study and performed the data analysis. TN collected the clinical data. ST, NH, YI, IM, NK, MO, KT, SN, and YT provided substantial revisions to the manuscript. All authors read and approved the final manuscript.

Competing interests
The authors declare that they have no competing interests.

Author details

[1]Sohbudai Nieren Clinic, Zama, Japan. [2]Department of Angiology and Cardiology, Kitasato University Graduate School of Medical Sciences, 1-15-1 Kitasato, Minami-ku, Sagamihara, Kanagawa, Japan. [3]Department of Rehabilitation Sciences, Kitasato University Graduate School of Medical Sciences, Sagamihara, Japan. [4]Division of Community and Family Medicine, Jichi Medical University, Tochigi, Japan. [5]Division of Nephrology, Department of Internal Medicine, Kitasato University School of Medicine, Sagamihara, Japan.

References

1. Miyata T, Wada Y, Cai Z, Iida Y, Horie K, Yasuda Y, et al. Implication of an increased oxidative stress in the formation of advanced glycation end products in patients with end-stage renal failure. Kidney Int. 1997; 51(4):1170–81.
2. Brownlee M, Cerami A, Vlassara H. Advanced glycosylation end products in tissue and the biochemical basis of diabetic complications. N Engl J Med. 1988;318(20):1315–21.
3. Miyata T, Ueda Y, Horie K, Nangaku M, Tanaka S, van Ypersele de Strihou C, et al. Renal catabolism of advanced glycation end products: the fate of pentosidine. Kidney Int. 1998;53(2):416–22.
4. Ueno H, Koyama H, Tanaka S, Fukumoto S, Shinohara K, Shoji T, et al. Skin autofluorescence, a marker for advanced glycation end product accumulation, is associated with arterial stiffness in patients with end-stage renal disease. Metabolism. 2008;57(10):1452–7.
5. Basta G, Schmidt AM, De Caterina R. Advanced glycation end products and vascular inflammation: implications for accelerated atherosclerosis in diabetes. Cardiovasc Res. 2004;63(4):582–92.
6. Vaz FM, Wanders RJ. Carnitine biosynthesis in mammals. Biochem J. 2002; 361(3):417–29.
7. Siliprandi N, Di Lisa F, Pieralisi G, Ripari P, Maccari F, Menabo R, et al. Metabolic changes induced by maximal exercise in human subjects following L-carnitine administration. Biochim Biophys Acta. 1990;1034(1):17–21.
8. Rajasekar P, Anuradha CV. L-carnitine inhibits protein glycation in vitro and in vivo: evidence for a role in diabetic management. Acta Diabetol. 2007; 44(2):83–90.
9. Cao Y, Qu HJ, Li P, Wang CB, Wang LX, Han ZW. Single dose administration of L-carnitine improves antioxidant activities in healthy subjects. Tohoku J Exp Med. 2011;224(3):209–13.
10. Sayed-Ahmed MM, Khattab MM, Gad MZ, Mostafa N. L-carnitine prevents the progression of atherosclerotic lesions in hypercholesterolaemic rabbits. Pharmacol Res. 2001;44(3):235–42.
11. Kalaiselvi T, Panneerselvam C. Effect of L-carnitine on the status of lipid peroxidation and antioxidants in aging rats. J Nutr Biochem. 1998;9(10):575–81.
12. Dayanandan A, Kumar P, Panneerselvam C. Protective role of L-carnitine on liver and heart lipid peroxidation in atherosclerotic rats. J Nutr Biochem. 2001;12(5):254–7.
13. Gomez-Amores L, Mate A, Miguel-Carrasco JL, Jimenez L, Jos A, Camean AM, et al. L-carnitine attenuates oxidative stress in hypertensive rats. J Nutr Biochem. 2007;18(8):533–40.
14. Evans A. Dialysis-related carnitine disorder and levocarnitine pharmacology. Am J Kidney Dis. 2003;41(4 Suppl 4):S13–26.
15. Payne RB, Little AJ, Williams RB, Milner JR. Interpretation of serum calcium in patients with abnormal serum proteins. Br Med J. 1973;4(5893):643–6.
16. Takahashi M, Ueda S, Misaki H, Sugiyama N, Matsumoto K, Matsuo N, et al. Carnitine determination by an enzymatic cycling method with carnitine dehydrogenase. Clin Chem. 1994;40(5):817–21.
17. Gotch FA, Sargent JA. A mechanistic analysis of the National Cooperative Dialysis Study (NCDS). Kidney Int. 1985;28(3):526–34.
18. Meerwaldt R, Hartog JW, Graaff R, Huisman RJ, Links TP, den Hollander NC, et al. Skin autofluorescence, a measure of cumulative metabolic stress and advanced glycation end products, predicts mortality in hemodialysis patients. J Am Soc Nephrol. 2005;16(12):3687–93.
19. Meerwaldt R, Graaff R, Oomen PH, Links TP, Jager JJ, Alderson NL, et al. Simple non-invasive assessment of advanced glycation endproduct accumulation. Diabetologia. 2004;47(7):1324–30.
20. Alain F, ENI Z, Chris S. Elphick: a protocol for data exploration to avoid common statistical problems. Methods Ecol Evol. 2010;1:3–14.
21. Adachi T, Fukami K, Yamagishi S, Kaida Y, Ando R, Sakai K, et al. Decreased serum carnitine is independently correlated with increased tissue accumulation levels of advanced glycation end products in haemodialysis patients. Nephrology (Carlton). 2012;17(8):689–94.
22. Fukami K, Yamagishi S, Sakai K, Kaida Y, Adachi T, Ando R, et al. Potential inhibitory effects of L-carnitine supplementation on tissue advanced glycation end products in patients with hemodialysis. Rejuvenation Res. 2013;16(6):460–6.
23. Nakao T, Inaba M, Abe M, Kaizu K, Shima K, Babazono T, et al. Best practice for diabetic patients on hemodialysis 2012. Ther Apher Dial. 2015;19:40–66.
24. Sarnak MJ, Levey AS, Schoolwerth AC, Coresh J, Culleton B, Hamm LL, et al. Kidney disease as a risk factor for development of cardiovascular disease: a statement from the American Heart Association councils on kidney in cardiovascular disease, high blood pressure research, clinical cardiology, and epidemiology and prevention. Hypertension. 2003;42(5):1050–65.
25. Savage T, Clarke AL, Giles M, Tomson CR, Raine AE. Calcified plaque is common in the carotid and femoral arteries of dialysis patients without clinical vascular disease. Nephrol Dial Transplant. 1998;13(8):2004–12.
26. Nakashima A, Yorioka N, Asakimori Y, Ito T, Masaki T, Shigemoto K, et al. Different risk factors for the maximum and the mean carotid intima-media thickness in hemodialysis patients. Intern Med. 2003;42(11):1095–9.
27. Nakai S, Masakane I, Akiba T, Shigematsu T, Yamagata K, Watanabe Y, et al. Overview of regular dialysis treatment in Japan as of 31 December 2006. Ther Apher Dial. 2008;12(6):428–56.
28. Higuchi T, Abe M, Yamazaki T, Mizuno M, Okawa E, Ando H, et al. Effects of levocarnitine on brachial-ankle pulse wave velocity in hemodialysis patients: a randomized controlled trial. Nutrients. 2014;6(12):5992–6004.
29. van Es A, Henny FC, Kooistra MP, Lobatto S, Scholte HR. Amelioration of cardiac function by L-carnitine administration in patients on haemodialysis. Contrib Nephrol. 1992;98:28–35.

31

L-carnitine in critically ill patients—a case series study

Takehiko Oami[1], Taku Oshima[1*], Noriyuki Hattori[1], Ayako Teratani[1], Saori Honda[2], Toshihiko Yoshida[2] and Shigeto Oda[1]

Abstract

Background: L-carnitine is essential for lipid metabolism, and lack of L-carnitine intake and loss by treatments lead to carnitine depletion causing muscle weakness, anemia, and immune dysfunction. Carnitine depletion occurs in critically ill patients after long treatments, but its epidemiology or the risk factors remain unclear. This study aims to investigate the prevalence and risk factors of L-carnitine depletion in critically ill patients.

Methods: Sixty-four patients were enrolled for the study. Total and free L-carnitine concentrations (t- and f-Carnitine) were measured at ICU admission and every 7 days afterward during hospitalization. Acylcarnitine- to f-Carnitine ratio (A/F Carnitine ratio) was analyzed in a subgroup of patients treated with continuous renal replacement therapy (CRRT). Acylcarnitine concentration was calculated as the difference between t- and f-Carnitine concentrations.

Results: Carnitine deficiency (f-Carnitine < 36 nmol/mL) was observed in 15 (23.4%) patients at ICU admission. Low body mass index (BMI < 19.5) was associated with a subsequent reduction of L-carnitine during the ICU stay (AUC = 0.81, $p < 0.01$). Sequential Organ Failure Assessment (SOFA) score was correlated with L-carnitine reduction but without a significant cutoff value. Patients treated with CRRT demonstrated elevated A/F Carnitine ratio ($p < 0.05$), possibly due to insufficient elimination or impaired metabolism of carnitine.

Conclusions: Less than one fourth of critically ill patients had carnitine deficiency at ICU admission, while low BMI and high SOFA scores were identified as potential risk factors for reduction of L-carnitine. Patients treated with CRRT presented signs of impaired carnitine metabolism. Further studies to investigate the potential benefits of L-carnitine supplementation may be warranted in these patients.

Keywords: Carnitine, Nutritional support, Critical care, Renal replacement therapy

Background

L-carnitine is an essential compound for energy utilization through lipid metabolism in the skeletal muscle [1]. It is mainly supplied through the regular diet, especially from animal meat and dairy products. It can also be synthesized endogenously from lysine and methionine in the liver and the kidneys. The endogenous composition of L-carnitine comprises of free carnitine and acylcarnitines (L-carnitine in the form of esters such as acetyl L-carnitine) [2, 3]. Carnitine deficiency can occur as a primary disorder due to the deficiency of L-carnitine cellular transporters, but it is more prevalent as secondary deficiency as a result of conditions such as insufficient intake, medical treatments promoting excretion, and excessive elimination by hemodialysis [2].

Critically ill patients are usually nourished artificially by enteral or parenteral feeding, which often leads to the lack of L-carnitine intake. The patients are also frequently treated with continuous renal replacement therapy (CRRT) that may cause L-carnitine depletion, in a similar way to hemodialysis. Lack of L-carnitine impairs the utilization of fatty acid as energy source and leads to muscle weakness and muscle loss due to catabolism, which leads to deterioration of patients' physical function.

* Correspondence: t_oshima@chiba-u.jp; oshima0528@gmail.com
[1]Department of Emergency and Critical Care Medicine, Chiba University Graduate School of Medicine, Chiba University Hospital, 1-8-1 Inohana Chuo-ku, Chiba, Chiba, Japan
Full list of author information is available at the end of the article

It is also suggested to lead to anemia and immune dysfunction [1, 4], leading to infectious complications.

While the prevalence of carnitine deficiency and the effect of supplementation have been studied previously in postoperative patients [5, 6], L-carnitine concentrations of patients admitted to the intensive care unit (ICU) for unscheduled treatments have not been well described. However, these patients are more likely to be treated longer [7] with higher risks of organ failure treatment [7]. Thus, these patients are more likely to develop carnitine depletion and possibly benefit from supplementation. The present study was conducted to define the prevalence of carnitine deficiency and risk factors of L-carnitine depletion in adult critically ill patients admitted to the ICU for unscheduled treatment and to identify the potential indications for supplementation of carnitine. Further analysis was conducted to determine the indication of carnitine supplementation in subgroup of patients who underwent CRRT [8].

Methods

Study design

A prospective observational study to analyze the total and free L-carnitine concentrations at ICU admission and during the hospital stay was conducted on adult critically ill patients. The primary objective was to define the prevalence of carnitine deficiency at the time of ICU admission. The secondary objectives were to define patient characteristics at ICU admission that indicate risks for future carnitine depletion and to define ICU treatments that influence L-carnitine concentrations. Patients were treated according to local treatment protocols and were not supplemented with L-carnitine as a part of their treatments. All patient samples were collected strictly from residual serum samples from routine blood analysis at ICU admission and during the hospital stay.

Patient selection

Adult patients admitted to the ICU of Chiba University Hospital, for unscheduled treatment from February 1, 2014, to March 30, 2014, were enrolled. Patients were excluded if they were under the age of 18 years, were admitted to the ICU for post elective surgery care, readmitted to the ICU, or were not expected to survive for more than 24 h at the time of screening for eligibility.

L-carnitine analysis

Residual serum samples were collected for L-carnitine analyses. Initial samples were collected from the routine blood evaluation at the time of ICU admission and followed every 7 days during the hospitalization for a maximum of 28 days. As sample collection relied on residual serum, follow-up samples collected within 1 day before or after the scheduled follow-up date were considered valid for evaluation.

All blood samples were centrifuged immediately after sampling at the central clinical laboratory of Chiba University Hospital and stored in serum form at 4 °C for no longer than 72 h. Samples were then collected and stored in the − 80 °C freezer until the analysis. L-carnitine concentrations were analyzed as total carnitine concentration (t-Carnitine) and free carnitine concentration (f-Carnitine) for all obtained samples. Acylcarnitine concentration was calculated as the difference of t-Carnitine and f-Carnitine concentrations (Acylcarnitine = t-Carnitine − f-Carnitine). t-Carnitine and f-Carnitine analyses were conducted by the enzyme cycling method (KAINOS laboratories Inc., Tokyo, Japan) [9] which uses carnitine dehydrogenase as the primary enzyme and thionicotinamide-adenine dinucleotide (thio-NAD+) and nicotinamide adenine dinucleotide (NADH) as the coenzymes. All samples were analyzed within 60 days from the sampling date. Preliminary tests were conducted to verify this procedure, which revealed no significant change in the measured results after 7-day storage at 4 ° C or after 60-day storage at − 80 °C, compared to immediate analysis after sample processing (data not shown). The lower and the upper reference values of f-Carnitine are 36 and 75 nmol/mL, respectively, according to the specification by the manufacturer.

Data collection

Patient characteristics consisting of age, height, weight, body mass index (BMI), Acute Physiology and Chronic Health Evaluation (APACHE) II score, Sequential Organ Failure Assessment (SOFA) score, origin of admission, and underlying medical conditions were recorded for evaluation of relative factors for the L-carnitine concentration on admission to the ICU. Post-ICU admission treatments such as antibiotic administration, nutrition, and CRRT were recorded for the assessment of factors that may relate to the change in L-carnitine concentrations after ICU admission.

Clinical outcomes were assessed as mortality during the ICU stay (ICU mortality), during the hospital stay (hospital mortality), and at 180 days after ICU admission (180 -day mortality).

Data analysis

For the primary analysis, patients were classified into two groups according to the L-carnitine concentration at ICU admission: low carnitine group, patients with f-Carnitine lower than the lower reference value (36 nmol/mL), and normal carnitine group, patients with f-Carnitine higher than the lower reference values. The patient background characteristics at the time of admission were also compared between the two groups to identify risk factors for carnitine depletion at the time of ICU admission.

For the secondary analyses, patients were classified into two groups according to the changes in L-carnitine concentrations from day 0 to day 14 of the hospital stay: carnitine reduction group (f-Carnitine at day 0 > f-Carnitine at day 14) or carnitine elevation group (f-Carnitine at day 0 ≤ f-Carnitine at day 14). Factors associated with the reduction or the elevation of L-carnitine concentrations were investigated by comparing the patient characteristics and treatments conducted after ICU admission.

Calculated acylcarnitine concentrations were studied as ratio to f-Carnitine (A/F Carnitine ratio) to evaluate the need for L-carnitine supplementation in patients treated with continuous renal replacement therapy for acute kidney injury (AKI).

Data are presented as mean ± standard deviation (SD), median and quartile, or absolute numbers and percentages as appropriate. We tested for differences between the two groups using an unpaired t test for continuous data and Fisher's exact test for categorical data. Receiver operating characteristics (ROC) curve analysis was conducted for potential risk factors using f-Carnitine reduction at day 14 as the dependent variable. The cutoff value was determined by Youden-Index. Statistical analyses were performed using the GraphPad Prism 6 (GraphPad Software, San Diego, CA, USA).

Results

Patient selection

During the study period, 338 patients were admitted to the ICU. Sixty-four patients were enrolled in the study after excluding 224 post surgery patients, two patients under the age of 18, six patients who were readmitted to the ICU, and five patients who were expected to die within 24 h, by the exclusion criteria. Also, 37 patients were lost for enrollment due to other reasons such as insufficient residual serum samples and admission during holidays when the initial sample processing was not possible (Additional file 1: Figure S1).

Primary outcome

The median t-Carnitine and f-Carnitine at the time of admission were 64.2 (50.5–102.3) nmol/mL and 50.5 (36.8–80.3) nmol/mL, respectively. Carnitine deficiency defined as f-Carnitine < 36 nmol/mL was observed in 15 (23.4%) patients (Table 1). No significant differences were found between the low carnitine group and the normal carnitine group age, sex, BMI, comorbidities, severity of the critical illness, or admission diagnoses (Table 1).

Secondary outcomes

Transition of carnitine concentrations

The median t-Carnitine and f-Carnitine at day 14, 71.7 (55.9–83.1) and 59.8 (46.0–69.1), respectively, were within the upper and lower reference values (Additional files 2 and 3).

Factors related to the reduction or the elevation of L-carnitine concentrations

Patients were divided into carnitine elevation group ($n = 14$, 48.3%) and carnitine reduction group ($n = 15$, 51.7%) according to the 14-day transition of f-Carnitine (Table 2). The 14-day transitions of f-Carnitine concentrations in the two groups are shown in Table 2 and Additional file 3: Figure S3 in the supplementary appendix. BMI was significantly lower in the carnitine reduction group compared with the carnitine elevation group (19.4 ± 2.9 and 22.4 ± 2.8, respectively, $p = 0.01$). No significant differences were found in the patient severity at ICU admission (SOFA score and APACHE II score). There were no significant differences in the rates of ICU treatments such as administration of artificial nutrition; CRRT for AKI was also not statistically significant (Table 2).

The association between the clinical factors and the degree of change in f-Carnitine from day 0 to day 14 (Δf-Carnitine) were further analyzed (Table 3). There was a significant negative correlation between the BMI and the Δf-Carnitine ($p = 0.01$). ROC curve analysis revealed a significant cutoff value of 19.5 (area under the curve (AUC) = 0.81, $p < 0.01$) (Fig. 1a).

Significantly positive correlation was observed between the SOFA score on ICU admission and the Δf-Carnitine ($p = 0.012$) (Additional file 4). However, a significant cutoff value was not defined by the ROC curve analysis (tentative cutoff value 8.5; AUC = 0.57, $p = 0.5$) (Fig. 1b).

Contribution of CRRT on the A/F Carnitine ratio

Patients treated with CRRT were compared with patients without CRRT. Although a significant difference of f-Carnitine concentrations was not found among patients with CRRT and without CRRT at day 14, A/F Carnitine ratio at day 14 was higher in CRRT patients compared with the patients without CRRT ($p = 0.012$, Fig. 2).

Discussion

In the present study, carnitine deficiency was observed in 23.4% of the critically ill patients admitted to the ICU for unexpected treatments. BMI lower than 19.5 was found to be a significant risk factor for L-carnitine reduction. SOFA score at the time of ICU admission was correlated with the subsequent decrease in L-carnitine concentrations, although a significant cutoff value was not defined.

Table 1 Primary outcome and patient characteristic at ICU admission

	All patients	f-Carnitine[‡] < 36	f-Carnitine[‡] > 36	p value
Patients (%)	64 (100.0)	15 (23.4)	49 (76.6)	
f-Carnitine[‡]	50.5 (36.8–80.3)	30.0 (25.5–34.2)	57.9 (46.0–100.3)	< 0.01
Age (year)	62.8 ± 17.4	60.1 ± 17.3	63.6 ± 17.5	0.49
Male (%)	41 (64.0)	7 (46.6)	34 (69.3)	0.13
Weight (kg)	57.4 ± 11.7	58.7 ± 9.6	56.7 ± 12.3	0.56
Body mass index	21.6 ± 3.8	23.3 ± 2.9	21.1 ± 3.9	0.06
Comorbidity				
Diabetes mellitus	10 (15.6)	3 (20.0)	7 (14.2)	0.68
Hyperlipidemia	3 (4.6)	0 (0)	3 (6.1)	1.0
Cirrhosis	4 (6.2)	1 (6.6)	3 (6.1)	1.0
Chronic kidney disease	5 (7.8)	2 (13.3)	3 (6.1)	0.3
Hemodialysis	4 (6.2)	2 (13.3)	2 (4.0)	0.23
APACHE II[¶] score	26.9 ± 10.4	25.5 ± 10.8	27.4 ± 10.3	0.56
SOFA[§] score	8.1 ± 4.8	6.1 ± 3.9	8.8 ± 5.0	0.06
Diagnosis, no. (%)				
Sepsis	18 (28.1)	2 (13.3)	16 (32.6)	0.19
Gastrointestinal disorder	13 (20.3)	5 (33.3)	8 (16.3)	0.16
Neurological disorder	9 (14.0)	3 (20)	6 (12.2)	0.42
Trauma	10 (15.6)	2 (13.3)	8 (16.3)	1.0
Patient origin				0.08
Emergency department	22 (34.3)	8 (53.3)	14 (28.5)	
General ward	17 (26.5)	1 (6.6)	16 (32.6)	
Other hospital	25 (39.0)	6 (40.0)	19 (38.7)	
Fasting duration (days)	1.1 ± 0.9	1.0 ± 0.6	1.2 ± 1.0	0.45
Artificial nutrition	5 (7.8)	1 (6.6)	4 (8.1)	1.0
Valproic acid treatment	2 (3.1)	0	2 (4.0)	1.0
Alb (g/dL)	2.9 ± 0.8	3.1 ± 0.7	2.8 ± 0.8	0.21
HbA1c (%)	6.4 ± 2.5	6.1 ± 2.3	6.4 ± 2.6	0.73

Data are presented as mean ± standard deviation, median (quartile), or absolute numbers and percentages (%) as appropriate

[‡]Free carnitine

[¶]Acute Physiology and Chronic Health Evaluation II

[§]Sequential Organ Failure Assessment

Carnitine deficiency in ICU patients

This study is the first epidemiological study to prospectively investigate the L-carnitine concentrations in critically ill patients who were admitted to the ICU for unscheduled treatment. Previous studies in postoperative patients have concluded that carnitine deficiency was rarely observed [5] and that the benefit of supplementation was limited [6, 10, 11]. Recent progress in ICU treatments including organ support therapies has enabled critically ill patients of various etiologies and severity to survive the critical illness and to endure long-term intensive treatments. However, little has been studied about carnitine concentrations and its roles in the current-day critically ill patients. Recent studies regarding carnitine concentrations have focused on non-critically ill patients [4, 12, 13] or critically ill patients already presenting symptoms of carnitine depletion [1, 14].

Indication for L-carnitine measurement and supplementation

There were no significant differences in the clinical outcomes such as length of ICU stay and mortality between patients with or without carnitine deficiency at the time of ICU admission (Additional file 5: Table S1). This observation suggests that carnitine deficiency at ICU admission does not immediately indicate the need for carnitine supplementation. However, long-term multidisciplinary treatments provided for current critically ill patients while lacking sufficient supplementation could increase the chance of carnitine depletion in the later

Table 2 Secondary outcomes

	Carnitine elevation group (n = 14)	Carnitine reduction group (n = 15)	p value
f-Carnitine[‡] change from day 0 to day 14 (Δf-Carnitine[‡])	12.2 (4.7~26.9)	− 22.3 (− 34.8~− 4.4)	< 0.01
Age	64.2 ± 17.0	61.8 ± 11.5	0.66
Body mass index	22.4 ± 2.8	19.4 ± 2.9	0.01
ICU duration	7.5 (3.0~13.7)	12.0 (5.0~21.0)	0.14
Sepsis during ICU stay	6 (40.0)	6 (42.8)	0.87
APACHE II[¶] score on admission	26.6 ± 8.7	29.4 ± 8.8	0.40
SOFA[§] score on admission	8.0 ± 3.6	9.0 ± 4.6	0.53
Mechanical ventilation during ICU stay	0.0 (0.0~2.0)	4.0 (0.0~8.0)	0.08
Artificial nutrition at day 14	7 (42.8)	8 (53.3)	1.0
Parenteral nutrition at day 14	3 (21.4)	0 (0)	0.1
Enteral nutrition at day 14	4 (28.5)	8 (53.3)	0.26
Calorie intake per weight at day 14	26.4 ± 9.2	28.8 ± 8.4	0.46
Renal replacement therapy during ICU stay	6 (42.8)	9 (60.0)	0.46

Data are presented as mean ± standard deviation, median (quartile), or absolute numbers and percentages (%) as appropriate
[‡]Free carnitine
[¶]Acute Physiology and Chronic Health Evaluation II
[§]Sequential Organ Failure Assessment

phase of the ICU stay. Although the median L-carnitine concentration for the ICU patients did not fall under the reference range during the 14-day study period, L-carnitine concentrations progressively declined in 51.7% of the patients. Medical treatments such as pivampicillin, valproic acid, and verapamil administration can lead to L-carnitine deficiency by either inhibiting cellular transporters or promoting L-carnitine excretion. Extended artificial nutrition is also a frequent cause of the depletion due to the lack of L-carnitine content in enteral or intravenous nutrition formula. L-carnitine is sufficiently pooled endogenously; thus, carnitine depletion usually occurs after more than 14 days of interrupted carnitine supply [14]. Evaluation over longer stay is likely to reveal further decrease of L-carnitine concentration, as

Table 3 Correlation between clinical factors and f-Carnitine[‡] change from day 0 to day 14 (Δf-Carnitine[‡])

	r[†]	p value
Body mass index	− 0.47	0.01
SOFA[§] score on admission	0.46	0.01
APACHE II[¶] score on admission	0.32	0.1
Length of renal replacement therapy	0.35	0.06
Mechanical ventilation during ICU stay	0.27	0.14
Calorie intake per weight at day 14	− 0.01	0.95
Serum Alb (g/dL) on admission	0.16	0.40
ICU length of stay	0.25	0.17

[‡]Free carnitine
[¶]Acute Physiology and Chronic Health Evaluation II
[§]Sequential Organ Failure Assessment
[†]Correlation analyzed with Spearman coefficient

demonstrated in some case reports of carnitine depletion [1, 14].

The relationship between BMI and decreased L-carnitine concentrations may be related to the fact that L-carnitine is mainly stored in the skeletal muscles, where it facilitates medium- and long-chain fatty acid transport from the cytosol into the mitochondria for β-oxidation and energy generation [1, 4]. Since muscle mass is frequently lost during the early phase of the critical illness due to catabolism [15], patients with smaller muscle mass, possibly reflected by low BMI, are likely to suffer loss of relatively greater portion of their carnitine pool, leading to decreased L-carnitine concentrations. However, more specific methods to evaluate muscle mass such as the body composition [16, 17] analysis or anatomical evaluations [18, 19] are needed to confirm this hypothesis. It should also be noted that the study population was limited to patients with relatively low BMI (mean ± SD 21.6 ± 3.8).

The mechanism behind carnitine reduction in patients with higher SOFA scores is not well defined. One explanation may be the metabolic load on mitochondrial function during severe illness [20]. One randomized controlled trial studied the effect of carnitine infusion in vasopressor-dependent septic shock patients based on this hypothesis [20]. Although carnitine concentrations were not measured in this study, early infusion of L-carnitine was related to reduced 28-day mortality without harmful effects, suggesting a potential benefit of L-carnitine infusion in this patient population. Despite the uncertainty of the mechanism, these findings warrant further investigation of L-carnitine concentrations in

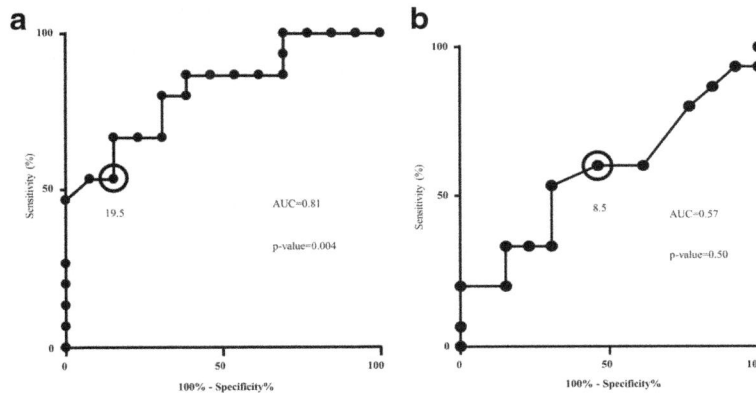

Fig. 1 ROC curve analysis for BMI and SOFA score associated with f-Carnitine reduction at day 14. Each plot depicts a relationship between sensitivity on the x-axis and 100-specificity on the y-axis. The cutoff value of BMI (**a**) was defined as 19.5, with the ROC curve depicting area under the curve (AUC) of 0.81 (95% confidence interval 0.66–0.97). A significant cutoff value was not defined for SOFA score (**b**) (tentative cutoff value 8.5; AUC = 0.57, 95% confidence interval 0.35–0.78)

relationship to the benefits of carnitine supplementation in patients with organ dysfunctions.

Patients treated with CRRT

Indication for supplementation of carnitine can also be determined by focusing on the accumulation of acylcarnitine by its ratio to free carnitine (A/F Carnitine ratio), as implemented in hemodialysis patients [8]. The accumulation of acylcarnitine in the blood indicates impaired mitochondrial metabolism, insufficient elimination by the kidney, or impaired transport of acylcarnitine due to the lack of L-carnitine supply and can lead to complications such as liver mitochondrial dysfunction [2]. The administration of L-carnitine in hemodialysis patients has been suggested to help the redistribution of acylcarnitine to eliminate potentially toxic acylcarnitines through hemodialysis [8]. The subgroup of patients

treated with CRRT presented elevated A/F Carnitine ratio, a finding consistent with hemodialysis patients [13]. The difference in the efficacy of RRT implicates a disparate mechanism affecting A/F Carnitine ratio in patients with CRRT compared to hemodialysis patients. In critically ill patients usually treated with CRRT, the relationship between mitochondrial dysfunction and severity has been shown in the previous reports [21, 22]. We speculate that not only insufficient elimination by kidneys but also impaired mitochondrial metabolism due to critical illness lead to accumulation of acylcarnitine. Although dialysis efficiency of CRRT is different from that of hemodialysis, carnitine supplementation in ICU patients treated with CRRT may help to avoid symptoms similar to dialysis-related complications such as anemia and muscle weakness [13].

Limitations

This study has some limitations, mainly related to the study design. The results obtained from limited patient enrollment in a single-center observation require external validation of the results. Valid patient follow-up was possible for only 14 days, while carnitine depletion is more likely to occur in long-term treatments [14]. Although we were able to identify the trend of carnitine reduction in patients with lower BMI and higher SOFA scores, the transition of carnitine concentrations were within the reference ranges. Longer follow-up in a larger patient population may have enabled more specific analyses, including the possibility of identifying other risk factors. The study design to use BMI as the only parameter for the estimation of endogenous carnitine supply is another limitation, as more specific methods are recommended to determine muscle mass [18, 19]. On the other hand, the contribution of carnitine metabolism on anemia and decreased cardiac performance, which is

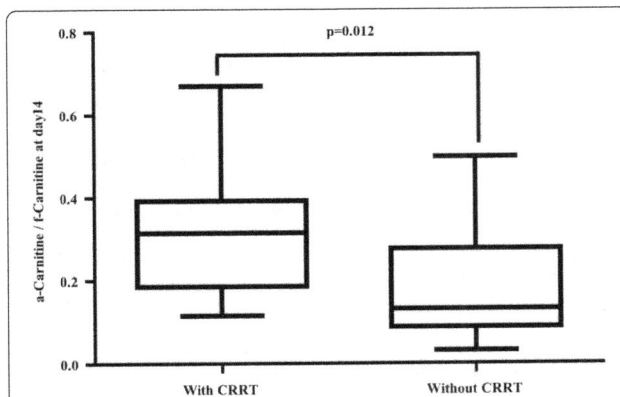

Fig. 2 Comparison of a-Carnitine/f-Carnitine ratio between the patients treated with or without CRRT. The box depicts the interquartile range and the line within the box indicating the median, respectively. The error bars indicate the 25th and 75th percentile range. The a-Carnitine/f-Carnitine ratio at day 14 was higher in patients with CRRT (p = 0.01)

known to be significant for hemodialysis patients [23], should be investigated in critically ill patients. Despite these limitations, the present study attempted to collect the epidemiological data on carnitine concentrations in modern critically ill patients and to identify the potential focuses for future studies.

Conclusions

Carnitine deficiency was observed in less than one fourth of critically ill patients at ICU admission. Low BMI (< 19.5) and high SOFA scores at ICU admission were identified as potential risk factors for carnitine depletion during extended ICU stay. Patients treated with CRRT presented signs of impaired carnitine metabolism. Further studies to investigate the potential benefits of carnitine supplementation may be warranted for these patients.

Additional files

Additional file 1: Figure S1. Flowchart of study enrollment.

Additional file 2: Figure S2. Distribution of carnitine concentrations on ICU admission. (a) The distribution of t-Carnitine on ICU admission is shown in the histogram. The mean t-Carnitine was 94.9 ± 79.6 nmol/mL, and the median t-Carnitine was 64.2 (50.5–102.3) nmol/mL. (b) The distribution of f-Carnitine on ICU admission is shown in the histogram. The mean f-Carnitine was 68.6 ± 51.2 nmol/mL, and the median f-Carnitine was 50.5 (36.8–80.3) nmol/mL.

Additional file 3: Figure S3. Comparison of f-Carnitine transition among the patients with f-Carnitine increased and decreased. The transition of f-Carnitine area for 14 days plotted at each sampling point. The round and square signs within the figure indicate the medians for f-Carnitine, and the error bars indicate 25th and 75th percentile range. The dotted lines indicate the upper and lower reference values for f-Carnitine. The patients whose data are lacking at day 7 or day 14 were excluded from this analysis.

Additional file 4: Figure S4. Correlation of BMI and SOFA score with the change in f-Carnitine from day 0 to day 14. (a) Each plot depicts a relationship between the BMI on the x-axis, and the change of f-Carnitine from day 0 to day 14 (Δ f-Carnitine) on the y-axis. There was a significant negative correlation between the BMI and the Δf-Carnitine ($r = -0.47$, $p = 0.01$), which suggests an association between lower BMI and larger decrease of f-Carnitine. (b) Each plot depicts a relationship between the SOFA score at the time of ICU admission on the x-axis, and the change of f-Carnitine from day 0 to day 14 (Δ f-Carnitine) on the y-axis. There was a significant correlation between the SOFA score on ICU admission and the Δf-Carnitine ($r = 0.46$, $p = 0.01$), which suggests an association between high SOFA score and larger decrease of f-Carnitine.

Additional file 5: Table S1. Clinical outcomes according to f-carnitine levels at ICU admission[a]

Abbreviations

AKI: Acute kidney injury; APACHE: Acute Physiology and Chronic Health Evaluation; BMI: Body mass index; CRRT: Continuous renal replacement therapy; f-Carnitine: Free carnitine concentration; ICU: Intensive care unit; NADH: Nicotinamide adenine dinucleotide; ROC: Receiver operating characteristics; SD: Standard deviation; SOFA: Sequential Organ Failure Assessment; t-Carnitine: Total carnitine concentration; thio-NAD[+]: Thionicotinamide-adenine dinucleotide

Acknowledgements
Not applicable

Funding
This research did not receive any specific grant from funding agencies in the public, commercial, or not-for-profit sectors.

Test reagents for t-Carnitine and f-Carnitine analyses were provided by KAINOS Laboratories Inc. (Tokyo, Japan) who had no involvement in the designing of the study, interpretation of the data, or the drafting of the manuscript. Carnitine analyses were conducted by the courtesy of the Central Clinical Testing Laboratory at Chiba University Hospital.

Authors' contributions
TO planned and conducted the study, analyzed the data, and drafted the manuscript. TOs planned and conducted the study and drafted the manuscript. NH made suggestions for the interpretation of the data and drafted the manuscript. AT recruited patients, collected patient samples, and critically revised the manuscript. SH and TY collected the samples, conducted the sample analysis, and critically revised the manuscript. SO supervised the study and drafted the manuscript. All authors gave the final approval for the final version of the manuscript prior to submission.

Competing interests
The authors declare that they have no competing interests.

Author details
[1]Department of Emergency and Critical Care Medicine, Chiba University Graduate School of Medicine, Chiba University Hospital, 1-8-1 Inohana Chuo-ku, Chiba, Chiba, Japan. [2]Clinical Laboratory, Chiba University Hospital, Chiba, Japan.

References
1. Hatamkhani S, Karimzadeh I, Elyasi S, Farsaie S, Khalili H. Carnitine and sepsis: a review of an old clinical dilemma. J Pharm Pharm Sci. 2013;16:414–23.
2. Reuter SE, Evans AM. Carnitine and acylcarnitines: pharmacokinetic, pharmacological and clinical aspects. Clin Pharmacokinet. 2012;51:553–72.
3. Cao Y, Wang YX, Liu CJ, Wang LX, Han ZW, Wang CB. Comparison of pharmacokinetics of L-carnitine, acetyl-L-carnitine and propionyl-L-carnitine after single oral administration of L-carnitine in healthy volunteers. Clin Invest Med. 2009;32:E13–9.
4. Calo LA, Vertolli U, Davis PA, Savica V. L carnitine in hemodialysis patients. Hemodial Int. 2012;16:428–34.
5. Wennberg A, Hyltander A, Sjoberg A, Arfvidsson B, Sandstrom R, Wickstrom I, Lundholm K. Prevalence of carnitine depletion in critically ill patients with undernutrition. Metabolism. 1992;41:165–71.
6. Pichard C, Roulet M, Schutz Y, Rossle C, Chiolero R, Temler E, Schindler C, Zurlo F, Furst P, Jequier E. Clinical relevance of L-carnitine-supplemented total parenteral nutrition in postoperative trauma. Metabolic effects of continuous or acute carnitine administration with special reference to fat oxidation and nitrogen utilization. Am J Clin Nutr. 1989;49:283–9.
7. Ostermann ME, Chang RW. Prognosis of acute renal failure: an evaluation of proposed consensus criteria. Intensive Care Med. 2005;31:250–6.
8. Vernez L, Dickenmann M, Steiger J, Wenk M, Krahenbuhl S. Effect of L-carnitine on the kinetics of carnitine, acylcarnitines and butyrobetaine in long-term haemodialysis. Nephrol Dial Transplant. 2006;21:450–8.
9. Takahashi M, Ueda S, Misaki H, Sugiyama N, Matsumoto K, Matsuo N, Murao S. Carnitine determination by an enzymatic cycling method with carnitine dehydrogenase. Clin Chem. 1994;40:817–21.
10. Roulet M, Pichard C, Rossle C, Bretenstein E, Schutz Y, Chiolero R, Furst P, Jequier E. Adverse effects of high dose carnitine supplementation of total parenteral nutrition on protein and fat oxidation in the critically ill. Clin Nutr. 1989;8:83–7.
11. Sandstedt S, Cederblad G, Lindholm M, Larsson J. The effect of carnitine supplemented total parenteral nutrition on lipid, energy and nitrogen metabolism in severely ill patients. Clin Nutr. 1991;10:97–104.
12. Ringseis R, Keller J, Eder K. Role of carnitine in the regulation of glucose homeostasis and insulin sensitivity: evidence from in vivo and in vitro studies with carnitine supplementation and carnitine deficiency. Eur J Nutr. 2012;51:1–18.
13. Evans AM, Faull RJ, Nation RL, Prasad S, Elias T, Reuter SE, Fornasini G. Impact of hemodialysis on endogenous plasma and muscle carnitine levels in patients with end-stage renal disease. Kidney Int. 2004;66:1527–34.

14. Bonafe L, Berger MM, Que YA, Mechanick JI. Carnitine deficiency in chronic critical illness. Curr Opin Clin Nutr Metab Care. 2014;17:200–9.

15. Puthucheary ZA, Rawal J, McPhail M, Connolly B, Ratnayake G, Chan P, Hopkinson NS, Phadke R, Dew T, Sidhu PS, et al. Acute skeletal muscle wasting in critical illness. JAMA. 2013;310:1591–600.

16. Ismael S, Savalle M, Trivin C, Gillaizeau F, D'Auzac C, Faisy C. The consequences of sudden fluid shifts on body composition in critically ill patients. Crit Care. 2014;18:R49.

17. Faisy C, Rabbat A, Kouchakji B, Laaban JP. Bioelectrical impedance analysis in estimating nutritional status and outcome of patients with chronic obstructive pulmonary disease and acute respiratory failure. Intensive Care Med. 2000;26:518–25.

18. Mourtzakis M, Wischmeyer P. Bedside ultrasound measurement of skeletal muscle. Curr Opin Clin Nutr Metab Care. 2014;17:389–95.

19. Moisey LL, Mourtzakis M, Cotton BA, Premji T, Heyland DK, Wade CE, Bulger E, Kozar RA. Skeletal muscle predicts ventilator-free days, ICU-free days, and mortality in elderly ICU patients. Crit Care. 2013;17:R206.

20. Puskarich MA, Kline JA, Krabill V, Claremont H, Jones AE. Preliminary safety and efficacy of L-carnitine infusion for the treatment of vasopressor-dependent septic shock: a randomized control trial. JPEN J Parenter Enteral Nutr. 2014;38:736–43.

21. Brealey D, Brand M, Hargreaves I, Heales S, Land J, Smolenski R, Davies NA, Cooper CE, Singer M. Association between mitochondrial dysfunction and severity and outcome of septic shock. Lancet. 2002;360:219–23.

22. Carre JE, Orban JC, Re L, Felsmann K, Iffert W, Bauer M, Suliman HB, Piantadosi CA, Mayhew TM, Breen P, et al. Survival in critical illness is associated with early activation of mitochondrial biogenesis. Am J Respir Crit Care Med. 2010;182:745–51.

23. Calvani M, Benatti P, Mancinelli A, D'Iddio S, Giordano V, Koverech A, Amato A, Brass EP. Carnitine replacement in end-stage renal disease and hemodialysis. Ann N Y Acad Sci. 2004;1033:52–66.

Permissions

List of Contributors

Norio Hanafusa
Department of Blood Purification, Kidney Center, Tokyo Women's Medical
University, 8-1 Kawada-cho, Shinjuku-ku, Tokyo 162-8666, Japan

Satoko Sakurai and Masaomi Nangaku
Division of Nephrology and Endocrinology, The University of Tokyo School of Medicine, Tokyo, Japan

Vui Eng Phui, Clare Hui Hong Tan, Kwek Foong Chew, Hock Hin Chua, Laura Lui Sian Ngu and Lawrence Wei Soon Hii
Department of Medicine, Sarawak General Hospital, Jalan Hospital, 93586 Kuching, Sarawak, Malaysia

Chee Kean Chen
Department of Anaesthesiology, Kuching Specialist Hospital, Kuching, Sarawak, Malaysia

Kee Hoe Lai
Department of Medicine, University Malaysia Sarawak, Kota Samarahan, Sarawak, Malaysia

Yukinao Sakai
Department of Nephrology, Nippon Medical School Musashikosugi Hospital, 1-396 kosugi-cho, Nakahara-ku, Kawasaki, Japan
Department of Nephrology, Graduate School of Medicine, Nippon Medical School, 1-1-5 Sendagi, Bunkyo-ku, Tokyo 113-8603, Japan

Saori Sakai
Department of Internal Medicine, Zenjinkai Maruko-Clinic, 1-840 Shinmaruko-higashi, Nakahara-ku, Kawasaki, Japan

Koji Mugishima, Anna Katayama, Yuichiro Sumi, Yusuke Otsuka and Tomoyuki Otsuka
Department of Nephrology, Nippon Medical School Musashikosugi Hospital, 1-396 kosugi-cho, Nakahara-ku, Kawasaki, Japan

Shuichi Tsuruoka
Department of Nephrology, Graduate School of Medicine, Nippon Medical School, 1-1-5 Sendagi, Bunkyo-ku, Tokyo 113-8603, Japan

Tomoyuki Kawano
Department of Medical Science and Cardiorenal Medicine, Yokohama City University Graduate School of Medicine and School of Medicine, Yokohama, Kanagawa, Japan
Kohsaikai Bunkojin Clinic, Yokohama, Kanagawa, Japan

Tadashi Kuji
Department of Medical Science and Cardiorenal Medicine, Yokohama City University Graduate School of Medicine and School of Medicine, Yokohama, Kanagawa, Japan
Yokodai Central Clinic, Yokohama, Kanagawa, Japan

Tetsuya Fujikawa
Department of Medical Science and Cardiorenal Medicine, Yokohama City University Graduate School of Medicine and School of Medicine, Yokohama, Kanagawa, Japan
Center for Health Service Sciences, Yokohama National University, Yokohama, Kanagawa, Japan

Eiko Ueda, Midori Shino, Kouichi Tamura, Nobuhito Hirawa and Yoshiyuki Toya
Department of Medical Science and Cardiorenal Medicine, Yokohama City University Graduate School of Medicine and School of Medicine, Yokohama, Kanagawa, Japan

Satoshi Yamaguchi
Kohsaikai Yokohama Jinsei Hospital, Yokohama, Kanagawa, Japan

Toshimasa Ohnishi
Kohsaikai Kamioooka Jinsei Clinic, Yokohama, Kanagawa, Japan

Jun Suzuki
Division of Infectious Diseases, Jichi Medical University Hospital, 3311-1 Yakushiji, Shimotsuke, Tochigi 329-0498, Japan

Tetsu Ohnuma and Masamitsu Sanui
Department of Anesthesiology and Critical Care Medicine, Jichi Medical University Saitama Medical Center, 1-847 Amanuma, Omiya-ku, Saitama City, Saitama 330-8503, Japan

Hidenori Sanayama
Division of General Medicine, The First Department of Comprehensive Medicine, Jichi Medical University Saitama Medical Center, 1-847 Amanuma, Omiya-ku, Saitama City, Saitama 330-8503, Japan

Kiyonori Ito
Division of Nephrology, The First Department of Comprehensive Medicine, Jichi Medical University Saitama Medical Center, 1-847 Amanuma, Omiya-ku, Saitama City, Saitama 330-8503, Japan

Takayuki Fujiwara
Division of Cardiology, The First Department of Comprehensive Medicine, Jichi Medical University Saitama Medical Center, 1-847 Amanuma, Omiya-ku, Saitama City, Saitama 330-8503, Japan

Hodaka Yamada
Division of Endocrinology and Metabolism, The First Department of Comprehensive Medicine, Jichi Medical University Saitama Medical Center, 1-847 Amanuma, Omiya-ku, Saitama City, Saitama 330-8503, Japan

Alan Kawarai Lefor
Department of Surgery, Jichi Medical University, 3311-1 Yakushiji, Shimotsuke, Tochigi 329-0498, Japan

Haruki Uojima
Department of Gastroenterology, Shonan Kamakura General Hospital, 1370-1 Okamoto, Kamakura, Kanagawa 247-8533, Japan
Department of Gastroenterology, Internal Medicine, Kitasato University School of Medicine, Sagamihara, Kanagawa, Japan

Shuzo Kobayashi, Takayasu Ohtake and Machiko Oka
Department of Kidney Disease and Transplant Center, Shonan Kamakura General Hospital, Kamakura, Kanagawa, Japan

Hisashi Hidaka
Department of Gastroenterology, Internal Medicine, Kitasato University School of Medicine, Sagamihara, Kanagawa, Japan

Shuichi Matsumoto
Department of General Internal Medicine, Fukuoka Tokushukai Medical Center, Kasuga, Fukuoka, Japan

Takeshi Kinbara, Ji Hyun Sung and Makoto Kako
Department of Gastroenterology, Shonan Kamakura General Hospital, 1370-1 Okamoto, Kamakura, Kanagawa 247-8533, Japan

Yasuhiro Yamanouchi
Department of Kidney Disease, Shinfuji Hospital, Fuji, Shizuoka, Japan

Takehiko Kunieda
Department of Kidney Disease, Shonan Clinic, Kamakura, Kanagawa, Japan

Hiroki Yamanoue
Department of General Internal Medicine, Shizuoka Tokushukai Hospital, Suruga, Shizuoka, Japan

Takayuki Kanemaru
Department of Surgery, Haibara General Hospital, Makinohara, Shizuoka, Japan

Kazuhiko Tsutsumi
Department of Surgery, Sanpoku Tokushukai Hospital, Murakami, Niigata, Japan

Tomoaki Fujikawa
Department of Gastroenterology, Shonan Fujisawa Tokushukai Hospital, Fujisawa, Kanagawa, Japan

Takeo Ishii
Internal Medicine, Zenjinkai group, Yokohama Daiichi Hospital, 2-5-15 Takashima Nishi-ku, Yokohama City, Kanagawa 220-0011, Japan
Department of Medical Science and Cardiorenal Medicine, Graduate School of Medicine,
Yokohama City University, Yokohama, Kanagawa, Japan

Yukiko Nakajima
Department of System and Safety, Zenjinkai group, 2-6-32 Takashima Nishi-ku, Yokohama
City, Kanagawa, Japan

Kunio Oyama
Internal Medicine, Zenjinkai group, Yokohama Daiichi Hospital, 2-5-15 Takashima Nishi-ku, Yokohama City, Kanagawa 220-0011, Japan

Fateme Shamekhi Amiri
Division of Nephrology, Imam Khomeini Hospital, Faculty of Medicine, Tehran University of Medical Sciences, Tehran, Iran

Makoto Harada, Kazuaki Fujii and Yukifumi Kurasawa
Department of Nephrology, Nagano Red Cross Hospital, 5-22-1, Wakasato, Nagano 380-8582, Japan
Department of Nephrology, Shinshu University School of Medicine, 3-1-1, Asahi, Matsumoto 390-8621, Japan

Takeshi Masubuchi
Department of Infection and Host Defense, Nagano Red Cross Hospital, 5-22-1, Wakasato,Nagano 380-8582, Japan
Department of Respiratory Medicine, Nagano Red Cross Hospital, 5-22-1, Wakasato, Nagano 380-8582, Japan

Tohru Ichikawa and Mamoru Kobayashi
Department of Nephrology, Nagano Red Cross Hospital, 5-22-1, Wakasato, Nagano 380-8582, Japan

Shinzo Kuzuhara
Department of Medicine, Kidney Center, Tokyo Women's Medical University, Tokyo, Japan
Department of Nephrology, Sekikawa Hospital, Tokyo, Japan

Shigeru Otsubo
Department of Medicine, Kidney Center, Tokyo Women's Medical University, Tokyo, Japan
Department of Blood Purification, Tohto Sangenjaya Clinic, 2-13-2 Taishido, Setagaya-ku, Tokyo 154-0004, Japan

Katsuya Kajimoto
Department of Cardiology, Sekikawa Hospital, Tokyo, Japan

Takashi Akiba
Department of Nephrology, Sekikawa Hospital, Tokyo, Japan

Kosaku Nitta
Department of Medicine, Kidney Center, Tokyo Women's Medical University, Tokyo, Japan

Chieko Takagi
Hidaka Hospital, Takasaki, Gunma, Japan
Dialysis Center, Ogo Clinic, 245-7, Motogi-machi, Maebashi-shi, Gunma 371-0232, Japan

Kumeo Ono
Ono Naika Clinic, Maebashi, Gunma, Japan

Hidenori Matsuo and Nobuo Nagano
Hidaka Hospital, Takasaki, Gunma, Japan

Yoshihisa Nojima
Department of Medicine and Clinical Science, Gunma University Graduate School of Medicine, Maebashi, Gunma, Japan

Kosaku Nitta
Department of Medicine, Kidney Center, Tokyo Women's Medical University, 8-1 Kawada-cho, Shinjuku-ku, Tokyo 162-8666, Japan

Norio Hanafusa and Ken Tsuchiya
Department of Blood Purification, Kidney Center, Tokyo Women's Medical University, Tokyo, Japan

Ikuto Masakane
Committee of Renal Data Registry (CRDR), Japanese Society for Dialysis Therapy (JSDT), Aramido Building 2F, 2-38-21 Hongo, Bunkyo-ku, Tokyo 113-0033, Japan
Department Nephrology, Yabuki Hospital, 4-4-5 Shima Kita, Yamagata City, Yamagata 990-0885, Japan

Takeshi Hasegawa
Subcommittee of Statical Analysis of CRDR, Japanese Society for Dialysis Therapy, Tokyo, Japan

Satoshi Ogata, Naoki Kimata, Shigeru Nakai, Norio Hanafusa, Takayuki Hamano, Kenji Wakai and Atsushi Wada
Committee of Renal Data Registry (CRDR), Japanese Society for Dialysis Therapy (JSDT), Aramido Building 2F, 2-38-21 Hongo, Bunkyo-ku, Tokyo 113-0033, Japan

Kosaku Nitta
Japanese Society for Dialysis Therapy, Tokyo, Japan

Saki Hasegawa, Shintaro Nakano, Jun Tanno, Shiro Iwanaga, Ritsushi Kato, Toshihiro Muramatsu, Takaaki Senbonmatsu and Shigeyuki Nishimura
Department of Cardiovascular Medicine, Saitama Medical University International Medical Center, 1397-1 Yamane, 350-1298 Hidaka, Saitama, Japan

Yusuke Watanabe and Hirokazu Okada
Department of Nephrology, Saitama Medical University, Saitama, Japan

Hidetomo Nakamoto
Department of General Internal Medicine, Saitama Medical University Hospital, Saitama, Japan

Jun Shiota
Department of Internal Medicine, Tsunashima Kidney Clinic, 1-10-4 Tsunashima-Higashi, Kohoku-ku, Yokohama 223-0052, Japan
Department of Internal Medicine, Kichijoji Asahi Hospital, Tokyo, Japan

Hitoshi Tagawa and Hitoshi Kasahara
Department of Internal Medicine, Kichijoji Asahi Hospital, Tokyo, Japan

Norihiko Ohura
Department of Plastic, Reconstructive and Aesthetic Surgery, Kyorin University School of Medicine, Tokyo, Japan

Yuka Kawate
Department of Nutrition, Kyoto Katsura Hospital, 17 Yamadahirao-cho Nishikyo-ku, Kyoto 615-8157, Japan

Hitomi Miyata
Department of Nephrology, Kyoto Katsura Hospital, 17 Yamadahirao-cho Nishikyo-ku, Kyoto 615-8157, Japan

Yusuke Kaida, Takatoshi Kambe, Ryo Yamamoto, Takuma Hazama, Yoshimi Takamiya, Ryo Shibata, Hidemi Nishida, Seiya Okuda and Kei Fukami
Division of Nephrology, Department of Medicine, Kurume University School of Medicine, 67 Asahi-machi, Kurume, Fukuoka 830-0011, Japan

Shintaro Kishimoto, Yusuke Koteda and Kenji Suda
Department of Pediatrics and Child Health, Kurume University School of Medicine, Kurume, Japan

Tetsurou Imai
Clinical Engineering Center, Kurume University Hospital, Kurume, Japan

Ibrahim Mousa, Raed Ataba and Khaled Al-ali
Department of Medicine, College of Medicine and Health Sciences, An-Najah National University, Nablus 44839, Palestine

Abdulsalam Alkaiyat
Public Health Department, College of Medicine and Health Sciences, An-Najah National University Hospital, An-Najah National University, Nablus 44839, Palestine

Sa'ed H. Zyoud
Poison Control and Drug Information Center (PCDIC), College of Medicine and Health Sciences, An-Najah National University, Nablus 44839, Palestine
Department of Clinical and Community Pharmacy, College of Medicine and Health Sciences, An-Najah National University, Nablus 44839, Palestine
Division of Clinical and Community Pharmacy, Department of Pharmacy, College of Medicine and Health Sciences, An-Najah National University, Nablus 44839, Palestine

Takahiro Shimoda, Kei Yoneki, Manae Harada, Takaaki Watanabe and Atsuhiko Matsunaga
Department of Rehabilitation Sciences, Graduate School of Medical Sciences, Kitasato University, 1-15-1 Kitasato, Sagamihara, Kanagawa 252-0373, Japan

Ryota Matsuzawa
Department of Rehabilitation, Kitasato University Hospital, Sagamihara, Japan

Keika Hoshi
Department of Hygiene, Kitasato University School of Medicine, Sagamihara, Japan

Kosuke Sekine
Department of Medical Engineer, Kameda Medical Center, Chiba, Japan

Takayuki Abe
Department of Preventive Medicine and Public Health, Keio University School of Medicine, Tokyo, Japan
Biostatistics Unit at Clinical and Translational Research Center, Keio University Hospital, Tokyo, Japan

Shinichiro Suzaki, Atsushi Katsumi, Naoshige Harada, Hidenori Higashi, Yuki Kishihara and Hidetaka Suzuki
Intensive Care Unit, Department of Emergency and Critical Care Medicine, Japanese Red Cross Musashino Hospital, Tokyo, Japan

Toru Takebayashi
Department of Preventive Medicine and Public Health, Keio University School of Medicine, Tokyo, Japan

Hideto Yasuda
Department of Intensive Care Unit, Kameda Medical Center, 929 Higashi-chou, Kamogawa-shi, Chiba 296-8602, Japan
Intensive Care Unit, Department of Emergency and Critical Care Medicine, Japanese Red Cross Musashino Hospital, Tokyo, Japan
Department of Preventive Medicine and Public Health, Keio University School of Medicine, Tokyo, Japan

Muhammad A. Siddiqui
Department of Research and Performance Support, Saskatchewan Health Authority, Regina, Saskatchewan, Canada
School of Health Sciences, Queen Margaret University, Edinburgh, UK

Suhel Ashraff
Department of Diabetes and Endocrinology, Royal Victoria Infirmary, Newcastle, UK

Derek Santos, Robert Rush and Thomas E. Carline
School of Health Sciences, Queen Margaret University, Edinburgh, UK

Zahid Raza
Department of Vascular Surgery, Royal Infirmary, Edinburgh, UK

Hidetomo Nakamoto
Department of General Internal Medicine, Saitama Medical University Hospital, 38 Morohongo, Moroyama-machi, Iruma-gun, Saitama 350-0495, Japan

Takanori Oh, Masahiro Shimamura and Eiji Iida
Pharmaceutical Clinical Research Department, Toray Industries Inc., 1-1, Nihonbashi muromachi 2-chome, Chuo-ku, Tokyo 103-8666, Japan

Sadanobu Moritake
Pharmaceuticals Business Department, Toray International (China) Co., Ltd, 1601 West Nanjing Road, Jing An District, Shanghai 200040, China

Kunihiro Ishioka, Takayasu Ohtake, Hidekazu Moriya, Yasuhiro Mochida, Machiko Oka, Kyoko Maesato, Sumi Hidaka and Shuzo Kobayashi
Kidney Disease and Transplant Center, Shonan Kamakura General Hospital, 1370-1 Okamoto, Kamakura 247-8533, Japan

Koichi Hayashi and Yusuke Sakamaki
Department of Internal Medicine, Tokyo Dental College Ichikawa General Hospital, 5-11-13 Sugano, Ichikawa, Chiba 272-8513, Japan

Toshihiko Suzuki and Shinsuke Ito
Department of Internal Medicine, Tokyo Bay Urayasu Ichikawa Medical Center, 3-4-32 Todaijima, Urayasu, Chiba 279-0001, Japan

Kentaro Tanaka
Department of Nephrology, School of Medicine, Faculty of Medicine, Toho University, 6-11-1 Omori-Nishi, Ota-ku, Tokyo 143-0015, Japan
Division of Diabetes and Metabolism, Institute for Adult Diseases, Asahi Life Foundation, Tokyo, Japan

Ken Sakai, Yasushi Ohashi, Masaki Muramatsu, Takeshi Kawamura, Seiichiro Shishido and Atsushi Aikawa
Department of Nephrology, School of Medicine, Faculty of Medicine, Toho University, 6-11-1 Omori-Nishi, Ota-ku, Tokyo 143-0015, Japan

Akifumi Kushiyam and Shigeko Hara
Division of Diabetes and Metabolism, Institute for Adult Diseases, Asahi Life Foundation, Tokyo, Japan

Masakazu Hattori
Division of Diabetes, Clinical Research Center for Endocrinology and Metabolic Diseases, National Hospital Organization Kyoto Medical Center, Kyoto, Japan

Kenji Tsuchida
Tsuchida Dialysis Access Clinic, 2-10-18, Fujiidera DH building 4F, Oka, Fujiidera-shi, Osaka 583-0027, Japan

Hirofumi Hashimoto
Yoshinogawa Medical Center, Nishichiejima 120, Kamojimachochiejima, Yoshinogawa-shi, Tokushima 776-8511, Japan

Kazuhiko Kawahara
Kamojima Kawashima Clinic, Fukui 396-3, Kamojimacho-inoo, Yoshinogawa-shi, Tokushima 776-0033, Japan

Ikuro Hayashi
Naruto Kawashima Clinic, Nishi 68-5, Otsuchodanzeki, Naruto-shi, Tokushima 772-0043, Japan

Yoshio Fukata
Wakimachi Kawashima Clinic, Tatejinja-shimominami 39-2, Ooaza-Inoshiri, Wakimachi, Mima-shi, Tokushima 779-3602, Japan

Munenori Kashiwagi
Seijukai Clinic, 4-5-16, Honcho, Chuo-ku, Osaka 541-0053, Japan

Akihiro C. Yamashita
Department of Chemical Science and Technology, Faculty of Bioscience and Applied Chemistry, Hosei University, 3-7-2, Kajinocho, Koganei-shi, Tokyo 184-8584, Japan

Michio Mineshima
Department of Clinical Engineering, Tokyo Women's Medical University, 8-1, Kawadacho, Shinjuku-ku, Tokyo 162-8666, Japan

Tadashi Tomo
Oita University Hospital Blood Purification Center, Idai-gaoka, 1-1, Hasama-machi, Yufu-shi, Oita 879-5593, Japan

Ikuto Masakane
Yabuki Hospital, 4-5-5, Shimakita, Yamagata 990-0885, Japan

Yoshiaki Takemoto
Department of Urology, Osaka City University, 1-4-3, Asahimachi, Abeno-ku, Osaka 545-0051, Japan

Hideki Kawanishi
Tsuchiya General Hospital, 3-30, Nakajimacho, Naka-ku, Hiroshima 730-8655, Japan

Kojiro Nagai and Jun Minakuchi
Kawashima Hospital, 1-39, Kitasakoichibancho, Tokushima-shi, Tokushima 770-0011, Japan

Akiko Takeshima, Hiroaki Ogata, Kei Asakura, Tadashi Kato, Yoshinori Saito, Kantaro Matsuzaka, Go Takahashi, Masanori Kato, Masahiro Yamamoto, Hidetoshi Ito and Eriko Kinugasa
Department of Internal Medicine, Showa University Northern Yokohama Hospital, 35-1 Chigasaki-chuo, Tsuzuki, Yokohama 2248503, Japan

Yoshiyuki Kadokura and Yoshihiro Yamada
Department of Otorhinolaryngology, Showa University Northern Yokohama Hospital, 35-1 Chigasaki-chuo, Tsuzuki, Yokohama 2248503, Japan

Tomohito Mizuno, Motonobu Nakamura, Nobuhiko Satoh and Hiroyuki Tsukada
Division of Nephrology and Endocrinology, The University of Tokyo Hospital, 7-3-1 Hongo, Bunkyo-ku, Tokyo 113-8655, Japan

Haruki Kume
Department of Urology, The University of Tokyo Hospital, 7-3-1 Hongo, Bunkyo-ku, Tokyo 113-8655, Japan

Akihiko Matsumoto
Department of Urology, The University of Tokyo Hospital, 7-3-1 Hongo, Bunkyo-ku, Tokyo 113-8655, Japan
Department of Hemodialysis and Apheresis, The University of Tokyo Hospital, 7-3-1 Hongo, Bunkyo-ku, Tokyo 113-8655, Japan

Yoshifumi Hamasaki and Masaomi Nangaku
Division of Nephrology and Endocrinology, The University of Tokyo Hospital, 7-3-1 Hongo, Bunkyo-ku, Tokyo 113-8655, Japan
Department of Hemodialysis and Apheresis, The University of Tokyo Hospital, 7-3-1 Hongo, Bunkyo-ku, Tokyo 113-8655, Japan

Kazuo Kimura
Department of Medicine, Kidney Center, Tokyo Women's Medical University, Tokyo, Japan
Department of Nephrology, Sekikawa Hospital, Tokyo, Japan

Katsuya Kajimoto
Department of Cardiology, Sekikawa Hospital, Tokyo, Japan

Shigeru Otsubo
Department of Medicine, Kidney Center, Tokyo Women's Medical University, Tokyo, Japan
Department of Blood Purification, Tohto Sangenjaya Clinic, 2-13-2 Taishido, Setagaya-ku, Tokyo 154-0004, Japan

Takashi Akiba
Department of Nephrology, Sekikawa Hospital, Tokyo, Japan

Kosaku Nitta
Department of Medicine, Kidney Center, Tokyo Women's Medical University, Tokyo, Japan

Yumi Kamada
Sohbudai Nieren Clinic, Zama, Japan
Department of Angiology and Cardiology, Kitasato University Graduate School of Medical Sciences, 1-15-1 Kitasato, Minami-ku, Sagamihara, Kanagawa, Japan

Takashi Masuda, Shinya Tanaka and Nobuaki Hamazaki
Department of Angiology and Cardiology, Kitasato University Graduate School of Medical Sciences, 1-15-1 Kitasato, Minami-ku, Sagamihara, Kanagawa, Japan

Kazuhiko Kotani
Division of Community and Family Medicine, Jichi Medical University, Tochigi, Japan

Takeshi Nakamura
Sohbudai Nieren Clinic, Zama, Japan
Department of Rehabilitation Sciences, Kitasato University Graduate School of Medical Sciences, Sagamihara, Japan

Yoko Itoh, Ibuki Moriguchi, Naoyuki Kobayashi and Michihito Okubo
Sohbudai Nieren Clinic, Zama, Japan

Kazuhiro Takeuchi, Shokichi Naito and Yasuo Takeuchi
Division of Nephrology, Department of Internal Medicine, Kitasato University School of Medicine, Sagamihara, Japan

Takehiko Oami, Taku Oshima, Noriyuki Hattori, Ayako Teratani and Shigeto Oda
Department of Emergency and Critical Care Medicine, Chiba University Graduate School of Medicine, Chiba University Hospital, 1-8-1 Inohana Chuo-ku, Chiba, Chiba, Japan

Saori Honda and Toshihiko Yoshida
Clinical Laboratory, Chiba University Hospital, Chiba, Japan

Index

www.ingramcontent.com/pod-product-compliance
Lightning Source LLC
Chambersburg PA
CBHW061330190326
41458CB00011B/3951